€70
'19
PPN

Stroke Revisited

This authoritative book series presents state of the art knowledge on the pathophysiology, prevention, diagnosis, and treatment of stroke, highlighting the many very important advances that have been achieved in recent years. Current issues in management are addressed in detail, equipping readers with an understanding of the rationale for particular approaches in different settings and with a sound knowledge of the role of modern imaging methods, surgical techniques, and medical treatments. The inclusion of numerous high-quality illustrations facilitates understanding of practical aspects and rapid retrieval of fundamental information. The series will be of value for stroke physicians, surgeons, other practitioners who care for patients with stroke, and students.

More information about this series at http://www.springer.com/series/15338

Seung-Hoon Lee
Editor

Stroke Revisited: Diagnosis and Treatment of Ischemic Stroke

Springer

Editor
Seung-Hoon Lee
Department of Neurology
Seoul National University Hospital
Department of Neurology
Seoul, South Korea

Stroke Revisited
ISBN 978-981-10-1423-9 ISBN 978-981-10-1424-6 (eBook)
DOI 10.1007/978-981-10-1424-6

Library of Congress Control Number: 2017949357

Printed on acid-free paper

This Springer imprint is published by Springer Nature
The registered company is Springer Nature Singapore Pte Ltd.
The registered company address is: 152 Beach Road, #21-01/04 Gateway East, Singapore 189721, Singapore

Preface

The most frequently used starting sentence in books or articles on stroke is: "stroke is a disease ranked 4th in worldwide mortality, and 1st in worldwide adult disabilities." Although I am personally sick of using this sentence and no longer use it when writing an article or a paper, there are still tons of papers and books that start with this sentence. Why is that? Do the readers not know the significance? Or is it to provide the readers with self-esteem, in that the disease you are reading about and treating is extremely important? Maybe both. Unfortunately, the importance of the disease is not emphasized enough or recognized by the public, probably due to the modesty of the clinicians and researchers treating and studying stroke. In most countries, both the patients and the medical staff have very low awareness of stroke compared to heart diseases, and the sizes of both the clinical and research workforce for stroke are incomparably small. The stroke unit is sometimes a part of the department of neurology and sometimes a part of internal medicine and rarely an independent department in many countries. Considering the severity and importance of the disease, this system is too inconsistent and insufficient. In addition to developing an integrated and systematic treatment protocol for stroke, the presence of a textbook that provides up-to-date knowledge and standard of treatment is essential.

I once had a meeting with the director of cardiovascular medicine in one of the biggest multinational pharmaceutical companies in the world. The director of the Europe-based company was an impressive, old, Caucasian madam. She said that the stroke department in her company was being managed entirely by the cardiovascular department. The meeting was held so that I could provide advice on research and development (R&D) in medications on stroke. Then, I was really puzzled about her lack of background knowledge on stroke. She graduated from a recognized medical school in Europe and practiced as a medical doctor in the cardiovascular division of the department of internal medicine. How could she know so little about stroke? She thought that stroke was simply another coronary artery disease that occurred in the brain, and I was the first person to tell her about stroke due to small vessel occlusion—which is an important subtype of stroke. Considering the fact that the head of R&D from a leading pharmaceutical company barely knew anything about stroke, it is not a surprise to see no medication or unsuccessful medication being developed for stroke treatment. Even now, I believe that the situation has not changed. If there was a textbook that provides a simple explanation of stroke and discusses the key differences between stroke and heart diseases, would the situation be any different?

Actually, there are not many textbooks that explain stroke in detail. During my residency and fellowship, there were only two or three books that I could read to study stroke. Even these books were not enough to fully appreciate the advancement in stroke treatment during 1990–2000. Brain imaging dramatically improved the quality of treatment by allowing immediate recognition of the continuously changing pathophysiology of the stroke patient. Nevertheless, majority of textbooks contain a big portion explaining outdated neurological examinations, providing no support for development in the practical field. Furthermore, most textbooks simply outlined the results from various studies and did not focus on helping readers to understand the key concepts or providing appropriate schemes for treatment protocols. Although the situation was probably similar for other fields, studying stroke during this period required extensive patience.

Recent development of smartphones and tablets allowed international communications through social media, and people now have access to extensive amount of information. Textbooks to deliver medical knowledge should also change to reflect the rapidly advancing modern technology and must focus on providing simple and clear explanations of key concepts. The content of each chapter should be minimized, and visual diagrams should be utilized to help the readers better understand key concepts. Listing unnecessary results from studies should be avoided, while standard treatment guidelines from various academic societies would be better to be collated and described. I decided to write such a textbook reflecting these changes and contacted Springer Nature. Springer Nature was very helpful and planned a new series of textbooks entitled *Stroke Revisited*. There are many difficulties, such as language barriers, for a Korean to contact a European publisher to plan and publish a series of textbooks. I would like to sincerely thank Springer Nature and its employees for their assistance in the publication of this textbook.

The target readers of this textbook are trainees such as residents and fellows, specialists in their early careers specializing in stroke treatment, and doctors and researchers from various fields who wish to understand stroke in more depth. Most individual chapters have a single focus and have minimal text so that it is convenient to read the entire chapter in a short period of time. Unnecessary text was not included, and the use of visual aids was maximized. Only the essential reference literature has been included. The key characteristic of this textbook is the presentation of treatment procedures in sequence, starting at the initial admission of stroke patient in the emergency room, diagnosis, treatment, up to discharge and/or preventive measures. Most textbooks are organized in the traditional literature form. Therefore, in practice, sorting and selecting the section to obtain the knowledge from is difficult and time--consuming. This textbook attempts to simulate the actual practice, providing simultaneous explanation of diagnosis and treatment. At the same time, I tried to provide the highest quality of academic depth and up-to-date information on stroke. I hope the readers can fully benefit from these efforts.

In order to ensure that this textbook provides cutting-edge, yet authoritative and reliable, knowledge on stroke, experts from different parts of the world were invited to write each chapter. I would like to thank all the authors who participated in writing this textbook. This textbook is the first part of the *Stroke Revisited* series, and I hope it provides a flavor for the parts to follow.

2017.1.17 Seung-Hoon Lee, M.D., Ph.D., F.A.H.A.

How to Read

To give readers practical information on stroke management, I tried to organize this book with a different style from conventional academic books. First, assuming that the readers are duty doctors in emergency units, the parts and chapters in this book were organized as time sequence after visit of stroke patients. Part I covers the establishment and organization of stroke units and centers, and Part II comprehensively describes the diagnosis and treatment of ischemic stroke in acute stage. Part III gives cutting-edge knowledge on certain but relatively frequent causes, and secondary prevention after stroke was fully illustrated in Part IV. Part V covering clinical practice guidelines, which play a critical role in current medical practice, delineates their history, usefulness, and disadvantages and suggests my improvement direction of the guidelines. In particular, Chap. 4 in Part II entitled "Overview of Patient Management Flow" summarizes contents of diagnosis and management in stroke unit, general ward, and rehabilitation center and indicates corresponding chapters with more detailed information. Accordingly, if you choose to read a chapter among them, you will easily find to learn its position from the whole stroke management flow. Second, if you read abstract in the beginning of each chapter, you can easily obtain essential summary of the whole content of the chapter. Third, I tried to provide a simple but conceptual diagram covering all aspects of contents as a figure in each chapter. You just look into the diagram, and you will find the essential points of the chapter. Finally, there are "suggestions from current clinical practice guidelines" in the final part of each chapter. This part briefly summarizes essential recommendations of clinical practice guidelines in the world, especially from the American Heart Association/American Stroke Association. Thus, you can easily get up-to-date recommendations and notice information gaps between cutting--edge knowledge and current guidelines.

As stated in the preface, I tried to convey real, practical, but cutting-edge knowledge of stroke management with the unique organization style. However, this book is not a manual nor a protocol on stroke management. This is because top-class authors in the world gathered together to organize the most up-to-date knowledge. I hope that this book will be a guide to better understanding of stroke, which is a better way to deal with stroke patients.

Seung-Hoon Lee, M.D., Ph.D., F.A.H.A.

Acknowledgments

Although I had an ideal model for a textbook in my brain, I rarely had an active conversation with publishers about my idea. This textbook was conceived in an e-mail proposal of the textbook after an unplanned meeting with Ms. Lauren Kim, the editor of Springer Nature. The editorial team and I have obtained manuscripts from renowned medical experts in the world and have edited the manuscripts according to the principles we have set for this textbook. Therefore, the contents of this book were completed only after tremendous efforts from the editorial team. I would like to thank Dr. Jung Min Kim, Dr. Tae-Jung Kim, and Ms. Eun-Sun Park for their effort in the editorial team. In addition, I would like to thank the executive members of edition who agreed with the philosophy behind this textbook and provided the title for this textbook series—*Stroke Revisited*—in addition to providing active support in publishing this book. Finally, I would like to thank the Cerebrovascular Research Society in Korea and its members for their financial and technical support.

Throughout my research career, I focused on publishing papers as an author and becoming a famous, prosperous scientist. I rarely thought of writing a textbook. I would like to express my love towards my wife, my children, and my family, for changing my selfish thoughts and helping me understand my responsibilities, that is, to help others and provide education to nurture future doctors.

2017.1.17 Seung-Hoon Lee, M.D., Ph.D., F.A.H.A.

Contents

List of Contributors

Abdulaziz S. Al Sultan University of Calgary, Calgary, AB, Canada

Ramana Appireddy Queen's University, Kingston, ON, Canada

Zarina Assis University of Calgary, Calgary, AB, Canada

Melissa Báez-Martínez IdiPAZ Health Research Institute, Madrid, Spain

Adam Brown Cleveland Clinic, Cleveland, USA

Jay Chol Choi Jeju National University, Jeju, South Korea

Muneer Eesa University of Calgary, Calgary, AB, Canada

Stefan T. Engelter University Hospital Basel, Basel, Switzerland

Mayank Goyal University of Calgary, Calgary, AB, Canada

Rula A. Hajj-Ali Cleveland Clinic, Cleveland, OH, USA

Stephen Honeybul Sir Charles Gairdner Hospital, Perth, WA, Australia

Keun-Sik Hong Inje University Ilsan Paik Hospital, Goyang, South Korea

Naohisa Hosomi Hoshigaoka Medical Center, Hiroshima, Japan

Han-Gil Jeong Seoul National Univeristy Hospital, Seoul, South Korea

Han-Young Jung Inha University College of Medicine, Incheon, South Korea

Timo Kahles Cantonal Hospital of Aarau, Aarau, Switzerland

Dong-Wan Kang Seoul National Univeristy Hospital, Seoul, South Korea

Beom Joon Kim Seoul National University Bundang Hospital, Seongnam, South Korea

Bum Joon Kim Kyung Hee University Hospital, Seoul, South Korea

Jeong-Min Kim Chung-Ang University Hospital, Seoul, South Korea

Jinkwon Kim CHA Bundang Medical Center, Seongnam, South Korea

Jong S. Kim Asan Medical Center, Seoul, South Korea

Yerim Kim Kangdong Sacred Heart Hospital, Seoul, South Korea

Young Seo Kim Hanyang University College of Medicine, Seoul, South Korea

Sang-Bae Ko Seoul National University Hospital, Seoul, South Korea

Tackeun Kim Seoul National University Bundang Hospital, Seongnam, South Korea

Tae-Jung Kim Seoul National University Hospital, Seoul, South Korea

Hyung-Min Kwon Seoul Metropolitan Government-Seoul National University Boramae Medical Center, Seoul, South Korea

Meng Lee Chang Gung University, Taoyuan, Taiwan

Seung-Hoon Lee Seoul National University Hospital, Seoul, South Korea

Jae-Sung Lim Hallym University Sacred Heart Hospital, Anyang, South Korea

Philippe A. Lyrer University Hospital Basel, Basel, Switzerland

Ángel Robles-Marhuenda IdiPAZ Health Research Institute, Madrid, Spain

Patricia Martinez-Sanchez IdiPAZ Health Research Institute, Madrid, Spain

Masayasu Matsumoto Hiroshima University Graduate School of Biomedical and Health Sciences, Hiroshima, Japan

Bijoy K. Menon University of Calgary, Calgary, AB, Canada

Kazuo Minematsu National Cerebral and Cardiovascular Center, Suita, Japan

Krassen Nedeltchev Cantonal Hospital of Aarau, Aarau, Switzerland

Tomohisa Nezu Hiroshima University Graduate School of Biomedical & Health Sciences, Hiroshima, Japan

Byung-Mo Oh Seoul National University Hospital, Seoul, South Korea

Chang Wan Oh Seoul National University Bundang Hospital, Seongnam, South Korea

Mi Sun Oh Hallym University Sacred Heart Hospital, Anyang, South Korea

Bruce Ovbiagele Medical University of South Carolina, Charleston, SC, USA

Joung-Ho Rha Inha University College of Medicine, Incheon, South Korea

Ana Rodríguez-Sanz IdiPAZ Health Research Institute, Madrid, Spain

Andreas Schweikert Cantonal Hospital of Aarau, Aarau, Switzerland

Han Gil Seo Seoul National University Hospital, Seoul, South Korea

Tae-Jin Song Ewha Womans University School of Medicine, Seoul, South Korea

Christopher Traenka University Hospital Basel, Basel, Switzerland

Toshiyuki Uehara Hyogo Brain and Heart Center, Himeji, Japan

Part I

Initial Assessment of Patients with Stroke-Like Symptoms

Stroke Center

1

Toshiyuki Uehara and Kazuo Minematsu

Abstract

Although intravenous recombinant tissue-type plasminogen activator therapy was approved for treating acute ischemic stroke within 3 h of symptom onset in 1996, less than 5% of patients with acute stroke were receiving this treatment. To facilitate adequate care for acute stroke patients, the Brain Attack Coalition (BAC) discussed the need to establish primary stroke centers (PSCs) where patients can receive emergency stroke care from qualified teams and developed recommendations with criteria for PSCs in 2000. A consensus statement from the BAC with extensive recommendations for comprehensive stroke centers (CSCs), a facility for stroke patients who require high-intensity medical and surgical care, was published in 2005. The Joint Commission began to certify PSCs in 2003 and CSCs in 2012. The "Get With The Guidelines®-Stroke" program, a popular database tool to record and track performance measures, was developed by the American Heart Association as a national quality improvement program. A third type of facility, the acute stroke-ready hospital (ASRH), is currently under development. An ASRH would have fewer capabilities than a PSC, but would be able to provide initial diagnostic services, stabilization, emergent care, and therapies to patients with acute stroke. This chapter introduces literature about stroke centers from the United States, Europe, and Japan and discusses the effectiveness and future challenges of stroke centers.

T. Uehara, M.D., Ph.D.
Hyogo Brain and Heart Center at Himeji,
Himeji, Japan

K. Minematsu, M.D., Ph.D. (✉)
National Cerebral and Cardiovascular Center,
5-7-1 Fujishirodai, Suita, Osaka 565-8565, Japan
e-mail: kminemat@ncvc.go.jp

In 1996, the Food and Drug Administration in the United States approved intravenous recombinant tissue-type plasminogen activator (rt-PA) administered within 3 h of symptom onset as a treatment for acute ischemic stroke. However, less than 5% of patients with acute stroke were receiving this treatment. To assist in ensuring adequate

S.-H. Lee (ed.), *Stroke Revisited: Diagnosis and Treatment of Ischemic Stroke*,
Stroke Revisited, DOI 10.1007/978-981-10-1424-6_1

care for acute stroke patients, in 2000, the Brain Attack Coalition (BAC) discussed the concept of stroke centers and proposed two levels: primary stroke centers (PSCs) to stabilize and provide emergency care for patients with acute stroke and comprehensive stroke centers (CSCs) to diagnose and treat stroke patients who require high-intensity medical and surgical care, specialized tests, or interventional therapies. The BAC developed recommendations with criteria for PSC in 2000 [1] and for CSC in 2005 [2] and updated recommendations for the establishment of PSCs in 2011 [3]. The concept is that stroke centers, by providing vital infrastructure, expertise, protocols, and monitoring care in accordance with nationally recognized guidelines and performance expectations, would provide improved care leading to better outcomes [4]. In an effort to improve the care of stroke patients nationally, a strong push has been made to develop care systems based on an organized hierarchy of stroke hospitals, similar to systems of trauma centers [1, 2]. In this chapter, we discuss components of PSCs and CSCs proposed by the BAC and evidence supporting the effectiveness of stroke centers.

1.1 Components of Stroke Centers Proposed by the BAC

1.1.1 PSCs

The recommendations for PSCs proposed by the BAC were organized around 11 major elements of stroke care. These elements were grouped into direct patient care areas and support services. Patient care areas included acute stroke teams, written care protocols, emergency medical services, emergency departments, stroke units, and neurosurgical services. Support services included commitment and support of a medical organization, a stroke center director, neuroimaging services, laboratory services, outcome and quality improvement activities, and continuing medical education [1]. A key message from the BAC recommendations was timely provision of acute stroke services and the resulting need for general laboratory services, electrocardiography, and chest X-rays to be available 24 h a day, 7 days a week (24/7); brain computed tomography (CT) on a 24/7 basis; and the availability of neurosurgical services within 2 h [5].

In 2011, the BAC revised and updated recommendations for the establishment of PSCs based on the past 10 years of experience and advances in medical care and technology [3]. The major elements of a PSC are shown in Table 1.1. Important revisions and additions are summarized in Table 1.2. Based on a literature review and local experience, the following areas were stressed in the revised, updated statement: (1) the importance of acute stroke teams to improve rapid diagnosis and treatment; (2) importance of stroke units with telemetry monitoring; (3) utilization of magnetic resonance imaging (MRI) with diffusion-weighted sequences; (4) MR angiography or CT angiography to assess the cerebral vasculature; (5) cardiac imaging studies, including transthoracic echocardiography, transesophageal echocardiography, and cardiac MRI assessment; (6)

Table 1.1 Major elements of a primary stroke center

Patient care elements
Acute stroke team
Written care protocols
Emergency medical services
Emergency department
Stroke unit
Neurosurgical services
Imaging services: brain, cerebral vasculature, cardiac
Laboratory services
Rehabilitation services
Administrative/support elements
Institutional commitment and support
Primary stroke center director, reimbursement for call
Stroke registry with outcomes and quality improvement components
Educational programs: public and professional
Support certification process
Participation in stroke system of care

Reproduced by permission of Stroke [3]

Table 1.2 Key revisions to primary stroke center recommendations

Service/element	Recommendation/revision	Comment
Acute stroke team	At least two members	At bedside within 15 min
Emergency medical services	Transport patient to nearest PSC	Class 1, Level B recommendation
Emergency department	Monitoring protocol for patients	Vital signs and neurologic status
Stroke unit	Multichannel telemetry; clinical monitoring protocol	Includes who to call and when to call for deterioration
Imaging	MRI, MRA, or CTA and cardiac imaging available	May not apply to all patients; not required in acute setting; performed within 6 h; read within 2 h of completion (for MRI/MRA/CTA)
Laboratory	HIV testing for admitted patients; toxicology screen	Centers for Disease Control and Prevention recommendation (HIV)
Rehabilitation	Early assessment and initiation	If patient clinically stable
Administrative support	Call pay consideration	May improve acute response
Center certification	Independent organization; performance measures	Self-certification not recommended

Reproduced by permission of Stroke [3]

importance of early initiation of rehabilitation therapy; and (7) independent local site certification, including site visits and disease performance measures [5].

1.1.2 CSCs

In 2005, the BAC developed recommendations for the establishment of CSCs [2]. These recommendations emphasized that service needs to deliver specialized care and included the following key components: (1) personnel with expertise, (2) diagnostic techniques, (3) surgical and interventional therapies, (4) infrastructure, and (5) educational/research programs (Table 1.3) [2]. The CSCs are the highest-level and well-equipped hospitals which can treat all types of stokes. The CSCs require infrastructures, highly qualified specialists, and specialized process for diagnosis and treatment of complex stroke patients who needed a high level of medical and surgical care, specialized intensive care unit (ICU) facilities such as neuroscience ICU, specialized tests, or intervention treatments. Moreover, the trained and expertise stroke team must be available 24/7 for surgical treatment or intervention therapies. Some stroke patients could benefit from CSCs treatment, those with stroke caused by unusual etiologies and demanding specialized testing, or multispecialty management. In addition, CSC would be to act as a resource center for other facilities in their region, such as PSCs. The CSCs could receive patients initially treated at a PSC and provide expertise about the diagnosis and management of particular patients, guidance for patient triage, and educational resource for other hospitals and healthcare professionals at a given geographical area [2]. In 2011, the American Heart Association (AHA)/American Stroke Association (ASA) proposed a set of metrics and related data elements covering the major aspects of specialized care for patients with ischemic stroke and nontraumatic subarachnoid and intracerebral hemorrhages at CSCs [6].

The BAC outlined the organization of stroke centers in a hospital network or geographical area in a consensus statement for CSCs [2]. In the current healthcare environment, hospital networks and systems are continuing to grow. Within such a network or system, one approach to acute stroke care might be to designate some hospitals as PSCs and others as CSCs (Fig. 1.1).

Table 1.3 Components of a comprehensive stroke center

Recommendation
Personnel with expertise in the following areas
Vascular neurology
Vascular neurosurgery
Advanced practice nurses
Vascular surgery
Diagnostic radiology/neuroradiology
Interventional/endovascular physician(s)
Critical care medicine
Physical medicine and rehabilitation
Rehabilitation therapy (physical, occupational, speech therapy)
Staff stroke nurse(s)
RT
Swallowing assessment
Diagnostic techniques
MRI with diffusion-weighted image
MRA/MRV
CTA
Digital cerebral angiography
TCD
Carotid duplex ultrasound
Transesophageal echo
Surgical and interventional therapies
Carotid endarterectomy
Clipping of intracranial aneurysm
Placement of ventriculostomy
Hematoma removal/draining
Placement of intracranial pressure transducer
Endovascular ablation of IAs/AVMs
IA reperfusion therapy
Endovascular therapy of vasospasm
Infrastructure
Stroke unit
ICU
Operating room staffed 24/7
Interventional services coverage 24/7
Stroke registry
Educational/research programs
Community education
Community prevention
Professional education
Patient education

Reproduced by permission of Stroke [2]

1.2 Certification of Stroke Centers

In 2003, the AHA/ASA and The Joint Commission (TJC) convened and agreed on a certification process for stroke through a Disease-Specific Certification program, including a voluntary evaluation process driven by demonstration of a consistent approach to the measurement of clinical outcomes and minimum standards for stroke care [7]. The three major requirements were necessary for Primary Stroke Center Certification. These three requirements were in compliance with the use of evidence-based guidelines, implementation of TJC standards, and measurement of clinical outcomes [7]. The stroke performance measures were developed to improve the quality of stroke. The stroke performance measures in ischemic stroke included deep venous thrombosis prophylaxis, acute treatment such as antithrombotic therapy and anticoagulation therapy at discharge in patients with atrial fibrillation, dysphagia screening, stroke education, smoking cessation advice/counseling, risk factor modification, and rehabilitation [8]. Furthermore, a subset of these stroke performance measures was included for hemorrhagic stroke patients [5]. In 2009, the stroke 8-measure set was approved as a core measure set (Table 1.4) [8].

The "Get With The Guidelines®-Stroke" (GWTG-Stroke) became a popular database tool to record and track performance measures. The GWTG-Stroke program was developed by the AHA as a national quality improvement program for hospitals to improve stroke care infrastructure utilizing a multidisciplinary team approach and incorporating elements such as patient management toolkits, multidisciplinary workshops, and stakeholder organizational meetings and offering data collection and decision support. The patient management tool measures seven achievement elements, including deep venous thrombosis prophylaxis, early antithrombotic administration, and time

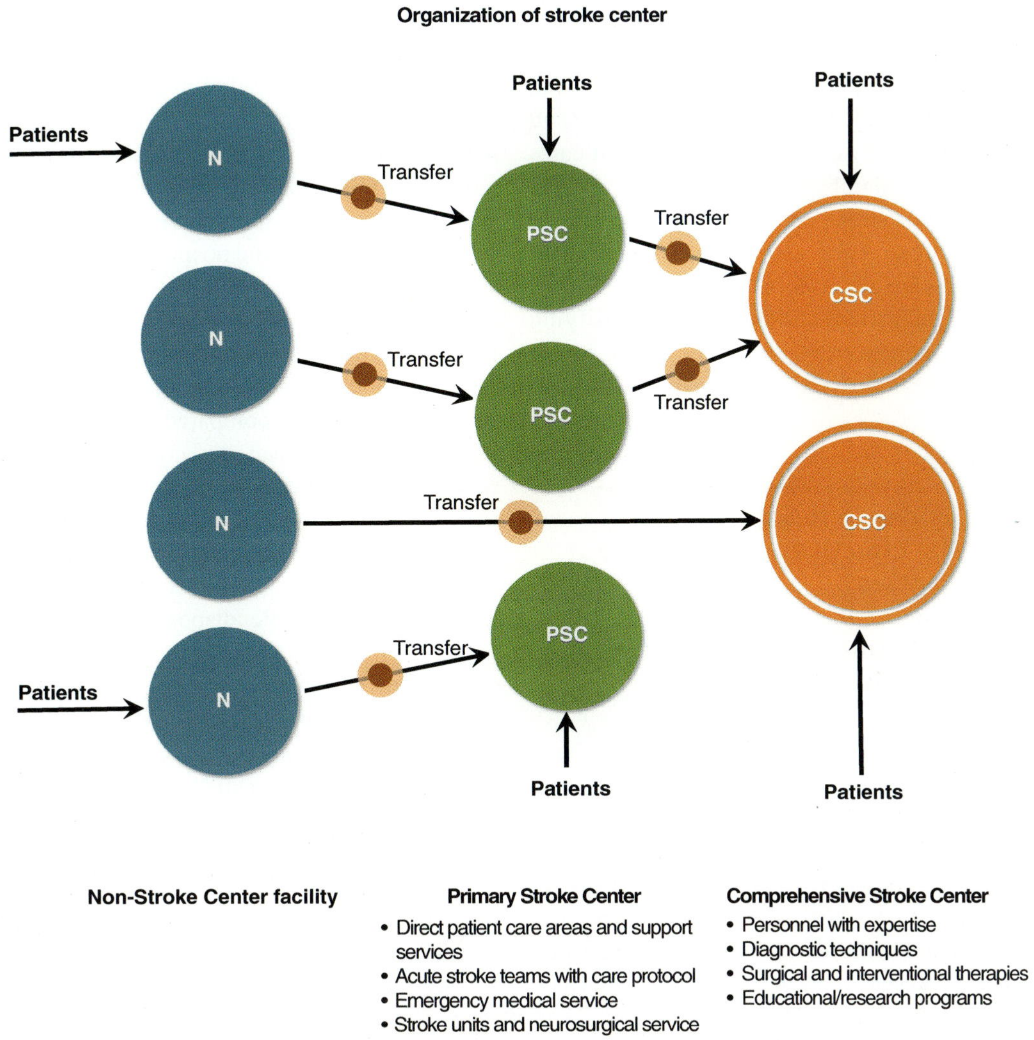

Fig. 1.1 Organization of stroke centers in a hospital network or geographical area. Representation of how various facilities caring for stroke patients could be organized based on a hospital network or defined geographical area. Patients can arrive at the various facilities via direct admission or transfer between facilities. *N* non-stroke center facility

Table 1.4 Stroke performance measures set

Prophylaxis against venous thromboembolism
Discharged on antithrombotic therapy
Anticoagulation therapy for atrial fibrillation/flutter
Thrombolytic therapy
Antithrombotic therapy by end of hospital day 2
Discharged on statin medication
Stroke education
Assessed for rehabilitation

Reproduced by permission of The Joint Commission [8]

to intravenous thrombolysis for eligible acute ischemic stroke patients [9]. After a pilot phase, hospitals began enrolling in GWTG-Stroke in April 2003.

The TJC established an advanced disease-specific care certification requirements for CSCs in 2012 [8]. This new requirements were designed to improve the substantial resources needed to establish and manage complex stroke and cerebrovascular cases. The certification requires centers to meet the following criteria: the program is in the United States and certified by TJC, uses standard methods to deliver clinical care and uses performance measures over time, and cares for a minimum number of patients [5].

The goal of stroke center certification was to improve stroke care and draw patients with stroke into capable centers. Since TJC and other entities/organizations started formally certifying and recognizing certain hospitals as PSCs, the number of such hospitals has increased dramatically [3].

1.3 Evidence to Support the Effectiveness of Stroke Centers

1.3.1 rt-PA Utilization and Quality of Stroke Care

Admission of certified stroke centers is associated with increased rates of rt-PA utilization and improvements in the quality of stroke care according to core measure adherence. Data from quality improvement programs such as GWTG-Stroke also showed that a PSC status improved compliance with and achievement of many disease performance measures. In recent studies, hospital participation in the GWTG-Stroke program was associated with increased achievement of process quality metrics, including increased frequency of acute pharmacological treatment (thrombolysis and early antithrombotic therapy), interventions to prevent early complications (deep venous thrombosis prophylaxis and swallowing assessments), and start of secondary stroke prevention before discharge (anticoagulation for atrial fibrillation and cholesterol reducing medication).

1.3.2 Functional Outcome

A nationwide observational register study of all patients with first-ever ischemic stroke treated in Finland showed an association between the level of acute stroke care and patient outcome. Admission to a PSC or CSC resulted in 1.5% and 2.4% reductions in mortality compared with admission to a general hospital (GH), respectively. The number needed to treat to allow one more patient to live at home 1 year after stroke was 40 for PSCs and 29 for CSCs when compared with GHs. For survival probability adjusted with Cox modeling for age, sex, comorbidities, previous medication and hospital use, and year of stroke, hazard ratios were 0.87 for CSCs and 0.90 for PSCs when compared with GHs (Fig. 1.2) [10]. A similar study in New York State also found significantly reduced mortality for patients cared for in a PSC compared with a non-PSC facility [11]. Lichtman et al. reported that TJC-certified status was associated in Medicare patients with decreased early mortality due to subarachnoid or intracerebral hemorrhage and with decreased early mortality, shorter hospitalization, and favorable disposition in ischemic stroke [12].

Song et al. found that patients hospitalized with acute ischemic stroke at GWTG-Stroke hospitals had greater improvement of clinical outcomes over time than at similar hospitals not participating in the GWTG-Stroke program. Compared with secular changes at control hospitals, GWTG-Stroke hospitals exhibited accelerated increases in the proportion of patients discharged to home and accelerated reductions in 30-day and 1-year mortality rates [9]. These findings indicate that hospital adoption of the GWTG-Stroke program is associated not only with improvements in the processes of care but also in improved functional outcome at discharge and reduced post-discharge mortality. One study indicated that care at a PSC for patients with acute ischemic stroke was cost-effective and improved outcomes [13].

1.4 Questionnaire Survey for Main Components of Stroke Centers in Europe and Japan

1.4.1 Europe

In 2007, the European Stroke Initiative Executive Committee reported the results of the European

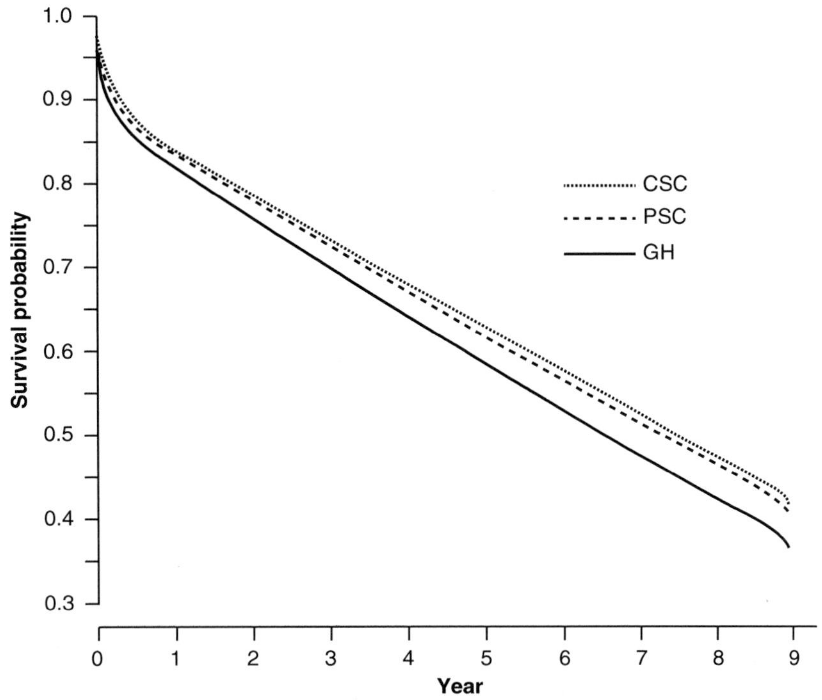

Fig. 1.2 Survival probability based on acute treating hospital facilities adjusted with a Cox model for age, sex, comorbidities, previous medication and hospital use, and year of stroke. Reproduced by permission of Stroke [10]

Expert Survey conducted to identify from expert opinions what the major components of stroke units should be [14]. This study showed the components considered "absolutely necessary" for CSCs and PSCs by 75% or more of directors of certified stroke teaching facilities. As a result, eight components were considered "absolutely necessary" by more than 75% of experts for both CSCs and PSCs: a multidisciplinary team, stroke-trained nurses, brain CT available 24/7, CT priority for stroke patients, extracranial Doppler sonography, automated electrocardiogram monitoring, intravenous rt-PA protocols available 24/7, and in-house emergency department. Eleven other components were considered necessary in CSCs by more than 75% of the experts: physiotherapy starting within 2 days, extracranial duplex sonography, transthoracic echocardiography, automated monitoring of pulse oximetry, automated monitoring of blood pressure, carotid surgery, angioplasty and stenting, collaboration with outside rehabilitation centers, stroke faculty, stroke pathways, and clinical research.

The AHA/ASA published a scientific statement of metrics for measuring quality of care in CSCs in 2011 [6]. However, the survey questionnaire conducted by the Executive Committee of the European Stroke Initiative demonstrated that less than 10% of European hospitals admitting acute stroke patients have optimal facilities and that even the minimum level was unavailable in 40% [15]. Recently, the European Stroke Organization (ESO) Stroke Unit Certification Committee published a special report of "ESO recommendations to establish a stroke unit and stroke center" [16]. The ESO Stroke Center is the coordinating body of the entire chain of care and covers prehospital care, emergency room assessment and diagnosis, emergency medical treatment, stroke unit care, ongoing rehabilitation and secondary prevention, and access to related neurosurgical and vascular intervention. A stroke unit is the most important component of the ESO Stroke Center [16].

1.4.2 Japan

In 2007, we conducted a questionnaire survey to identify the essential components of stroke centers in Japan and compared our results with the European Expert Survey [17]. Compared with the European Expert Survey, our results of surveys in Japan showed the following characteristics: (1) neurosurgical treatments were more likely to be emphasized; (2) MRI and MR angiography were better recognized than carotid and transcranial ultrasonography; and (3) a multidisciplinary stroke team and stroke-trained nurses in the category of personnel and stroke pathway, community stroke awareness programs, and prevention programs in the category of protocols and procedures were less likely to be emphasized. Approximately three-quarters of respondents were neurosurgeons in our survey, whereas most European stroke experts were neurologists. Given the results of separately analyzed responses from neurosurgeons and neurologists in our study, the differences in results between the surveys in Europe and Japan may be partly explained by the different proportions of neurologists and neurosurgeons.

1.5 Future Challenges for Establishing Stroke Center Systems

Significant geographic disparities exist in access to PSCs. Access is limited in suburban and rural areas. Demographic factors are strongly associated with access to care in smaller cities, but were found to have little impact elsewhere, including in major cities [18]. Currently, a 3-tier system has been proposed, consisting of acute stroke-ready hospitals (ASRHs), PSCs, and CSCs, in order of increasing resources/capabilities [19]. The AHA/ASA has published policy recommendations for stroke systems of care, some of which are applicable to the operations of the ASRH [4]. ASRHs would have fewer capabilities than PSCs, but would be able to provide initial diagnostic services, emergent care and therapies, and inducing stabilization in patients with stroke in their emergency department. They then transferred appropriate patients to another hospital, such as PSCs or CSCs for advanced medical services and definitive care. After the acute event has resolved, most patients are expected to return to their local facilities and healthcare professionals for outpatient care and perhaps rehabilitation [4].

Mullen et al. found that 36.9% of the US population, approximately 114 million people, would be unable to access a CSC within 60 min by ground transportation, even if CSCs are optimally located throughout the United States [19]. A British study showed that stroke interventional endovascular services were available in only a small number of hospitals and only about 50% of those with no endovascular service available for stroke had transfer plans with a center that did provide those services [20]. Systems planning and policy initiatives that incentivize certification of selected hospitals should be considered to ensure maximum population benefit. A systems planner will need to carefully assess the local need in rural areas to determine whether a CSC is justified. If not, alternative strategies such as PSCs and ASRHs may be used to provide basic stroke care, with telemedicine and a rapid transfer protocol linking these hospitals to more distant CSCs [19].

With the advent of new diagnostic and therapeutic options, as well as the evaluation of evidence-based guidelines, stroke care systems will continue to be further improved and refined.

Suggestions from Clinical Practice Guidelines Establishment of primary stroke centers (PSCs) or regional acute stroke-ready hospital (ASRH) is needed to provide emergency care to acute stroke patients, which is based upon local resources. These systems should be closely associated with comprehensive stroke centers (CSCs). The centers or hospitals for acute stroke care should have a multidisciplinary committee to monitor stroke care quality and outcomes and are needed to be certified by an independent external institution.

References

1. Alberts MJ, Hademenos G, Latchaw RE, et al. Recommendations for the establishment of primary stroke centers. JAMA. 2000;283:3102–9.
2. Alberts MJ, Latchaw RE, Selman WR, et al. Recommendation for comprehensive stroke center:

a consensus statement from the Brain Attack Coalition. Stroke. 2005;36:1597–618.
3. Alberts MJ, Latchaw RE, Jagoda A, et al. Revised and updated recommendations for the establishment of primary stroke centers: a summary statement from the brain attack coalition. Stroke. 2011;42:2651–65.
4. Alberts MJ, Wechsler LR, Lee Jensen ME, et al. Formation and function of acute stroke-ready hospitals within a stroke system of care recommendations from the Brain Attack Coalition. Stroke. 2013;44:3382–93.
5. Gorelick PB. Primary and comprehensive stroke centers: history, value and certification criteria. J Stroke. 2013;15:78–89.
6. Leifer D, Bravata DM, Connors JJ 3rd, et al. Metrics for measuring quality of care in comprehensive stroke centers: detailed follow-up to Brain Attack Coalition comprehensive stroke center recommendations: a statement for healthcare professionals from the American Heart Association/American Stroke Association. Stroke. 2011;42:849–77.
7. Fedder W. National and international quality initiatives to improve stroke care. Neurol Clin. 2008;26:1191–207.
8. The Joint Commission Web site. http://www.jointcommission.org. Accessed 20 Sep 2016.
9. Song S, Fonarow GC, Olson DM, et al. Association of Get the Guideline-Stroke Program participation and clinical outcomes for Medicare beneficiaries with ischemic stroke. Stroke. 2016;47:1294–302.
10. Meretoja A, Roine RO, Kaste M, et al. Effectiveness of primary and comprehensive stroke centers PERFECT stroke: a nationwide observational study from Finland. Stroke. 2010;41:1102–7.
11. Gropen TI, Gagliano PJ, Blake CA, et al. Quality improvement in acute stroke: the New York state stroke center designation project. Neurology. 2006;67:88–93.
12. Lichtman JH, Jones SB, Leifheit-Limson EC, et al. 30-day mortality and readmission after hemorrhagic stroke among Medicare beneficiaries in joint commission primary stroke center-certified and noncertified hospitals. Stroke. 2011;42:3387–91.
13. Guzauskas GF, Boudreau DM, Villa KF, et al. The cost-effectiveness of primary stroke centers for acute stroke care. Stroke. 2012;43:1617–23.
14. Leys D, Ringelstein EB, Kaste M, et al. The main components of stroke unit care: results of a European expert survey. Cerebrovasc Dis. 2007;23:344–52.
15. Leys D, Ringelstein EB, Kaste M, et al. Facilities available in European hospitals treating stroke patients. Stroke. 2007;38:2985–91.
16. Ringelstein EB, Chamorro A, Kaste M, et al. European stroke organisation recommendations to establish a stroke unit and stroke center. Stroke. 2013;44:828–40.
17. Uehara T, Yasui N, Okada Y, et al. Which should be the essential components of stroke centers in Japan? Questionnaire survey to directors of facilities certified by the Japan stroke society. Cerebrovasc Dis. 2014;37:409–16.
18. Mullen MT, Wiebe DJ, Bowman A, et al. Disparities in accessibility of certified primary stroke centers. Stroke. 2014;45:3381–8.
19. Mullen MT, Branas CC, Kasner SE, et al. Optimization modeling to maximize population access to comprehensive stroke centers. Neurology. 2015;84:1196–205.
20. Sanyal R, Barrick J, Bhalla A, et al. 2010 British association of stroke physicians survey of interventional treatments for stroke in the United Kingdom. Int J Stroke. 2013;8:62–8.

Stroke Unit

2

Joung-Ho Rha

Abstract

A stroke unit is an organized in-hospital care for acute stroke. It was first conceptualized in the 1960s but has become the mainstream of acute stroke treatment in the twenty-first century. It consists of stroke team, stroke ward with monitoring function, and operating protocol. Other medical supports such as emergency room, laboratory, and neuroradiology service are also required. Its effect is comparable to other proven treatments of acute stroke, and as the evidence accumulates, it has become key element of acute stroke care organization, and now most guidelines state that an acute stroke patient should be cared in a stroke unit with a high grade of recommendation. Nationwide effort to disseminate stroke unit to afford most stroke patients is required to lessen the death and disability, which also leads to decreased total medical cost, as a stroke unit is cost-effective. Recently, a mobile stroke unit, which is an ambulance with CT and telemedicine support, is being established so that hyperacute stroke treatment can be started even faster at prehospital stage.

A stroke unit is a specialized in-hospital treatment unit which is designed for optimized acute stroke care (Fig. 2.1). It is not only confined to hardware facility but also includes stroke team and clinical pathway. Since its evidence of efficacy and usefulness accumulates continuously, establishment of a stroke unit is getting more and more popular in stroke care hospital, and nowadays it has become the essential component of stroke care organization.

Regarding the term "stroke unit," there is a little disparity between the American and European side, probably due to the difference in medical system. American physicians use the term more confined way, as one of the essential components of stroke center. On the other hand, European physicians use the term more broadly, sometimes to mean the stroke center including the rehabilitation unit. In this chapter, stroke unit is used strictly to refer the former to avoid

J.-H. Rha
Department of Neurology, Inha University College of Medicine, Incheon, South Korea
e-mail: jhrha@inha.ac.kr

S.-H. Lee (ed.), *Stroke Revisited: Diagnosis and Treatment of Ischemic Stroke*,
Stroke Revisited, DOI 10.1007/978-981-10-1424-6_2

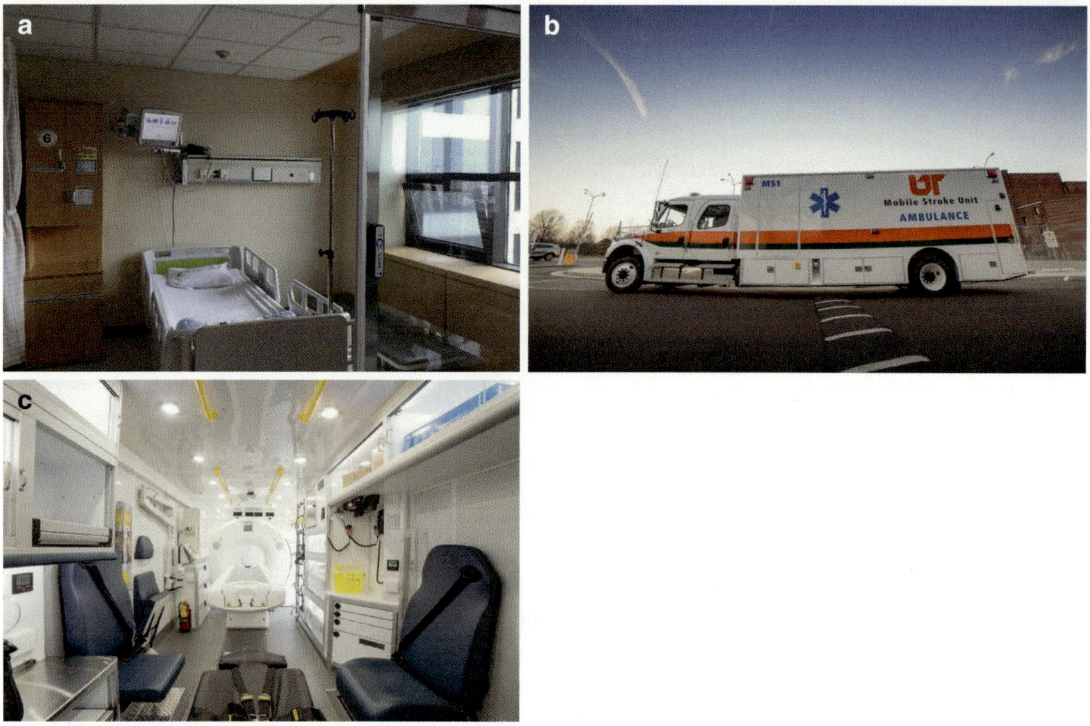

Fig. 2.1 Stroke unit. Interior view of stroke unit (**a**); exterior (**b**) and interior (**c**) view of mobile stroke unit. Reproduced by permission of Business Wire (University of Tennessee Web Site, http://www.businesswire.com/news/home/20160322005420/en/University-Tennessee-College-Medicine-Launches-World%E2%80%99s-Mobile)

confusion, and there is a separate chapter for stroke center in this textbook.

2.1 Historical Perspective

The term "stroke unit" first appeared in 1969 from medical literature [1], but the concept of dedicated in-hospital ward for stroke traces back to 1962 in New York, where the investigator evaluated rehabilitation ward for hemiplegic patient. At that time, most studies compared the dedicated rehabilitation ward for stroke to the other general ward. The first study to investigate modern concept of stroke unit [2], which is an organized inpatient care for acute stroke, would be the Edinburgh study in 1980 [3], which is a randomized controlled study with 311 acute stroke patients to compare stroke unit versus general medical ward. After then, a series of controlled trials followed to investigate the efficacy of a comprehensive stroke unit, mostly performed in the 1990s. Among them, the Trondheim study is most representative, which is a randomized controlled trial comparing stroke unit versus general medical ward in 220 acute stroke patients and showed big success in reducing death and dependency with an odds ratio of 0.36 (95% confidence interval (CI) = 0.21 ~ 0.61) [4]. As the evidences of stroke unit accumulate, stroke unit became one of the essential components of stroke carc organization in the twenty-first century [5], and now most clinical practice guidelines in the world state that the acute stroke patient should be treated in the stroke unit with a high grade of recommendation.

2.2 Stroke Unit Efficacy

According to the latest systematic Cochrane review (Stroke Unit Trialists' Collaboration, 2013), a comprehensive stroke unit is estimated

Table 2.1 Efficacy of proven acute stroke treatment by reducing death and dependency

Modality	Background	RRR	ARR	NNT
Stroke unit	Stroke Unit Trialists' Collaboration, 2013	6.9%	4.0%	25
Aspirin	IST, 1997	2.6%	1.2%	83
Intravenous tPA	NINDS, 1995	9.8%	5.5%	18
Endovascular thrombectomy	HERMES Consortium, 2016	32.8%	10.6%	10
Decompression craniectomy	Pooled analysis, 2007	48.8%	23.0%	4

IST International Stroke Trial, *NINDS* National Institute of Neurological Disorder and Stroke, *HERMES* Highly Effective Reperfusion evaluated in Multiple Endovascular Stroke Trials, *RRR* relative risk reduction, *ARR* absolute risk reduction, *NNT* numbers needed to treatment

to reduce death and dependency by an odds ratio of 0.82 (95% CI 0.68 ~ 0.98) [6]. When we compare this result to other proven treatments of acute stroke [7], through indirect comparison by death and dependency, the efficacy of a stroke unit exceeds that of acute aspirin use and is almost comparable to that of intravenous tPA (Table 2.1). This rather unexpectedly big effect made stroke unit a mainstream of acute stroke care as important as thrombolytic treatment. Another study showed that this effect does not fade away as time goes by but lasts more than 10 years of follow-up [8, 9].

2.3 Mechanism of Efficacy

There can be many reasons for the abovementioned efficacy, but the biggest should be attributed to close monitoring and early intervention of patient status, such as vital signs, neurological status, and electrocardiogram, which leads to better management of blood pressure, prompt detection of early neurological deterioration or paroxysmal atrial fibrillation, and effective prevention of possible complications [10]. Optimized clinical pathway by written care protocol according to guideline and early rehabilitation can also accelerate in-hospital process and thus contribute to better outcomes. But all these effects are abolished in the general ward or other types of care, even though applying the same clinical pathway or protocol, probably because the caregiver is not dedicated to stroke care [11].

2.4 Component of Stroke Unit

To be a functionally effective stroke unit, many components are needed, either as human resources, facilities, or operating protocols [12, 13]. These components can be different from hospital to hospital, and many regional variations also exist. In some countries there are criteria to be certified by academic or government authority. However, there are essential components which are almost uniform in most stroke units (Table 2.2).

First of all, there must be an organization of multidisciplinary stroke team to operate a stroke unit. This team is composed of a doctor, nurse, and coordinator. Stroke team doctors are usually neurologist or neurosurgeons with their subspecialty in stroke. The attending duty schedule and emergency hotline are also required. A stroke nurse is a specially trained nurse for a dedicated stroke patient care, receiving continuous education for neurological monitoring and stroke care protocol. In some institution, certification of neurological scale such as the National Institute of Health Stroke Scale (NIHSS) is required. A stroke coordinator is a person who takes an important role to facilitate all the administrative and in-hospital process to be in proper order and time. They notify the stroke team to be ready for the next process, so that most of the in-hospital performance index such as door-to-imaging or door-to-needle/puncture time can be shortened. They also inform the patient or family for better understanding of in-hospital process and later educate them for effective secondary prevention and stroke awareness. Their contribu-

Table 2.2 Essential component of stroke unit

Component		Comment
Stroke team	Neurologist, neurosurgeon with stroke subspecialty regular meeting	By trained program, academic activity, and clinical experience
	Stroke nurse, coordinator	Dedicated for stroke care
	Neuroradiologist, neurointerventionist	Angio-suite team
	Rehabilitation physician social worker	Early rehabilitation
Written care protocol	Operation manual	Admission/discharge criteria
		Neurological flow sheet
	Clinical pathway	
Facility	Stroke ward	Monitoring devices
	Emergency service	
	Neuroradiology Stroke priority fast track laboratory support 24/7	CT, MR with DWI Vessel imaging (CTA, MRA, DSA)
Quality improvement	Regular quality assessment regular education	Set target index to improve stroke team patient and public

DWI Diffusion-weighted image, *CTA* CT angiography, *MRA* MR angiography, *DSA* digital subtraction angiography

tion for good outcome of stroke patient is usually greater than expected and very efficient in the aspect of time and cost. A neuroradiologist or neurointerventionist is also a member of the stroke team, with angio-suite technicians and nurses. A rehabilitation doctor in the stroke team evaluates the patient and conducts early rehabilitation. Regular meeting and education program for a stroke team is recommended for inside communication and quality improvement. Sometimes, a social worker joins the stroke team to provide social service to patients if necessary.

The treatment in the stroke unit can be individualized, but the principle should follow the evidence-based guidelines, and for this purpose written care protocol is required as the operation manual of stroke unit. Also, every stroke unit is recommended to have its own clinical pathway optimized to the hospital. This can contribute to select the right patient for intervention without missing and also to accelerate intrahospital performance such as door-to-needle time. A stroke unit also needs to provide its own flow sheet which can record the patient's neurological status. Most hospitals now adopt electronic medical record and order system, and clinical pathway can be incorporated into it, with an automated notification system which alerts the stroke team by mobile communication and alarming function for fast track investigation and treatment.

The protocol should also describe which patient to admit to the stroke unit and when to discharge. Each stroke unit can set its own criteria, but usually acute stroke patient within 48 or 72 h after onset is the target patient, especially post-thrombolysis or thrombectomy patient. Besides unstable stroke or transient ischemic attack (TIA) patient with fluctuating or progressive neurological status, patient before and after neurovascular intervention such as stent insertion, but not just for diagnostic angiography, can also be a subject of stroke unit admission. Some stroke units also admit acute hemorrhagic stroke patient who needs critical care. But when the stroke patient is comatose and postsurgical status or vital sign is unstable with intubation and ventilator control, admission to intensive care unit is necessary for critical care. Patient moves to general ward when neurological status is stable for 48 to 72 h.

In the aspect of facility, stroke unit ward and monitoring devices are required. The stroke unit ward needs to be spacious enough for each bed, and close monitoring should be possible directly from the nursing station at all times. A stroke unit needs to be equipped with monitoring devices for blood pressure, electrocardiogram, and O_2 saturation and respiration, and all of these should be always available when needed. Because of the emergency characteristic of acute stroke, the emergency department service of the hospital is necessary. Laboratory service also should be available 24/7. Neuroradiology service with CT, MR with diffusion-weighted image, and noninvasive or conventional angiography also should be supported, and stroke priority of CT/MR fast track is recommended to shorten door-to-imaging time.

Once a stroke unit is established, continuous effort to improve its performance is necessary, and to accomplish this, quality assessment and improvement activity should persist. After a careful setup of practical target index to improve, the entire stroke team needs to communicate and make effort to that goal, thus making a better stroke unit every year. Finally, it is recommended that stroke team members educate the patient and public for stroke awareness and prevention to serve the neighboring community.

2.5 Mobile Stroke Unit

Recently the term "mobile stroke unit" is used to refer to an ambulance equipped with CT and telemedicine device inside (Fig. 2.1b, c), so that early neurological evaluation and intravenous tPA administration during transfer are possible. This treatment paradigm is especially suitable for low hospital density area, and mobile stroke unit is now actively being set up in many countries including the United States [14].

2.6 Cost-Effectiveness

Establishing stroke unit takes costs, both for facility and human resources, and thus needs more payment. But because the patient outcome gets better with less disability, the length of hospital stay shortens, and the total medical cost is reduced [15]. As a whole, the costs for stroke care without stroke unit much exceed those with stroke unit, so it can be said that stroke unit is cost-effective, which was verified by many studies [16]. So the stroke unit is demanded not only by patient group but also by health insurance providers. From this point of view, the government needs to encourage the establishment of as many stroke units as possible so all stroke patients can benefit, to lessen not only the burden of death and disability but also to decrease the whole national medical expense, among which the portion by stroke is enormous.

2.7 Current Status

As the evidence of stroke unit efficacy accumulates, most developed countries are making effort to establish and disseminate stroke units. In the United States, more than 1200 stroke units are currently running in 2016, though the density varies area by area. Germany is running more than 200 certified stroke units, which are evenly distributed throughout the country, and total bed numbers of 1200 are estimated to cover 60% of all acute stroke patients. Other countries are also planning to increase the proportion of stroke unit care, until every stroke patient is treated in the stroke unit finally.

Suggestions from Clinical Practice Guidelines The centers should run a comprehensive specialized stroke care (stroke unit), which incorporates rehabilitation. The stroke unit should have its own standardized protocols on acute stroke care.

References

1. Haerer AF, Smith RR, Currier RD. UMC stroke unit: review of the first 100 cases. J Miss State Med Assoc. 1969;10:237–41.
2. Marshall AM. The stroke unit—a new concept. J Neurosurg Nurs. 1971;3:153–6.
3. Garraway WM, Akhtar AJ, Hockey L, et al. Management of acute stroke in elderly: follow up of a controlled trial. Br Med J. 1980;281:827–9.
4. Indredavik B, Bakke F, Solberg R, et al. Benefit of stroke unit: a randomised controlled trial. Stroke. 1991;22:1026–31.
5. Ringelstein EB, Chamorro A, Kaste M, et al. European stroke organisation recommendations to establish a stroke unit and stroke center. Stroke. 2013;44:828–40.
6. Stroke Unit Trialists Collaboration. Organised inpatient (stroke unit) care for stroke. Cochrane Database Syst Rev. 2013;9:CD000197. doi:10.1002/14651858.CD000197.pub3.
7. Donnan GA, Fisher M, Macleod M, et al. Stroke. Lancet. 2008;371:1612–23.

8. Drummond AE, Pearson B, Lincoln NB, et al. Ten year follow-up of a randomised controlled trial of care in a stroke rehabilitation unit. BMJ. 2005;331:491–2.
9. Candelise L, Gattinoni M, Bersano A, et al. Stroke-unit care for acute stroke patients: an observational follow-up study. Lancet. 2007;369:299–305.
10. Choi HY, Seo JH, Yang JH, et al. Beneficial effects of stroke-unit care in stroke patients with atrial fibrillation. Yonsei Med J. 2013;54:301–5.
11. Langhorne P, Dey P, Woodman M, et al. Is stroke unit care portable? A systematic review of the clinical trials. Age Ageing. 2005;34:324–30.
12. Langhorne P, Pollock A, Stroke Unit Trialists' Collaboration. What are the components of effective stroke unit care? Age Ageing. 2002;31:365–71.
13. Leys D, Ringelstein EB, Kaste M, et al. The main components of stroke unit care: results of a European expert survey. Cerebrovasc Dis. 2007;23:344–52.
14. Parker SA, Bowry R, Wu TC, et al. Establishing the first mobile stroke unit in the United States. Stroke. 2015;46:1384–91.
15. Saka O, Serra V, Samyshkin Y, et al. Cost-effectiveness of stroke unit care followed by early supported discharge. Stroke. 2009;40:24–9.
16. Te Ao BJ, Brown PM, Feigin VL, et al. Are stroke units cost effective? Evidence from a New Zealand stroke incidence and population-based study. Int J Stroke. 2012;7:623–30.

Initial Assessment and Differential Diagnosis

3

Jeong-Min Kim

Abstract

Stroke diagnosis should be performed in a prompt and efficient manner with two major objectives: first, to rule out other potential causes of neurological deficit than stroke and, second, to confirm stroke diagnosis and estimate initial onset time to determine whether the patient could receive recanalization treatment. There are several situations where initial diagnosis of stroke can be difficult. The risk of missed diagnosis seems to be substantial in the following conditions: (1) posterior circulation stroke, especially when initial symptom is isolated vertigo or loss of consciousness, and (2) a patient with young onset age. Prompt and careful patient history taking, physical and neurological examination, and laboratory studies including appropriate brain imaging modalities are paramount in the initial assessment and differential diagnosis for the stroke suspected patients. Multidisciplinary approach should be implemented for prompt diagnostic and therapeutic procedures for the acute stroke patients.

Stroke results from abrupt onset neurological deficits due to impaired cerebral blood flow. It can be easily detectable by the public or medical personnel if relatively well-known stroke-related symptoms, such as sudden facial palsy, unilateral arm weakness, or speech difficulty, are the initial manifestation. These well-known symptoms are useful for public education and therefore constitute the worldwide FAST (face, arms, speech, time) campaign to detect acute cerebral infarction. However, initial diagnosis of stroke is not a simple task in some cases, and general physicians or internists, and even neurologists or stroke specialists, could overlook initial symptom or signs of hyperacute stroke. It is especially critical in clinical situations where patients visit emergency clinic complaining of neurological symptom developed within time window of reperfusion treatment, because "time is brain." The efficacy of

J.-M. Kim, M.D., Ph.D.
Department of Neurology, Chung-Ang University Hospital, Seoul, South Korea
e-mail: bellokim1@gmail.com

S.-H. Lee (ed.), *Stroke Revisited: Diagnosis and Treatment of Ischemic Stroke*, Stroke Revisited, DOI 10.1007/978-981-10-1424-6_3

recanalization therapy would be maximized and the risk of complication such as symptomatic hemorrhage minimized when the treatment is initiated as fast as possible.

There are two major undesirable but probable consequences in the assessment of patients suspected of acute stroke in emergency setting: the first is to proceed reperfusion treatment to the patient who did not actually have stroke, but stroke mimic, such as brain tumor, abscess, nonconvulsive seizure, metabolic encephalopathy, or psychogenic weakness; the other condition is not to treat stroke patient with acute onset because stroke diagnosis was missed at the initial evaluation. Both conditions are critical for patients as well as doctors, since thrombolytic treatment is a potentially dangerous treatment modality due to hemorrhagic risk. Stroke patients who were overlooked for treatment by recanalization therapy eventually lose the chance of successful recovery by reperfusion of occluded artery. Therefore, prompt and careful patient history taking, physical and neurological examination, and laboratory studies including appropriate brain imaging modalities are paramount in the initial assessment and differential diagnosis for the stroke suspected patients. At the same time, multidisciplinary approach should be emphasized for the prompt diagnostic and therapeutic practice for the acute stroke patients.

3.1 Initial Evaluation of Stroke Patients

Initial evaluation and assessment of stroke usually takes place in the emergency department. The two major objectives in the assessment of suspected stroke patients are, first, to detect other potential causes of neurological deficit and, second, to confirm stroke diagnosis and estimate initial onset time to decide if the patient could receive recanalization treatment. There are several scoring systems to define stroke or transient ischemia attack diagnosis in emergency settings, although its usefulness in real clinical situation remains questionable [1, 2].

3.1.1 History

Cerebral infarction is a medical emergency just like acute coronary syndrome. However, unlike myocardial infarction associated with typical chest pain which aids the diagnosis of coronary artery disease with high sensitivity and specificity, it is far more difficult to derive a prompt and definite diagnosis of cerebral infarction in emergency setting by patient history taking because highly diverse neurological symptoms and sign can be presented according to involved cerebral arteries, and many neurological and non-neurological diseases can mimic stroke symptom. The single most important information is initial symptom and its onset time from patient history. The time of onset is defined as when the patient was at the symptom-free state or previous baseline or when the patient was last known to be symptom-free [3]. The onset time is obtained from a patient, but when not possible, neurologists should interview bystanders or family witnesses and emergency medical service personnel to get as precise information as possible within a short time [3]. Combined vascular risk factors, previous medical history, and current medication profile needs to be reviewed before considering reperfusion treatment.

3.1.2 Physical and Neurological Examination

The general examination is to identify other potential causes of the patient's neurological symptoms, potential causes of stroke, and coexisting medical conditions and issues that may impact the management of acute stroke [3].

Airway, breathing, and circulation should be maintained from the initial evaluation. Vital sign with blood pressure, heart rate, and body temperature assessment is essential and should be monitored if necessary. Cardiovascular examination including chest auscultation and peripheral artery palpation may disclose potential cardioembolic source and systemic atherosclerosis burden. The initial neurological examination should be brief but thorough, and in cases of suggestive of stroke, the use of formal stroke scoring systems, such as the National Institute of Health Stroke Scale, is recommended to quantify neurological deficit, facilitate communication among medical teams, and establish therapeutic strategy [3].

3.1.3 Laboratory and Imaging Studies

Several laboratory and imaging studies are routinely performed in emergency setting in the patients suspected of stroke to exclude alternative diagnoses such as hemorrhagic stroke, to identify combined serious medical condition, and to select eligible patients for thrombolysis treatment (Table 3.1 and Fig. 3.1). Serum glucose test is important because both hyper- and hypoglycemia could result in focal neurological deficit, and both conditions result in secondary neuronal damage and are related to poor prognosis in acute stroke. Complete blood count especially platelet count, as well as coagulation battery, provides an essential information regarding whether this patient could be a candidate of intravenous thrombolysis treatment or not. Increased serum D-dimer could, in some situations, suggest less well-known stroke etiology associated with occult cancer, although its incidence is increasing due mostly to rapidly aging society. Serum cardiac markers, electrocardiogram, and chest radiography provide combined cardiologic problems such as coronary artery disease, congestive heart failure, and cardiac arrhythmia, although these data should not delay the initiation of reperfusion treatment.

Table 3.1 Immediate diagnostic studies for evaluating a patient with suspected acute stroke

For all patients
Noncontrast brain CT or brain MRI (followed by angiography)
Blood glucose
Oxygen saturation
Blood pressure and pulse rate
Serum electrolyte/renal function test
Hepatic function test
Complete blood count (especially platelet count)
Cardiac ischemia markers
Electrocardiogram
Coagulation tests including prothrombin time, activated partial thromboplastin time, and D-dimers
Chest radiography
For selected patients
Toxicology screening
Blood alcohol level
Pregnancy test
Arterial blood gas tests
Lumbar puncture
Electroencephalogram

Noncontrast brain CT has been recommended as an initial imaging modality to rule out hemorrhagic stroke and to initiate intravenous thrombolysis. Recent advance of endovascular thrombectomy among acute ischemic stroke patients confirmed therapeutic efficacy and safety from multiple large randomized clinical trials; therefore, prompt evaluation of cerebral arteries is getting more critical among the patients with suspected major intracranial arterial occlusion (Fig. 3.2). So far, there exists a wide variation of brain imaging protocols for acute stroke patients among stroke centers. Further research needs to be performed to determine appropriate imaging protocol beyond noncontrast brain CT to select optimal additional imaging modalities among CT angiography, brain MRI, or perfusion imaging and also to prioritize among additional imaging studies and intravenous thrombolysis.

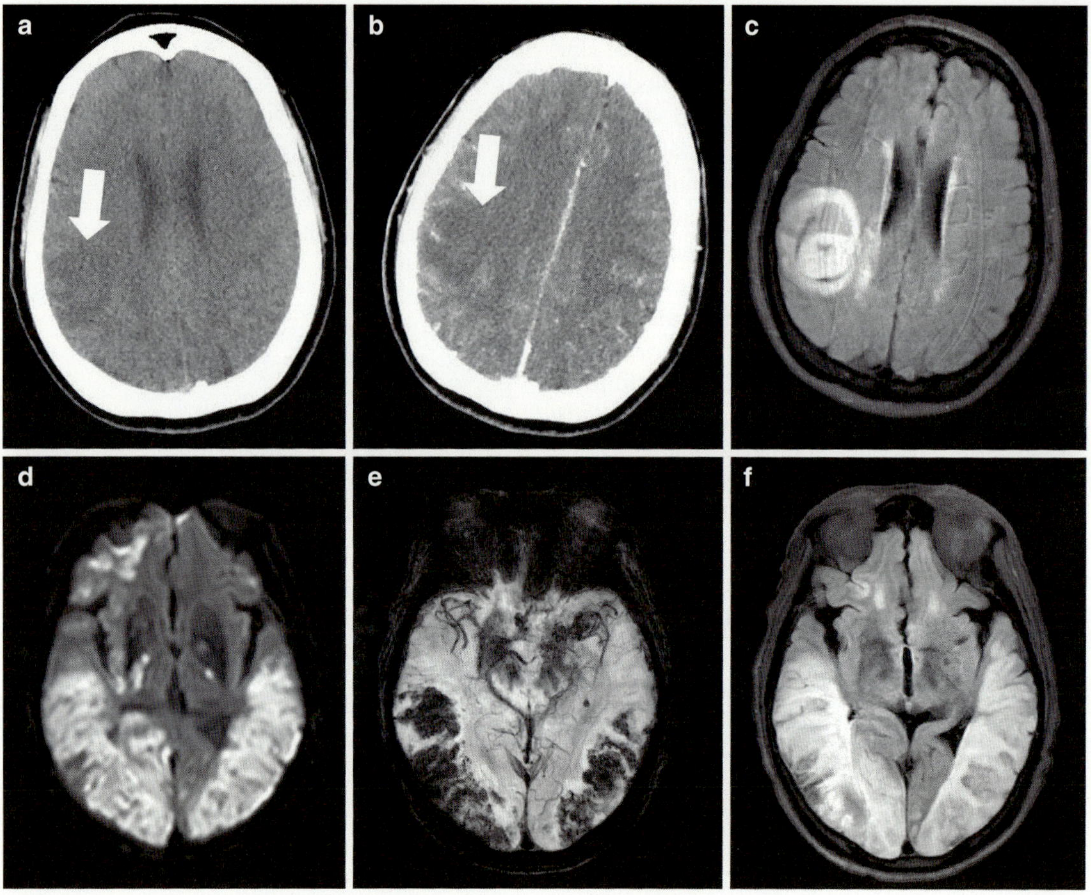

Fig. 3.1 Representative cases of stroke mimics. The first case (**a–c**) is a 65-year-old woman who complained of sudden onset left-side weakness and hypesthesia. Initial pre- and post-gadolinium (**a**, **b**) brain CT showed low-attenuated lesion involving right postcentral gyrus without enhancement (*white arrow*). Since initial symptom onset was within 3 h, she was treated by intravenous thrombolysis, but weakness progressed thereafter. Subsequent brain MR imaging (MRI) with T2-based fluid-attenuated inversion recovery protocol showed edematous mass lesion with heterogeneous signal intensity and fluid-fluid level. Further evaluation with serial brain MRI and biopsy revealed brain abscess as a final diagnosis. The second case (**d–f**) is a 62-year-old woman who was found to be in a comatose state at home. Initial neurological examination revealed semicomatose mental status and left-side dominant weakness with extensor Babinski reflex. Brain MR imaging showed diffuse high-signal intensity from diffusion-weighted image and low-signal intensity from susceptibility-weighted image mainly involving both parietal and occipital cortices. Admission serum glucose level and osmolality at admission were significantly elevated, and she was diagnosed as hyperosmolar hyperglycemic coma

Fig. 3.2 A case of missed stroke diagnosis. An 85-year-old man with lost consciousness was transferred from general hospital. Neurologist was delayed 4 h after symptom onset because primary assessment was syncope, but recovery of mentality was delayed. Initial neurological examination revealed semicomatose mental status with decorticated posture and bilateral extensor Babinski reflex. Brain MR imaging with diffusion-weighted image showed slight increased signal intensity involving both cerebral hemispheres (**a**). MR angiography revealed the occlusion of left middle cerebral artery and right internal carotid artery at petrous segment (**b**, **c**). Emergent endovascular thrombectomy successfully recanalized both occlude vessels (**d**, **e**) and extracted red thrombi (**f**), but his mentation was not recovered and followed brain CT revealed massive brain edema and hemorrhagic transformation involving both cerebral hemispheres (**g**, **h**). He died 5 days after symptom onset

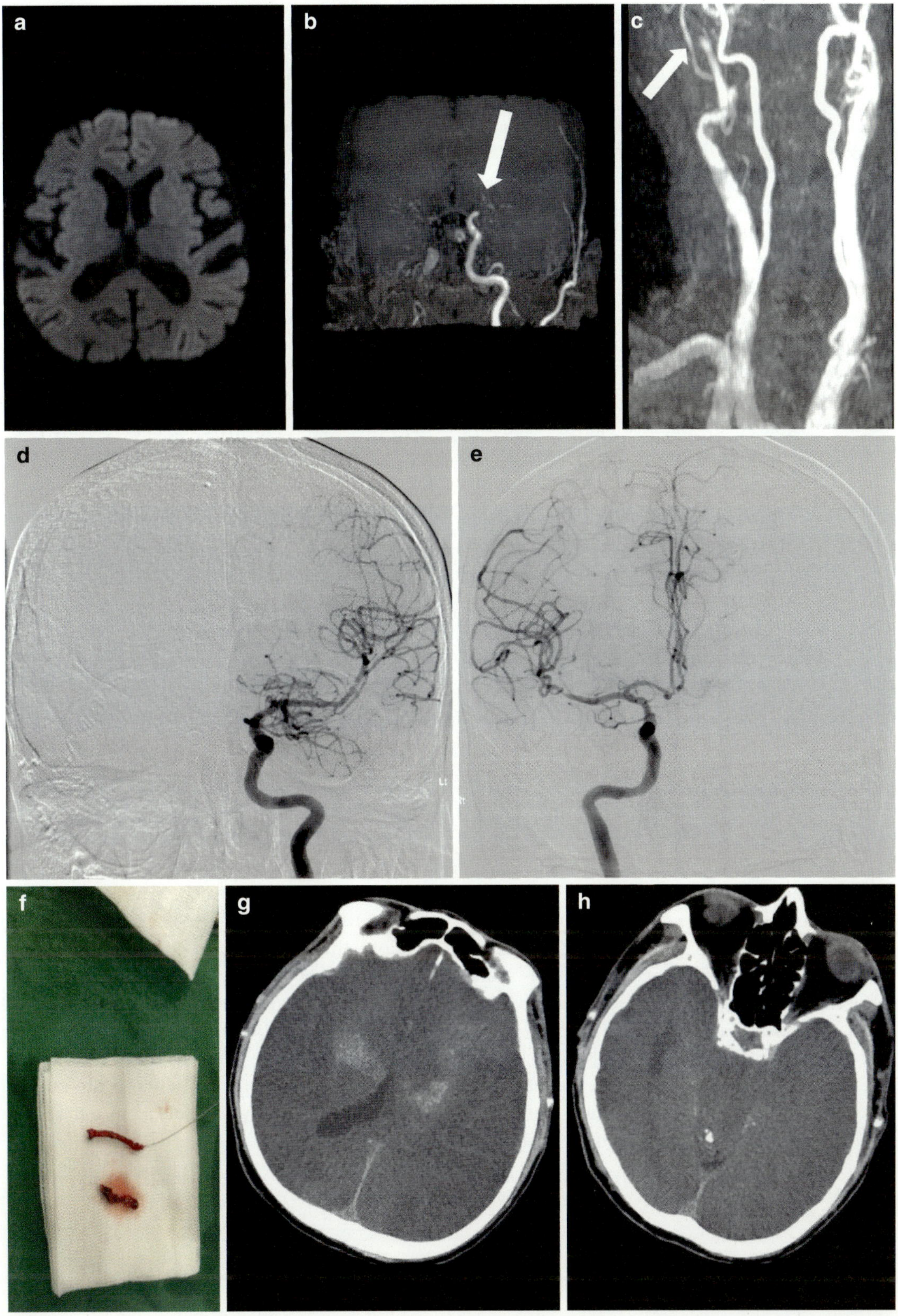
a
b
c
d
e
f
g
h

3.2 Cases with High Risk of Missed Diagnosis of Stroke

Missed stroke diagnosis in emergency setting could result in catastrophic consequence because of delayed reperfusion treatment or missed opportunity for secondary prevention with antithrombotics. The length of stay is increased, and the neurological deficit at discharge and mortality rate is higher among missed stroke victims than those without missed diagnosis. Several retrospective studies show that initial misdiagnosis occurs in up to 20% of stroke patients, without significant differences between emergency department of academic center where neurologist primarily deals with the suspected stroke patient and community hospital where general physician manages stroke suspects [4]. Based on several hospital-based cohort studies, the risk of missed diagnosis is greatest in the following conditions: (1) posterior circulation stroke, especially when initial symptom was isolated vertigo or loss of consciousness, and (2) a patient with young onset age.

Isolated vertigo by small brainstem infarction, vertigo with hearing loss after anterior inferior cerebellar artery infarction, or recurrent vertigo due to vertebrobasilar insufficiency are well-known situations in which general physicians or even neurologists frequently miss the right diagnosis. Brain CT with or without angiography is commonly performed in emergency department among patients with dizziness to rule out so-called central origin, which is not an ideal imaging modality in detecting acute brainstem or cerebellar stroke. Brain MRI with diffusion-weighted image should be considered among the patients with suspected central vertigo, although it can also miss acute vertigo due to small lesion in up to 20% of isolated acute vertigo patients [5]. Recently serial neuro-ophthalmological examinations including gaze-evoked nystagmus, horizontal vestibulo-ocular reflex, and ocular tilt reaction (viz., HINTS, head impulse, nystagmus, test of skew) were studied among the patients with acute vestibular syndrome, and it showed that HINTS examination could detect vertigo after medullary or pontine infarction with higher sensitivity and specificity than brain MRI taken 24–48 h after symptom (Fig. 3.3) [6]. The dangerous signs can also be remembered using the acronym INFARCT (impulse normal, fast-phase alternating, refixation on cover test). Although neurologists in these days have become increasingly dependent on brain MRI for acute stroke diagnosis, this result emphasizes the importance of careful bedside examination and maintaining patient contact for the right diagnosis.

Stroke is uncommon among young adults but its incidence has been rising over recent decades. When a neurologist is confronted with a young patient complaining of sudden onset neurological deficit, the list of initial differential diagnosis may include complicated migraine, seizure attack, demyelinating encephalitis such as multiple sclerosis, and conversion disorder, and stroke would be less appreciated as a primary suspect. The young stroke patients are distinct group of patients which have different clinical characteristics and stroke mechanism compared to the "general" stroke population [7]. Currently several prospective cohort studies are underway to disclose the risk factors, etiologies, and outcomes of ischemic stroke among young population. It is desirable to perform additional brain imaging including vascular evaluation to derive a definite diagnosis or to exclude stroke among young patients with sudden onset focal neurological deficit in emergency setting.

Fig. 3.3 Bedside oculomotor examination in the acute vestibular syndrome to detect stroke. Bedside oculomotor examinations including ocular alignment from ocular tilt reaction and horizontal head impulse test of vestibulo-ocular reflex, along with gaze-evoked nystagmus, could differentiate stroke among the patients with acute vestibular syndrome, which is known to be more sensitive than early brain MR imaging. Reproduced by permission of Journal of Clinical Neurology [5]

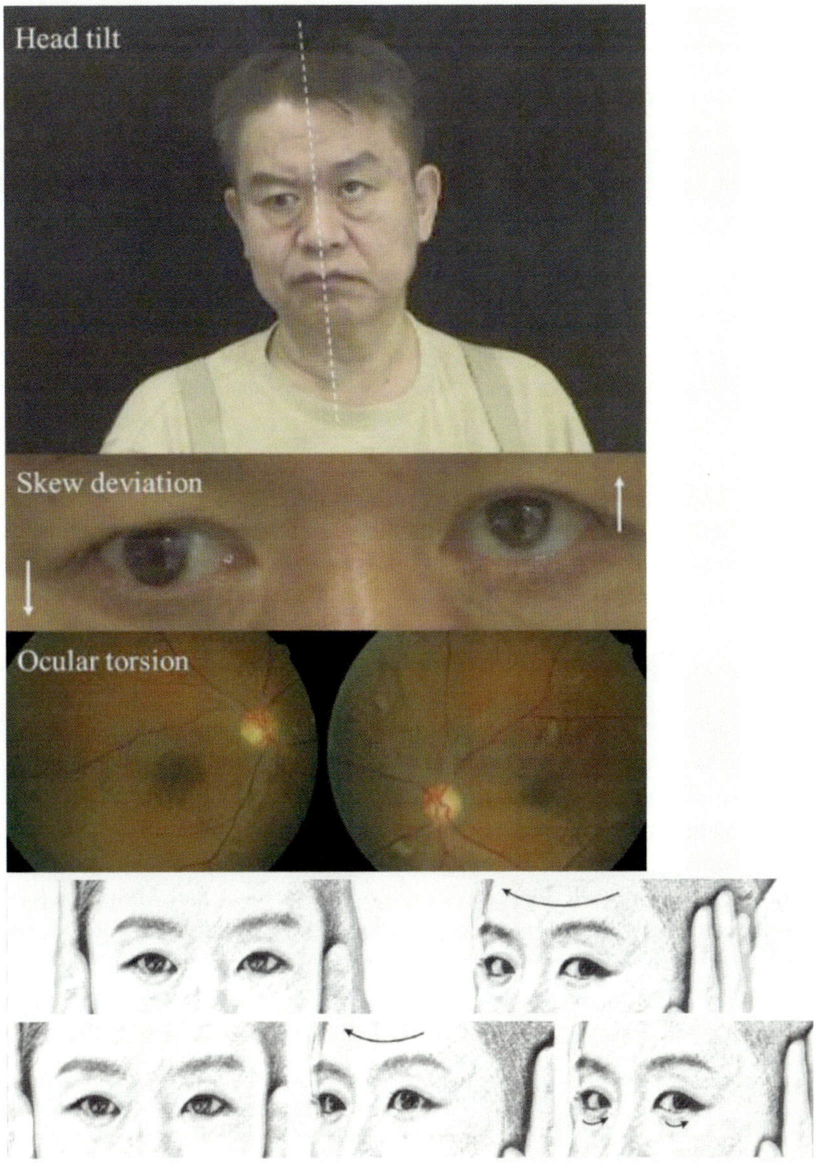

3.3 Stroke Mimics Treated by Thrombolysis

Several neurological and non-neurological disorders could mimic stroke. Central nervous system tumor or abscess is known to be associated with more insidious symptom onset and gradual progression, but their initial symptom onset could be as sudden as stroke in several special situations such as acute bleeding within tumor or focal seizure elicited by mass effect. Hemiplegic migraine and other

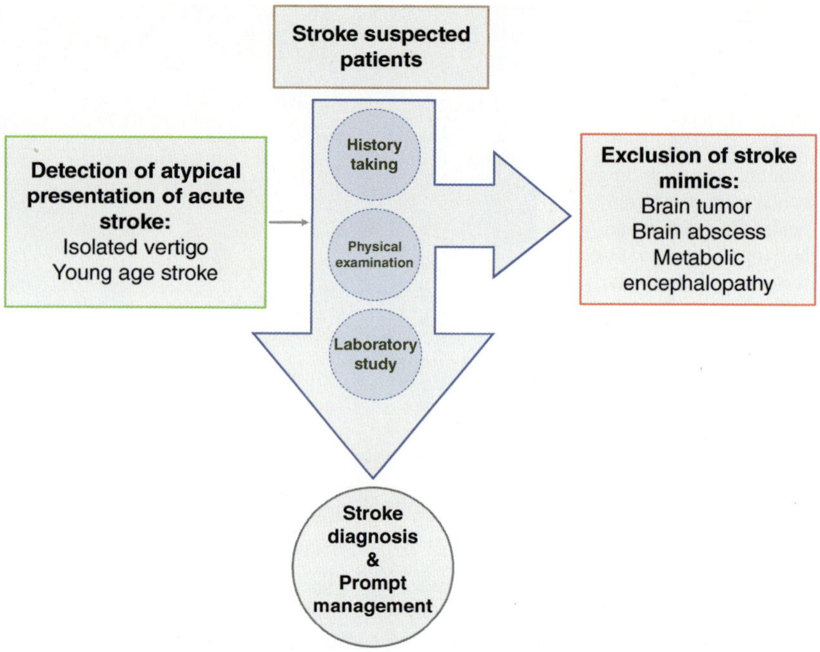

Fig. 3.4 A schematic diagram showing initial diagnostic process of stroke suspected patients

complicated migraine are neurological disorders which cause sudden onset neurological deficit which is reversible by nature. Alcohol intoxication, Wernicke's encephalopathy, and drug toxicity should be considered when a patient had a previous history of alcohol abuse or medication history which could suppress central nervous system. Hypertensive encephalopathy and glycemic disorders (both hyper- and hypoglycemia) are well-known diseases affecting CNS to cause decreased mental status and focal neurological deficit in selected cases. Psychogenic weakness such as conversion disorder is another clinical situation which distresses emergency medical personnel to rule out structural lesion in the brain.

These conditions should be excluded at initial evaluation step by patient history, physical/neurological examination, and laboratory studies (Fig. 3.4). However in some cases stroke mimics are treated as acute stroke, including intravenous thrombolysis because stroke specialists have to make a decision based on limited clinical information within a short period of time. One recent study revealed that among 512 patients treated by thrombolysis after diagnosis of stroke, 14% were later determined to be stroke mimics, including seizure, complicated migraines, and conversion disorders [8]. Based on their finding that 87% of stroke mimics were functionally independent at discharge and none experienced hemorrhagic complication, they suggested safety of administering intravenous thrombolysis to patients with suspected cerebral infarction even when the diagnosis is not stroke [8]. However it is undeniable that highest care must be taken not to implement thrombolytic treatment for those patients without stroke at emergency setting.

Suggestions from Clinical Practice Guidelines
An emergency unit for acute stroke should have a standardized protocol for neurological evaluation of patients with suspected stroke. Intravenous fibrinolysis using the recombinant tissue plasminogen activator is recommended to begin within 60 min after the patient's visit. A team for acute stroke care must be organized as multidisciplinary including stroke physicians, surgeons, nurses, and angiographic interventionists.

References

1. Kidwell CS, Starkman S, Eckstein M, et al. Identifying stroke in the field. Prospective validation of the Los Angeles prehospital stroke screen (LAPSS). Stroke. 2000;31:71–6.
2. Goldstein LB, Simel DL. Is this patient having a stroke? JAMA. 2005;293:2391–402.
3. Jauch EC, Saver JL, Adams HP Jr, et al. Guidelines for the early management of patients with acute ischemic stroke: a guideline for healthcare professionals from the American Heart Association/American Stroke Association. Stroke. 2013;44:870–947.
4. Richoz B, Hugli O, Dami F, et al. Acute stroke chameleons in a university hospital: risk factors, circumstances, and outcomes. Neurology. 2015;85:505–11.
5. Huh YE, Kim JS. Bedside evaluation of dizzy patients. J Clin Neurol. 2013;9:203–13.
6. Kattah JC, Talkad AV, Wang DZ, et al. HINTS to diagnose stroke in the acute vestibular syndrome. Stroke. 2009;40:3504–10.
7. Kwon HS, Kim C, Lee SH, et al. Protocol of the stroke in Korean young adults study: a multicenter case-control study and prospective cohort study. J Stroke Cerebrovasc Dis. 2016;25:1503–8.
8. Chernyshev OY, Martin-Schild S, Albright KC, et al. Safety of tPA in stroke mimics and neuroimaging-negative cerebral ischemia. Neurology. 2010;74:1340–5.

Part II

Diagnosis and Treatment of Stroke: Acute Stage

Overview of Patient Management Flow

4

Seung-Hoon Lee

Abstract

Treatment of patients suspected to have had a stroke begins as soon as the patient arrives at the emergency room. This chapter summarizes the sequence of procedures followed from diagnosis to treatment of these patients, starting with the arrival of the patient. Explanation of patient care is further divided into emergency unit, stroke unit, intensive care unit, general ward, rehabilitation ward, and discharge planning. More detailed contents are designed to introduce the future chapters.

Patients who are in a critical condition are transported to a medical center capable of providing adequate treatment according to the emergency patient delivery system of the country. Since each country has its own optimized system, this topic will not be discussed here. The contents to be discussed in this chapter include the treatment of suspected stroke patients in each center's emergency unit, e.g., stroke unit for acute medical care, general ward for general medical care, and rehabilitation unit for rehabilitation. This chapter describes the most important aspect of this book, the sequence of events (Fig. 4.1) from admission to discharge of patients suspected to have had a stroke in the physicians' point of view. Only the key points related to each aspect have been outlined in this chapter, which will act as a guide to the future chapters containing more detailed explanations. Further reading of the subsequent chapters after reading this introductory chapter will provide a comprehensive and thorough understanding of treatment of acute stroke.

4.1 Care in the Emergency Unit

Treatment of suspected stroke patients in the emergency room is a battle against time. The ischemic core is rapidly growing after the ischemic stroke occurs. Faster recanalization of the occluded vessel results in a higher chance of recovery of the ischemic tissue. Therefore, a clear and quick diagnosis of the patient followed by focusing all available personnel of the center on the recanalization procedure is essential.

S.-H. Lee, M.D., Ph.D., F.A.H.A.
Department of Neurology, Seoul National University Hospital, Seoul, South Korea
e-mail: sb0516@snu.ac.kr

S.-H. Lee (ed.), *Stroke Revisited: Diagnosis and Treatment of Ischemic Stroke*, Stroke Revisited, DOI 10.1007/978-981-10-1424-6_4

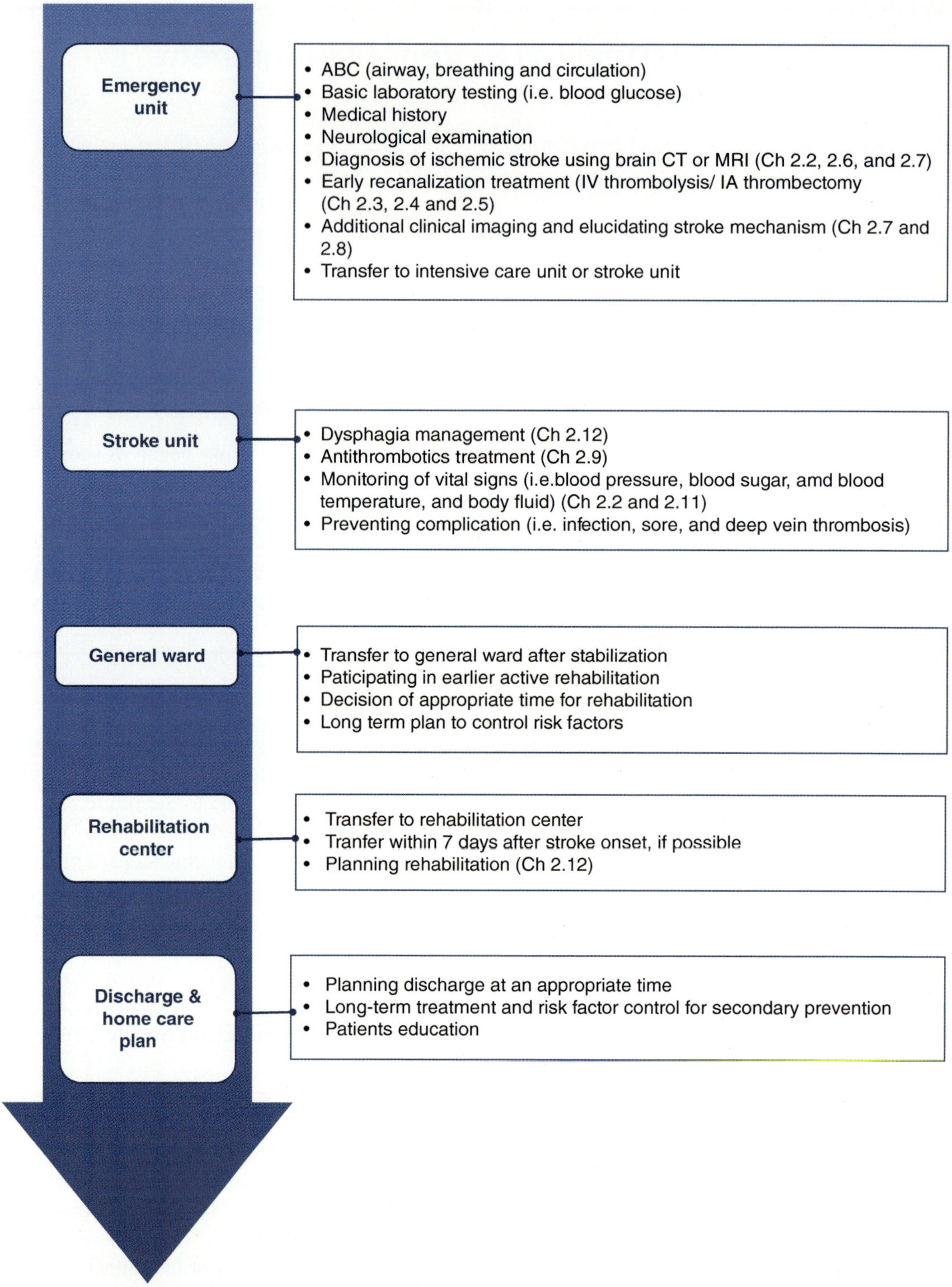

Fig. 4.1 A schematic diagram showing patient management flow (*CT* computed tomography, *MRI* magnetic resonance imaging, *IV* intravenous, *IA* intra-arterial)

While these procedures should not be extemporaneous, they must follow an automated, protocol-based system that controls all the processes. This is essential especially because the patients admitted due to acute stroke tend to come in during night hours and holidays, as opposed to just during regular shift hours and working days. Therefore, the emergency room medical staffs responsible for acute stroke should always prepare for admission of acute stroke patients.

4.1.1 Diagnosis and Basic Treatment of Suspected Acute Stroke Patients

When most patients enter the emergency room, in most cases the medical staff already knows whether or not the patient has had an acute stroke. The patient may already have knowledge and may have informed the staff when making a phone call to emergency system, or the emergency medical technicians in an ambulance may observe the patient and inform the emergency room medical staff before arrival, although this varies between countries based on their systems. Even if the information is not provided prior to the arrival, the emergency medical technicians should consider the patients that show sudden focal neurological deficits as stroke patients. In most cases, the suspected patient is indeed suffering from stroke, and even if misdiagnosed, it has little effect on the patient's prognosis.

When treating a stroke patient, the emergency ABC (airway, breathing, and circulation) assessment should first be in order. After securing the airway, and checking the breathing and circulation of the patient, necessary treatment should be administered. If aspiration of vomit is present in the bronchus or the respiration is unstable, immediate endotracheal intubation may be necessary. In most cases, the patients have elevated blood pressure (BP), but intervention to reduce the BP is not immediately applied and the BP is monitored unless the systolic and diastolic blood pressures (SBP and DBP) are above 220 and 120, respectively. The need for oxygen supply and Levin tube insertion should be checked, and blood sampling as well as the establishment of an intravenous (IV) route with a large bore needle should be performed. Basic laboratory testing should be performed immediately with the obtained blood sample, while the blood glucose level should be confirmed using the fingertip to identify potential hypoglycemia. Normal saline should be infused intravenously through the obtained IV route, but the infusion should be just enough to maintain euvolemia before the diagnosis is confirmed. If needed, a Foley catheter should be inserted. Concurrently, the medical history should be obtained from the patient, guardians, or family members, and a basic physical examination with neurological examination should be performed to confirm the initial neurological status in an early stage. The National Institutes of Health Stroke Scale (NIHSS) scoring is the standard index that is widely used. The neurological physicians should try to perform all the above tasks within 10 min of the patient's arrival.

4.1.2 Confirmation of Acute Ischemic Stroke: Clinical Imaging

As the neurological physicians perform the above procedures, they should also prepare to perform brain computed tomography (CT). The brain CT result should not be delayed due to the above procedures; therefore, they should ensure the fast completion of the above procedures. Brain CT is an extremely useful examination to distinguish whether or not the patient's symptom presentation is due to hemorrhagic stroke. The sensitivity and specificity of brain CT in the diagnosis of hemorrhagic stroke are very high, and a majority of hemorrhagic stroke patients are identified from this examination. If the patient has a brain hemorrhage, the patient is treated accordingly. The treatment details are outlined in Sect. 3.3. If the brain CT results are normal or the patient shows initial ischemic change, there is a very high chance that the patient has suffered from an ischemic stroke. A detailed explanation is outlined in Chap. 5. In most cases, a non-contrast brain CT is sufficient, although some centers perform CT angiography or magnetic resonance imaging (MRI) for a more detailed initial diagnosis. While both approaches have their own advantages and disadvantages, a plain CT should be sufficient to distinguish hemorrhage in the centers with experienced physicians, since the time is the most important factor in the early stages of treating stroke. Both general and professional aspects of performing CT are outlined in Chap. 9.

4.1.3 Performing IV Thrombolysis and/or Intra-Arterial (IA) Thrombectomy

Soon after performing the CT, if the patient can be treated with IV thrombolysis using recombinant tissue plasminogen activator (rt-PA), the physicians should immediately treat the patient after obtaining consent from the patient or the guardian. This treatment is available only for those patients who had their initial symptoms less than 4.5 h prior to the treatment. If the patient shows a sign of recovery immediately after IV thrombolysis, the patient is treated after transferring to the stroke unit. If the patient shows no sign of recovery or if the patient requires treatment after 4.5 h of showing initial symptoms, IA mechanical thrombectomy can be used. This will be discussed in detail in Chaps. 6 and 8.

4.1.4 Additional Clinical Imaging and Elucidating the Stroke Mechanism

Whether the patient undergoes early recanalization treatment or does not undergo treatment for various reasons, a brain MRI must be performed in order to correctly identify the mechanism of stroke in these patients. Although health insurance coverage systems are different in the world, MRI has obvious advantages over CT for stroke diagnosis and should be performed if possible. However, MRI prevents patient monitoring for 20–30 min. Thus, for the patients in a critical condition, MRI should be performed only after their conditions become stable. Diffusion-weighted imaging (DWI), perfusion-weighted imaging (PWI), fluid-attenuated inversion recovery (FLAIR) imaging, and MR angiography (MRA) provide information about the patient's ischemic conditions and reopening of the occluded vessels. Therefore, these imaging modalities are extremely useful in gaining an insight into the mechanism of the stroke. A detailed explanation is outlined in Chap. 10.

4.1.5 Decision About the Treatment Strategy for Acute Patients and Transfer to the Stroke Unit or the ICU

The patient, when admitted to the emergency room, should be treated in the stroke unit immediately. However, each center has a different triage system after admission, and admission to the stroke unit soon after initial and recanalization treatment in emergency room is not a bad strategy. This should be decided by the centers according to their optimized protocol and equipment settings. If the patient's condition is not stable enough to treat in the stroke unit, the patient can be immediately transferred to the intensive care unit (ICU) for subsequent treatment.

4.2 Care in the Stroke Unit

4.2.1 Dysphagia Management

In addition to the vital signs, the first thing to check in a patient who is admitted to the stroke unit is the presence and degree of dysphagia. Since aspiration pneumonia has a great impact on the prognosis of stroke patients, the proper treatment in early stages can prevent a bad outcome. Therefore, identification of dysphagia is critical. A detailed explanation is outlined in Chap. 15.

4.2.2 Use of Antithrombotics

Antithrombotics are not allowed to be administered for 24 h if the patient has undergone the IV thrombolysis treatment. Subsequently, a decision about the appropriate treatment course is made, i.e., whether or not antiplatelet drug or anticoagulants should be used and which would be the more appropriate option for the patient. A detailed explanation is outlined in Chap. 12.

4.2.3 Blood Pressure, Blood Sugar, Body Fluids, and Body Temperature

The primary purpose of treatment in a majority of the stroke units is to continuously monitor vital signs and immediately recognize any change in the patient's neurological status, in order to prevent potential delays in treatment and produce the best possible medical treatment outcome. A detailed explanation is outlined in Chaps. 5 and 14.

4.2.4 Complication Prevention and Management: Infection, Pressure Sores, etc.

One of the most fundamental treatments in the stroke unit is to prevent complications from stroke. Unless otherwise indicated, the Foley catheter should be immediately removed in order to prevent urinary tract infections and/or bladder atony. Insertion of a Levin tube should be considered, and air mattresses and physical therapy should be considered to prevent pressure sores. Other considerations include preventing deep vein thrombosis, injuries from fall, and other possible complications that can occur.

4.3 Care in the General Ward or the Rehabilitation Ward

When the patient is stable, he or she can be transferred to the general ward. However, this depends on the center's protocol; there are cases in which stroke patients stay in the stroke unit throughout their hospitalized period. Although this allows better monitoring of the patients, it also largely limits the physical activity of the patient, which causes discomfort to the patient and hinders the rehabilitation procedure. It is better that patients who do not require extensive monitoring are transferred to the general ward in order to participate in active rehabilitation. Although how early the rehabilitation should be performed is under controversy, it is better to start earlier if the patient can handle the rehabilitation. Therefore, identifying the time at which rehabilitation can begin in different patients is also a key responsibility of the physicians. Moreover, the risk factors in the stroke should be carefully analyzed, and a long-term plan should be made to control the risk factors.

4.4 Care in the Rehabilitation Center

Patients with mild symptoms may not need to be transferred to the rehabilitation center; however, active rehabilitation treatment can greatly improve the patients' conditions in most cases. The timing of transfer to the rehabilitation center can vary among centers and countries, although it is best to transfer the patient within 7 days if the patient is suffering from a stroke without further complications. If the stroke is severe or complicated by other conditions, the transfer timing should be decided after monitoring the patient's condition. Rehabilitation can be performed in both inpatient and outpatient setting. Further explanation on rehabilitation is outlined in Chap. 15.

4.5 Discharge and Home Care Plan

When the treatment is complete, the patient should be discharged and encouraged to go back to his or her normal life. While early return to normal life is better for the patient's quality of life, a hasty discharge can result in recurrence or worsening of the stroke. Therefore, a decision on discharge should be made with careful consideration for each patient. As mentioned before, risk factors should be carefully analyzed to provide appropriate treatment and select adequate long-term antithrombotic intervention. The most important thing is to educate the patient and the guardians to take measures to prevent a recurrence in the future. Providing education on risk factors and drug compliance according to appropriate protocols for each center is essential. If the patient has hypertension or diabetes, the patient should be able to self-monitor the blood pressure and blood sugar levels.

Conclusion

Although stroke is a topic of study that should be clinically understood by physicians, it is a matter of life or death for the patients. Traditional textbooks focus heavily on the academic aspect of the disease and are published as a manual by clinically inexperienced physicians. The author of this book focuses on explaining the disease from both academic and clinical aspects. The sequence of procedures from initial transfer of stroke patients by the emergency transfer system to the start of the treatment and discharge was explained in this chapter. A diagram depicting this flow is provided to assist the readers (Fig. 4.1), as only the key factors are mentioned for conceptual understanding. Detailed explanation of each aspect is provided in the future chapters indicated in each section. This chapter will hopefully provide a rough treatment guideline for inexperienced physicians when they treat a stroke patient for the first time.

Suggestions from Current Clinical Practice Guidelines Not applicable to this chapter.

5 Initial Diagnosis and Management of Acute Ischemic Stroke

Young Seo Kim

Abstract

After the onset of an ischemic stroke, every minute is important for reducing ischemic brain injury. Patients with suspected ischemic stroke require rapid and efficient evaluation to identify those who are eligible for time-sensitive reperfusion therapies. Establishing the exact time of stroke onset is of utmost importance. After taking the history of the patient, a rapid physical and neurologic examination including stroke scale is necessary. In patients with stable vital signs, emergent non-contrast-enhanced computed tomography (NECT) should be performed to exclude intracerebral hemorrhage. If NECT is interpreted as an ischemic stroke, immediately obtaining a computed tomography angiography (CTA) and perfusion CT may aid in making therapeutic decisions for intra-arterial thrombectomy without time delay. Laboratory and cardiac evaluations should also be performed as soon as possible to exclude conditions that mimic strokes by examining metabolic abnormalities and to confirm exclusion criteria for intravenous thrombolysis. To ensure timely treatment after arrival to the emergency department, the cooperation of the stroke teams, including emergency medical physicians, neurologists, intervention team, nursing staff, and medical technicians, is important. Since intra-arterial thrombectomy has been successful in patients with middle cerebral artery or internal carotid artery occlusion, reducing the time from door to groin puncture is another key component of acute treatment for ischemic stroke. This chapter emphasizes the rapid management of patients with suspected ischemic stroke and focuses on what physicians should do during this stage. Additional medical management techniques specific to the emergency department will be discussed briefly.

Y.S. Kim, M.D., Ph.D.
Department of Neurology, College of Medicine,
Hanyang University, Seoul, South Korea
e-mail: aescula@hanmail.net

S.-H. Lee (ed.), *Stroke Revisited: Diagnosis and Treatment of Ischemic Stroke*,
Stroke Revisited, DOI 10.1007/978-981-10-1424-6_5

Table 5.1 Guidelines for rapid evaluation of the patient with acute stroke

Period measured	Optimal time (min)
From ED arrival to emergency physician evaluation	10
From ED arrival to CT scan initiation	25
From ED arrival to CT scan interpretation	45
From ED arrival to initiation of therapy (80% compliance)[a]	60

Reproduced by permission of Stroke [1]
ED emergency department, *CT* computed tomography
[a]Target should be compliance with these guidelines in at least 80% of cases

The first few hours after the onset of stroke symptoms provide a crucial intervention window to prevent permanent disability or death. The major goal in this hyperacute stage is to reduce infarct volume and to minimize neurologic deficits. If the occluded vessels are successfully recanalized, the patients will improve and penumbral zones will be normalized. With no recanalization, penumbral tissues will turn into areas of permanent infarction with severe symptoms persisting. Because earlier recanalization results in a better outcome, a systematic approach to reduce time delay should be emphasized in this stage by the collaboration of stroke teams. A consensus panel convened by the National Institutes of Neurological Disorders and Stroke (NINDS) established goals for time frames in the evaluation of stroke patients in the emergency department (Table 5.1) [1]. However, stroke teams may not satisfy to meet the recommended time frame and should make every effort to reduce time delays.

5.1 Establishing Time of Stroke Onset and History Taking

If stroke symptoms are recognized by emergency physicians, "stroke code" should be activated immediately. In some well-developed areas, emergency medical service (EMS) personnel are trained to identify stroke symptoms, and the stroke team could be alerted on the way to the hospital. Following stroke code activation, the exact time of symptom onset should be determined because time-dependent treatments are performed based on this information. Physicians should ask patients when the stroke symptoms began. However, the patient may not be able to talk about their symptoms or onset status due to neurologic deficits or comorbidities. In this situation, obtaining a detailed history from family members, witnesses who observed the onset of the stroke, and emergency medical personnel can provide valuable information. In addition, any observations of the patient during daily activities might be evaluated with cautious history taking, as a patient's daily routine may aid in providing a stroke onset time. Cellular phone recordings could also verify the normal status of the patient. Because therapeutic intervention in this stage carries risk and requires rapid decision, the physician may contact responsible family members or a legally authorized representative to discuss the possible risks or benefits of the intervention.

Additional history about the patient should also be obtained quickly. Risk factors such as hypertension, diabetes mellitus, dyslipidemia, and cardiac disease, as well as migraine, seizure, trauma, drug abuse, alcohol abuse, pregnancy, and previous stroke history, should be noted. Medication history including the use of antithrombotics should be obtained. Intravenous thrombolysis exclusion criteria should be assessed in a timely manner. In addition, the patient's weight is needed to determine the dose of recombinant tissue plasminogen activator (rtPA).

5.2 Physical Examination

After the airway, breathing, and circulation of the patient have been assessed and vital signs including blood pressure, heart rate, oxygen saturation, and temperature have been recorded, a more detailed physical examination should be performed. A general physical examination is important to identify possible etiologic factors for ischemic stroke as well as possible complications and coexisting comorbidities. Examination of the face and head may reveal signs of trauma. Auscultation of the neck and chest may reveal carotid bruits and cardiac murmurs, arrhythmias, and rales, respectively. Skin and extremity examination may reveal a few signs specific to coagulopathies, platelet disorders, trauma, or embolic lesions. Because acute comorbidities may influence the selection of an acute treatment, a thorough but brief examination is necessary.

5.3 Neurologic Examination and Stroke Scales

The neurological evaluation of an acute stroke patient must be brief and efficient. An experienced neurologist should immediately assess the level of consciousness and breathing patterns. If patients are alert and able to respond to verbal stimuli, neurological examinations should be performed based on common stroke scales, such as the National Institutes of Health Stroke Scale (NIHSS) (Table 5.2). The scales have

Table 5.2 National Institutes of Health Stroke Scale

Tested Item	Responses	Score
1a. Level of consciousness	Alert	0
	Not alert, but arousable with minimal stimulation	1
	Not alert, requires repeated stimulation to attend	2
	Coma/unresponsiveness	3
1b. LOC questions (Ask patient the month and their age)	Answers both correctly	0
	Answers one correctly	1
	Both incorrect	2
1c. LOC commands (Ask patient to open and close eyes, make fist/let go)	Obeys both correctly	0
	Obeys one correctly	1
	Both incorrect	2
2. Best gaze (only horizontal movement)	Normal	0
	Partial gaze palsy	1
	Forced deviation	2
3. Visual fields testing	No visual field loss	0
	Partial hemianopia	1
	Complete hemianopia	2
	Bilateral hemianopia (blind including cortical blindness)	3
4. Facial palsies (ask patient to show teeth or raise eyebrows and close eyes tightly)	Normal symmetrical movement	0
	Minor paralysis (flattened nasolabial fold)	1
	Partial paralysis (total or near-total paralysis of lower face)	2
	Complete paralysis of one or both sides (absence of facial movement)	3
5. Motor function—arm (left, right)	Normal (extends arms 90 for 10 s without drift)	0
	Drift	1
	Some effort against gravity	2
	No efforts against gravity	3
	No movement	4
	Untestable (joint fused or limb amputated)	9

(continued)

Table 5.2 (continued)

Tested Item	Responses	Score
6. Motor function—leg (left, right)	Normal (hold leg 30° for 5 s without drift)	0
	Drift	1
	Some effort against gravity	2
	No efforts against gravity	3
	No movement	4
	Untestable (joint fused or limb amputated)	9
7. Limb ataxia	No ataxia	0
	Present in one limb	1
	Present in two limb	2
8. Sensory (use pinprick to test arms, legs, trunk, and face—compare side to side)	Normal	0
	Mild to moderate decrease in sensation	1
	Severe to total sensory loss	2
9. Best language (describe picture, name items, read sentences)	No aphasia	0
	Mild to moderate aphasia	1
	Severe aphasia	2
	Mute	3
10. Dysarthria (read several words)	Normal articulation	0
	Mild to moderate slurring of words	1
	Near unintelligible or unable to speak	2
	Intubated or other physical barrier	9
11. Extinction and inattention	Normal	0
	Inattention or extinction to bilateral simultaneous stimulation in one of the sensory modalities	1
	Severe hemi-inattention or hemi-inattention to more than one modality	2
	Total score	

demonstrated their utility and can be administered by a broad spectrum of health providers [2]. Use of a standard stroke scale helps quantify the degree of neurological deficits and facilitate communication among stroke teams. When a patient's consciousness is impaired, neurologists should uncover localizing and lateralizing signs. Deviation of the eyes or head, air-escaping pattern of the face, asymmetric withdrawal response to noxious stimuli, asymmetric brainstem reflexes, and asymmetric pathologic reflexes are examples of brain damage. A thorough neurological examination is necessary in patients who are unconscious to rule out conditions that may mimic stroke. Although intravenous rtPA use in stroke mimics does not show harmful effects, thrombolytic treatment of stroke mimics should be under 3% based on non-contrast-enhanced computed tomography (NECT) alone [3].

5.4 Emergency Management of Stroke Patients

5.4.1 Brain and Vascular Imaging

Imaging of the brain with NECT is crucial to confirm the diagnosis of cerebral hemorrhage, which appears as an area of high density. It is widely used in almost all hospitals because it is inexpensive, noninvasive, and easily accessible. It is the single most important imaging modality because a decision of intravenous thrombolysis can be easily made, and it can also reveal brain tumors, which would be a contraindication to thrombolysis. NECT may show early signs of infarction such as a loss of gray-white matter interface among the nuclei of the basal ganglia and insular cortex. Cortical swelling by cerebral ischemia may produce sulcal effacement, and early arterial occlusion may show signs of a hyperdense vessel. When these signs of early infarct are present, the degree of ischemia will be more profound and the outcome will be poor [4].

Diffusion-weighted imaging (DWI) of the brain is the most sensitive and specific imaging for acute infarct even in the early stages of a stroke. It can differentiate an old infarction from a recent infarction and detect relatively small lesions in the brainstem, which are poorly visualized with NECT. In the hyperacute stage of ischemic stroke, visible diffusion lesions will include both regions of irreversible infarctions with more severe apparent diffusion coefficient (ADC) changes and regions of salvageable penumbra with less severe ADC changes. Standard MRI sequences (T1-weighted, T2-weighted, fluid-attenuated inversion recovery [FLAIR]) are relatively insensitive to acute stroke but may be useful to diagnose stroke mimics such as seizure and metabolic abnormalities. DWI/FLAIR mismatch has been recently suggested, especially in patients with unclear onset or wake-up stroke. It is a concept based on DWI changes beginning with the onset of stroke and FLAIR changes that are apparent after 3 h. However, it should only be used in specific conditions and on an individual basis [5]. Susceptibility-weighted imaging (SWI) and gradient echo imaging (GRE) are able to detect very small amounts of deoxyhemoglobin and intracerebral hemorrhages and microbleeds. Based on these MRI findings, they could be used as an initial imaging modality to evaluate acute stroke patients. However, if MRI scans are not readily available for 24 h, as in most hospitals, time should not be wasted waiting for MRI results.

Vascular imaging in the state of hyperacute stroke is an emerging field because intra-arterial thrombectomy of middle cerebral artery (MCA) or internal carotid artery (ICA) occlusions has been associated with improved functional outcomes and higher rates of recanalization without the increase of symptomatic intracranial hemorrhage [6]. Helical CT angiography (CTA) is a quick, noninvasive method to evaluate the intracranial and extracranial vasculature in the acute stroke stage with high sensitivity and specificity. Since a CTA could be acquired immediately after NECT and lasts less than 5 min, a time-saving decision could be made to perform a CTA while in the CT room. In the presence of large artery occlusions such as MCA or ICA, an intervention team alert for endovascular thrombectomy is necessary at this time. MR angiography (MRA) or Doppler ultrasound can also evaluate intracranial vasculature. However, important limitations include a long acquisition time and less accuracy. Conventional angiography is rarely required during the hyperacute phase of stroke evaluation. It should be reserved for situations where intra-arterial thrombectomy is required.

Perfusion CT or MRI that reveal parenchymal perfusion of the patient may provide additional information to identify potentially salvageable brain tissue. This will better identify those patients who are most likely to benefit from reperfusion therapy, which is especially useful in patients with an unclear stroke onset. Brain perfusion imaging provides information about regional cerebral hemodynamics such as cerebral blood flow (CBF), cerebral blood volume (CBV), mean transit time (MTT), and time to peak (TTP). It can delineate an infarct core and penumbral tissue by using CBF-CBV mismatched areas on a perfusion imaging. On the other hand, the penumbra is indicated as DWI-perfusion-weighted imaging in mismatched areas on a perfusion MRI. There is a growing body of reports that those mismatched areas are potentially salvageable and are an ideal target for neuroprotection or reperfusion therapies [7]. However, the acquisition of additional imaging should not delay treatment with intravenous thrombolysis and should be performed only in a hospital where rapid processing is possible. Recent advances in CT machines and software enable angiography and perfusion imaging to be obtained simultaneously after NECT (Fig. 5.1).

After an intravenous rtPA is administered based on the CT or MRI, patients with large artery occlusions (MCA, ICA) should perform conventional angiography. In this situation, a conventional angiography with intra-arterial thrombectomy should be readied by interventional teams. If the conventional angiography still

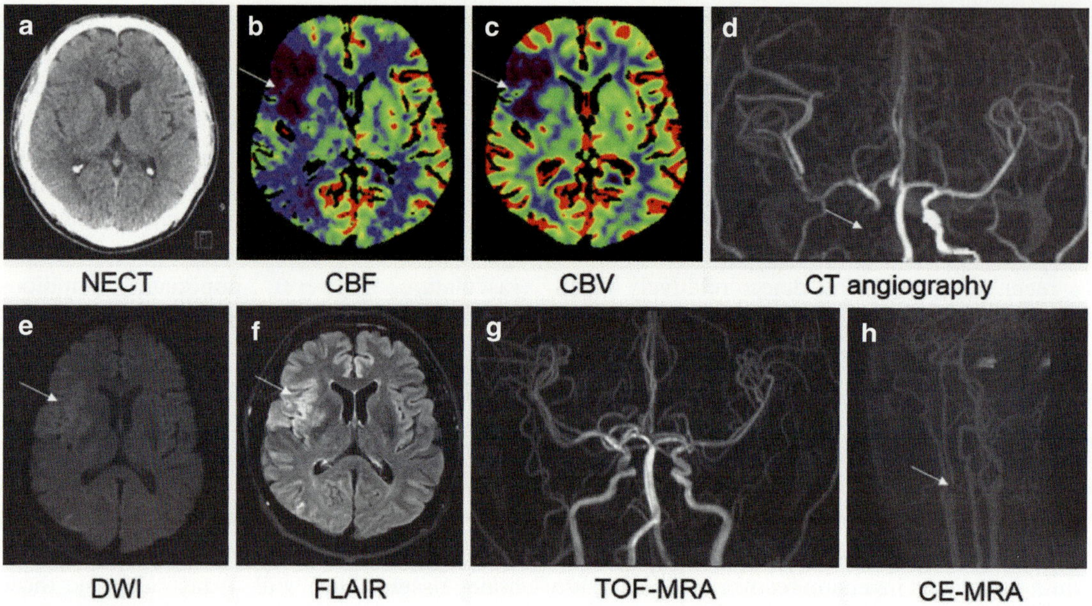

Fig. 5.1 CT and MRI images from a 55-year-old man with the sudden onset of dysarthria and left-sided weakness 60 min earlier. NECT appears normal without early ischemic changes (**a**). Perfusion CT was immediately obtained after NECT and shows CBF (**b**) and CBV (**c**) mismatch (*arrows*). Reconstructed angiography based on perfusion CT shows obstruction of the internal carotid artery (**d**). Intravenous rtPA was administered and patient symptoms subsided except for mild dysarthria. Brain MRI was performed 24 h after initial symptoms. DWI (**e**) and FLAIR (**f**) show permanent infarction (*arrows*), and TOF-MRA (**g**) shows recanalization of internal carotid artery. Contrast-enhanced MRA showed severe stenosis at the proximal internal carotid artery (*arrow*) (**h**). *CT* computed tomography, *MRI* magnetic resonance image, *NECT* non-contrast-enhanced computed tomography, *CBF* cerebral blood flow, *CBV* cerebral blood volume, *rtPA* recombinant tissue plasminogen activator, *DWI* diffusion-weighted image, *FLAIR* fluid-attenuated inversion recovery, *TOF-MRA* time-of-flight magnetic resonance angiography

shows a large artery occlusion, mechanical thrombectomy with Solitaire or Trevo should be used to recanalize the occluded artery [6]. When intravenous thrombolysis is contraindicated in a patient, intra-arterial thrombectomy can be performed independently. Detailed methods and evidence will be dealt with in subsequent chapters.

5.4.2 Ancillary Laboratory Tests

A few laboratory tests are routinely required during the initial evaluation of patients who have a suspected stroke. The results of these tests may provide information about serious comorbid diseases and conditions that can mimic stroke and possible stroke etiology. These tests may assist with therapeutic decision-making, especially to identify if intravenous thrombolysis is contraindicated. This is extremely valuable when the patient's history is vague or inconclusive. Routine laboratory tests should include blood glucose, electrolytes with renal function tests, complete blood count with platelet count, liver function tests, prothrombin time (PT), international normalized ratio (INR), activated partial thromboplastin time (aPTT), and cardiac enzymes (creatine kinase (CK), CK-MB, troponin). In addition, a chest radiograph should be obtained in all stroke patients. It may show a widened mediastinum indicative of an aortic dissection that can mimic stroke, cardiomegaly, or pulmonary edema, which is indicative of heart failure. An electrocardiogram (ECG) should also be performed in all patients to determine the cause of the stroke and to optimize immediate and long-term management. Due to the close association between stroke and cardiac abnormalities, it is important to assess the cardiovascular status of patients presenting with acute stroke. Baseline ECG, chest radiograph, and cardiac biomarkers may identify concurrent myocardial ischemia or cardiac arrhythmias. These routine laboratory tests might be performed in the emergency department setting, if possible, so as not to delay administration of intravenous rtPA.

Some laboratory tests are not routine during a hyperacute stroke evaluation but may be considered in certain patients. Due to the increasing number of patients who are using direct thrombin inhibitors (dabigatran) and direct factor Xa inhibitors (rivaroxaban, apixaban, and edoxaban), it is important to understand what studies may assist in determining anticoagulant effects. The PT/INR is not helpful in determining the anticoagulant effect of those types of medicines. A thrombin time (TT) and ecarin clotting time (ECT) may demonstrate direct thrombin activity. However, it takes a long time to obtain the results [8]. Unfortunately, there is no specific assay for direct factor Xa inhibitor. In young patients, toxicology screening for sympathomimetic drugs (cocaine, methamphetamine, etc.) may identify the underlying cause of the stroke. In women of childbearing age, a pregnancy test is needed because it can affect overall management protocols.

Because time is critical, a limited number of essential diagnostic tests are recommended. Stroke protocols and critical pathways should be clearly defined in all hospitals (Fig. 5.2). Mandatory and selected laboratory tests are described in Table 5.3.

5.5 General Medical Managements in Hyperacute Stage of Ischemic Stroke

In the hyperacute stages of ischemic stroke, management should be focused on reperfusion within the critical period. However, physicians should not neglect management of life-threatening comorbid conditions. Initial assessment of the airway, breathing, and circulation is necessary in the emergency department, and a constant reassessment is required to avoid oxygen desaturation, respiratory compromise, and hypotension. Because patients often suffer a fall after a stroke, the physician should look for traumatic injuries and the neck should be stabilized. In addition, temperature, blood pressure, and blood glucose should be managed properly in the hyperacute stage.

5.5.1 Airway and Oxygen

Hypoxia frequently occurs after stroke. Common causes of hypoxia are partial airway obstruction, hypoventilation, aspiration, atelectasis, and pneumonia. Patients with a severe stroke presenting with diminished levels of consciousness or brainstem dysfunction may have an increased risk of airway compromise due to impaired oropharyngeal mobility and sensation and loss of protective reflexes. Patients with these conditions or with frequent vomiting may need intubation to protect the airway from aspiration of gastric contents. In addition, prior to the swallowing evaluation, strict avoidance of oral intake is imperative. However, in patients with mild to moderate stroke, routine oxygen supplementation did not show beneficial effects [9]. If patients have less than 94% oxygen saturation, noninvasive oxygen therapy with nasal cannula or with a Venturi mask is recommended [1]. Patients can better maintain oxygen saturation and cerebral perfusion when lying flat in a supine position.

5.5.2 Intravenous Fluids

Patients with acute ischemic stroke are sometimes hypovolemic, especially those with severe stroke. Hypovolemia should be avoided because it may predispose them to cerebral hypoperfusion and exacerbate brain edema, increased myocardial stress, and renal impairments. Therefore, maintaining iso-osmolar and euvolemic states with isotonic solutions, such as 0.9% saline, is required for patients with acute ischemic stroke. Hypotonic solutions, such as 5% dextrose or 0.45% saline, may distribute into the intracellular spaces and may exacerbate ischemic brain edema. In addition, dextrose-containing fluid

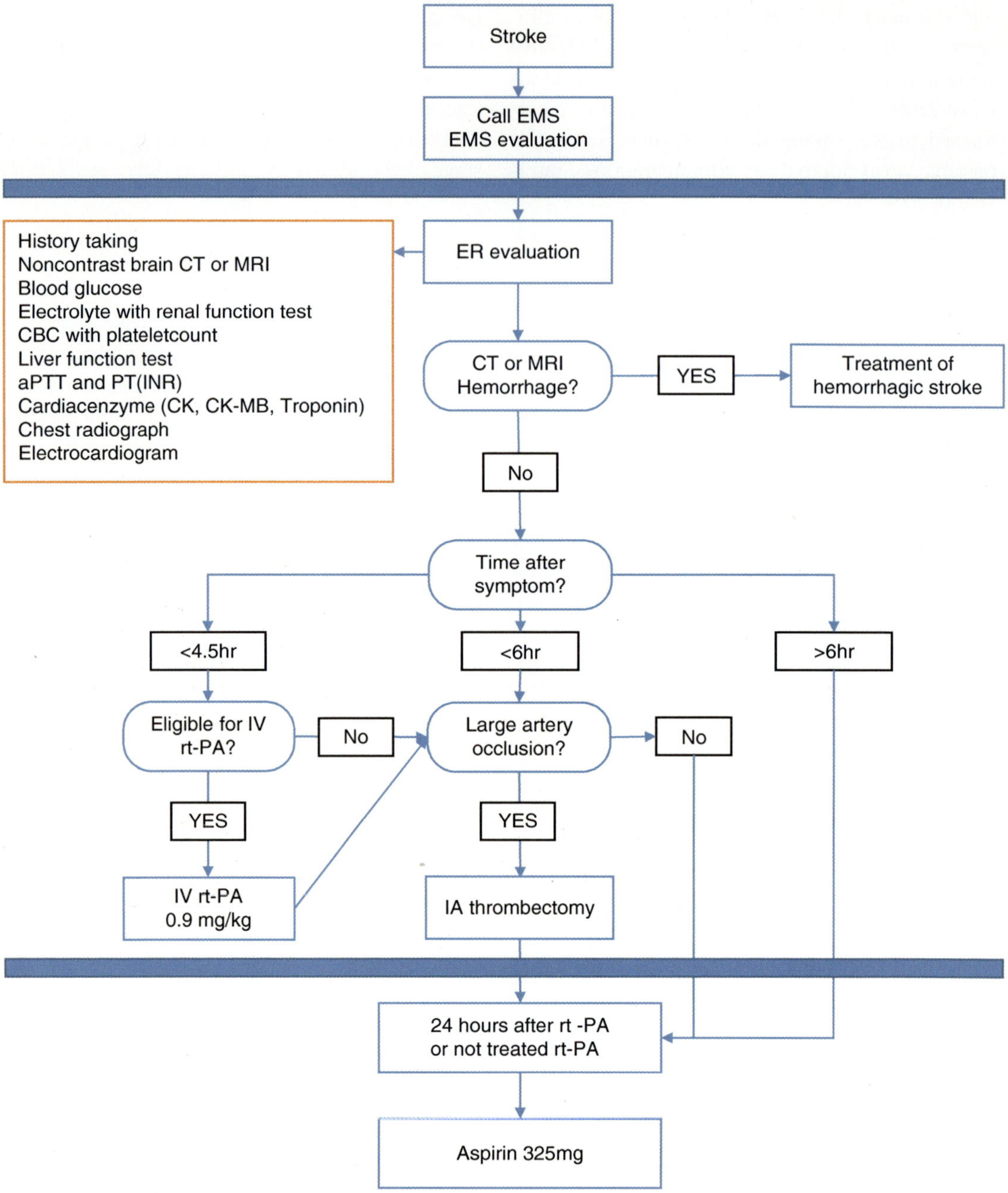

Fig. 5.2 Example for stroke protocol and critical pathway. Algorithm for initial diagnosis and treatment should be clearly defined in all acute stroke care hospitals

Table 5.3 Immediate ancillary laboratory studies

Mandatory tests
Blood glucose
Electrolytes with renal function tests
Complete blood count with platelet count
Liver function tests
Prothrombin time with international normalized ratio
Activated partial thromboplastin time
Cardiac enzymes (CK, CK-MB, troponin)
Chest radiographs
Electrocardiogram
Selected tests
Thrombin time and/or Ecarine clotting time (dabigatran taking patients)
Toxicology screening
Blood alcohol level
Routine urinalysis with pregnancy screening
Arterial blood gas tests (hypoxia-suspected patients)
Lumbar puncture (subarachnoid hemorrhage-suspected patients with normal CT)
Electroencephalogram (seizure-suspected patients)

Reproduced by permission of Stroke [1]
CK creatine kinase, *CT* computed tomography

may also exacerbate ischemic brain injury. In some patients who have a predisposed vulnerability to intravascular volume overload, such as renal or heart failure, volume replacement should be performed cautiously.

5.5.3 Temperature

Hyperthermia (above 37.6 °C) is observed in about one third of acute stroke patients. It is associated with stroke severity, infarct size, mortality rate, and a worsened outcome [10]. Thus, lowering the temperature with antipyretics may be beneficial to acute stroke patients. In some situations with occult infections, such as pneumonia, urinary tract infection (UTI), sepsis, and infective endocarditis, patients should be managed with empirical antibiotics.

5.5.4 Blood Pressure

Arterial blood pressure is commonly increased after an acute ischemic stroke and starts to spontaneously decrease after 90 min of stroke symptoms. Moderately increased blood pressure may augment the delivery of blood to the ischemic area and should be treated conservatively because it can be advantageous to the patient. However, extreme hypertension is clearly harmful because it leads to hypertensive encephalopathy, cardiac complications, renal insufficiency, and hemorrhagic transformation of an ischemic brain. Unfortunately, an ideal blood pressure range has not been scientifically determined. The blood pressure range during an acute ischemic stroke will depend on the stroke subtype and other patient-specific comorbidities. Some conditions, such as myocardial ischemia, aortic dissection, and heart failure, accompany acute ischemic stroke and may be exacerbated by arterial hypertension. However, most guidelines recommend that blood pressure should remain untreated unless the systolic pressure is above 220 mmHg or the diastolic above 120 mmHg. Reasonable blood pressure control should be implemented on a case-by-case basis.

Specific blood pressure management recommendations have been established for acute ischemic stroke patients being considered for thrombolysis therapy (Table 5.4) [1]. These recommendations include a gentle approach to bring the pressure below 185/110 mmHg to qualify for fibrinolytic therapy with intravenous rtPA. Once intravenous rtPA is administered, the blood pressure must be maintained below 180/105 mmHg to reduce the risk of intracerebral hemorrhage. Blood pressure control in the hyperacute stage may be performed by intravenous antihypertensive agents rather than with a single pill medication. It would be beneficial to use short-acting, titratable agents such as labetalol, nicardipine, and esmolol. In patients undergoing intra-arterial

Table 5.4 Blood pressure control in hyperacute stage

Patient eligible for acute reperfusion therapy with BP >185/110 mmHg
• Labetalol 10–20 mg IV over 1–2 min, may repeat one time
• Nicardipine 5 mg/h IV, titrate up by 2.5 mg/h every 5–15 min, maximum 15 mg/h
• Other agents (hydralazine, enalapril, etc.) may be considered when appropriate
If BP is not maintained at or below 185/110 mmHg, do not administer rtPA
Management of BP during and after rtPA or other acute reperfusion therapy to maintain BP at or below 180/105 mmHg
• Monitor BP every 15 min for 2 h from the start of rtPA therapy, then every 30 min for 6 h, and then every hour for 16 h
• If systolic BP >180–230 mmHg or diastolic BP >105–120 mmHg
– Labetalol 10 mg IV over 1–2 min, followed by continuous IV infusion 2–8 mg/min, or nicardipine 5 mg/h IV, titrate up to desired effect by 2.5 mg/h every 5–15 min, maximum 15 mg/h
• If BP not controlled or diastolic BP >140 mmHg, consider IV sodium nitroprusside

Reproduced by permission of Stroke [1]
BP blood pressure, *rtPA* recombinant tissue plasminogen activator

thrombectomy, blood pressure should be lowered to prevent reperfusion injury and hemorrhagic transformation. However, the proper range of blood pressure has not yet been determined.

Hypotension should also be avoided because it may decrease cerebral perfusion pressure and increase cerebral edema. To maintain cerebral perfusion, head down, intravenous fluid, inotropic agents, and vasopressors can be used. Since hypotension after an ischemic stroke is rare, physicians should explore medical causes such as myocardial infarction, gastrointestinal bleeding, aortic dissection, and sepsis.

5.5.5 Blood Glucose

Hypoglycemia is uncommon during the hyperacute stage of ischemic stroke and it is likely to be associated with antidiabetic medications. Hypoglycemia may cause neurological symptoms, including stroke mimics and seizures. These symptoms may be reversible if the hypoglycemia is rapidly corrected. However, severe and prolonged hypoglycemia can result in permanent brain damage. Therefore, blood glucose should be measured as soon as possible in patients with acute ischemic stroke, and low glucose lower than 60 mg/dL should be corrected immediately with a dextrose solution (50% DW).

Hyperglycemia is common during acute ischemic stroke. This increase in blood glucose levels may be associated in part with a nonfasting state and in part to a stress reaction with impaired glucose metabolism. Although a cause and effect relationship could not be determined, many observational studies have found an association between admission hyperglycemia and worsened outcome of strokes [11]. Currently there is no clear target for blood glucose levels during an acute ischemic stroke. It is best to control blood glucose levels with subcutaneous insulin below 180 mg/dL in acute stroke patients. Physicians should monitor glucose to reduce hypoglycemic events that commonly occur after normal correction of hyperglycemia.

Conclusion

A predetermined system for rapid and precise assessment is essential in patients with acute ischemic strokes. The acute stroke teams should be able to perform their own tasks in a parallel manner with minimal delay (Table 5.5). Coordination of these stroke team members in the hyperacute stage may enable them to achieve the main goal of ischemic stroke treatment, which may reduce brain damage and improve outcome.

Suggestions from Clinical Practice Guidelines
For initial evaluation of acute stroke patients, a stroke rating scale such as the National Institutes of Health Stroke Scale (NIHSS) needs to be used. Several laboratory tests including hematologic, coagulation, and biochemistry tests are helpful for emergency care, but blood glucose should be immediately analyzed using a fingertip glucose test. Hypoglycemia (blood glucose level <60 mg/dL) should be normalized by bolus injection of high-dose dextrose solution. Blood pressure is

Table 5.5 Time schedule of each member of stroke team after emergency department arrival

Stroke team member	Time (minute)			
	0–15	15–30	30–60	60–120
Emergency nurse	Check vital signs Check glucose level IV fluid (0.9% N/S) administration Blood sampling for laboratory tests Monitor ECG Monitor oxygen saturation Prepare patient for transport to CT	Check blood pressure Prepare infusion pump and rtPA for intravenous administration	Monitor patient Line connection of rtPA for IV administration	
Emergency physician	Assess airway, breathing, circulation Assess stroke symptoms (if patient have ambiguous symptoms, call stroke physician) Stroke code activation Determine onset time of stroke History taking Physical examination ECG interpretation	Medical care (airway, oxygen, IV fluids, temperature, blood pressure, blood glucose) Collaborate with stroke physician		
Stroke physician	Confirm stroke symptoms Neurologic examination briefly Transport patient to CT room Interpretation of CT Obtain perfusion CT and angiography (ischemic stroke patient)	NIHSS scoring Review contraindication of IV thrombolysis Explain harm and benefit of thrombolysis to patient and family Consider surgery for intracranial hemorrhage	Review laboratory findings IV rtPA administration in patient without contraindication Notify intervention team for IA thrombectomy if large artery occlusion is noted Correct coagulation abnormality in patient with hemorrhagic stroke	Review neuroimaging with intervention physician Therapeutic decision-making for IA thrombectomy Transport patient to angio-room
CT technician	Prepare and obtain CT Reconstruction of CT angiography			
Intervention technician			Prepare conventional angiography	
Intervention physician				Conventional angiography IA thrombectomy
Stroke unit nurse				Ready for admission

IV intravenous, *ECG* electrocardiogram, *CT* computed tomography, *rtPA* recombinant tissue plasminogen activator, *IA* intra-arterial generally observed without control if not reaching 220/120 mmHg. However, if the patient is eligible for intravenous fibrinolysis, the blood pressure should be lowered slowly to <185/110 mmHg. Brain imaging is indispensable for stroke diagnosis in emergency setting. Non-enhanced brain computed tomography should be performed for initial and differential diagnosis of stroke.

References

1. Jauch EC, Saver JL, Adams HP Jr, et al. Guidelines for the early management of patients with acute ischemic stroke: a guideline for healthcare professionals from the American Heart Association/American Stroke Association. Stroke. 2013;44:870–947.
2. Lyden P, Raman R, Liu L, et al. National Institutes of Health stroke scale certification is reliable across multiple venues. Stroke. 2009;40:2507–11.
3. Chernyshev OY, Martin-Schild S, Albright KC, et al. Safety of tPA in stroke mimics and neuroimaging-negative cerebral ischemia. Neurology. 2010;74:1340–5.
4. Wardlaw JM, Mielke O. Early signs of brain infarction at CT: observer reliability and outcome after thrombolytic treatment—systematic review. Radiology. 2005;235:444–53.
5. Wouters A, Lemmens R, Dupont P, et al. Wake-up stroke and stroke of unknown onset: a critical review. Front Neurol. 2014;5:153.
6. Badhiwala JH, Nassiri F, Alhazzani W, et al. Endovascular thrombectomy for acute ischemic stroke: a meta-analysis. JAMA. 2015;314:1832–43.
7. Scalzo F, Nour M, Liebeskind DS. Data science of stroke imaging and enlightenment of the penumbra. Front Neurol. 2015;6:8.
8. Blommel ML, Blommel AL. Dabigatran etexilate: a novel oral direct thrombin inhibitor. Am J Health Syst Pharm. 2011;68:1506–19.
9. Ronning OM, Guldvog B. Should stroke victims routinely receive supplemental oxygen? A quasi-randomized controlled trial. Stroke. 1999;30:2033–7.
10. Hajat C, Hajat S, Sharma P. Effects of poststroke pyrexia on stroke outcome: a meta-analysis of studies in patients. Stroke. 2010;31:410–4.
11. Capes SE, Hunt D, Malmberg K, et al. Stress hyperglycemia and prognosis of stroke in nondiabetic and diabetic patients: a systematic overview. Stroke. 2001;32:2426–32.

Intravenous Thrombolysis for Acute Ischemic Stroke

6

Andreas Schweikert, Timo Kahles, and Krassen Nedeltchev

Abstract

Despite extensive research efforts, treatment options for acute ischemic stroke were limited until the mid-1990s. Since then, two major therapeutic developments—both aiming at restoration of cerebral blood flow within hours of symptom onset—have been made. The first was the introduction of intravenous thrombolytic therapy in the clinical routine following the publication of the National Institute of Neurological Disorders and Stroke trial in 1995. Intravenous thrombolysis with recombinant tissue plasminogen activator (r-tPA) proved to be safe and significantly improved the clinical outcome when used within 3 h after symptom onset. For the following 20 years, it would—with some refinements in use—remain the only reperfusion therapy for acute ischemic stroke with proven benefit. Recently—in 2015—endovascular thrombectomy demonstrated impressive efficacy in several large clinical trials and broadened treatment options, especially for strokes with proximal vessel occlusions. Together, these two treatments have contributed to a substantial improvement in clinical outcome. In this chapter we will focus on intravenous thrombolysis in acute ischemic stroke.

Over the last decades, remarkable advances in the management of acute ischemic stroke have been achieved. The shared strategy of all successful therapeutic interventions is the restoration of sufficient cerebral blood perfusion in order to limit permanent ischemic damage. Favorable clinical outcome is therefore extremely time-dependent, regardless by what means it is pursued. Currently, the only treatment strategies with proven efficacy in improving clinical outcome are intravenous recombinant tissue plasminogen activator (r-tPA) [1] and endovascular thrombectomy [2]. Both have been shown to achieve fast cerebral reperfusion at a fairly low bleeding risk. From many points of view, the introduction of rapid clot dissolution with r-tPA in the mid-1990s was a milestone. Its approval by

A. Schweikert • T. Kahles • K. Nedeltchev, M.D., F.E.S.O., F.E.S.C. (✉)
Department of Neurology, Cantonal Hospital of Aarau, CH-5001 Aarau, Switzerland
e-mail: krassen.nedeltchev@ksa.ch

S.-H. Lee (ed.), *Stroke Revisited: Diagnosis and Treatment of Ischemic Stroke*, Stroke Revisited, DOI 10.1007/978-981-10-1424-6_6

the Food and Drug Administration (FDA) and its adaption into clinical routine have resulted in a significant reduction of disability after stroke. Up to date, despite many attempts of introducing new methods or agents, r-tPA remains the only FDA-approved pharmacological therapy in acute ischemic stroke. Here we discuss the evolution, evidence, clinical use, and shortcomings of thrombolytic therapy and its significance in the era of endovascular thrombectomy.

6.1 Pathophysiology of Thrombus Formation

Thrombus formation is the result of blood coagulation. The term embolus refers to a thrombus that has been dislocated from its source (i.e., heart, carotid stenosis) and lodged in a downstream vascular bed, blocking flow into the affected organ (i.e., a portion of the brain). Thrombus formation is a complex multistep process, which is usually initiated by endothelial injury.

The injured endothelium activates adhesive proteins (i.e., von Willebrand factor) that act as connector between the subendothelial matrix (i.e., collagen) and platelets by binding to their membrane receptor glycoproteins Ib and Ic/IIa (GP1b and GP 1c/2a). In the next step, activated platelets express membrane receptor glycoprotein IIb/IIIa (GP2b3a) facilitating direct interconnection between them and leading to rapid platelet aggregation, ultimately building up a mass. Platelet apposition at the site of the endothelium injury further accelerates the coagulation cascade.

Thrombin is the key clotting factor in the formation of a thrombus, as it cleaves fibrinogen to fibrin. Assisted by other coagulation factors, fibrin monomers then polymerize and thereby stabilize the aggregated platelets, eventually forming the thrombus. The relative platelet/fibrin content of a specific thrombus is depending on blood flow and shear forces. In arterial flow, thrombi tend to be predominantly platelet-rich, while in venous flow they contain more fibrin. Composition of a clot also changes over time: older thrombi usually exhibit more fibrin cross-linking, making them more difficult to lyse.

6.2 Thrombolytics

Thrombolytics have in common that they all target the web-like fibrin structure of the thrombus.

The plasminogen activators (PA) react with endogenous plasminogen to generate plasmin, a proteolytic enzyme, which disrupts the cross-linkage between fibrin molecules. PAs are naturally expressed in different tissues, e.g., vascular endothelial cells. Mass production and altering specific properties of PAs are possible with molecular biological recombination technics. Substances derived from other sources (i.e., bacteria, saliva of the vampire bat) can also act as PAs. While direct PAs (i.e., alteplase, tenecteplase, reteplase) are serine proteases specifically cleaving an arginine-valine amino acid bond on plasminogen, indirect PAs (i.e., streptokinase, desmoteplase) are complexing with plasminogen to convert additional plasminogen to plasmin. Fibrinolytics reacting directly with fibrin (i.e., plasmin, microplasmin) have also been studied.

All the aforementioned substances can be further characterized as being fibrin-specific (i.e., alteplase, tenecteplase, reteplase, desmoteplase, plasmin) or non-fibrin-specific (i.e., streptokinase, urokinase). Along with fibrin specificity, *half-life* and *antigenicity* (i.e., the induction of neutralizing antibodies) are further features influencing the efficacy and safety of a specific thrombolytic drug.

Although there are several intrinsic inhibitors of the fibrinolytic cascade (i.e., thrombin), their concentration is in general too low to exert a substantial effect on pharmacological fibrinolysis.

6.3 Recombinant Tissue Plasminogen Activator (r-tPA) for Acute Ischemic Stroke

While streptokinase was widely established for treatment of acute myocardial infarction by the late 1970s, it took another two decades until alteplase—a recombinant tissue plasminogen activator (r-tPA)—finally proved effective in improving the chances of good clinical outcome after acute ischemic stroke [3]. Consecutively, alteplase was approved by the Food and Drug Administration (FDA) for the treatment of acute ischemic stroke at a 0.9 mg/kg dose applied within 3 h of symptom onset. Since its introduction into clinical practice, few modifications regarding its use have been made, such as expanding the time window to 4.5 h [4]. Regardless of this expansion, numerous trials as well as clinical experience have shown that treatment success is extremely time-dependent, demanding fast diagnostic procedures to ensure rapid application of the drug. The most feared complication of treatment using alteplase is cerebral hemorrhage, warranting cautious handling.

6.3.1 History

Research on thrombolytics reaches back to 1933 when Tillet and Garner observed that a blood clot added to cultured beta-hemolytic streptococci would dissolve. They correctly assumed that a certain substance (originally named fibrinolysin, later called streptokinase) produced by the bacteria was responsible for this effect. Subsequently, streptokinase was therapeutically used to treat bleeding complications like hemothorax. Intravenous streptokinase was first tested in humans in 1958 in order to treat acute myocardial infarction (AMI). Twenty years of tenacious research documented the benefit of streptokinase for treatment of AMI until it finally found its way into the clinical routine.

Streptokinase has some major disadvantages. It is a non-fibrin-specific indirect PA, potentially causing anaphylactic-type allergic reactions and often inducing high levels of neutralizing antibodies. Hence, its second use within 6 months can be problematic. The disadvantages led to the development of a second generation of thrombolytics. In the 1980s, when molecular biological advances allowed the production of recombinant molecules, r-tPA (alteplase) was introduced into clinical practice. Due to its high fibrin specificity, its activity is increased 400-fold in the presence of fibrin. Furthermore, it is identical to human tissue-type plasminogen activator; thus, antigenicity is not a relevant issue.

For numerous reasons, the path to routine thrombolytic therapy for acute stroke was stonier than for coronary artery disease. The use of the first-generation thrombolytic drugs (streptokinase, urokinase) was not recommended by the National Institutes of Health in 1980, mostly due to the apprehension of an increased risk of intracerebral hemorrhage. Furthermore, shortcomings in the design of the early thrombolytic studies further delayed clinical breakthrough. Two of those delaying factors that should be kept in mind for today's practice included the choice of a too large time window and the allowance for combination with other anticoagulants.

Those limitations were ultimately overcome by the National Institute of Neurological Disorders and Stroke (NINDS) r-tPA stroke trial (Fig. 6.1). In this study, patients were randomized into two groups, with patients receiving placebo in one arm vs. 0.9 mg/kg of alteplase in the other within 3 h of symptom onset. Although negative for the primary endpoint defined as National Institutes of Health Stroke Scale (NIHSS) reduction greater than 4 points within 24 h, the secondary endpoint defined by the 3-month outcome was positive. This result was subsequently confirmed by the second part of the same study, showing that—compared to the placebo group—13% more patients in the alteplase group had no disability at 3 months, even though in these patients significantly more symptomatic ICHs (6.4% vs. 0.6%) had occurred. Subgroup analysis showed that this effect was independent of age, severity, and stroke subtype. Notably, in an analysis including only those patients that were treated within the first 2 h of symptom onset, the positive treatment effect on the outcome was highest. Based on these findings, the FDA approved alteplase for acute ischemic stroke within 3 h of symptom onset in 1996. Post hoc analysis of two other major clinical studies, the European Cooperative Acute Stroke Study (ECASS) and ECASS-II trials, and pooled analysis of the aforementioned trials (ECASS, NINDS, ECASS-II) plus the Alteplase Thrombolysis for Acute Noninterventional Therapy in Ischemic Stroke (ATLANTIS) trial also confirmed that tPA treatment was effective [5].

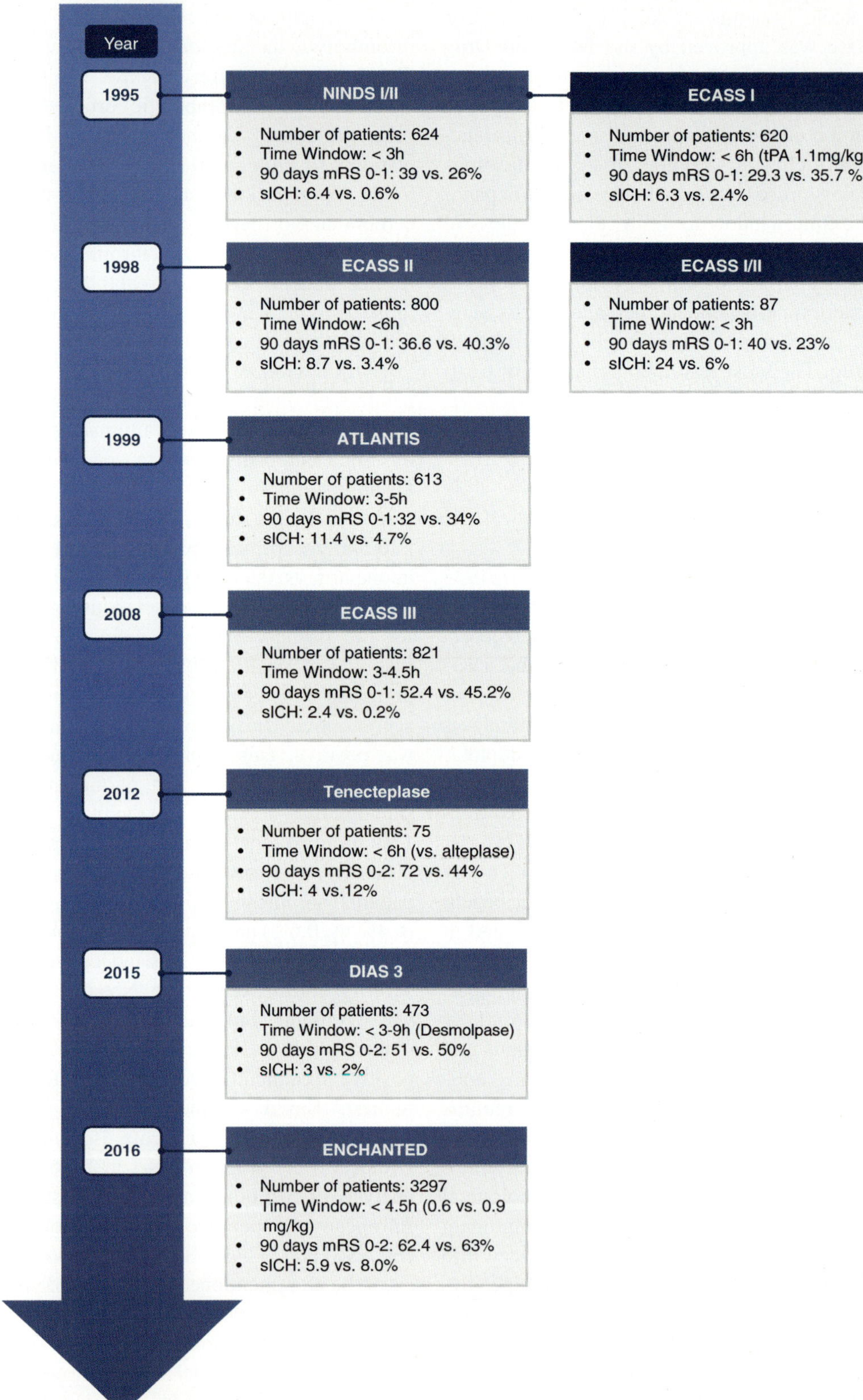

Fig. 6.1 History of clinical trials of IV thrombolysis

Finally, following the publication of the ECASS-III study in 2008, the time window for administration of intravenous (IV) thrombolysis was expanded from 3 to 4.5 h of symptom onset. It has to be emphasized that even though patients treated within 3 to 4.5 h after symptom onset benefit from r-tPA therapy, their outcome was worse than those treated within 3 h underlining once more the time dependency of the treatment.

6.3.2 Clinical Use

IV thrombolysis is usually only administered in hospitals. Within 10–20 min after arrival, the stroke-suspected patient should be sent for emergency imaging. Most centers use CT of the brain for exclusion of hemorrhage. The decision for IV thrombolysis is based on the result of the laboratory test, given that the time from symptom onset is less than 4.5 h, and potential contraindications regarding the use of IV thrombolysis have been ruled out. Contraindications against r-tPA use are discussed below (see Contraindications). Once the decision is made, treatment should be applied immediately on-site, striving for a "door-to-needle time" of less than 60 min. A CT angiography or other means of vascular imaging are not required for IV thrombolysis. Perfusion imaging will be helpful under special conditions, e.g., wake-up stroke, but it is also not mandatory. If performed, none of these should delay administration of treatment.

6.3.3 Dosage and Application

Alteplase[1] is the only preparation of r-tPA available for clinical use. Up to 100 kg body weight (BW), dosage is weight-dependent (0.9 mg r-tPA/kgBW; maximum dose: 90 mg). Ten percent of the calculated dose is given as a bolus, and the rest is continuously infused over 1 h. The infusible solution has to be prepared right before IV—delivery by dissolving lyophilized r-tPA in a solution containing L-arginine. In Japan, r-tPA was approved only for the dosing of 0.6 mg/kgBW. Recent study failed to demonstrate the non-inferiority of 0.6 mg r-tPA/kgBW compared to 0.9 mg r-tPA/kgBW [6]. For this reason, there are no general recommendations regarding the use of this lower dosage in the USA and Europe.

6.3.4 Contraindications

There are numerous formal contraindications to the utilization of IV r-tPA. Most of them were coined in analogy to the exclusion criteria defined by experts in the NINDS trial. Some of these criteria, as suitable as they may have been in the context of a clinical trial, have been shown to unreasonably limit the use of alteplase in clinical practice. For this reason, guidelines established by major stroke societies have been developed and adjusted over the last decades. The following section will give a short overview over some of the most relevant contraindications. For a comprehensive and more detailed review, it is strongly advised to consult national and/or international guidelines (e.g., American Heart Association/American Stroke Association [7], German Neurological Society [8], Japan Stroke Society [9]) (Table 6.1).

6.3.4.1 Intracranial Hemorrhage

Acute intracranial hemorrhage of any kind is an absolute contraindication to IV thrombolysis. Likewise, the history of ICH formally is an absolute contraindication. IV thrombolysis may be considered in these patients based on clinical judgment bearing in mind relevant factors (e.g., time passed since ICH, cause of ICH, extension of residual defect, recurrence of bleeding).

6.3.4.2 Severe Hypertension

Systolic blood pressure over 185 mm Hg and diastolic blood pressure over 110 mm Hg are contraindications to IV r-tPA therapy. If the blood pressure can be controlled and lowered below the

[1] Brand names: ***Activase***, ***Cathflo Activase***, Genentech (San Francisco, USA); ***Actilyse***, Boehringer Ingelheim International (Ingelheim, Germany); ***Cathflo***, Roche (Mississauga, Canada); ***Activacin***, Kyowa Hakko Kirin (Tokyo, Japan); ***Grtpa***, Tanabe Mitsubishi Pharma (Osaka, Japan).

Table 6.1 Contraindications of administration IV r-tPA

	Exclusion criteria
Patients with acute stroke within 3 h from symptom onset	History of intracranial hemorrhage
	Severe hypertension (systolic > 185 mm Hg or diastolic > 110 mm Hg)
	Previous serious head trauma in previous 3 months
	Prior ischemic stroke in previous 3 months (AHA/ASA) or 1 month (Japan Stroke Society)
	Coagulopathy/thrombocytopenia
	• Coagulopathy: INR > 1.7, aPTT > 40 s, or PT > 15 s
	• Thrombocytopenia: a low platelet count (<100,000/mm^3)
	Use of anticoagulants
	• Current use of vitamin K antagonist with an INR > 1.7
	• Heparin received within 48 h, with elevated aPTT
	• Current use of LMWH within 24 h
	• Current use of direct thrombin inhibitors or factor Xa inhibitors within 48 h, with elevated coagulation tests (such as aPTT, INR, platelet count, and ECT; TT; or appropriate factor Xa activity assays)
	Severe hypoglycemia or hyperglycemia
	• Blood glucose concentration <50 mg/dL (2.7 mmol/L) but considerable if symptoms do not improve rapidly after correction of glucose level
	Extensive hypoattenuation on CT scan (>1/3 cerebral hemisphere)
	Only minor or rapidly improving stroke symptoms (clearing spontaneously)
Additional criteria of patients with acute stroke within 3–4.5 h from symptom onset	Advanced age (>80 years)
	Severe stroke (NIHSS > 25)
	Current use of oral anticoagulant regardless of INR
	History of both diabetes and prior ischemic stroke

defined thresholds prior to application, the use of alteplase can be considered safe.

6.3.4.3 Previous Serious Head Trauma

IV thrombolysis is not recommended by the AHA/ASA guidelines in patients with serious head trauma within the preceding 3 months.

6.3.4.4 Previous Stroke

IV thrombolysis is not recommended by the AHA/ASA guidelines in patients with ischemic stroke within the last 3 months and by the guidelines of the Japan Stroke Society within 1 month after the index event.

6.3.4.5 Coagulopathy/Thrombocytopenia/Use of Anticoagulants

IV thrombolysis is not recommended in patients with platelet counts <100,000/mm^3, INR > 1.7, aPTT > 40 s, or PT > 15 s as safety and efficacy of treatment is unknown in this population. IV thrombolysis is also contraindicated in patients with a low platelet count (<100,000/mm^3). The evidence supporting this is very weak as there are only few published case reports. As unsuspected abnormal platelet counts seems to be extremely unlikely, it is not recommended to postpone IV thrombolysis waiting for the results of the platelet count. Regarding those patients taking vitamin K antagonist, current AHA/ASA guidelines suggest an INR of 1.7 as cutoff for IV thrombolysis: while in patients with an INR ≤ 1.7 treatment might be justified, it is contraindicated in those with an INR > 1.7. IV thrombolysis is not recommended by the AHA/ASA in patients who received LMWH for anticoagulation purpose in the last 24 h.

6.3.4.6 Oral Direct Thrombin Inhibitors and Factor Xa Inhibitors

Direct oral anticoagulants (DOAC) have shown to be at least as effective as warfarin in the prevention of stroke in patients with atrial fibrillation. Together with the simpler handling, this has led to a rapid increase of their prescription over the past years. Unfortunately, there is still no standardized way of addressing some of the major problems that come with their use. Most importantly, standard coagulation test (INR, Quick, aPTT) are not reliable enough to discriminate if the DOAC is still active or not. Even though direct Xa inhibitors may alter prothrombin time (PT) and activated partial thromboplastin time (aPTT) and direct thrombin inhibitors pTT and INR, there are no cutoffs defined. Furthermore, in patients with renal failure, the elimination half-life of oral direct thrombin inhibitors as well as factor Xa inhibitors is increased. Thrombin time may be a sensitive indicator for ongoing direct thrombin inhibitor activity. Similarly, assays directly measuring factor Xa activity may be useful in the case of factor Xa inhibitors [10].

For this reason, ASA guidelines recommend IV thrombolysis in patients receiving the aforementioned anticoagulants only on the basis of normal coagulation tests (aPTT, INR, platelet count, ecarin clotting time, thrombin time, or appropriate factor Xa activity assay) or if the patient has not received the DOAC > 48 h, provided the renal function is normal. Until further studies have been performed, we recommend establishing a feasible pathway together with the hospitals' laboratory based on current guidelines and the availability of coagulation tests in the emergency setting. Regarding the use of antidotes (e.g., idarucizumab for dabigatran) prior to IV thrombolysis, there is also an ongoing debate. Due to the uncertainties regarding its use, we recommend to include patients in trials assessing its efficacy.

6.3.4.7 Severe Hypoglycemia or Hyperglycemia

Severe alterations of glucose level may mimic acute stroke. Nevertheless, severe hypoglycemia or hyperglycemia should not be considered as contraindication for IV thrombolysis per se. Therapy should be considered if symptoms do not improve rapidly after correction of glucose level.

6.3.4.8 Early Radiographic Ischemic Changes (EIC) vs. Extensive Hypoattenuation on CT

Indistinction between gray and white matter, edema, mass effect, or midline shift are considered to be early infarct signs on a cranial CT scan. IV thrombolysis is recommended in the setting of EICs of mild to moderate extent. On the other hand, in patients with extensive hypoattenuation (=frank hypodensity) on cranial CT scan, IV thrombolysis is not recommended.

6.3.4.9 Advanced Age

Patients' age of 80 years or more was considered a relative contraindication to IV thrombolysis. AHA/ASA guidelines do not anymore recommend withholding therapy form these patients within a 3 h time window. Other guidelines including those of the ESO recommend treating older patients even in a 4.5 h time window.

6.3.4.10 Mild or Improving Stroke Symptoms

AHA/ASA guidelines specify disabling (not mild) deficits as follows: complete hemianopia (≥2 on NIHSS, question 3) or severe aphasia (≥2 on NIHSS, question 9) or visual or sensory extinction (≥1 on NIHSS, question 11) or any weakness limiting sustained effort against gravity (≥2 on NIHSS, question 5 and 6) or any deficits that lead to a total NIHSS score > 5, or any remaining deficit considered potentially disabling in the view of the patient and the treating practitioner. Patients with improving symptoms after severe initial neurological deficits, who were not treated with IV thrombolysis, frequently suffer from an unfavorable outcome [11]. It is recommended that patients with moderate/disabling symptoms should receive IV thrombolysis and that improving stroke symptoms should not postpone IV thrombolysis as the outcome is extremely time-dependent.

6.3.5 Complications

6.3.5.1 Intracerebral Hemorrhage

Intracerebral hemorrhage (ICH) is the most feared and a potentially life-threatening complication following IV thrombolysis as it is associated with a bad outcome. The first 36 h after application of r-tPA are considered critical. Studies show that ICH is more common in patients treated with IV r-tPA than in the placebo-treated controls. The NINDS trial reported ICH within the first 36 h after stroke onset in 6.4% of the patients in the r-tPA group and in 0.6% of the patients in the placebo group ($p < 0.001$). Despite these results, there was no significant increase in overall mortality in the group of patients receiving IV thrombolysis. This was subsequently demonstrated for r-tPA treatment initiated within 4.5 h. Nevertheless, due to the concerns regarding ICH, the approval of treatment with alteplase by the EMA was granted on the terms that treatment outcome was prospectively registered. This is carried out by the Safe Implementation of Thrombolysis in Stroke—International Stroke Thrombolysis Register (SITS-ISTR). It surveyed ICH rates of 1.5% within a 3 h, 1.8% within a 3–4.5 h, and 2.6% within a 4.5–6 h time window [12].

Several risk factors for ICH development in patients treated with IV r-tPA have been reported including age, early ischemic changes in CT, prior antiplatelet therapy, or extent of neurological deficits at presentation. But despite higher incidence of ICH in those patients, the benefit of r-tPA treatment still outweighs its risks and is not justifying withholding the thrombolytic therapy.

ICH should be considered in all patients whose neurologic conditions worsen during or after thrombolysis. For diagnosis, emergency cranial CT is the image modality of choice. Treatment is symptomatic and similar to spontaneous ICH including the evaluation of the necessity of a neurosurgical intervention.

6.3.5.2 Extracranial Hemorrhage

Extracranial hemorrhage after IV thrombolysis most often occurs if a trauma (e.g., fall) has foregone. Hemorrhage in "compressible" body parts (e.g., arms, legs, face) can usually be well controlled by compression and cooling the site of hemorrhage. Ongoing IV thrombolysis can in some cases be continued to be administered depending on the clinical judgment of the treating physician. Complications like excessive blood loss or the development of a compartment syndrome might warrant close observation or further action. If major bleeding (e.g., gastrointestinal or retroperitoneal bleeding) is suspected, thrombolytic therapy should be immediately discontinued. Urgent CT of the suspected site of bleeding should be performed, blood typed, and crossmatched. Further steps should be evaluated depending on the site of bleeding.

6.3.5.3 Reperfusion Injury

Another rare complication following successful recanalization of an occluded vascular territory is cerebral reperfusion injury with edema (also called hyper- or reperfusion syndrome). It is not only seen in the context of IV thrombolysis but also carotid endarterectomy (CEA), stenting, or even spontaneous revascularization.

6.3.5.4 Orolingual Angioedema

Orolingual angioedema (OLAE) is a relatively rare complication of IV r-tPA treatment, affecting about 2–8% of patients. Few studies indicate that OLAE might be more common in patients being treated with angiotensin-converting enzyme inhibitors. About half of the patients develop symptoms during the infusion, the other half shortly after it. Patients usually show mild, transient, and unilateral swelling and edema of the tongue or the lips. Ten percent of all OLAE cases can be life-threatening due to upper airway obstruction requiring urgent intubation. Treatment options include discontinuation of lytic therapy, application of oxygen, and administration of corticosteroids, antihistamines, and epinephrine. The use of the B2 bradykinin receptor antagonist icatibant (Firazyr®) might be considered in severe cases of orolingual edema. Up to date its application is off-label, and clinical experience is limited and mainly based on case reports.

6.3.5.5 Neurotoxicity

Apart from the beneficial effects of tPA in acute ischemic stroke in terms of clot lysis, prolonged ischemic periods, which are usually associated with blood-brain barrier disruption, result in extravasation of exogenous tPA and subsequently might lead to neurotoxicity. The detrimental properties of tPA are mediated by interaction with NMDA receptors and free radical generation among others [13]. Thus, early restoration of cerebral blood flow is crucial in preventing ischemic injury and is known to promote good functional outcome [14]. There is an open discussion about neurotoxic effects of alteplase itself, possibly (and rarely) resulting in seizures or even worsening of ischemia. It remains unclear whether those effects are mediated by r-tPA itself or by L-arginine which is part of the solution the former is dissolved in. Treatment in any case is symptomatic.

Conclusion

In acute ischemic stroke, IV thrombolysis is a well-established therapy within a 4.5 h time window from symptom onset. In the hands of an experienced stroke team, it can substantially improve a patient's functional outcome at a relatively low risk. It is highly important that the treatment is initiated as fast as possible, as time is brain. Contraindications of IV thrombolysis have been constantly refined according to the state of knowledge. Patient's age and stroke severity should not be a reason to withhold IV thrombolysis anymore. With the introduction of endovascular thrombectomy, new challenges have emerged regarding the use of IV thrombolysis that calls for further research efforts.

Suggestions from Clinical Practice Guidelines Eligible patients for intravenous (IV) fibrinolysis (recombinant tissue plasminogen activator, 0.9 mg/kg, maximum dose 90 mg) are selected among the patients along the established inclusion/exclusion criteria. IV fibrinolysis should be begun within 4.5 h after symptom onset, and an ideal door-to-needle time (from patient's visit time to time of bolus administration) is within 60 min. Accordingly, IV fibrinolysis-related sequence in the emergency unit is conducted as quickly as possible. If blood pressure of the eligible patient for intravenous fibrinolysis is more than 185/110 mm Hg, the blood pressure should be lowered slowly to <185/110 mm Hg.

References

1. Wardlaw JM, Murray V, Berge E, et al. Thrombolysis for acute ischaemic stroke. Cochrane Database Syst Rev. 2014;7:CD000213.
2. Goyal M, Menon BK, van Zwam WH, et al. Endovascular thrombectomy after large-vessel ischaemic stroke: a meta-analysis of individual patient data from five randomised trials. Lancet. 2016;387:1723–31.
3. The National Institute of Neurological Disorders Stroke rtPA Stroke Study Group Nal. Tissue plasminogen activator for acute ischemic stroke. N Engl J Med. 1995;333:1581–8.
4. Hacke W, Kaste M, Bluhmki E, et al. Thrombolysis with alteplase 3 to 4.5 hours after acute ischemic stroke. N Engl J Med. 2008;359:1317–29.
5. Hlavica M, Diepers M, Garcia-Esperon C, et al. Pharmacological recanalization therapy in acute ischemic stroke – evolution, current state and perspectives of intravenous and intra-arterial thrombolysis. J Neuroradiol. 2015;42:30–46.
6. Anderson CS, Robinson T, Lindley RI, et al. Low-dose versus standard-dose intravenous alteplase in acute ischemic stroke. N Engl J Med. 2016;374:2313–23.
7. Jauch EC, Saver JL, Adams HP Jr, et al. Guidelines for the early management of patients with acute ischemic stroke: a guideline for healthcare professionals from the American Heart Association/American Stroke Association. Stroke. 2013;44:870–947.
8. Ringleb P, Hamann G, Roether J, et al. Akuttherapie des ischämischen Schlaganfalls – Rekanalisierende Therapien. Akt Neurol. 2016;43:82–91.
9. Minematsu K, Toyoda K, Hirano T, et al. Guidelines for the intravenous application of recombinant tissue-type plasminogen activator (alteplase), the second edition, October 2012: a guideline from the Japan Stroke Society. J Stroke Cerebrovasc Dis. 2013;22:571–600.
10. Steiner T. Neue direkte orale Antiokoagulantien – was im Notfall zu beachten ist. Dtsch Ärzteblatt. 2012;109:1928–30.
11. Nedeltchev K, Schwegler B, Haefeli T, et al. Outcome of stroke with mild or rapidly improving symptoms. Stroke. 2007;38:2531–5.

12. Ahmed N, Kellert L, Lees KR, et al. Results of intravenous thrombolysis within 4.5 to 6 hours and updated results within 3 to 4.5 hours of onset of acute ischemic stroke recorded in the Safe Implementation of Treatment in Stroke International Stroke Thrombolysis Register (SITS-ISTR): an observational study. JAMA Neurol. 2013;70:837–84.
13. Kaur J, Zhao Z, Klein GM, et al. The neurotoxicity of tissue plasminogen activator? J Cereb Blood Flow Metab. 2004;24:945–63.
14. Lees KR, Bluhmki E, von Kummer R, et al. Time to treatment with intravenous alteplase and outcome in stroke: an updated pooled analysis of ECASS, ATLANTIS, NINDS, and EPITHET trials. Lancet. 2010;375:1695–703.

History of Intra-arterial Thrombolysis

7

Mi Sun Oh

Abstract

Timely recanalization of the occluded vessels may restore cerebral perfusion of still-salvageable, infarcted brain tissue, thereby possibly improving clinical outcome in patients with acute ischemic stroke (AIS). The administration of intravenous recombinant tissue plasminogen activator (IV rt-PA) within 4.5 h of symptom onset is the only US Food and Drug Administration-approved medical treatment in AIS. However, most patients with AIS present more than the time window for IV rt-PA. In addition, IV rt-PA often fails to recanalize large proximal arteries. Therefore, the numerous recanalization therapies for AIS patients have been developed substantially over the past decades, which include the use of intra-arterial fibrinolysis, the bridging of intravenous with intra-arterial thrombolysis, and the use of multimodal approaches to recanalization therapy including thrombectomy and thromboaspiration with different available devices. In this chapter, we outlined the brief history of endovascular stroke management.

Intravenous recombinant tissue plasminogen activator (IV rt-PA) is the standard therapy for acute ischemic stroke (AIS) patients presenting up to 4.5 h after symptom onset. However, the majority of AIS patients arrive beyond the guideline-recommended time window for the administration of IV rt-PA. Additionally, the low rate of recanalization of large artery occlusion of IV rt-PA and contraindications for its use has limited the impact of IV rt-PA. This has led to over the past decade attempt continuing the development of a multimodal intra-arterial thrombolysis (IAT) approaches in order to improve recanalization rates and extend the time window of recanalization therapy in AIS patients. The alternative strategies of IAT include not only local IAT using thrombolytic agents but also mechanical IAT using various devices.

M.S. Oh, M.D.
Department of Neurology, Hallym University Sacred Heart Hospital, Hallym University College of Medicine, Anyang, South Korea
e-mail: iyyar@hallym.ac.kr

S.-H. Lee (ed.), *Stroke Revisited: Diagnosis and Treatment of Ischemic Stroke*, Stroke Revisited, DOI 10.1007/978-981-10-1424-6_7

The strategies of IAT are as follows:

- Chemical IAT
- Combined IVT and IAT (the bridging therapy) with/without mechanical clot disruption
- Endovascular mechanical IAT: mechanical clot retriever (MERCI, Multi-MERCI), thromboaspiration (Penumbra), stent retriever (Solitaire, Trevo), balloon angioplasty, and stenting

Devices and techniques for the endovascular stroke therapy have been evolving rapidly, making the execution of randomized clinical trials. In this chapter, the history of IAT for the recanalization therapy in AIS patients, including both local IAT using thrombolytic agents and mechanical interventions, are briefly outlined with reviewing the landmark trials (Fig. 7.1 and Table 7.1).

7.1 History of Local Chemical IAT

Earlier endovascular therapies attempted using IAT with thrombolytic agents. IA application of thrombolytic agents can deliver a higher dose of drug directly into the clot, thus increasing the chances for recanalization. The lower systemic exposure and smaller dose of thrombolytic agents used with IAT makes treatment possible in ineligible patients for treatment of IV rt-PA. Other advantages of IAT include direct angiographic

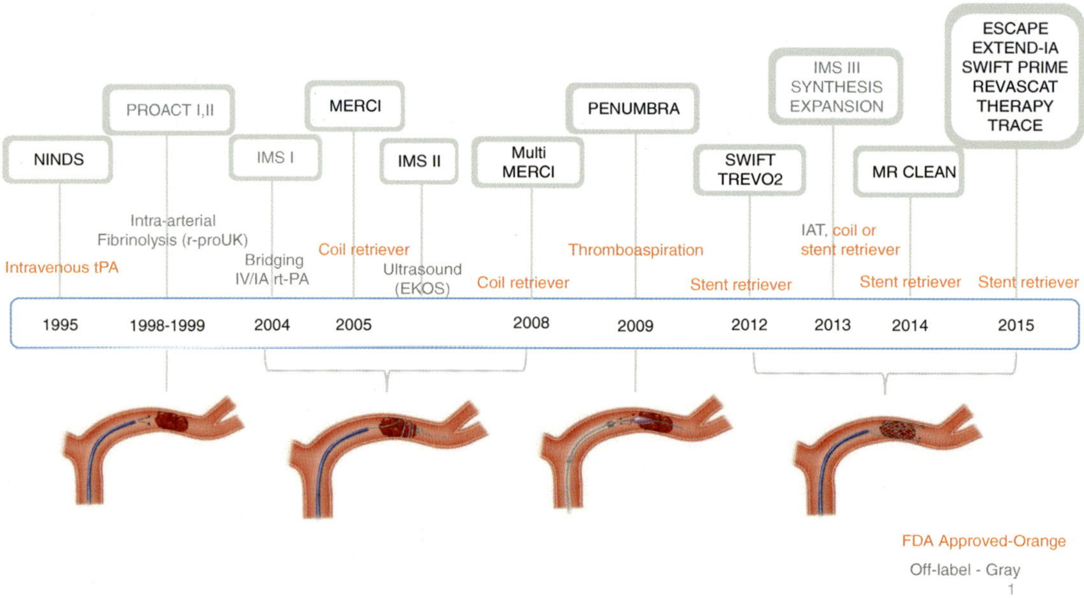

Fig. 7.1 The history of thrombolysis. Prolyse in Acute Cerebral Thromboembolism (PROACT) II trial; The Mechanical Embolus Removal in Cerebral Ischemia (MERCI); Interventional Management of Stroke [IMS] III; Local Versus Systemic Thrombolysis for Acute Ischemic Stroke [SYNTHESIS] Expansion; Mechanical Retrieval and Recanalization of Stroke Clots Using Embolectomy [MR RESCUE]; Multicenter Randomized Clinical Trial of Endovascular Treatment for Acute Ischemic Stroke in the Netherlands [MR CLEAN]; Evaluation Study of Congestive Heart Failure and Pulmonary Artery Catheterization Effectiveness [ESCAPE]; Extending the Time for Thrombolysis in Emergency Neurological Deficits–Intra-Arterial [EXTEND-IA]; Solitaire With the Intention For Thrombectomy as Primary Endovascular Treatment [SWIFT PRIME]; Endovascular Revascularization With Solitaire Device Versus Best Medical Therapy in Anterior Circulation Stroke Within 8 h [REVASCAT]

Table 7.1 Summary of landmark trials of endovascular therapy for AIS

	Number, active group	Study design	Occluded vessels	Duration of symptoms (h)	Baseline NIHSS, median	Successful recanalization TIMI 2–3/TICI 2b–3 (%)	Good clinical outcomes, 90-day mRS 0–2 (%)	Mortality at 90 days (%)	sHT (%)
IAT with thrombolytic agent									
PROACT I	26	RCT, IA pro UK + IV heparin vs. IV heparin	MCA (M1/M2)	<6	17	58	58	27	15
PROACT II	121	RCT, IA pro UK + IV heparin vs. IV heparin	MCA (M1/M2)	<6	17	66	40	25	10
MELT	57	RCT, IA UK vs. control	MCA (M1/M2)	<6	14	NA	49	5	9
Combined IV and IA thrombolysis (bridging therapy)									
EMS	17	RCT, IV rt-PA + IA rt-PA vs. IA rt-PA	MCA (M1/M2), ICA	<3	16	54	NA	29	12
IMS I	62	Single-arm study, IV rt-PA + IA rt-PA	MCA (M1/M2), ICA, VBA	<3	18	56	43	16	6
IMS II	55	Single-arm study, IV rt-PA + IA rt-PA/EKOS	MCA (M1/M2), ICA, VBA	<3	19	58	46	16	10
IMS III	434	RCT, IV rt-PA + EVT/IA rt-PA vs. IV rt-PA	MCA (M1/M2), ICA, VBA	<3	17	65–81	41	19	6
Endovascular mechanical IAT									
MERCI	151	Single-arm study, IA MERCI, IAT	MCA (M1/M2), ICA, VBA	<8	22	46	28	44	8
Multi-MERCI	164	Single arm, IA MERCI, IAT + IV rt-PA	MCA (M1/M2), ICA, VBA	<8	19	68	36	34	10
Penumbra pivotal trial	125	Single arm, IA Penumbra, IV rt-PA	MCA (M1/M2), ICA, VBA	<8	18	82	25	33	11
SWIFT (Solitaire)	58	RCT, Solitaire vs. MERCI	MCA (M1/M2), ICA, VBA	<8	17	83	36	17	2
TREVO 2 (TREVO)	88	TREVO vs. MERCI	MCA (M1/M2), ICA, VBA	<8	19	85	40	33	7
SYNTHESIS	181	RCT, ET vs. IV rt-PA	NA	<4.5	13	NA	42	8	6
MR-RESCUE[a]	34; 30	RCT, ET vs. medical therapy	MCA (M1/M2), ICA	<8	17;19	67;77	21;17	18;20	9;0

Abbreviations: *NIHSS* National Institutes of Health Stroke Scale score, *TICI* thrombolysis in cerebral infarction, *TIMI* thrombolysis in myocardial infarction, *mRS* modified Rankin Scale, *SHT* symptomatic hemorrhagic transformation, *RCT* randomized controlled trial, *Pro-UK* pro-urokinase, *IV rt-PA* intravenous recombinant tissue plasminogen activator, *IAT* intra-arterial thrombolysis, *MCA* middle cerebral artery, *VBA* vertebrobasilar artery, *ICA* internal carotid artery, *NA* not available

[a]Embolectomy patients with good penumbral pattern on magnetic resonance imaging (MRI); embolectomy in patients without good penumbral pattern on MRI

visual assessment of treatment efficacy and the extension of the time window. The thrombolytic agents for IAT in AIS include urokinase (UK), pro-urokinase (pro-UK), streptokinase, alteplase, and reteplase [1].

7.1.1 The Prolyse in Acute Cerebral Thromboembolism (PROACT) (1998, *N* = 46)

The PROACT I study was a phase II, double-blind, randomized, placebo-controlled trial that compared IA r-pro-UK (6 mg) and low-dose IV heparin with IA placebo and low-dose IV heparin for symptomatic M1 and M2 middle cerebral artery (MCA) occlusion within 6 h of stroke onset [2]. The PROACT I trial was terminated early because the Food and Drug Administration (FDA) approved IV rt-PA. A total of 40 patients were recruited before premature termination. The recanalization of an occluded vessel, defined as a Thrombolysis in Myocardial Infarction (TIMI) score of 2 or 3, was significantly more likely in the pro-UK group versus the placebo group (57.7% vs. 14.3%, respectively). The overall risk of symptomatic hemorrhagic transformation (SHT) was also higher in the pro-UK group to 15.4% compared to 7.1% in the placebo group.

7.1.2 The PROACT II (1999, *N* = 180)

The PROACT II study was a phase III, open-label, randomized controlled trial of assessing the efficacy and safety of IA pro-UK (9 mg) plus IV heparin compared with IV heparin alone in patients presenting within 6 h of stroke onset and with angiographically confirmed MCA occlusions [3]. In PROACT II trial, the primary clinical outcome of a modified Rankin Scale (mRS) score of 0–2 at 90 days was achieved in a higher percentage of the IA pro-UK group (40%) compared with the heparin-only control group (25%). The successful recanalization, defined as TIMI grade 3, was also higher in the pro-UK group (19%) compared to the control group (4%) [3]. SHT was increased in the pro-UK group (10% vs. 2%), but these increases of SHT did not affect mortality rates (25% in the pro-UK group vs. 27% in the control group) [3].

7.1.3 The Middle Cerebral Artery Embolism Local Fibrinolytic Intervention (MELT) (2007, *N* = 114)

The Japanese MELT study was a randomized, controlled trial examining the safety and efficacy of IA infusion of UK in patients with symptomatic M1 or M2 MCA occlusion of less than 6 h of stroke onset [4]. This trial was terminated after the approval of IV rt-PA in Japan. In the MELT trial, preliminary results did not show significance in primary efficacy outcome (mRS score 0–2) at 90 days. However, there was significantly more patients with excellent functional outcome (mRS score of 1 less) and the National Institute of Health Stroke Scale (NIHSS) score 0 or 1 at 3 months in the UK group than the control group.

The PROACT II trial is the only randomized controlled trial of IA thrombolytic agents to date, which verified statistically significant clinical benefit. Because of the small size and marginal significance, The FDA did not approve a stroke label for IA r-pro-UK and requested a confirmatory efficacy trial that has not yet been conducted. Furthermore, there have been no direct comparative trials to examining the safety and efficacy of IAT versus IV rt-PA in AIS. The disadvantages of IAT include additional time required to activate the interventional team and to transport patients to the specialized hospitals available to IAT.

7.2 History of Combined IV and IA Thrombolysis (Bridging Therapy)

Several studies have investigated the feasibility, safety, and efficacy of combined IV rt-PA and IAT in AIS patients. The rationale for combined IVT and IAT came from the concern that the delayed time of initiation with the IAT may negate the potential benefits of more efficacious recanalization as well as that proximal intracranial artery occlusions with larger clot burdens may benefit most from IAT. The bridging therapy came from the efforts of the combined advantages of IVT (wide availability, fast administration) and IAT (higher recanalization, extended time window).

7.2.1 Combined IV and IA Administration of rt-PA

7.2.1.1 The Emergency Management of Stroke (EMS) Bridging Trial (1999, *N* = 34)

The EMS was a double-blind, randomized, placebo-controlled, multicenter phase I pilot trial, which randomized patients to the IV/IA group [low-dose IV rt-PA (0.6 mg/kg) followed by local IA rt-PA via microcatheter] or the placebo/IA group (IV placebo followed local IA of rt-PA via microcatheter) [5]. Based on the subanalysis of the 22 patients with a persistent clot on angiography, the IV/IA bridging approach yielded significantly higher rates of recanalization (54% vs. 10%, respectively) but no difference in the clinical and functional outcomes [5]. The rates of death, SHT, and the life-threatening extracranial bleeding complications were higher in the IV/IA group than in the placebo/IA group but not statistical significance [5].

7.2.1.2 The International Management of Stroke (IMS) I (2004, *N* = 80)

The IMS I and II studies were a prospective, multicenter, open-label, single-arm pilot trial, with the aim of assessing the feasibility and safety of a combined low-dose IV rt-PA and IA rt-PA administered in patients with persistent clot after the bolus of IV rt-PA [6]. These IMS studies included patients with intracranial internal carotid artery (ICA) occlusion, vertebrobasilar artery (VBA) occlusion, as well as M1 and M2 MCA occlusion [6]. In IMS I, 34 (43%) of the 80 enrolled patients achieved an mRS $\leq$ 2 at 90 days compared with 39% and 28% of the patients in the rt-PA and placebo groups of the National Institute of Neurological Disorders and Stroke (NINDS) trial, respectively [6]. The partial or complete recanalization, defined as TIMI 2–3, was achieved in 35 (56%) of the 62 patients who underwent combined IVT and IAT. The rate of SHT (6.3%) in IMS subjects was comparable with the IV rt-PA group (6.6%) but higher than the rate in the placebo group (1.0%) in the NINDS trial. The 90-day mortality in IMS subjects (16%) was lower but not statistically different from the mortality rate of the rt-PA group (21%) or the placebo group (24%) in the NINDS trial [6].

7.2.2 The IV and IA Bridging Therapy with Mechanical Clot Disruption

7.2.2.1 The IMS II (2007, *N* = 81)

In IMS II, the mechanical clot disruption using an ultrasound-based thrombolysis augmentation device, MicroLysUS microinfusion catheter (EKOS, Bothell, WA), to deliver the rt-PA into the clot was employed [7]. Of the 81 enrolled patients receiving IV rt-PA, 55 patients received both IV and IA rt-PA via either the EKOS microinfusion catheter (n = 36) or a standard microcatheter (n = 19). Recanalization to TIMI 2–3 was achieved 60% in IMS II, with rates appearing higher in patients who were additionally treated with the EKOS [7]. Good functional outcome, defined as an mRS score of 0–2, at 90 days (46%) and mortality at 90 days (16%) in IMS II subjects were significantly improved compared with the placebo group of the NINDS study (28% and 24%, respectively); however, there was no significant improvement in outcome or mortality compared with the IV rt-PA group of the NINDS study (39% and 21%, respectively). The rate of SHT (9.9%) in IMS subjects was higher compared with that of placebo group (1%) but not significantly different from that of rt-PA group (6.6%) in the NINDS trial.

These results, taken together, suggest that the bridging therapy is promising, as recanalization rates and clinical outcomes seem to be similar or higher than those achieved via the IVT alone and the IAT alone. Especially, the bridging approach that permitted mechanical clot disruption may improve the efficacy of thrombolytic therapy, as the mechanical device can disrupt the clot and macerate the occluding thrombus, thus increasing the surface area on which fibrinolytic agents can act. In the absence of more sophisticated devices, early experiment of mechanical clot disruption used repeated passage of the microguidewire or microcatheter through thrombus. One of the more successful methods to mechanical clot disruption has been to use ultrasonic energy, such as the EKOS system used in the IMS II study. The IMS III trial was then designed to compare combined low-dose IV rt-PA and endovascular therapy to standard-dose IV rt-PA alone, with all eligible patients receiving IV rt-PA within 3 h or stroke onset. Endovascular therapy approaches used in the study included IA rt-PA with or without EKOS, Merci, Penumbra, or Solitaire devices [8]. The published results of these trials were presented in the next chapter (Chap. 8). Other devices that used laser technologies such as endovascular photoacoustic recanalization device (EndoVasix, Belmont, CA) and neurolaser thrombolysis system (LaTIS, MN, USA) were employed but have been less frequently used, with a relatively unsuccessful pilot studies.

7.3 History of Endovascular Mechanical Thrombectomy

Endovascular mechanical thrombectomy have several potential advantages over IAT with thrombolytic agents, including higher rates of recanalization, rapid achievement of recanalization, lower risk of thrombolytics-associated hemorrhage, revascularization of large artery occlusions, and a longer treatment time window. Additionally, compared with the disrupting clot, endovascular mechanical clot removal leads to rapid recanalization and lower rates of distal embolization secondary to clot fragmentation. Several devices have been designed to directly retrieve or aspirate the occluding thrombus. There are currently four devices approved by the FDA for recanalization of large arterial occlusion in AIS patients.

7.3.1 First-Generation Mechanical Thrombectomy: The Mechanical Embolus Removal in Cerebral Ischemia (MERCI) Retrieval Device (FDA Approval in 2004)

The first FDA-approved mechanical thrombectomy device for the treatment of AIS was the MERCI retriever system (Concentric Medical Inc., CA, USA), which is designed as corkscrew-shaped device consisting of a flexible nitinol wire in five helical loops. The balloon of the guiding catheter is blown up distally from the occluding thrombus to achieve anterograde blood flow arrest and prevent distal embolization. By deploying a corkscrew-like retrieval device, it retracted into the clot and is then pulled back into the catheter with the clot ensnared. Once the clot is removed, the procedure is completed by deflating the occluding proximal balloon and rapidly restoring circulation.

7.3.2 Landmark Trials: The MERCI (2005, *N* = 151) Trial

The MERCI study was a prospective, multicenter, single-arm trial to explore the safety and efficacy of the MERCI device compared with the control group of the PROCT II trial as a historical control [9]. The MERCI trial included patients ineligible for IV rt-PA within 8 h of stroke onset. The mean onset time to treatment (OTT) was 4.3 ± 1.7 h, and the mean procedure duration was 2.1 h [9]. The rate of recanalization (TIMI 2–3) was significantly higher than that in the control group of the PROACT II trial as a historical control (46% vs. 18%, respectively), but lower than that in the IAT group of the PROACT II trial (66%) [9]. After adjunctive therapy (IA rt-PA/UK, angioplasty, snare), the rate of recanalization increased to 60.3%. The overall rate of patients achieving good neurological outcome (mRS score ≤ 2) at 90 days was comparable to that in the control group in the PROACT II trial (23% vs. 25%, respectively). In contrast, the mortality rate of 44% was significantly higher than in the previous trials of the treatment of AIS. Of the 141 patients treated with the device, clinically significant procedural complications and SHT occurred in 7% and 8% of the patients, respectively. Good neurologic outcomes at 90 days were more frequent (46% vs. 10%), and mortality rates were lower (32% vs. 54%) with successful compared with unsuccessful recanalization [9].

7.3.3 The Multi-MERCI Trial (2008, *N* = 164)

The Multi-MERCI study was a prospective single-arm trial to test both first-generation (X5 and X6) and second-generation (L4, L5, and L6) MERCI devices [10]. Patients met the same inclusion criteria as in the first MERCI trial, but patients who had failed recanalization after IV rt-PA were also included. In the Multi-MERCI part I (*N* = 111), the prior treatment with IV rt-PA, mechanical clot disruption, IA rt-PA, and other adjunctive therapies were allowed. Mean OTT was 4.3 h, and mean onset time to reperfusion (OTR) was 5.9 h. The rates of recanalization (TIMI 2–3) were higher in patients receiving adjunctive therapies after the retriever than in those treated with the retriever alone (68% vs. 55%, respectively). Rates of recanalization were 86% in the posterior circulation (*N* = 14), 65% in the ICA terminus (*N* = 52), 61% in M1 (*n* = 77), and 91% in M2 (*N* = 21) [10]. The overall rate of good neurological outcome (mRS score ≤ 2) at 90 days was achieved in 36% of patients, whereas 34% of patients died. SHT occurred in 16 patients (10%), with 2% having parenchymal hematoma type II. Clinically significant procedural complications occurred in nine patients (6%). Of note, there was no difference in the rate of SHT or procedural complications between patients with IV rt-PA prior to MERCI device deployment and those without [10]. When analyzed according to recanalization status, successful recanalization was associated with good neurological outcome and lower mortality rates at 90 days. Despite high rates of recanalization in the MECI and Multi-MERCI trials, clinical efficacy was not proven compared with the previous major trials of IVT and IAT.

7.3.4 Endovascular Thromboaspiration: The Penumbra System (FDA Approval in 2007)

The Penumbra system is based on an aspiration platform, which is developed to provide a more rapid recanalization and is reliable than mechanical thrombectomy with a lower risk of fragmentation or distal embolization. The Penumbra Stroke System (Penumbra, CF, USA) consists of two different revascularization parts: a reperfusion microcatheter to debulk and aspirate the occluding thrombus and a ring retriever to extract the remnant thrombus.

7.3.5 The Penumbra Pivotal Stroke System Trial (2009, *N* = 125)

The Penumbral pivotal study was a prospective, multicenter, single-arm trial, which used the data of the MERCI trial as historical control [11]. In this trial, the enrolled 125 patients either are ineligible for IV rt-PA or have failed recanalization after IV rt-PA within 8 h of stroke onset and have NIHSS scores ≥8 and large artery occlusion on angiography. Recanalization (TIMI 2–3) was obtained in 82% of patients. The rate of HT was 28% of patients, 11% of whom were symptomatic. Overall good neurological outcome (mRS score ≤ 2) was seen in 25% of patients, and 33% of patients died. Although the rate of recanalization using the Penumbra device was the highest of the prospective trials (compared with 55% in the Multi-MERCI trial and 66% in the PROACT II trial), the neurological outcome was comparable or lower (25% with mRS 0–2, vs. 36% in the Multi-MERCI trial and 40% in the PROACT II trial) [11]. The investigators attribute this disparity to the lack of sufficient power and higher baseline NIHSS score.

The Randomized, Concurrent Controlled Trial to Assess the Penumbra System's Safety and Effectiveness in the Treatment of Acute Stroke (THERAPY) (2016, $N = 108$) was a prospective, multicenter, randomized, open-label, blinded end point, concurrent controlled trial of the Penumbra with IV rt-PA compared with IV rt-PA alone in AIS patients with LA thrombus length ≥ 8 mm.

7.3.6 Balloon Angioplasty and Stenting

The urgent balloon angioplasty, with or without stent replacement, has been a useful technique in treating atherothrombotic AIS causing in situ thrombosis rather than embolic occlusions. There were only a few studies investigating the feasibility and efficacy of intracranial stents for the urgent treatment of AIS. The Stent-Assisted Recanalization in Acute Ischemic Stroke (SARIS) (2009, $N = 20$) study was a prospective, single-arm trial aimed to evaluate the safety of stent deployment as a primary therapeutic intervention for acute stroke [12]. The investigators used the Wingspan (Boston Scientific, Natick, MA) and the Enterprise (Cordis, Bridgewater, NJ) intracranial self-expanding stents. Twenty patients who were either ineligible for IV rt-PA or failed treatment to IV rt-PA were enrolled. Recanalization (TIMI 2–3) was achieved in all patients, SHT occurred in 5%, and fair or better functional outcomes (mRS score 0–3) at 30 days were seen in 60%. There was no procedure-related complication. The main limitation of stent-assisted recanalization is the theoretical risk of intracranial stent failure and complications related to placement of a permanent intracranial implant, such as the risk of delayed in-stent stenosis and the need for an aggressive antithrombotic regimen.

7.4 New-Generation Mechanical Thrombectomy: Stent Retriever

Stent retriever attempts to maintain the advantages of a stent platform, including fast device delivery and rapid restoration of blood flow without the disadvantages of permanent intracranial implant. The self-expanding stents are partially deployed within symptomatic intracranial thrombus; the thrombus is captured between the stent and the vessel wall. The thrombus is retrieved when the stent is removed. Removal of the stent eliminates the need for acute dual antiplatelet therapy, as is needed for permanent stent implant (Fig. 7.2).

7.4.1 Solitaire FR Device (FDA Approval in 2012)

The Solitaire FR stent (ev3, Irvine, CA, USA) was the first to be released and the most to be tested for the treatment of AIS patients. It was originally developed for the intervention of cerebral aneurysm. The Solitaire FR With the Intention For Thrombectomy (SWIFT) (2012, $N = 113$) study was a prospective, multicenter, randomized, open-label trial to test the safety and efficacy of the Solitaire FR stent platform-based clot retriever and to compare it with the MERCI retrieval system [13]. The Rates of recanalization (TIMI 2–3) were significantly higher in the Solitaire group than in the MERCI group (83% vs. 48% when assessed by the local investigator and 69% vs. 30% when assessed by the central laboratory). More patients had good clinical outcomes (mRS ≤ 2) at 90 days with Solitaire than with Merci (58% vs. 33%). Mortality rates were also found to be lower in the Solitaire group than the Merci group (17% vs. 38%).

7.4.2 Thrombectomy Revascularization of Large Vessel Occlusion in Acute Ischemic Stroke (TREVO) Device (FDA Approval in 2012)

The TREVO device (Concentric Medical Inc.) is being studied in the open-label Thrombectomy Revascularization of Large Vessel Occlusions in Acute Ischemic Stroke (TREVO) study (2012, $N = 178$) [14]. The TREVO 2 trial compared the TREVO stent retriever with the MERCI device in

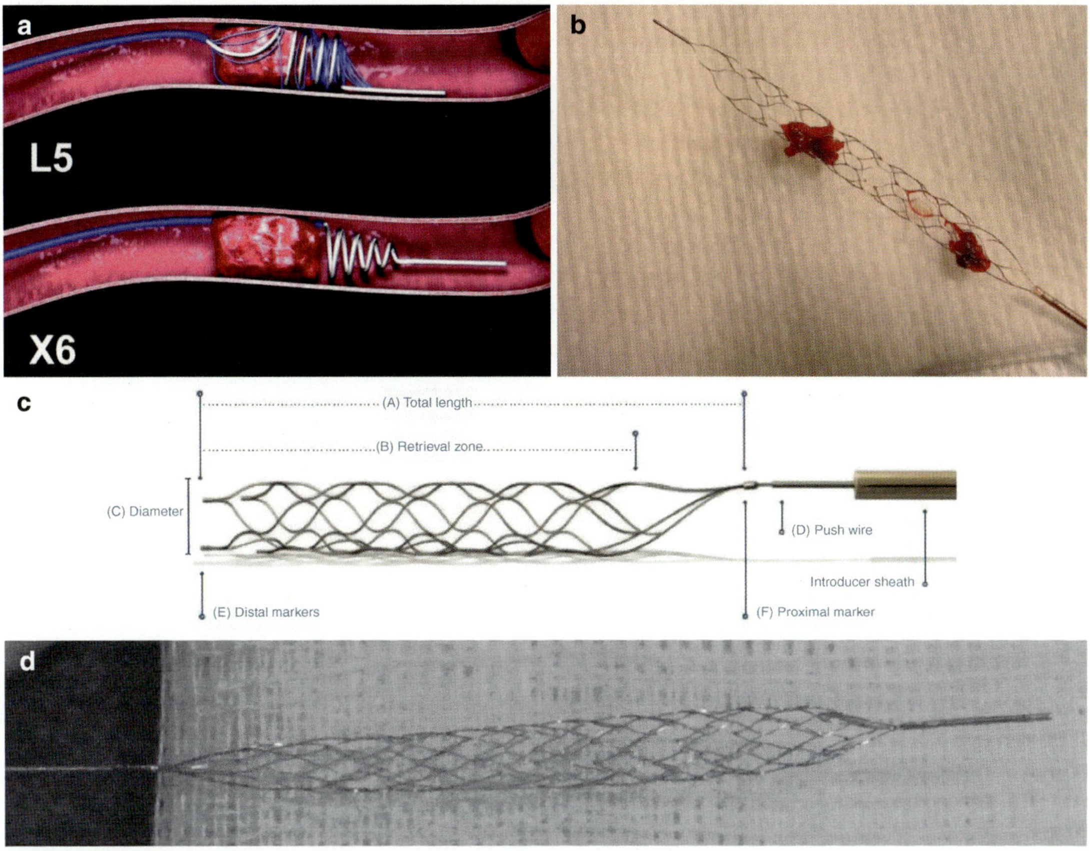

Fig. 7.2 Mechanical devices for intra-arterial thrombectomy. (**a**) Mechanical thrombectomy with the Merci® retriever works by wrapping around and capturing the clot. Reproduced by permission of Stroke (Smith WS et al. Stroke. 2008;39:1205–1212). (**b**) TREVO® stent retriever. Reproduced by permission of Stroke (Román LS et al. Stroke. 2012;43:1657–1659). (**c**) Solitaire® stent retriever. Reproduced by permission of Medtronic Inc. (**d**) The Revive SE clot retrieval device consists of a self-expanding nitinol basket with a closed distal end. Reproduced by permission of Stroke (Rohde S et al. Stroke. 2011;42:2954–2956)

AIS patients with acute intracranial artery occlusions within 8 h. The primary efficacy end point, TICI 2 to 3 reperfusion assessed by a central laboratory, was achieved significantly more often in the TREVO-treated patients compared with the MERCI -treated patients (86% vs. 60%, respectively). The primary safety end point, a composite of procedure-related complications, was comparable for the two groups (15% vs. 23%). Good functional outcome (mRS $\leq$ 2) was also more common in patients treated with the stent retriever (40% vs. 22%).

Two randomized preliminary trials with stent retriever have been encouraging, showing unprecedented recanalization rates and better functional outcomes than ever reported with other interventions including endovascular mechanical thrombectomy with the MERCI device. New trials are designed to investigate the clinical efficacy of endovascular treatment, in particular thrombectomy with stent retriever, compared with the standard medical care including IV rt-PA began, and the results of these trials have been published in 2014–2016 (Table 7.2).

Table 7.2 Advantages and disadvantages of endovascular therapies

	Advantages	Disadvantages	Guidelines (2013, 2015 AHA/ ASA)
All endovascular therapies	• Higher rate of recanalization vs. IV rt-PA • Direct angiographic visualization of clot burden, collateral circulation, immediate assessment of treatment effect (recanalization status) • Extension of the time window • Combination approaches (possible use of mechanical means to disrupt the clot with use of the guide wire, microcatheter, or other devices) • Addressing early reocclusion or underlying stenosis • Lower systemic hemorrhagic complication	• Only appropriate for large vessel occlusions • Delay to initiation of therapy • Periprocedural complications • Specialized infrastructure and expertise needed limiting access and raising cost	• Patients eligible for IV rt-PA should receive IV rt-PA even if IAT are being considered *(class I; level of evidence A)* • IAT or mechanical thrombectomy is reasonable in patients who have contraindications to the use of IV rt-PA (class IIa; level of evidence C)
IAT with thrombolytics	• Direct infusion of the higher-dose fibrinolysis into the occluding thrombus • Lower systemic concentration of thrombolytic agent with less risk of extracranial hemorrhagic complications vs. IV rt-PA	• Not FDA approved • Additional time delays required for the preparations of the procedure • Higher rate of SHT (PROCT II) vs. IV rt-PA in the NINDS study • Additional risks of the endovascular procedure itself: arterial dissection, perforation, distal embolization, subarachnoid hemorrhage, hemorrhagic infarction, retroperitoneal hematoma, and groin hematoma • Limited efficacy demonstrated in RCT (PROCT II)	• IA fibrinolysis is beneficial for treatment of carefully selected patients with major ischemic strokes of <6 h caused by MCA occlusion who are not otherwise candidates for IV rt-PA *(class I; level of evidence B)* • The optimal dose of IA rt-PA is not well established, and rt-PA does not have FDA approval for IA use.
Combined IV and IAT	• Without delaying initiation therapy vs. IAT • Higher recanalization rate vs. IV rt-PA	• Not FDA approved • No improved outcomes vs. IV rt-PA • Higher hemorrhagic transformation vs. IV rt-PA	
Mechanical clot disruption	• Significant outcomes benefit vs. IV rt-PA alone at up to 6 h from onset of symptoms • Significant recanalization benefit vs. standard IAT	• Not FDA approved • Fewer accessible occlusions than IAT • Significantly increased rate of SICH vs. NINDS placebo but not vs. NINDS IV rt-PA alone • Possible increased risk of distal embolization	

Table 7.2 (continued)

	Advantages	Disadvantages	Guidelines (2013, 2015 AHA/ASA)
Mechanical thrombectomy with Merci retrieval system	• FDA approved • Successful recanalization of MCA, ICA, and BA/VA occlusions • Possible treatment for the patients who excluded from IV rt-PA (e.g., after surgery and increased INR) or who failed to recanalization with IV rt-PA • Possible treatment for the calcified thrombus	• Difficult to reach the thrombus in sclerotic arteries • Broken-off pieces of the thrombus into parts and distal occlusion	• The Merci, Penumbra System, Solitaire FR, and Trevo thrombectomy devices can be useful in achieving recanalization alone or in combination with IV rt-PA in carefully selected patients (class IIa; level of evidence B) • When mechanical thrombectomy is pursued, stent retrievers such as Solitaire FR and Trevo are generally preferred to coil retrievers such as Merci (class I; level of evidence A) • Patients should receive endovascular therapy with a stent retriever if they meet all the following criteria (class I; level of evidence A). (2015): • Pre-stroke mRS score 0 to 1 • AIS receiving IV • rt-PA within 4.5 h of onset • Causative occlusion of the ICA or proximal MCA (M1) • Age ≥ 18 years • NIHSS score of ≥6 • ASPECTS of ≥6 • Treatment can be initiated (groin puncture) within 6 h of onset
Thromboaspiration	• FDA approved • Higher rates of recanalization • Possible lower rate of distal embolization than mechanical thrombectomy or clot disruption	• Unclear outcomes benefit	
Stent retriever	• FDA approved • Clear outcome benefits in RCTs • Successful recanalization of MCA and ICA occlusions	• No data of BA/VA occlusion • Difficult access of tortuous vessel • Poor rate of recanalization of atherosclerotic steno-occlusion	

Abbreviations: *NIHSS* National Institutes of Health Stroke Scale score, *TICI* thrombolysis in cerebral infarction, *TIMI* thrombolysis in myocardial infarction, *mRS* modified Rankin Scale, *SHT* symptomatic hemorrhagic transformation, *RCT* randomized controlled trial, *Pro-UK* pro-urokinase, *IV rt-PA* intravenous recombinant tissue plasminogen activator, *IAT* intra-arterial thrombolysis, *MCA* middle cerebral artery, *VBA* vertebrobasilar artery, cerebral artery

7.4.3 Recent Randomized Controlled Comparison Trials of Endovascular Mechanical Thrombectomy Versus the Standard Medical Care with or Without IV rt-PA (2013–2015)

Three neutral trials of endovascular approaches were published in 2013: a bridging therapy of low-dose IV rt-PA followed by clot retrieval or IA rt-PA versus IV rt-PA alone for stroke (IMS III) [8], direct comparison of IVT versus endovascular treatment for AIS (Systemic Thrombolysis for Acute Ischemic Stroke, SYNTHESIS Expansion), and a trial of imaging selection and endovascular treatment for AIS (The Mechanical Retrieval and Recanalization of Stroke Clots Using Embolectomy, MR RESCUE) [15]. These trials were confounded by a lack of confirmation of large artery occlusion using a noninvasive angiography, a delay of initiating thrombolysis in the IA or bridging group, and use of first-generation devices.

However, the published or presented trials in 2015, including MR CLEAN, ESCAPE, EXTEND-IA, SWIFT PRIME, REVASCAT, THERAPY, and THRACE, have proven the efficacy of endovascular mechanical thrombectomy in AIS caused by occlusion of large artery in anterior circulation. Compared with the earlier three trials, the recently positive clinical trials used the newer-generation stent retriever devices, confirmed a proximal artery occlusion as a target therapy on noninvasive angiography before enrollment, and reduced onset-to-reperfusion time. Thus, these differences raised the rates of successful recanalization and substantially good neurological outcomes in patients treated with the endovascular therapy. In the next chapter (Chap. 8), the results of these recent trials were presented in detail.

Conclusions

Clinical trials have demonstrated a benefit of IAT in the selected AIS patients who present beyond the time window for IV rt-PA, who fail to improve with IV rt-PA, or who do not meet the inclusion criteria for IV rt-PA. The evidence of novel endovascular therapy, especially stent retrievers in AIS, has been proven by recent randomized clinical trials. Stent-based thrombectomy has rapidly affected clinical practice and promises to revolutionize the endovascular treatment of disabling AIS. Much work remains to select appropriate AIS patients for endovascular treatment and to shorten the time to reperfusion in order to result in timely restoration of perfusion of still-salvageable, infarcted brain tissue.

Suggestions from Clinical Practice Guidelines Not applicable to this chapter.

References

1. Nogueira RG, Schwamm LH, Hirsch JA. Endovascular approaches to acute stroke, part 1: drugs, devices, and data. AJNR Am J Neuroradiol. 2009;30:649–61.
2. del Zoppo GJ, Higashida RT, Furlan AJ, et al. PROACT: a phase II randomized trial of recombinant pro-urokinase by direct arterial delivery in acute middle cerebral artery stroke. PROACT investigators. Prolyse in Acute cerebral Thromboembolism. Stroke. 1998;29:4–11.
3. Furlan A, Higashida R, Wechsler L, et al. Intra-arterial prourokinase for acute ischemic stroke: the PROACT II study: a randomized controlled trial. JAMA. 1999;282:2003–11.
4. Ogawa A, Mori E, Minematsu K, et al. Randomized trial of intraarterial infusion of urokinase within 6 hours of middle cerebral artery stroke: the middle cerebral artery embolism local fibrinolytic intervention trial (MELT) Japan. Stroke. 2007;38:2633–9.
5. Lewandowski CA, Frankel M, Tomsick TA, et al. Combined intravenous and intra-arterial r-TPA versus intra-arterial therapy of acute ischemic stroke: Emergency Management of Stroke (EMS) bridging trial. Stroke. 1999;30:2598–605.
6. The IMS Study Investigators. Combined intravenous and intra-arterial recanalization for acute ischemic stroke: the interventional management of stroke study. Stroke. 2004;35:904–11.
7. IMS II Trial Investigators. The interventional Management of Stroke (IMS) II study. Stroke. 2007;38:2127–35.
8. Broderick JP, Palesch YY, Demchuk AM, et al. Endovascular therapy after intravenous t-PA versus t-PA alone for stroke. N Engl J Med. 2013;368: 893–903.
9. Smith WS, Sung G, Starkman S, et al. Safety and efficacy of mechanical embolectomy in acute ischemic stroke: results of the MERCI trial. Stroke. 2005;36:1432–8.
10. Smith WS, Sung G, Saver J, et al. Mechanical thrombectomy for acute ischemic stroke: final results of the multi MERCI trial. Stroke. 2008;39:1205–12.
11. Penumbra Pivotal Stroke Trial Investigators. The penumbra pivotal stroke trial: safety and effectiveness of a new generation of mechanical devices for clot removal in intracranial large vessel occlusive disease. Stroke. 2009;40:2761–8.
12. Levy EI, Siddiqui AH, Crumlish A, et al. First Food and Drug Administration-approved prospective trial of primary intracranial stenting for acute stroke: SARIS (stent-assisted recanalization in acute ischemic stroke). Stroke. 2009;40:3552–6.
13. Saver JL, Jahan R, Levy EI, et al. Solitaire flow restoration device versus the Merci retriever in patients with acute ischaemic stroke (SWIFT): a randomised, parallel-group, non-inferiority trial. Lancet. 2012;380:1241–9.
14. Nogueira RG, Lutsep HL, Gupta R, et al. Trevo versus Merci retrievers for thrombectomy revascularisation of large vessel occlusions in acute ischaemic stroke (TREVO 2): a randomised trial. Lancet. 2012;380:1231–40.
15. Kidwell CS, Jahan R, Gornbein J, et al. A trial of imaging selection and endovascular treatment for ischemic stroke. N Engl J Med. 2013;368:914–23.

Mechanical Thrombectomy: New Era of Stent Retriever

8

Ramana Appireddy, Zarina Assis,
and Mayank Goyal

Abstract

In the previous chapters, the intravenous (IV) as well as intra-arterial (IA) thrombolysis for acute ischemic stroke (AIS) have been discussed. In this chapter, we will move on to discuss mechanical thrombectomy for acute ischemic stroke. Mechanical thrombectomy has been around for over a decade now. There have been tremendous advances in the device technology over this time. We will discuss briefly mechanical thrombectomy and its evolution over the last few years especially in the field of stent technology in mechanical thrombectomy for AIS. We will then briefly discuss the current evidence for mechanical thrombectomy in AIS and then move on to discuss the general principles and the technique and practical considerations of stent retriever thrombectomy. The words "mechanical thrombectomy" and "endovascular thrombectomy" are used interchangeably in this chapter.

Mechanical thrombectomy involves the use of mechanical devices to aid in achieving recanalization of an occluded vessel. The mechanical thrombectomy can be done as a primary or secondary modality of treatment for acute ischemic stroke. Based on the location of the device with respect to thrombus at the time of thrombectomy, they can

R. Appireddy
Department of Medicine, Queen's University/
Kingston General Hospital,
Room # 703, Connel 7, 76 Stuart Street, Kingston,
ON K7L2V7, Canada
e-mail: appiredm@kgh.kari.net

Z. Assis
Diagnostic and Interventional Neuroradiology,
Cumming School of Medicine, University of Calgary,
Foothills Medical Centre,
1403 29th St NW, Calgary, AB T2N 2T9, Canada

M. Goyal, M.D. (✉)
Department of Diagnostic Imaging, Seaman Family
MR Research Centre, Foothills Medical Centre,
1403 29th St NW, Calgary, AB T2N 2T9, Canada
e-mail: mgoyal@ucalgary.ca

S.-H. Lee (ed.), *Stroke Revisited: Diagnosis and Treatment of Ischemic Stroke*,
Stroke Revisited, DOI 10.1007/978-981-10-1424-6_8

be classified into proximal systems (Penumbra, AngioJet), distal systems (MERCI, Catch, Lazarus, etc.), and on the spot systems (stents, stent retrievers).

The chief advantages of mechanical thrombectomy include their ability to achieve faster and more efficient revascularization in addition to having an extended therapeutic time window from symptom onset compared to IV/IA thrombolytics alone. The chief disadvantages of the mechanical thrombectomy include the additional cost of the devices, setup, the need for skilled interventionist and the support staff, and the increased risk of procedural complications like vascular perforation, fragmentation and distal migration of thrombus, etc. In the following sections, we will discuss the evolution of the mechanical thrombectomy for AIS followed by the use of stents during mechanical thrombectomy in AIS.

8.1 Evolution of Mechanical Thrombectomy

The biggest advance in the field of stroke care has been the introduction of IV tissue plasminogen activator (tPA) for AIS in 1995. Since then further advances have been happening in the intra-arterial therapy and mechanical thrombectomy for AIS over the last two decades. Manipulation of the thrombus using a micro guidewire is probably the first form of mechanical thrombectomy.

The evolution of mechanical thrombectomy for AIS can be divided distinctly into three phases based on the treatment strategies (Table 8.1). During the initial years, the device development influenced the treatment approach. A better understanding of the stroke pathophysiology, and the endovascular stroke therapy led to the identification of the best treatment strategy which in turn resulted in further refinement of the device technology culminating in the current generation of stent retriever-based mechanical thrombectomy. This highlights the constant interplay between the understanding of the disease pathophysiology and technological evolution. Over the years multiple devices of varying shapes and sizes, physical properties, and treatment strategies have been introduced. Some of them like MERCI concentric retriever and Penumbra are notable for the important role they played in the advancement of the endovascular thrombectomy and will be briefly discussed below.

The concentric retriever (Concentric Medical, Mountain View, Calif., USA) better known as MERCI retriever is a flexible nitinol wire which takes the shape of a spiral when deployed beyond the thrombus trapping it. Retrieval of the device leads to successful

Table 8.1 Mechanical thrombectomy: phases, principles, and devices

Phase	Strategy	Devices
Phase 1	Thrombectomy + recanalization	Concentric retrieve Penumbra aspiration system Snare
Phase 2	Recanalization only	Balloon-mounted stents Self-expanding unretrievable stents (Wingspan, Enterprise, Neuroform)
Phase 3	Thrombectomy + recanalization	Stent retrievers (Solitaire, Trevo, Retrieve, pREset)

thrombectomy. The rates of recanalization with the concentric retriever varied from 40 to 60% depending on the location of the occlusion as well as the clinical series. After demonstrating success for thrombectomy in the clinical trials (MERCI and Multi MERCI trials), it was approved by the FDA in 2004 for clinical use in acute ischemic stroke.

The Penumbra aspiration system was the second device to obtain FDA approval in 2008 for flow restoration in acute ischemic stroke. The device consists of two components—a mechanical disruptor and an aspiration system. The system works by initial debulking of the thrombus with the continuous aspiration of the thrombus. Penumbra pivotal stroke trial was a prospective, multicenter, single-arm study in which the Penumbra aspiration system achieved around 82% TIMI grade 2–3 recanalization.

Both the concentric retriever and Penumbra aspiration system often have low and variable recanalization rates in routine clinical practice. The rigidity of the systems also affected the ease of navigability and had safety concerns when handling the often delicate cerebral vasculature. However, these systems remained the mainstay of therapy for AIS revascularization for some time. The next era of mechanical thrombectomy had begun with the introduction of stents for the treatment of acute ischemic stroke and will be discussed below.

8.2 Evolution of Stent Technology for Mechanical Thrombectomy

Stents are hollow tubular structures with mesh-like wall usually made of *nitinol (an alloy of nickel and titanium)*. In general, the stents are navigated into an arterial segment of interest under fluoroscopic guidance. The stent is then deployed at the location of interest. As the stent expands, it pushes the thrombus and/or the underlying plaque against the vessel wall, thus trapping the thrombus. The various stents differ based on their physical properties, design, technique of deployment as well as retrievability, and vasculature used. Depending on the method of stent deployment, they are divided into balloon-mounted or self-expanding stents, which will be discussed later on.

8.2.1 Stents Used in Endovascular Stroke Therapy

During the initial few years, the technique of stent-assisted revascularization to manage acute ischemic stroke was directly adopted from cardiology with little modification. Subsequently, with growing experience and better understanding, the stent technology was adopted with some amendments and finally led to the development of dedicated neurovascular stents. In the following section, we will discuss the evolution of stent technology beginning with balloon-mounted stent moving on to self-expanding stents and then to stent retrievers.

Balloon-mounted cardiology stents were first used for revascularization in acute ischemic stroke. The stent was mounted on a balloon which could be expanded to the desired size. Despite the initial encouraging results, it was soon realized that the balloon-mounted stents were not optimal for cerebral vasculature. The degree and pressure of the balloon deployment were the main concerns. Often the lack of adequate information on the vessel diameter can lead to inappropriate over inflation of the balloon with the risk of vascular injury or underinflation resulting in incomplete stent deployment. The pressure of the balloon inflation could lead to arterial rupture or dissection irrespective of the degree of inflation. Other factors like deliverability, trackability, and conformability of the balloon-mounted stent system in the often tortuous cerebral vasculature posed technical challenges and safety concerns.

The next phase started with the development and use of self-expanding stents (SES). These stents were primarily used during treatment of cerebral aneurysms as well as intracranial stenosis.

Many centers used these stents as off-label for revascularization in acute ischemic stroke. The self-expanding stents are sheathed and designed to self-expand to a predetermined size when unsheathed. The ability to self-expand obviated the need for a balloon-assisted expansion and the resulting vascular complications. A microcatheter along with the enclosed stent is positioned just beyond the thrombus location. The stent is then slowly unsheathed allowing for the stent to self-expand and compress the thrombus against the vessel wall resulting in recanalization. Some of the self-expanding stents include *Wingspan* (Stryker, Natick, MA, USA), *Enterprise* (Cordis Neurovascular, Miami Lakes, FL, USA), and *Neuroform system* (Stryker, Natick, MA, USA).

Though the balloon-mounted stents and the self-expanding stents were never FDA approved for mechanical thrombectomy in acute ischemic stroke, they were used off-label for this purpose. Also, both the stents had to be left behind in the cerebral vasculature which needed immediate and long-term antiplatelets to prevent acute as well as in situ stent thrombosis later on. Though this is a standard of care in cardiology with a high safety margin, the use of antithrombotics (antiplatelets/GpIIb/IIIa antagonists) is risky in AIS because of the additional risk of intracerebral hemorrhage when used in conjunction with IV tPA. Also, hemorrhagic transformation of infarct can lead to a worse prognosis in the presence of antithrombotics. The big breakthrough happened when the retrievable stents were introduced which will be discussed below.

An entirely retrievable stent was initially developed as a revascularization device to be used during aneurysmal coiling in 2003. Though the potential utility of these new stent retrievers in mechanical thrombectomy was hinted at, it was not until a few years later when the first successful reports were published. Coupled with suboptimal results using the then approved mechanical thrombectomy devices and the need for more fast and efficient revascularization, the stent retrievers took the center stage for experimentation in mechanical thrombectomy for ischemic stroke opening up an entirely exciting field of stroke therapeutics which led to the innovation and further development of the stent retriever technology and multiple multicenter randomized clinical trials culminating in successful demonstration of an effective endovascular stroke therapy for AIS.

These stent retrievers are similar to the self-expanding stents described earlier with regard to unsheathing and deployment (self-expanding); in addition, they remain attached to a wire at their proximal end and which in some cases could be electrolytically detached. As of 2016, some of the stent retrievers available in the market include *Solitaire FR* (Covidien/Medtronic), *Trevo XP* (Stryker Neurovascular), *REVIVE SE* (Codman Neurovascular), and *pREset & pREset Lite* (Phenox). Though all of them have a similar physical shape, they differ from one another in the cell design, radial force exerted by the stent, orientation of the struts, radiopaqueness, size available, detachability, etc. A detailed description of the individual stents and their properties is beyond the scope of the current chapter, and a few salient features of the stents are provided below (Table 8.2). In Fig. 8.1, an image of the *Trevo stent retriever* is shown demonstrating its use.

Table 8.2 Stent retrievers currently available and their salient features

Stent retriever	Sizes available (mm) (Diameter–stent length)	Features
Solitaire FR	4–15 4–20 6–20 6–30	One proximal marker Three distal markers
Trevo XP ProVue Retriever	3–20 4–20 6–25	Fully radiopaque
REVIVE SE	4.5–22 Single size only	Distal basket closed Distal and proximal radiopaque marker Not available in the USA Permanently attached to proximal wire
pREset	4–20 6–30	Helical-shaped slits Proximal closed-ring design One proximal Two distal markers
pREset Lite	4–20 3–20	

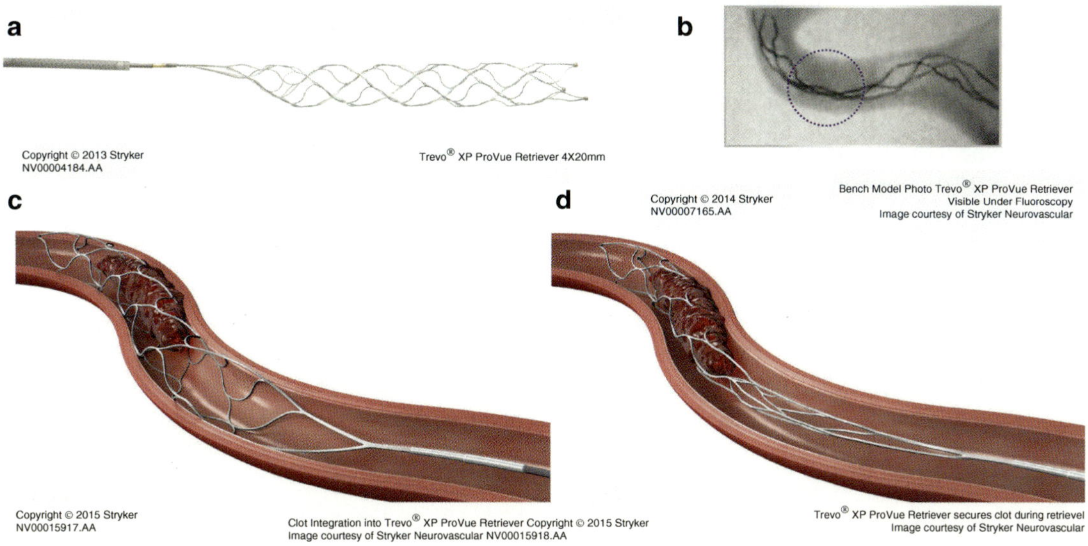

Fig. 8.1 Trevo stent retriever. (**a**) Trevo stent retriever, (**b**) radiopaque design of the Trevo stent retriever, (**c**) Trevo stent retriever deployed at the location of the thrombus, and (**d**) Trevo stent retriever trapping the thrombus as it is being retrieved. Reproduced by permission of Stryker Inc.

8.3 Current Evidence on Stent Retrievers

8.3.1 Initial Evidence on Stent Retrievers

The first reported use of the Solitaire AB (aneurysmal bridging) stent retriever for ischemic stroke was in 2009 when it was successfully used for mechanical thrombectomy of a middle cerebral artery M1 segment occlusion after a failed attempt with the MERCI retriever. This was soon followed by multiple case series (involving approximately 280 patients) reporting the use of Solitaire AB stent retriever for mechanical thrombectomy. In these case series, the Solitaire stent retriever was used both as a primary device and the rescue treatment when other modalities like IV tPA and/or mechanical thrombectomy using other devices failed.

Simultaneously, another stent retriever, Trevo (Stryker Neurovascular), was developed for the treatment of mechanical thrombectomy in acute ischemic stroke. After initial animal studies which showed safety and efficacy, a small case series and the Trevo study showed the feasibility, safety, and utility of the Trevo stent retriever in mechanical thrombectomy of acute ischemic stroke.

These initial encouraging results, the suboptimal performance of the then existent mechanical thrombectomy devices, led to the first-generation randomized clinical trials of the stent retrievers against the MERCI concentric retriever—SWIFT and TREVO2 which will be discussed below.

SWIFT was a randomized, parallel group noninferiority trial in which 113 patients with moderate to severe ischemic stroke were randomized to the Solitaire FR (flow restoration) stent retriever (n = 58) or MERCI retriever (n = 55) [1]. The trial recruitment was halted by DSMB after an interim efficacy analysis during which the pre-specified criteria for trial termination were met. The primary end point of successful recanalization (with the assigned study device and not needing rescue treatment) without symptomatic intracranial hemorrhage occurred in 61% with Solitaire FR stent retriever compared to 24% with MERCI retriever. Core lab-assessed rates of angiographic recanalization with Solitaire FR stent retriever was 69% compared to 30% with the MERCI retriever. The need for rescue treatment was also lower in the Solitaire FR group (21%) compared to the MERCI retriever (44%). Good neurological outcome at 90 days (modified Rankin scale of 2 or less, NIHSS score improvement of 10 points) was seen in 58% with Solitaire FR stent retriever compared to 33% with MERCI retriever. The safety end points (study device related, symptomatic ICH, death from any cause at 90 days) were also lower in the Solitaire FR group (9%, 2%, 17%, respectively) compared to the MERCI retriever (16%, 11%, 38%, respectively).

TREVO2 was also an open-label randomized non-inferiority trial in which 178 patients were randomized to the Trevo retriever (n = 88) or MERCI retriever (n = 90) [2]. The primary efficacy end point of TICI $\geq$ 2 reperfusion (using assigned device—as determined by core lab) was 86% with the Trevo retriever compared to 60% with the MERCI retriever. There was a non-statistically significant difference in the need for rescue therapy in the Trevo retriever compared to the MERCI retriever (18% vs. 31%, $p = 0.0851$). Good clinical outcome at 90 days (mRS 0–2) is seen in 40% with Trevo retriever and 22% with MERCI retriever. Despite meeting some of the efficacy end point, the composite safety primary end point and mortality at 90 days were not statistically different between Trevo retriever and MERCI retriever (15% vs. 23%, $p = 0.18$ and 22% vs. 24%, $p = 0.18$, respectively).

Following these trails, FDA approved both the stent retrievers for mechanical thrombectomy in acute ischemic stroke in 2012. The three major randomized trials (IMS III, SYNTHESIS, and MR RESCUE) that were finished in 2012 failed to show the expected superiority of the endovascular stroke therapy compared to intravenous thrombolysis with tPA alone. In addition to other reasons, the use of older generation devices with their drawbacks and very limited use of these novel stent retrievers in these trials contributed to the negative trial results. With a better understanding of the reasons for failure and availability of technologically advanced mechanical thrombectomy devices, researchers around the world embarked on multiple randomized controlled trials pitting the endovascular stroke therapy (predominantly using the novel stent retrievers) against standard IV thrombolysis using tPA which will be discussed below.

8.3.2 Recent Randomized Controlled Trials

The role of stent retrievers in achieving high rates of recanalization with speed and safety has been demonstrated in five recent endovascular trials—MR CLEAN, ESCAPE, SWIFT PRIME, EXTEND-IA, and REVASCAT [3–7]. MR CLEAN is the first trial to have successfully shown the superiority of the endovascular treatment, the results of which were presented at the World Stroke Congress in October 2014. Following the release of the MR CLEAN trial results, two of the other trials ESCAPE and EXTEND-IA temporarily withheld the trial recruitment and planned interim analysis. SWIFT PRIME followed suit after a few days. The trial results of ESCAPE, SWIFT PRIME, and EXTEND-IA were subsequently presented at the International Stroke Conference in February 2015 followed by the release of the results of REVASCAT trial a few months later. The overwhelming positivity of all the five trials, consistent results across trials in various health systems across the globe, led to a long overdue paradigm shift in stroke care. We will discuss individual trials followed by pooled analysis of patient-level data from all the five trials.

8.3.3 MR CLEAN

Multicenter randomized clinical trial of endovascular treatment for acute ischemic stroke in the Netherlands (MR CLEAN) was a multicenter prospective randomized open-label blinded end point evaluation clinical trial run at 17 centers in the Netherlands comparing intra-arterial treatment versus no intra-arterial treatment for acute ischemic stroke [3]. The trial design was pragmatic and closely resembles the routine clinical practice. The investigators sought out to explore if any form of intra-arterial therapy (IAT) was superior to usual care (control, including the use of IV tPA) in acute ischemic stroke with proximal anterior circulation occlusion. All modalities of intra-arterial treatment (thrombolysis using tPA, urokinase, MERCI retriever, Penumbra aspiration system, sonolysis, stent retrievers) were approved to be used in the trial, and there was no restriction on the use of multiple modalities for a patient in whom one modality fails. Also, the need for performance of an acute cervical carotid stenting during thrombectomy was left to the discretion of the local interventionist. Patients were eligible to be randomized into the trial irrespective of their status with regard to eligibility, contraindications, treatment status, and response to IV tPA. The trial enrolled 500 patients with 233 (46.4%) randomized to the intra-arterial treatment. Despite approval of a broad range of the IA treatment modalities, 81.5% (190/233) of the patients in the trial were treated with stent retrievers. The exclusive use of other modalities like IA thrombolysis (1/233), MERCI retriever (2/233), and thromboaspiration (1/233) was very limited. The use of IV tPA was comparable across the intervention (87.1%) and control groups (90.6%). 90-day median mRS was chosen as the primary outcome for the trial which was lower in the intervention group with an adjusted common odds ratio of 1.67. Shift analysis of the mRS scores also favored the intervention for mRS groups 0–5; there was, however, no mortality benefit between both the groups. All the clinical and imaging secondary outcomes also favored the intervention group. Despite minor limitations of the trial, MR CLEAN trial results closely resemble the complex situations seen in routine clinical practice, thus increasing the generalizability of the trial results. The trial design, baseline demographic characteristics, imaging features and time metrics, and the trial results are presented in Tables 8.3, 8.4, 8.5 and 8.6, respectively.

8.3.4 ESCAPE

Endovascular treatment for small core and anterior circulation proximal occlusion with emphasis on minimizing CT to recanalization times (ESCAPE) was a prospective, multicenter randomized, open-label, controlled trial with blinded outcome evaluation [4]. The trial was run worldwide at 22 centers, predominantly in Canada. The trial recruitment was kept on hold after the results of the MR CLEAN trial were released. The data safety monitoring board advised the trial to be stopped due to efficacy after the unplanned interim analysis. At that point, the trial had enrolled 316 patients out of an initial target sample size of 500. The trial compared the endovascular treatment along with the usual standard of care (intervention) with the usual standard of care alone (control) in acute ischemic stroke patients older than 18 years with an NIHSS > 5 and an occlusion in the proximal anterior circulation and small ischemic core and large penumbra. Though the use of any mechanical thrombectomy devices as per local site availability was allowed, the emphasis was placed on the use of retrievable stents by the trial investigators. Similar to the MR CLEAN trial, patients were eligible to participate in the trial irrespective of their eligibility or treatment status with respect to IV tPA. Some of the unique features of the trial included the extended time window, emphasis on patient selection, and workflow during the trial execution. Patients were eligible to be enrolled up to 12 h from symptom onset. There was a trend toward a better outcome in the patients enrolled beyond 6 h from symptom onset. However, the numbers were not sufficient to achieve statistical significance. The trial investigators aimed to select patients with good premorbid function coming in with an acute moderate-severe disabling ischemic stroke with demonstrable occlusion in the proximal anterior circulation with a small ischemic core and ability to initiate rapid endovascular treatment after stroke imaging. To achieve this goal, patients were carefully selected using various clinical (modified Barthel index) and imaging tools (CT

Table 8.3 Design features of the five clinical trials of endovascular stroke therapy

	MR CLEAN	ESCAPE	SWIFT PRIME	REVASCAT	EXTEND-IA
Design feature					
Age range (years)	≥18	≥18	≥18–85	≥18–85[a]	≥18
Time window (h)[b]	6	12	6	8	6
NIHSS eligibility	≥2	≥6	≥8 and <30	≥6	None
Premorbid functional status	None	mBI > 90	mRS ≤ 1	mRS ≤ 1	mRS ≤ 1
Imaging modalities					
Parenchymal imaging	NCCT or MRI	NCCT or MRI MRI discouraged	NCCT or MRI	NCCT or MRI	NCCT/MRI
Vascular imaging	CTA or MRA or DSA	CTA	CTA or MRA	CTA or MRA	CTA/MRA
Perfusion imaging	None	CTP	CTP or MRI-PWI	None	CTP or MRI-PWI
Imaging eligibility criteria					
Parenchymal non-contrast	None	ASPECTS ≥ 6	ASPECTS ≥ 6	CT ASPECTS ≥ 7 or MRI ASPECTS ≥ 6	None
Vascular occlusion	• Distal ICA • MCA M1/M2 • ACA A1	• Carotid T/L • MCA M1 • MCA–2/more M2s • Moderate to good collaterals	• Intracranial ICA • MCA M1	• Distal ICA • MCA M1 • Tandem (proximal ICA + M1)	• ICA • MCA M1or M2
Treatments					
Control arm	SOC ± IV tPA	SOC ± IV tPA	SOC + IV tPA in all	SOC ± IV tPA	SOC + IV tPA in all
Intervention arm	SOC ± IV tPA + IAT *IAT—IA thrombolysis ± Mechanical thrombectomy (aspiration, retraction, stent retrieval, wire disruption)*	SOC ± IV tPA + mechanical thrombectomy using available and approved device. *Solitaire stent retriever was recommended*	SOC + IV tPA + mechanical thrombectomy using Solitaire stent retriever only	SOC ± IV tPA + mechanical thrombectomy using Solitaire stent retriever only	SOC + IV tPA + mechanical thrombectomy using Solitaire stent retriever only

SOC standard of care, *IAT* intra-arterial therapy, *IV tPA* intravenous tissue plasminogen activator, *ICA* internal carotid artery, *MCA* middle cerebral artery, *M1* first segment of MCA, *M2* second segment of MCA, *ACA* anterior cerebral artery, *mBI* modified Barthel index, *mRS* modified Rankin scale, *CTA* CT angiography, *MRA* MR angiography, *DSA* digital subtraction angiography, *NCCT* non-contrast CT, *MRI* magnetic resonance imaging, *CTP* CT perfusion, *MRI-PWI* MRI perfusion-weighted imaging, *ASPECTS* Alberta stroke program early CT score

[a]The upper age limit was 80 initially and later expanded up to 85 with an ASPECTS cutoff of 8

[b]The time from onset of symptoms to start of the endovascular therapy

ASPECTS scoring, CT angiography, multiphase CT angiography, CT perfusion). A lot of emphases was placed on achieving target metrics during the patient care workflow during the trial recruitment and execution. The investigators adopted target metrics of 60 min for study CT-to-groin puncture and 90 min for study CT-to-first reperfusion to be achieved for the patients enrolled in the trial. Constant weekly monitoring of the quality of the participant recruitment and workflow metrics at individual sites during trial recruitment was done, and appropriate feedback was provided to the individual sites. The investigators emphasized the role of parallel processing of the clinical and imaging information as well as parallel decision making with the goal to achieve the fastest reperfusion by the endovascular route. The above mentioned components of the ESCAPE trial design were crucial to its success. The trial design, baseline demographic characteristics, imaging features and time metrics, and the trial results are presented in Tables 8.3, 8.4, 8.5 and 8.6 respectively.

8.3.5 SWIFT PRIME

Solitaire with the intention for thrombectomy as primary endovascular treatment (SWIFT PRIME) trial was an international multicenter, prospective, randomized, open-label, blinded end point evaluation trial that was run in 39 centers across the USA and Europe [5]. The trial compared the combined use of endovascular thrombectomy using Solitaire stent retriever and IV tPA (intervention) versus IV tPA alone (control) in AIS patients (18–85 years) with a moderate to severe stroke (NIHSS ≥ 8) and intracranial ICA and/or MCA occlusion with a target mismatch penumbral pattern who received tPA within 6 h of onset

Table 8.4 Baseline demographic characteristics of the population in the five clinical trials of endovascular stroke therapy

	MR CLEAN		ESCAPE		SWIFT PRIME		REVASCAT		EXTEND-IA	
Character	Active	Control	Active	Control	Active	Control	Active	Control	Active	Control
Number randomized	233	267	165	150	98	98	103	103	35	35
Number treated			151 (91.5%)		87	98	98		27[a]	35
Age	65.8[b]	65.7[b]	71[b]	70[b]	65.0[c]	66.3[c]	65.7 ± 11.3[c]	67.2 ± 9.5[c]	68.6 ± 12.3[c]	70.2 ± 11.8[c]
Male sex %	57.9	58.8	47.9	47.3	55	47	53.4	52.4	49	49
NIHSS median (IQR)	17 (14–21)	18 (14–22)	16 (13–20)	17 (12–20)	17	17	17	17	17 (13–20)	13 (9–19)
NIHSS range	3–30	4–38			13–20	13–19				
IV tPA (%)	87.1	90.6	72.7	78.7	100	100	68	78	100	100
AFib (%)	28.3	25.8	37	40	36	39	34.0	35.9	34	31
Diabetes (%)	14.6	12.7	20	26	12	15	21.4	18.4	6	23
Past stroke (%)	12.4	9.4	10.3	11.3	3.1	1.0	12	18		
HTN (%)	42.1	48.3	63.6	72	67	58	60.2	69.9	60	66

NA not available

[a]2/35 did not receive angiogram and in 6/33 *Solitaire* stent was not deployed

[b]Median

[c]Mean ± SD

Table 8.5 Baseline imaging characteristics and time metrics of the five clinical trials of endovascular stroke therapy

	MR CLEAN		ESCAPE		SWIFT PRIME		REVASCAT		EXTEND-IA	
Character	Active	Control	Active	Control	Active	Control	Active	Control	Active	Control
Imaging										
ASPECTS (median)	9	9	9	9	9	9	7	8		
ASPECTS (IQR)	7–10	8–10	8–10	8–10	7–10	8–10	6–9	6–9		
Location of occlusion (%)[a]										
Intracranial ICA	0.4	1.1			18	16	0	1		
Extracranial/cervical ICA	32.3	26.3	12.7	12.7			18.6	12.9	31[b]	31[b]
ICA with M1	25.3	28.2	27.6	26.5			25.5	26.7		
M1	66.1	62	68.1	71.4	67	77	64.7	64.4	57	51
M2 only	7.7	7.9	3.7	2.0	14	6	9.8	7.9	11	17
A1/A2	0.4	0.8								
Ischemic core volume at baseline (ml)[c]	NR	NR	NR	NR					18.9 ± 18.5	19.6 ± 17.4
Perfusion lesion volume (ml)[d]	NR	NR	NR	NR					105 ± 39	116 ± 48
General anesthesia (%)	37.8		9.1		37%		6.8		36%	
Time metrics (median minutes)										
Onset to randomization	204	196	169	172	190.5	188	223	226		
Onset to randomization (<3 h)%	NR	NR	53.3%	52.0%			31.1	30.1		
IV tPA to randomization	NR	NR	24	20.5					29	36
Onset to study CT			134	136			192[e]	183[e]		
Onset to IV tPA	85	87	110	125	110.5	117	117.5	105.0	127	145
Study CT-to-groin puncture			51		57		67		93	
Study CT-to-first reperfusion			84							
Stroke onset to reperfusion			241[f]		252[g]	NA	355		248[h]	
Stroke onset to groin puncture	260	–			224	NA	269		210	
Groin puncture to reperfusion			30[f]		24[g]		59		43[h]	
Door t IV tPA									43	46
IV tPA to groin puncture			50.5		77				74	
ED door to groin puncture					90		109		113	
Use of retrievable stents	81.5%		86.1%		100%				100%	100%

[a]The classification of vascular occlusion varied from trial to trial. Hence multiple groups are mentioned and the results provided as per the trial results
[b]Does not specify the exact location of the internal carotid artery
[c]Ischemic core was defined as cerebral blood flow of less than 30% of that in normal tissue
[d]Perfusion lesion was defined as one with a time to maximum (Tmax) delay of more than 6 s on CT perfusion imaging
[e]Corresponds to the imaging performed before randomization at least 30 min after the initiation of IV tPA (in patients in whom the drug was administered)
[f]First reperfusion
[g]First deployment of stent retriever
[h]TICI2b or 3 or completion of procedure

Table 8.6 Results of efficacy and safety of the five clinical trials of endovascular stroke therapy

	MR CLEAN		ESCAPE		SWIFT PRIME		REVASCAT		EXTEND-IA	
Character	Active	Control	Active	Control	Active	Control	Active	Control	Active	Control
Efficacy										
mRS score at 90 days (median)	3	4			2	3			1	3
Odds of mRS (0–2) with intervention	1.67[a]		3.1		[a]		1.7[a]		4.2[b]	
mRS (0–1) at 90 days (%)	11.6	6.0							51%	29%
mRS (0–2) at 90 days (%)	32.6	19.1	53	29.3	60	35	43.7	28.2	71	40
NIHSS (24 h) (median)	13	16	6	13						
NIHSS (90 day) (median)			2	8	1	5	2	6		
Early neurological improvement									80%	37%
mTICI 2b or 3 at final angiography	58.7%		72.4%		88%		65.7		86%	
mAOL score 2–3 at 24 h (%)	84.0	57.5	NA	31.2%						
Reperfusion at 24 h[c] (%)	75.4	32.9							100%	37%
Complete recanalization at 24 h	75.4	32.9			83[d]	40[d]			94%	43%
Safety										
Death (7 days) %	11.6	12.4					9.7	4.9		
Death (30 days) %	18.9	18.4								
Death (90 days) %	NR	NR	10.4	19	9	12	18.4	15.5	8.6	20
Any serious adverse events	47.2	42.3	21.7	18.1	36	31				
Symptomatic ICH										
• Any %	7.7	6.4	3.6	2.7	0	3	1.9[f]	1.9[f]	0	5.7
• PH1%	0	0.7	3.0	2.0	4	3	2.9	3.9		
• PH2%	6	5.2	2.4	2.0	1	4	2.9	1.9		
New stroke in a different territory %	5.6	0.4								
Embolization into another vascular territory[g] (%)	8.6						4.9		5.7%	

(continued)

Table 8.6 (continued)

	MR CLEAN		ESCAPE		SWIFT PRIME		REVASCAT		EXTEND-IA	
Character	Active	Control	Active	Control	Active	Control	Active	Control	Active	Control
Vascular dissections (%)	1.7		0.6				3.9			
Vascular perforation (%)	0.9		0.6		2.3[h]		4.9			

mAOL modified arterial occlusive lesion, *TICI* thrombolysis in cerebral infarction, *CTA* CT angiography, *NR* not reported
[a]Adjusted common odds ratio
[b]Adjusted odds ratio
[c]24 h CTA recanalization data was available in 394 of the 500 patients
[d]NIHSS at 27 h
[e]Based on SITS-MOST criteria
[f]Neither patient had clinical symptoms as a result
[g]2 patients of 87 treated had SAH and contrast extravasation. They had resolved without any sequelae

of stroke. As per initial trial design and protocol, perfusion imaging was used to identify the target mismatch penumbral pattern. This was done by the RAPID software which was an automated operator independent post-processing system. Criteria were defined to identify the core infarct, severe hypoperfusion, and ischemic penumbra. After enrolling 71 patients, the imaging criteria for moderate-to-large core were modified to be able to exclude patients with an ASPECTS score of <6 on NCCT or DWI-MRI alone without the need for perfusion imaging. This was chiefly done to simplify as well as increase the recruitment at centers not familiar with perfusion imaging.

Similar to EXTEND-IA and REVASCAT trials discussed, later on, the *Solitaire* stent retriever was exclusively used, and all patients had to be treated with IV tPA. However, there was no need to wait for a response to IV tPA. Similar to the emphasis on workflow metrics of the ESCAPE trial, the investigators targeted a time of 90 min for the picture (CTA/MRA) to groin puncture time. Also, the patients had to be treated with endovascular therapy within 6 h of onset. Patients with evidence of carotid dissection or complete occlusion of the carotid artery were excluded in the trial. similarly, patients with evidence of preexisting carotid pathology that precludes safe delivery, deployment and retrieval of the stent retriever were excluded from being enrolled in the trial. The trial design, baseline demographic characteristics, imaging features and time metrics, and the trial results are presented in Tables 8.3, 8.4, 8.5 and 8.6 respectively.

8.3.6 EXTEND-IA

Extending the time for thrombolysis in emergency neurological deficits with intra-arterial therapy (EXTEND-IA) was a multicenter, prospective, randomized, open-label, blinded end point study run in 14 centers in Australia and New Zealand [6]. It was a small phase 2b trial that enrolled 70 patients of the 100 initially planned. Similar to the ESCAPE trial, its recruitment was withheld for interim analysis following the announcement of MR CLEAN results. The trial tested if early endovascular thrombectomy using Solitaire FR stent retriever along with IV tPA (intervention) was superior to IV tPA alone (control) for AIS patients with proximal anterior circulation occlusion and salvageable brain tissue on perfusion imaging within 4.5 h after onset of symptoms. Similar to the SWIFT PRIME and REVASCAT (discussed below), all patients needed to be treated with IV tPA, and Solitaire stent retriever was exclusively used for the mechanical thrombectomy. All the patients had to have a groin puncture within 6 h from the onset, and thrombectomy had to be completed within 8 h from onset of stroke. Certain features that distinguish EXTEND-IA from the other trials include the compulsory use of perfusion imaging to select patients, assessment of reperfusion using CT/MRI at 24 h, and early neurological improvement measures at day 3 as co-primary clinical outcomes. The trial investigators chose CT/MRI for the perfusion imaging-based selection. However, the CT imaging was exclusively used for all the patients during the actual enrollment. Automated processing of perfusion imaging data (CT/MRI) was done using RAPID software. Time to maximum (Tmax) of more than 6 s and relative cerebral blood flow (CBF) of <30% of the normal tissue was used to identify the ischemic penumbra and core respectively on perfusion imaging. The reperfusion was defined as the percentage reduction in the perfusion lesion volume between first imaging and imaging at 24 h, and early neurologic improvement was defined as a decrease of 8 points or more on the NIHSS or a score of 0 or 1 at 3 days. The proportion of patients achieving independent mRS (score 0–2) is highest in this trial (71%) compared to other trials. The selection of patients in the earliest time window could have contributed to these results, again highlighting the role of treating patients in the shortest time windows. The trial used a novel metric called "median home time" which is defined as the number of days spent at home during the first 90 days after the diagnosis of stroke. The median home time adjusted for the NIHSS score and age at the baseline was 73 and 15 days for the intervention and control arm, respectively. Complications specifically related to the use of the stent retriever were not observed during the trial. There was no mortality difference between the groups. Though the use of perfusion imaging helps in the better patient selection, the variable nature of the imaging depending on the vendor and the lack of consensus on the most appropriate perfusion imaging parameter to predict penumbra and core have to be considered. Other notable limitations include the smaller sample size in this trial. The trial design, baseline demographic characteristics, imaging features and time metrics, and the trial results are presented in Tables 8.3, 8.4, 8.5 and 8.6 respectively.

8.3.7 REVASCAT

Randomized trial of revascularization with Solitaire FR device versus best medical therapy in the treatment of acute stroke due to anterior circulation large vessel occlusion presenting within 8 h of symptom onset (REVASCAT) was a multicenter, prospective, randomized, sequential, open-label phase 3 study with blinded evaluation [7]. It was run in 4 centers in Catalonia, Spain, and enrolled 206 patients in total. The trial was also terminated midway due to loss of equipoise following the results of four trials mentioned above. The trial tested if endovascular thrombectomy using the *Solitaire* stent retriever with usual care (with or without IV tPA) was superior to usual care (with or without IV tPA) for AIS patients >18 years, NIHSS >6, and target occlusion.

A distinguishing feature of the trial design includes the requirement to wait for an angiographic response to IV tPA. As per the trial protocol, IV tPA eligible patients had to show a qualifying occlusion by CTA/MRA after 30 min of tPA infusion. This would have helped partially in selecting the patients with refractory clots. However, the shorter window of 30 min would not have been sufficient to choose a genuinely IV tPA refractory patients. Moreover, this approach might lead to additional delays in the patient care pathway which is evident by the longer door to reperfusion times in the trial results. Also, because of exclusion of the patients with IV tPA responsive thrombi, the proportion of patients with TICI 2b-3 reperfusion were smaller compared to the other trials. Similar to SWIFT PRIME, only patients with high-functioning baseline (mRS $\leq$ 1) were eligible to participate in the trial. Both the intervention and control arms had most patients with very high-functioning baseline (mRS = 0) with 83.5% and 80.6%, respectively. In addition, the trial did not allow for any other rescue intra-arterial therapy, and a maximum of 6 passes of the stent retriever was allowed. The trial design, baseline demographic characteristics, imaging features and time metrics, and the trial results are presented in Tables 8.3, 8.4, 8.5 and 8.6 respectively.

8.3.8 HERMES Collaboration

Highly effective reperfusion evaluated in multiple endovascular stroke trials (HERMES) collaboration is a collaborative group formed to assess patient-level data from all the five abovementioned randomized controlled trials (MR CLEAN, ESCAPE, SWIFT PRIME, EXTEND-IA, REVASCAT) [8]. The analysis of individual patient-level data across these trials makes for a valid assessment. There are also many similarities in between these trials. These include the emphasis placed on faster treatment, use of imaging-based criteria to select patients, exclusive or predominant use of stent retrievers with high recanalization rates, and lower complications. All the trials also tested the endovascular therapy (with or without standard care) against standard care alone.

The pooling of patient-level data of 1287 patients (634 in the endovascular thrombectomy arm and 653 in the control arm) showed that for the pre-specified primary outcome of mRS at 90 days, the adjusted common odds ratio (acOR) was 2.49 (95% CI 1.76–3.53) for improvement of 1 point on the mRS with endovascular therapy (Fig. 8.2). The number needed to treat for at least 1 patient to have a 1 point reduction of the mRS score was 2.6. All the pre-specified secondary efficacy outcomes were higher in the endovascular therapy group (mRS of 0–1 at 90 days-acOR = 2.72, mRS score 0–2 at 90 days-acOR = 2.71, NIHSS score 0–2 at 24 h-acOR = 3.77, early neurological recovery

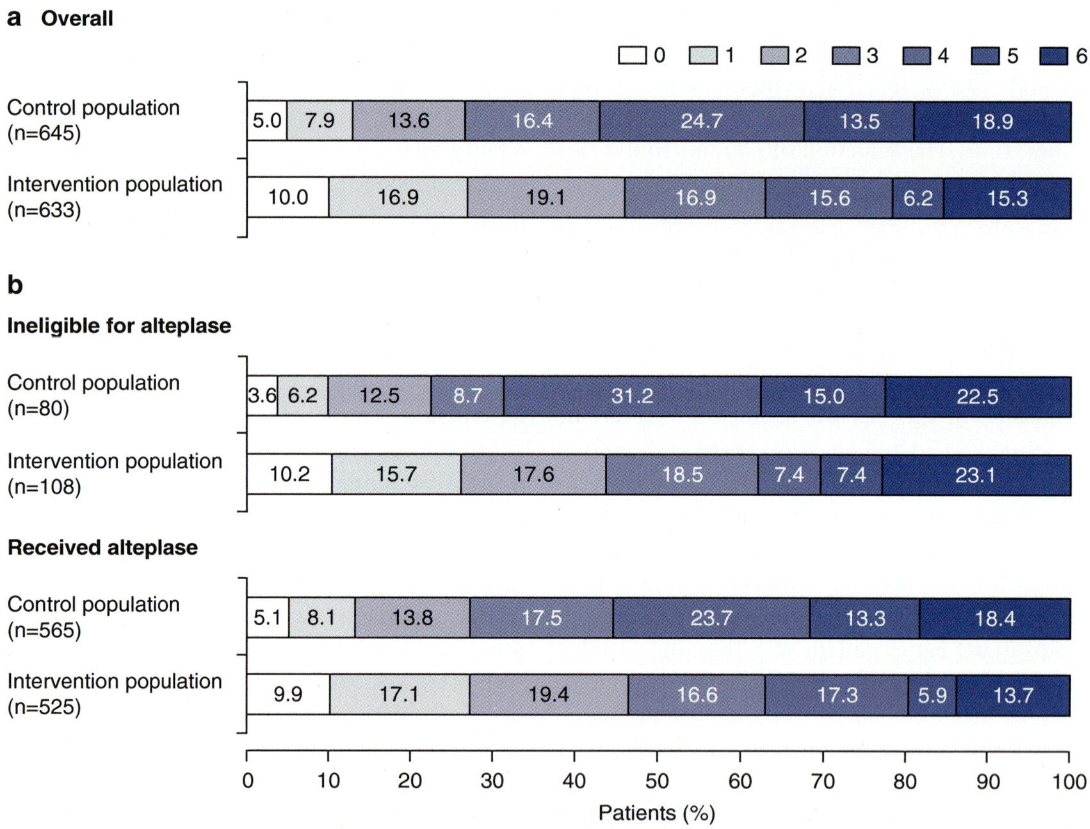

Fig. 8.2 Distribution of 90 day modified Ranking Scale score in the control and intervention arms in the HERMES pooled analysis (**a**) Distribution of score at 90 days in the intervention and control groups in the overall trial population. (**b**) Distribution of scores at 90 days in the intervention and control groups for patients treated with or ineligible for IV tPA. Reproduced by permission of Lancet [8]

at 24 h-acOR = 4.36). The mortality at 90 days and risk of parenchymal hematoma type 2 and symptomatic intracranial hemorrhage were similar between both the groups. The data showed benefit of endovascular therapy for mRS distribution shift at 90 days across all the pre-specified variables like age, sex, baseline NIHSS, location of vascular occlusion, and eligibility/treatment status with respect to IV tPA, ASPECTS score, and time from onset to randomization. The beneficial effect of endovascular therapy was also seen in elderly patients (>80 years), patients randomized after 5 h from onset, as well as those not receiving IV tPA (Fig. 8.3). The baseline demographic characteristics and results of the individual patient-level pooled analysis are presented in Tables 8.7 and 8.8 respectively

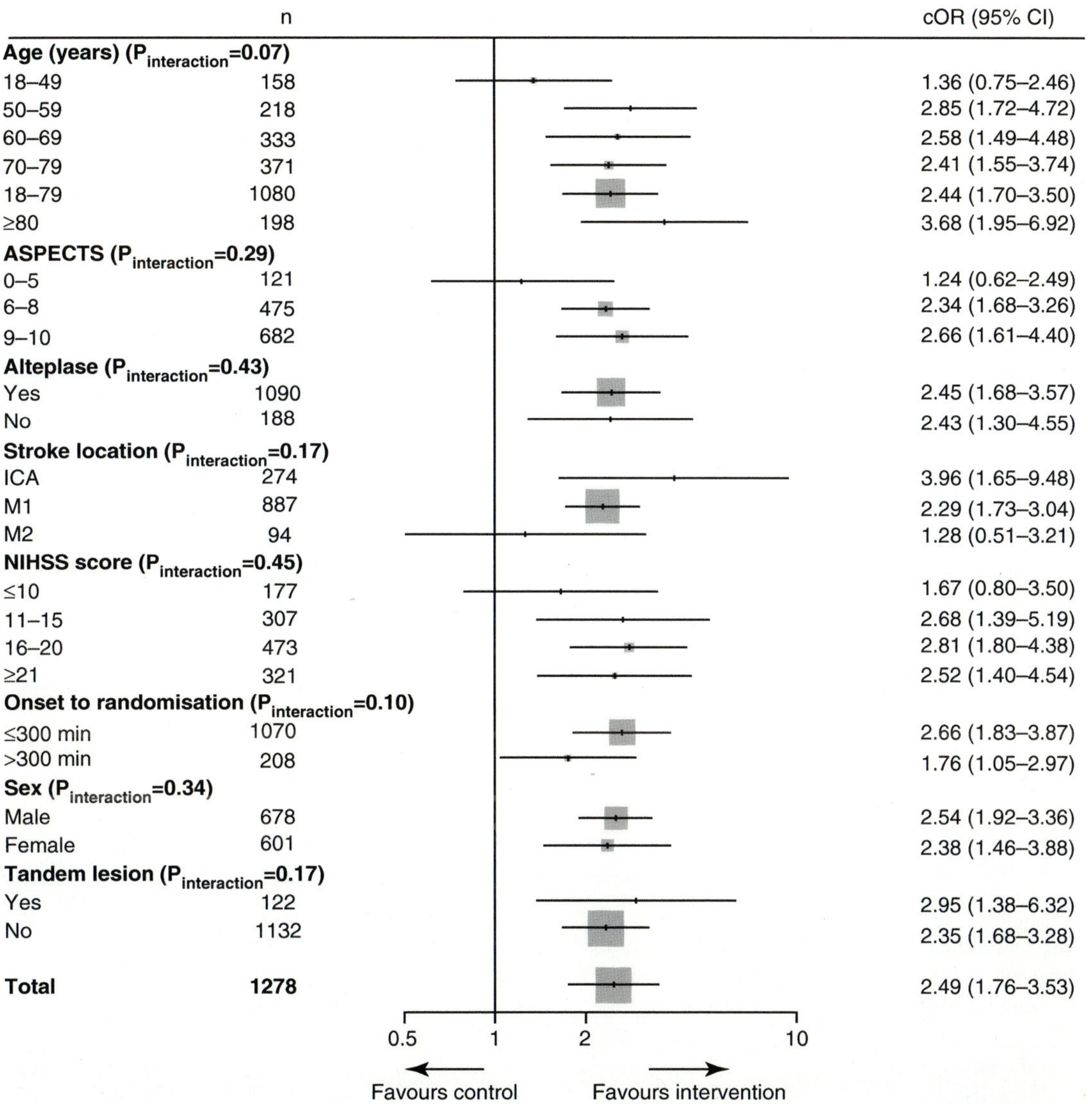

Fig. 8.3 Forest plot showing adjusted treatment effect for mRS at 90 days in pre-specified subgroups with *p* values for heterogeneity across subgroups. *cOR* common odds ratio, *mRS* modified Rankin scale, *ASPECTS* Alberta stroke program early CT score, *ICA* internal carotid artery, *M1* M1 segment of middle cerebral artery, *M2* M2 segment of middle cerebral artery, *NIHSS* National Institutes of Health Stroke Scale. Reproduced by permission of Lancet [8]

Table 8.7 Baseline demographic characteristics of the individual patient level meta-analysis by the HERMES collaboration

	Intervention (endovascular ± standard care) (*n* = 634)	Control (standard care alone) (*n* = 653)
Demographic and clinical features		
Median age (years)	68 (57–77)	68 (59–76)
Male (%)	52%	54%
Hypertension	56%	59%
Atrial fibrillation	33%	33%
Smoking (recent/current)	31%	32%
Baseline NIHSS (range)	17 (14–20)	17 (13–21)
Baseline imaging		
Baseline ASPECTS	9 (7–10)	9 (8–10)
Location of occlusion		
ICA	21%	22%
M1 MCA	69%	69%
M2 MCA	8%	7%
Other	2%	2%
Treatment		
IV tPA	83%	87%
IV tPA within 180 mins	70%	71%
Time metrics (min)		
Onset to randomization	195.5	196
Onset to IV tPA	100	100
Onset to reperfusion	285	NA

Standard care—standard care is usually medical care ± IV tPA

Table 8.8 Safety and efficacy results of the individual patient level meta-analysis of the HERMES collaboration

	Intervention	Control	Odds ratio (95%CI)[ab]	Adjusted odds ratio (95%CI)[ab]
Efficacy				
mRS score reduction (shift analysis, primary outcome)			2.26 (1.67 to 3.06)	2.49 (1.76 to 3.53)
mRS score 0–1 at 90 days	26.9%	12.9%	2.49 (184 to 3.35) $p < 0.0001$	2.71 (1.99 to 3.71)
mRS score 0–2 at 90 days	46%	26.5%	2.35 (1.85 to 2.98)	2.71 (2.07 to 3.55)
NIHSS score 0–2 at 24 h	21%	8.3%	2.66 (2.06 to 4.12)	3.77 (2.49 to 5.71)
NIHSS at 24 h (mean score)	10.4 (8.7)[c]	14.2 (7.8)[c]		
NIHSS at 24 h (median score)	8 (3 to 16)	15 (9 to 19)		
Change in NIHSS from baseline to 24 h (mean change)	−6.4 (8.2)[d]	−2.6 (6.6)[d]		
Change in NIHSS from baseline to 24 h (median change)	−7 (−12 to −1)	−2 (−6 to 1)		
Safety				
Symptomatic ICH[e]	4.4%	4.3%	1.07 (0.62 to 1.83)[f]	1.07 90.62 to 1.84)[f]
PH type 2[e]	5.1%	5.3%	0.99 (0.60 to 1.63)[f]	1.04 (0.63 to 1.72)[f]
Mortality[e]	15.3%	18.9%	0.77 (0.54 to 1.10)[f]	0.73 (0.47 to 1.13)[f]

mRS modified Rankin scale, *NIHSS* National Institute of Health Stroke Scale
[a]Common odds ratio indicating the odds of improvement of 1 point on the mRS
[b]$p < 0.0001$
[c]Adjusted beta coefficient is 3.8 with a $p < 0.0001$
[d]Adjusted beta coefficient is 3.9 with a $p < 0.0001$
[e]Statistically no difference in the "risk difference," "rate ratio," "odds ratio," and "adjusted odds ratio" between both the groups
[f]$p > 0.05$—not statistically significant

8.4 Translating the Evidence into Standard of Care

Endovascular stroke therapy needs a collaborative endeavor from various health-care professionals, administrators, and other involved members to be effective in replicating the results of the clinical trials. The three key components for successful endovascular stroke therapy are appropriate patient selection, optimized endovascular workflow, and efficient endovascular setup to achieve fast reperfusion. Also, other important factors like prehospital stroke triaging, transport, and the role of primary stroke centers play a significant role and are discussed elsewhere [9]. In the following paragraphs, we will discuss further the abovementioned key components that lead to a successful endovascular stroke therapy.

The major challenge in the treatment of acute ischemic stroke is appropriate patient selection trying to balance the benefits and risks. This apparently simple process involves consideration of many clinical, imaging characteristics for decision making in a timely fashion. To begin with, selecting patients with ideal demographic features and good baseline function is important.

8.4.1 Demographic and Baseline Features

8.4.1.1 Age

All the five trials included patients more than 18 years old. In the REVASCAT and SWIFT PRIME trials, upper age cutoff was 85 whereas, in the rest of the three trials, there was no upper age cutoff. The median age of the patients from the patient-level pooled analysis was 68 (57–77) years and 68 (59–76) in the intervention and control arms, respectively. Patients in the age groups 60–79 and ≥80 years constituted 55.1 and 15.5% of the total trial population. The pooled analysis suggested consistent benefit across all the age subgroups including the octogenarians. Age remains a strong predictor of outcome at the patient-level pooled analysis. Endovascular therapy should not be withheld for any patient solely based on the age if all other eligible criteria are met.

8.4.1.2 Sex

In all the five endovascular trials, both the genders were well represented. In the patient-level pooled analysis, the proportion of males was 52 and 54% in the intervention and control arms, respectively. There was no heterogeneity in treatment effect across the sexes. Hence, patients with AIS should be considered for endovascular therapy irrespective of their sex.

8.4.1.3 Premorbid Function

All the trials except MR CLEAN had used a valid measure of premorbid functional status to determine patient's trial eligibility. In the ESCAPE trial, modified Barthel index of >90 was a prerequisite for trial eligibility. Patients were excluded from the trial enrollment if their modified Rankin score was >2 for the EXTEND-IA trial and >1 for the REVASCAT and SWIFT PRIME trial. The selection of a patient with a good baseline functional status influences his/her ability to withstand the stress of a major medical illness and its treatment as well as participation in rehabilitation.

Despite MR CLEAN trial not having any premorbid functional status eligibility criteria for enrollment in the trial, the baseline mRS score was 0 in 81.5% and 80.1% of intervention and control arms, respectively. The overall proportion of patients with an mRS of ≤2 in the MR CLEAN trial was 95.7 and 95.9% in the intervention and control arms, respectively. In the SWIFT PRIME, 83% of the patients in either arm had an mRS of 0; 99 and 98% of patients had an mRS of 0–1 in the control and intervention arms, respectively. In the REVASCAT trial, 83.5 and 80.6% of patients had an mRS of 0 in the intervention and control arms, respectively.

Overall, all the trials had selected patients with good baseline functional status. To replicate the results of these trials in routine clinical practice, physicians should strictly adhere to randomized clinical trial eligibility criteria during patient selection. Due to this selective enrollment, questions remain on the utility of this therapy in patients with intermediate and poor baseline function. One should exercise caution and make a judicious call when selecting patients with an intermediate or poor baseline functional status for the endovascular thrombectomy if they meet other eligibility criteria.

8.4.2 Imaging-Based Selection

All the five randomized trials had used imaging to determine trial eligibility as well as for follow-up imaging to determine recanalization. Mandatory vascular imaging to identify target occlusion in all the trials and selecting patients with small ischemic core and large penumbra is a crucial reason for the success of the second-generation trials. Though the studies differed in their individual imaging-based selection criteria, the underlying central principles remained the same: "selecting patients with a favorable ischemic pattern due to a proximal arterial occlusion." In the following section, we will discuss further the individual components of the imaging.

8.4.2.1 CT Versus MRI

All the trial designs permitted the use of CT/MRI as initial imaging modality for trial eligibility. However, CT technology was predominantly used for selecting patients at baseline. Due to the widespread availability, speed of acquisition, low cost, ease of operation, ease of patient monitoring, and safety profile in patient's medical implants/devices, CT imaging trumps as the tool for urgent neurovascular imaging in most of the centers across the world. We do not discourage from using MRI; however, centers adopting MRI for acute stroke protocols should pay proper attention to the impact of the MR screening in their hospital/health system workflow. For estimating infarct volume at early and late follow-up, MRI would have better image resolution. In the following discussion, we will focus primarily on CT-based imaging.

8.4.2.2 Favorable Ischemic Pattern

The favorable ischemic pattern is the presence of small ischemic core and significant salvageable brain tissue. This pattern can be identified using both plain (non-contrast imaging) and perfusion imaging.

8.4.2.3 Non-Contrast CT

Alberta stroke program early CT score (ASPECTS) is a well-validated measure of quantifying the early ischemic changes in the MCA territory. It is a 10-point hierarchical scale. The MCA territory is divided into ten regions with a score of 1 assigned to each. The presence of early ischemic changes in a region is assigned a score of 0. Thus, the higher the score, the more limited is the extent of the early ischemic changes. The score had been well validated and the ability of ASPECTS to predict clinical outcome had been well demonstrated in the past. APECTS is a simple risk stratification tool that can be used widely in the emergency setting using a NCCT scan. The necessary training for interpretation and score using the ASPECTS score is provided on the website www.aspectsinstroke.com.

The ESCAPE and SWIFT PRIME trials used an ASPECTS score of ≥6 for the trial eligibility criteria. Similarly, in the REVASCAT trial, an ASPECTS score ≥7 on CT and ASPECTS score ≥6 on MRI are used for selecting eligible patients. In the MR CLEAN trial, neither ASPECTS criteria nor another estimate of the extent of early ischemic changes was used as criteria for study enrollment. In the EXTEND-IA trial, as mentioned earlier perfusion imaging was used to select patients into the trial using mismatch criteria for penumbra and ischemic core.

The median ASPECTS in the patient-level pooled analysis was 9 in both the intervention and control arms indicating that the trial population had very limited ischemic changes on baseline imaging.

8.4.3 Perfusion Imaging

The perfusion imaging can be used to identify the ischemic core (irreversible brain damage) and ischemic penumbra (potentially salvageable brain tissue). The use of perfusion imaging to select patients likely to benefit from an acute stroke therapy has been there for many years. The variability in the imaging protocols, smaller sample size, insufficient evidence, and mostly the lack of a highly effective treatment for large vessel occlusion has limited the understanding, utility, and validation of the perfusion imaging. Data from perfusion imaging and its utility in endovascular thrombectomy decision making from MR CLEAN and SWIFT PRIME trials will be discussed below.

8.4.3.1 MR CLEAN Perfusion Imaging

The MR CLEAN investigators have looked if the CT perfusion imaging parameters had any effect on the outcome as well as any interaction with the treatment effect of IAT [10]. The data from 175 patients of the total of 500 patients was analyzed. The ischemic penumbra was defined as a relative mean transit time (MTT) 45% higher than that of the contralateral hemisphere (relative MTT >1.45) and a cerebral blood volume (CBV) >2.0 mL/100 g. Ischemic core was defined as a relative MTT >1.45 and a CBV <2.0 mL/100 g. The two CTP parameters that were significantly associated with the functional outcome were the CTP-derived ischemic-core volume and percentage ischemic core. Penumbra volume was not associated with functional outcome. Other CTP-derived parameters like ischemic-core volume, Penumbra volume, and percentage ischemic core did not have interaction with the treatment effect (IAT). From the analysis, it appears that the larger CTP ischemic-core volume is associated with worse functional outcome. The perfusion imaging was done in multiple centers using different scanners and different protocols (acquisition times, brain coverage, and software for processing) which again are an inherent drawback of perfusion imaging. The authors concluded that the use of CTP-based selection of AIS otherwise eligible for IAT is not supported.

8.4.3.2 SWIFT PRIME Perfusion Imaging

The data from 161 of the 196 patients enrolled in the SWIFT PRIME trial was analyzed to assess if the early CT perfusion imaging can predict the size of the ischemic core and the volume of critically hypoperfused tissue as well as if these two parameters can predict the infarct volume [11]. The ischemic core identified by the baseline CT perfusion imaging predicted the 27 h infarct volumes in both the endovascular and tPA alone groups. Also, baseline showing areas with Tmax >6 s (hypoperfused tissue) strongly correlated with the 27 h infarct volume in non-reperfusers.

8.4.4 Vascular Occlusion

One of the biggest drawbacks of the previous generation endovascular trials (IMS III, SYNTHESIS, MR RESCUE) was that vascular imaging to select patients was used to a very minimal extent. This has led to inclusion of patients without vascular occlusion in those endovascular trials. All the recent five trials mentioned above have used one or the other modality of vascular imaging to select patients with a proximal occlusion in the anterior circulation. Though the trials differed slightly in the eligible vascular occlusions, in the patient-level pooled analysis, around 20% of the occlusions were in the intracranial ICA (with or without extracranial occlusion—tandem occlusion), and 70% were in the M1 segment of the MCA. The M2 segment constituted only 7–8% of the cases in the pooled analysis. Patients with intracranial ICA occlusion benefitted from endovascular thrombectomy with or without extracranial ICA occlusion and irrespective of the treatment modality. The authors concluded that because of the different treatment options employed to deal with extracranial occlusion, further clinical trial data addressing the tandem occlusions is needed to identify the best modality to deal with the extracranial occlusion. The MCA M2 occlusions are another population which are underrepresented in the pooled analysis. This is because three of the five trials excluded MCA M2 occlusions, and the remaining two trials enrolled only a few of them. There are a couple of issues with identification and the severity of clinical deficits following an MCA M2 occlusion. Often, it is difficult to differentiate an M1 segment from an M2 segment owing to early branching of the MCA main trunk as well as prominent MCA M2 branch. The potential for misclassification is reflected in the enrollment of a few MCA M2 occlusions which are mistaken for an MCA M1 segment. Occlusion of an M2 branch can result in a significant neurological deficit, thus mimicking as an M1 occlusion clinically. Often, these M2 branches tend to be of larger diameter, thus making them suitable and safe for mechanical thrombectomy. Even occlusion of a smaller caliber M2 can lead to significant neurological deficit owing to the eloquence of the supplied brain parenchyma. There is no good randomized clinical trial data to support the safety and efficacy of mechanical thrombectomy for distal occlusions. Based on data from these trials and other published literature, mechanical thrombectomy using smaller stent retrievers can be attempted in these cases with reasonable safety by experienced interventionists.

8.4.5 Optimization of Endovascular Workflow

All patients with moderate to severe strokes should be considered eligible for endovascular therapy unless proved otherwise by imaging and/or clinical features. With this assumption, the endovascular team should be prenotified for all incoming moderate to major strokes. After a brief and focused neurological examination, patients with suspected stroke should undergo a complete and fast neurovascular imaging to determine eligibility for endovascular treatment. The vascular imaging should include the aortic arch to the vertex with additional collateral imaging, preferably multiphase CTA. The inclusion of perfusion imaging should depend on local center's preference and expertise. Parallel processing of the imaging data as it becomes available to determine rtPA, as well as endovascular eligibility, should be done. All acute ischemic stroke patients eligible for endovascular thrombectomy should be rushed to the intervention radiology suite after appropriate discussion with the neurointerventionists. Some of the processes that had significant impact on our endovascular workflow at Calgary include rapid decision making using advanced imaging, considering patient's premorbid clinical status, having remote imaging access for the interventionist, avoiding other redundancy in clinical decision making and workflow, rapid patient transport to the intervention radiology suite often not waiting for designated porters, fast patient transfer on to the angio-lab table, and prepping the patient for the intervention. Generally, the on-call endovascular team is not physically present in the hospital after hours and needs to come in. Patient preparation by the stroke neurology team can help in saving valuable time. Workflow and treatment times along the acute stroke care pathway play a pivotal role in determining the patient outcomes. The impact of the time on the outcome as well as various nuances with regard to the time metrics has been looked in the recent RCTs as well as the HERMES pooled analysis and will be discussed below.

8.4.5.1 ESCAPE

The core philosophy of the ESCAPE trial investigators was that AIS patients with large vessel occlusion and small to moderate infarct core and moderate to good collaterals would benefit from rapid endovascular thrombectomy if the reperfusion was achieved quickly after the imaging [12]. The ESCAPE trial investigators analyzed the impact of time on clinical outcome and the effect of patient, hospital, and health system characteristics on workflow within the trial. The direct transfer patients (endovascular capable hospital) had shorter onset to imaging time (34 min) and ED arrival to imaging times (8 min) compared to the drip and ship protocol patients. Similarly, the direct transfer patients treated during routine daytime hours had shorter CT-to-groin puncture (8 min) compared to after hours. Of the 109 patients who received both IV tPA and endovascular thrombectomy, the CT-to-groin puncture was longer on an average by 24 min when treated at remote hospitals (drip and ship protocol) compared to direct transfer to an endovascular center. General anesthesia was associated with a 22-min average prolongation of the CT-to-groin puncture time. Every 30-min increase in time from qualifying CT to reperfusion was associated with an absolute decrease in the probability of functionally independent outcome (mRS 0–2 at 90 days) by 8.3%, after adjusting for age, sex, baseline National Institutes of Health Stroke Scale, occlusion site, baseline ASPECTS, intravenous alteplase administration, and time from onset to qualifying CT ($p = 0.006$). A modest relation was found between achieving a functionally independent outcome (mRS 0–2) and symptom onset-to-reperfusion time, and no association was found with stroke onset to CT time. Use of the post imaging time metrics like the imaging to puncture as well as imaging to reperfusion as performance metrics and benchmarks for administering endovascular therapy is highly recommended.

8.4.5.2 SWIFT PRIME

Similar to ESCAPE, the analysis of workflow in the SWIFT PRIME trial was done [13]. All the workflow time metrics (qualifying imaging to groin puncture, ED arrival to groin puncture, ED arrival to perfusion) were longer in the patients presenting directly to the endovascular capable center (ECC). However, the symptom onset to ED arrival as well as the symptom onset to device deployment was significantly shorter in the patient group presenting directly to the ECC (65 and 203 min, respectively) than the patients transferred from another center to an ECC (214.5 and 299 min, respectively).

The probability of achieving an mRS of 0–2 (functional independence) was 91% if reperfusion was achieved at 150 min from symptom onset, and it decreased by approximately 10% (absolute) over the next 60 min and then 20% (absolute) with every subsequent 60-min delay. The trial population was divided into two subgroups to determine the effect of time on the outcome—the patient group who presented directly to the endovascular capable center (ECC) and the patient group who presented to a non-endovascular capable center and then were transferred to an ECC. For the ECC group, the rates of achieving a functional independence among patients with reperfusion in the stent retriever group declined with increasing symptom onset to reperfusion time as well as qualifying imaging to reperfusion time. 1–1.5/100 patients treated with stent retrievers will not have a functionally independent outcome at 90 days for every 6-min delay in the symptom onset to reperfusion. Similarly, 9/10 patients treated will have a functional independent outcome at 90 days if reperfused within 2.5 h of onset.

8.4.5.3 Hermes

As discussed earlier, endovascular intervention was associated with a substantially lower degree of patient disability at 3 months, with mRS scores of 2.9 (95% CI, 2.7–3.1) in the endovascular group and 3.6 (95% CI, 3.5–3.8) in the medical therapy group. The cOR of a less-disabled outcome with endovascular therapy was 2.49 (95% CI, 1.76–3.53), and the absolute risk difference (ARD) was 38.1% ($p < 0.001$), with earlier treatment associated with greater magnitude of benefit. The amount of benefit from the thrombectomy declined as the time from symptom onset to arterial puncture increased. There was a benefit from endovascular thrombectomy seen up to 418 min (7 h and 18 min) from symptom onset to expected arterial puncture. Of the 634 patients randomized to the endovascular group, 607 (95.7%) underwent arterial puncture, and in 563 (88.8%) thrombectomy intervention was done [14]. Substantial reperfusion was achieved in 390 (71.0%) of the 549 patients who underwent an endovascular thrombectomy. The median time from symptom onset to arterial puncture was 238 min and from symptom onset to reperfusion 301 min in the 607 patients who underwent arterial puncture. Emergency department to treatment times had a significant treatment effect modification compared to the symptom onset to ED arrival times. In the HERMES analysis, there was no interaction among the treatment groups for excellent outcome (mRS 0–1), symptomatic hemorrhage, and major parenchymal hematoma between these two major time intervals.

Symptom onset to reperfusion time significantly impacts the 3-month disability for the endovascular thrombectomy group. Delay in symptom onset to reperfusion time was associated with increased levels of disability at 3 months among the endovascular group. Every 9-min delay in the symptom onset-to-good reperfusion would lead to higher 3-month mRS (by 1 or more points) for 1 out of 100 patients treated. For symptom onset to reperfusion time of 180 min, the probability of functional independence (mRS 0–2) at 3 months was 64.1% compared to 46.1% with symptom onset-to-reperfusion time of 480 min. The effect of symptom onset to reperfusion times on 3-month outcome was seen in subgroups analyzed by age, baseline NIHSS, clot location, baseline ASPECTS score, mode of patient arrival (direct ED arrival or transfer), and time from symptom onset to IV tPA.

For every 4-min delay in emergency department door-to-reperfusion time, 1 of every 100 treated patients had a worse disability outcome. Among direct arrival patients, functional independence at 3 months was more frequent both with faster emergency department door-to-reperfusion and brain imaging-to-reperfusion times. Rates of mortality, symptomatic intracranial hemorrhage, and major parenchymal hematoma did not significantly change with longer delay to reperfusion. A 15-min decrease in the ED to reperfusion time would lead to 39 patients not having a disabled outcome, and 25 of these 39 would have functional independence for every 1000 successfully reperfused patients. Based on the HERMES meta-analysis, the benefit of the endovascular thrombectomy ± medical therapy is maximal in the first 2 h from symptom onset and persisted up to 7.3 h. Earlier treatment is associated with a better 3-month outcome.

8.4.6 Time Epochs in Stroke Care

The imaging correlates (occlusion, small to moderate core, and moderate-good collaterals) that predict success of the endovascular therapy are a surrogate marker for "perfect" brain physiology, and the lack of these imaging correlates can indicate an "imperfect" or "suboptimal" brain physiology for endovascular stroke therapy. There are two main epochs with regard to acute stroke care—epoch 1, onset to imaging, and epoch 2, imaging to reperfusion.

In the analysis mentioned before, significant relation was consistently seen with timings in the epoch 2. However, this does not downplay the significance of epoch 1. The ESCAPE trial population consists of patients with "perfect" physiology identified by the imaging during the second epoch. Patients make a transition from epoch 1 to epoch 2 at the time of imaging. Various known and unknown factors influence a patient's state of brain physiology as well as the speed and degree of transition from a "perfect" to an "imperfect" brain physiological state. Depending on various factors, a patient with the "perfect" physiology may develop an "imperfect" physiology as the time from symptom onset increases.

As the clinical decision making happens at the interface of these time epochs, decreasing the duration of epoch 1 may help capture more patients with "ideal" brain physiology. The single biggest factor that influences such transition is "time" itself in addition to other factors like penumbral perfusion (denoted by collaterals, CT perfusion parameters), brain physiology, neuronal vulnerability, etc. Other factors that influence the transition both physiologically and pharmacologically need to be studied to be able to extend the benefit of the endovascular therapy. Also, system issues related to the patient workflow, referral systems, and transport should be optimized to decrease the duration of the epoch 1. These system changes will have a population impact in potentially increasing the volumes of patients that are identified with "perfect" physiology in epoch 2.

8.4.7 Efficient Endovascular Setup

The second critical component involves the need to have an organized endovascular setup geared to perform effective and safe endovascular therapy promptly. As mentioned earlier, prenotification of the endovascular team, remote imaging access can help in increasing the speed of the whole process. Endovascular manpower consisting of the interventionist, support staff is a crucial component of the whole operation. The single biggest challenge in many centers around the world is the availability of access to the endovascular suite and a neuro-interventionist 24/7. The problem is further amplified in the developing world where the burden of stroke is already high and projected to increase further. Trying to keep a balance between providing round-the-clock neuro-intervention support and the logistic/financial challenges of such operation is a tough act for health systems across the world. Other problems include training next-generation neuro-interventionists. Guidelines regarding training of the neuro-interventionists and maintenance of the necessary skill have been recently proposed by an international expert panel [15]. In the section below, we have discussed further about some of the practices that can be adopted to increase the efficiency of the endovascular workflow.

A couple of illustrative cases below will highlight the various points discussed in the above sections (Figs. 8.4, 8.5, and 8.6). The

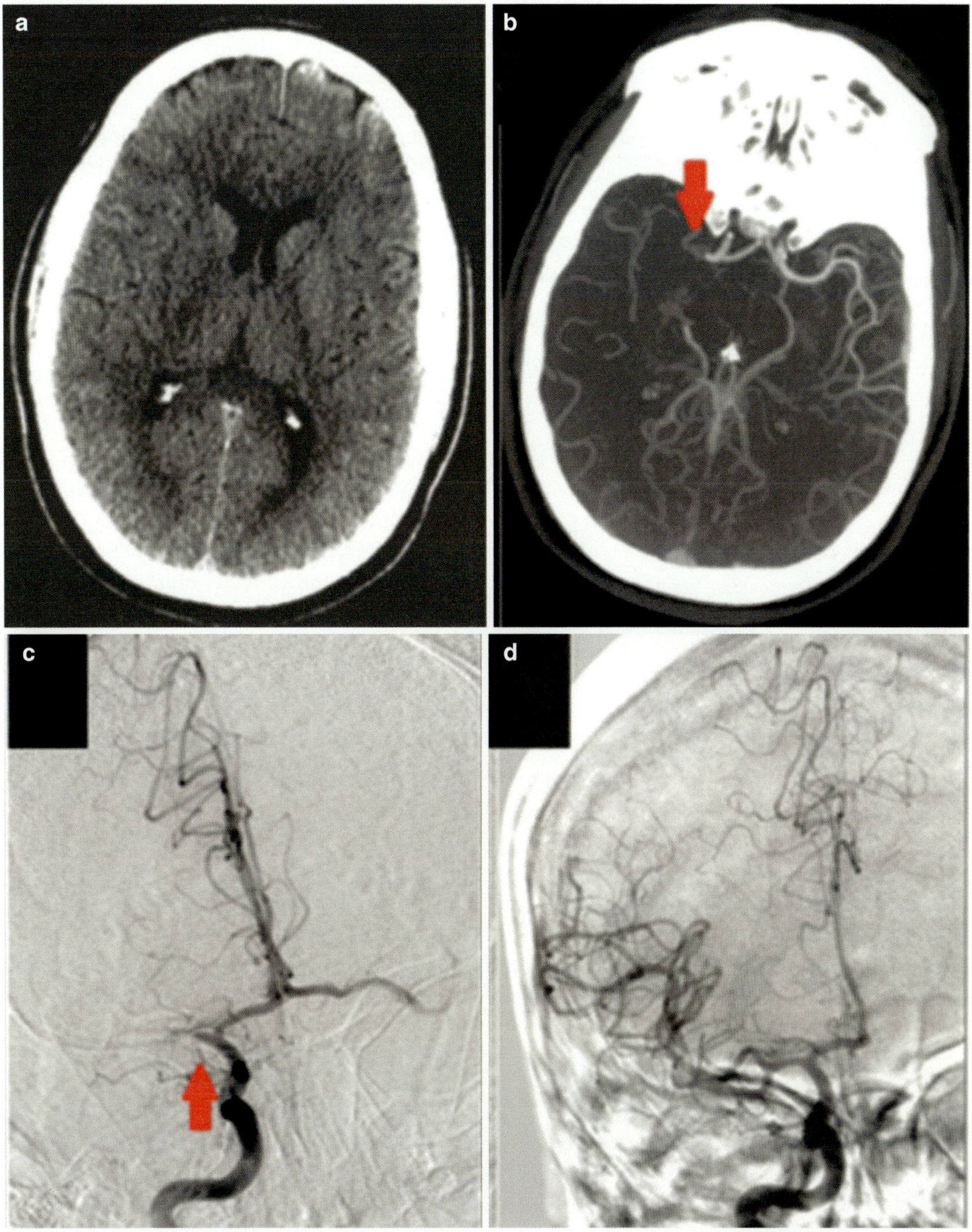

Fig. 8.4 This is a case of wake-up stroke (last seen normal 12 h earlier) with right MCA occlusion treated with endovascular thrombectomy. This case highlights the role of careful selection of patients using appropriate clinical and imaging tools. (**a**) Initial CT head. ASPECTS = 8; early ischemic changes seen in lentiform nucleus and insular cortex. (**b**) CTA showing right MCA M1 segment occlusion at its origin. Multiphase CTA demonstrated good collaterals (not shown here). (**c**) First angiography run showing right MCA M1 occlusion. (**d**) Final angiography run showing complete recanalization of the MCA M1 segment. (**e**) MRI on day 2 showing a small infarct in the right lentiform nucleus. Reproduced by permission of current atherosclerosis reports [9]

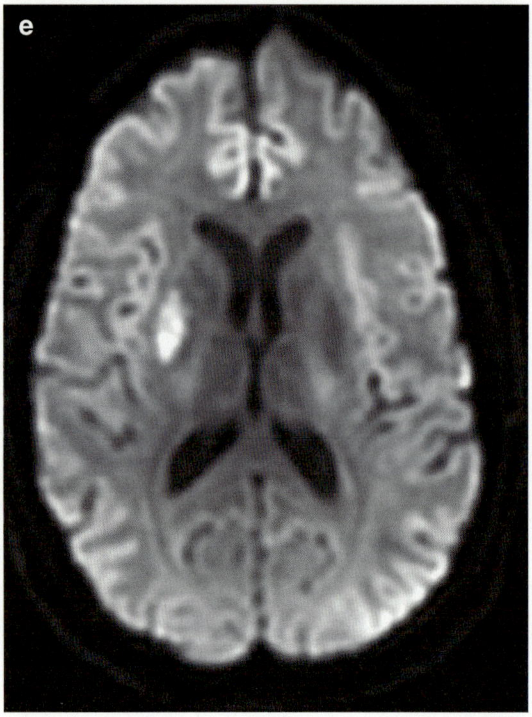

Fig. 8.4 (continued)

above case demonstrates that rapid endovascular stroke therapy can be delivered in safe and efficient manner resulting in very good clinical outcomes. This requires careful planning and organization of prehospital care, optimization of the acute stroke care pathways in the emergency department, imaging services, and the endovascular workflow.

8.5 Technique of Stent Retriever Thrombectomy at the Calgary Stroke Program

Though there is no universally accepted technique for stent thrombectomy, we describe the general principles adopted at the Calgary Stroke Program, Foothills Medical Center, University of Calgary, Canada. Also, we discuss other procedure-related issues like reasons for the failure of the stent thrombectomy and possible complications and how to avoid them. The following section serves only as a general guide mainly for centers that are starting their endovascular program. Other experienced centers adopt different techniques/use different equipment based on their experience and preference. Whatever is the technique used, fast, effective, and safe recanalization should be the goal.

8.5.1 Patient Selection and Decision Making

At the Calgary Stroke Program, we choose patients carefully based on the ESCAPE trial criteria. All the AIS patients get a NCCT, multiphase CTA ± CT perfusion. Patients transferred from another center either directly or by drip and ship protocol may get repeat imaging (NCCT ± CTA) depending on the time from arrival to initial imaging as well as the neurological status of the patient. Patients with good baseline function and having an occlusion in the proximal anterior circulation with good collaterals and small ischemic core and large penumbra are chosen. The decision to treat with IV tPA is made soon after imaging, and the IV tPA is usually administered just outside the CT scanner unless the patient clinical situation warrants transfer to a monitored bed in the emergency department. If the patient is eligible for endovascular thrombectomy, the interventionist and the intervention radiology staff are made aware of this, and the patient is transferred from the CT scanner to the intervention radiology suite directly most of the times. At our center, a patient's IV tPA treatment status does not influence the endovascular decision making, and in cases who received IV tPA, we do not wait for the therapeutic response. A lot of emphasis is placed on parallel processing and decision making as the information becomes available.

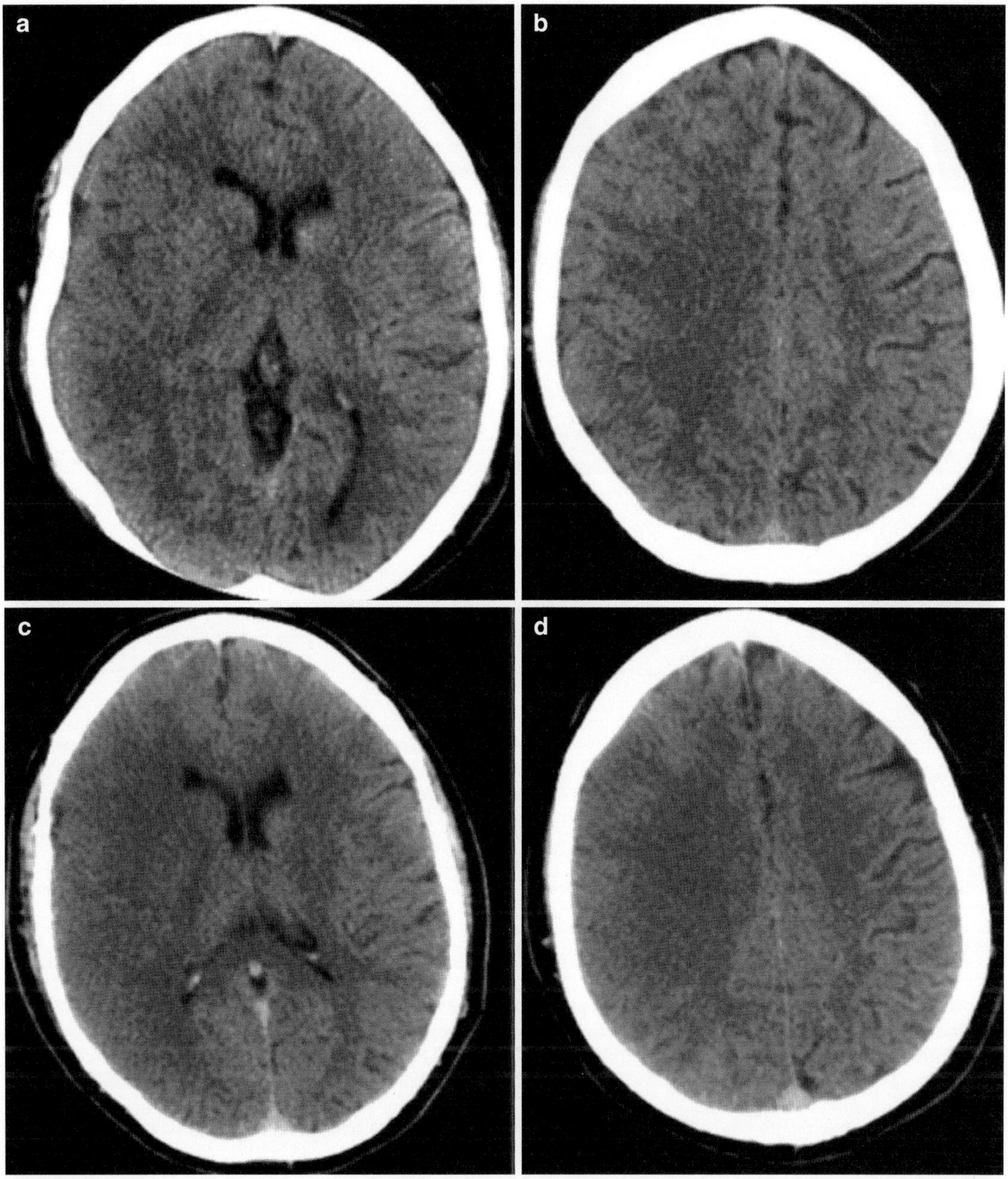

Fig. 8.5 This is a case highlighting the time-dependent tissue fate in AIS. This is a case of acute ischemic stroke due to right ICA occlusion on CTA (not shown here). (**a** and **b**) First NCCT done at 11:30 pm in the primary stroke center showing very early but limited ischemic changes in the right MCA territory. Patient was transported to the comprehensive stroke center as he was eligible for endovascular thrombectomy. (**c** and **d**) Second NCCT done after the patient is transferred to the comprehensive stroke center. The repeat scans done at 3:00 am (3.5 h later) showed fairly well-established extensive changes making him unsuitable for thrombectomy. Reproduced by permission of current atherosclerosis reports [9]

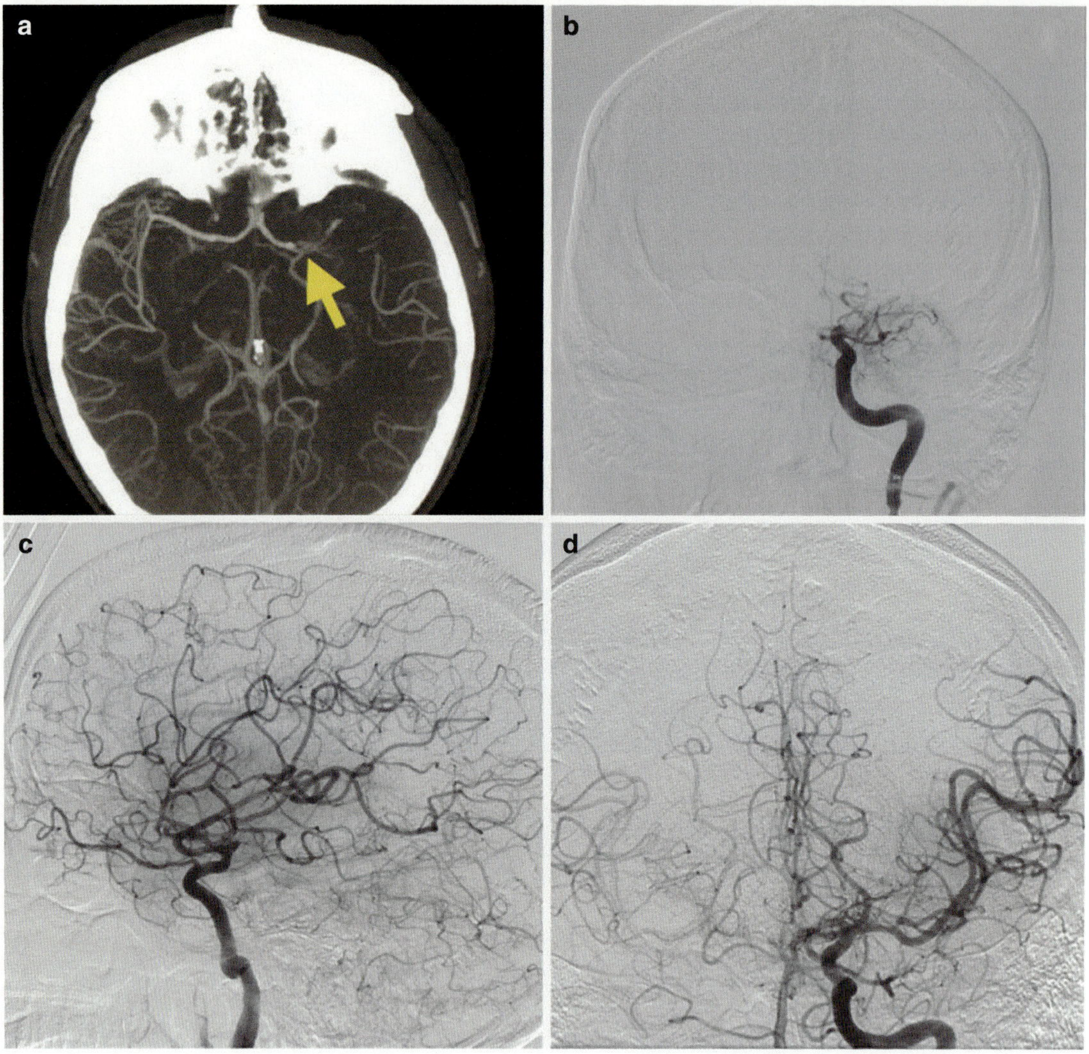

Fig. 8.6 A 30-year-old male on Warfarin for a previous cardiac thrombus comes with AIS. The time line below demonstrates the patient's endovascular stroke therapy workflow:

- 3:00 pm—Symptom onset—right hemiparesis + aphasia—witnessed by family
- 3:43 pm—Arrival at ED. NIHSS—25
- 3:51 pm—NCCT/CTA—ASPECTS: 10; left MCA1 occlusion. Good collaterals (not shown)
- 4:11 pm—Groin puncture
- 4:20 pm—First angio run
- 4:28 pm—Complete revascularization
- Day 3—Discharge home, NIHSS—0

8.5.2 General Anesthesia

The use of the general anesthesia (GA) during endovascular thrombectomy has been a controversial topic earlier with both advocates as well as opponents. The use of GA in the recent five trials has been limited. The use of GA was associated with a significant effect modification (p = 0.011) resulting in 51% estimated decrease in the treatment effect compared to the non-GA in the MR CLEAN trial [16]. The chief disadvantages with using GA for endovascular thrombectomy include anesthetic-induced hypotension, increased imaging to reperfusion times logistic issues with regard to the manpower, availability, coverage, cost, etc.

8.5.3 Endovascular Equipment and Setup

It is ideal to have a prearranged stroke tray ready for use in the angiogram suite at all times, so that the procedure can be initiated without any delay. In our center, a stroke kit (BRISK, Brisk Recanalization Ischemic Stroke Kit) is always ready to be used with emphasis on using standardized techniques and devices as much as possible (Fig. 8.7). The prearranged stroke tray should contain:

1. Sterile drapes, sponge sticks for skin preparation, needles, preloaded local anesthetic, surgical blade, etc.
2. Stroke kit (prepacked, to be opened at the time of the procedure) containing puncture needle (18 G), introducer J-wire, 8 Fr femoral arterial sheath, Terumo wire (035″ Terumo 180 cm long wire), syringes (5 cc, 10 cc, and 60 cc), catheter tubings to be connected to pressurized system for saline flushing (at least three in number), fiber-free wipes.
3. Other devices to be kept handy, preferably in the lower shelf of the sterile stroke tray are 8 Fr balloon guide catheter, a few commonly used inner select catheters for arch access (like H1, angled, Simmonds, etc.), 021″ microcatheter, non-traumatic curved 014″–016″ micro-guide wires, and vessel closure devices.

In addition to having a stroke ready set, the whole team (interventionists, nurses, and technologists) should be aware of the availability and location of the chief and auxiliary equipment/devices. These include the stent retrievers, alternate microcatheter system, aspiration tubing system, heparinized saline bags, contrast, etc. Cross-training of the intervention radiology staff (nurses and the technicians) is also crucial. Having this training and knowledge will help in quickly starting the procedure especially during after hours.

8.5.4 Technique of Thrombectomy

8.5.4.1 Puncture and Access

Almost all our anterior circulation stroke patients end up having an 8 French femoral sheath with an 8 French balloon guide catheter (parked in the internal carotid artery; the level is decided on the basis of tortuosity and can usually be determined on the CTA), appropriate coaxial selective inner catheter for arch access, and a stent retriever (by default a 4 × 40 mm size stent retriever for

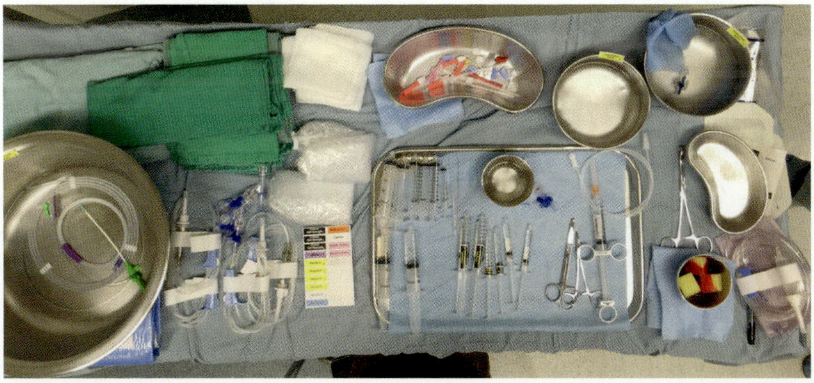

Fig. 8.7 BRISK set—Brisk Recanalization Ischemic Stroke Kit. All the "cheap" stuff ready to go, pre-organized in terms of what is needed first. The "expensive stuff" which consists of 5–6 packets can be opened when the case is started. This is very useful especially in the middle of the night and avoids delay due to waiting for endovascular staff to arrive

M1 occlusions) with appropriate microcatheter (021″ size microcatheter). A 021″ microcatheter is taken over 016 micro-guide wire (with tip shaped to give a non-traumatic "J" configuration) into the occluded MCA and carefully navigated distal to the site of the thrombus (proximal M2 segment).

8.5.4.2 Choosing the Appropriate Stent and Size

The appropriate stent selection depends on the location of the vascular occlusion as well as the diameter of the vessel. It is not uncommon to have an early MCA branching with an MCA M2 branch as large as the MCA M1 main trunk. The diameter of the occluded artery can be easily assessed from the CTA images. An estimate of the length of the occluded segment can also be made from the multiphase CTA imaging, especially if there is retrograde collateral filling of the occluded vessel on the delayed phase of the multiphase CTA.

By default, we almost always use a standard 4 mm diameter stent for an M1 segment occlusion. However, in case of M2 or ACA occlusions, a smaller stent size (e.g., 3 mm diameter) is recommended. More proximal occlusions, like terminal ICA occlusion, may warrant the use of larger caliber stents (5–6 mm diameter).

8.5.5 Stent Deployment and Retrieval

8.5.5.1 Location and Duration of Deployment

The stent retriever is deployed immediately distal to the occluded segment, to capture the entire length of the clot/thrombus. After withdrawing the microwire, a check microcatheter injection is performed to confirm the correct positioning of the distal end of the microcatheter, as well as to rule out any iatrogenic microwire perforations (this injection is done as a run using a very small amount of contrast with just enough injection pressure to allow for visualization). An appropriate-sized stent retriever is then carefully deployed across the occluded segment. After the deployment of the stent retriever, an angiographic run is performed. This is done to primarily assess the immediate bypass effect after stent deployment.

Soon after initial stent deployment and confirming the immediate bypass effect, the stent is left in situ anywhere from 5 to 10 min for integration of the thrombus into the stent struts. At this stage, the balloon guide catheter in the proximal ICA is gradually inflated just to occlude the parent vessel and block antegrade blood flow. The stent retriever is then slowly pulled back with consistent moderate force along with the microcatheter while applying moderate consistent negative suction pressure through the side port of the Y-connector connected to the balloon guide using a 60 cc syringe. The stent is then inspected for the trapped thrombus.

The balloon is then deflated to allow for forward blood flow while performing aspiration through the guide catheter to look for good backflow of blood. If the stent does not demonstrate entrapped clot or debris, and there is no back flow through the guide, then the possibility of the clot stuck within the guide catheter or femoral sheath hub should be considered. In such instances aspiration should be continued through the guide catheter using a 60 cc syringe. If unsuccessful, it is advised to withdraw the guide catheter out under negative suction, to prevent distal embolization of the retrieved clot. After checking the guide for a trapped clot and flushing the system, the selected vessel can be recatheterized as prior.

An angiographic run is obtained to look for any residual thrombus. If there is adequate recanalization, the procedure is terminated. If there is still residual thrombus, the stent retriever is again introduced into the occluded artery and deployed again, and the same procedure is repeated. This is usually done up to three to four passes. If there is no success after three to four attempts, the procedure is terminated. It has been found that higher number of stent passes is associated with less likelihood of good outcome.

8.5.5.2 Lack of Recanalization After Stent Deployment: Why and What to Do Further

In case there is absolutely no bypass effect after stent deployment, there are a couple of possibilities:

1. The stent retriever is not in the correct position and is covering only part of the clot. The exact location of the clot/thrombus is relatively easy to determine on the source images of the multiphase CTA: the proximal end of the clot can be determined on the first phase, while the distal end of the clot can be seen on the second or third phase. In this case, without waiting further, the stent retriever is repositioned.
2. There is complete capture of the clot: the clot has come through the interstices of the stent and is ready to be pulled out.
3. The clot is firm and the stent retriever has no impact on the clot. The differentiation between 2 and 3 is difficult, and very often the only way to differentiate is to actually remove the stent and see if the clot is captured.

8.5.6 Safety of Stent Retriever Thrombectomy

The stent retriever thrombectomy is a relatively safe technique. However, one must watch out for potential complications. Some of these rare complications include the risk of arterial dissection and arterial perforation.

8.5.6.1 Arterial Dissection and Perforations

Arterial dissection is an uncommon complication, especially encountered when dealing with extremely tortuous vasculature, underlying vasculopathy (like collagen vascular disorders), severe atheromatous disease, or absence of a good road map (especially in case of tandem occlusions of cervical ICA with no distal opacification, and the wire is navigated blindly through the path of least resistance). This can be prevented by selecting optimal devices (long femoral sheaths, less sturdy/rigid guide catheters, non-traumatic guide wires, etc.) and being cautious when intervening on an agitated/restless patient. Intracranial arterial perforation is also an uncommon complication seen when navigating a markedly tortuous intracranial circulation or while dealing with an agitated/restless patient. This can also happen when there are intracranial aneurysms along the access route. The use of conscious sedation (preferred) or general anesthesia in agitated patients can markedly improve the safety of the intervention. Careful inspection of CTA images should be performed to rule out any incidental vascular malformations like aneurysms before starting the procedure. The reported rates of these complications in both the MR CLEAN and ESCAPE trial are <2%.

Conclusion

Mechanical thrombectomy has markedly transformed the care of acute ischemic stroke due to large vessel occlusion. The evidence is very compelling and has been demonstrated in health systems across the world. The pace of accumulation of this evidence has been very rapid. The health-care professionals as well as the health systems around the world have been suddenly faced with the challenge to elevate their standard of care to match the current evidence. Multiple and often unique challenges are faced in implementing the mechanical thrombectomy for acute ischemic stroke. Now more than ever is the need for close collaboration and partnership among the stroke fraternity to bring this promising therapy to the people that need it the most in a timely, safe, and effective manner.

Suggestions from Clinical Practice Guidelines

Endovascular mechanical thrombectomy with stent retrievers is the first-line option over intra-arterial fibrinolysis. However, intravenous (IV) fibrinolysis with recombinant tissue plasminogen activator should be first considered among the patients who arrive within 4.5 h. If patients' symptoms are relieved after IV fibrinolysis, mechanical thrombectomy is not needed, but if not, mechanical thrombectomy should be conducted as quickly as possible. Observing patients after IV fibrinolysis to evaluate clinical improvement before conducting mechanical thrombectomy is not desirable. Mechanical thrombectomy should be considered as the next option even in patients who are not eligible for IV fibrinolysis. Mechanical thrombectomy should be done at an experienced stroke care center with qualified angiographic interventionists.

References

1. Saver JL, Jahan R, Levy EI, et al. Solitaire flow restoration device versus the Merci retriever in patients with acute ischaemic stroke (SWIFT): a randomized, parallel-group, non-inferiority trial. Lancet. 2012;380:1241–9.
2. Nogueira RG, Lutsep HL, Gupta R, et al. Trevo versus Merci retrievers for thrombectomy revascularisation of large vessel occlusions in acute ischaemic stroke (TREVO 2): a randomized trial. Lancet. 2012;380:1231–40.
3. Berkhemer OA, Fransen PS, Beumer D, et al. A randomized trial of intraarterial treatment for acute ischemic stroke. N Engl J Med. 2015;372:11–20.
4. Goyal M, Demchuk AM, Menon BK, et al. Randomized assessment of rapid endovascular treatment of ischemic stroke. N Engl J Med. 2015;372:1019–30.
5. Saver JL, Goyal M, Bonafe A, et al. Stent-retriever thrombectomy after intravenous t-PA vs. t-PA alone in stroke. N Engl J Med. 2015;372:2285–95.
6. Campbell BC, Mitchell PJ, Kleinig TJ, et al. Endovascular therapy for ischemic stroke with perfusion-imaging selection. N Engl J Med. 2015;372:1009–18.
7. Jovin TG, Chamorro A, Cobo E, et al. Thrombectomy within 8 hours after symptom onset in ischemic stroke. N Engl J Med. 2015;372:2296–306.
8. Goyal M, Menon BK, van Zwam WH, et al. Endovascular thrombectomy after large-vessel ischaemic stroke: a meta-analysis of individual patient data from five randomised trials. Lancet. 2016;387:1723–31.
9. Appireddy R, Zerna C, Menon BK, et al. Endovascular interventions in acute ischemic stroke: recent evidence, current challenges, and future prospects. Curr Atheroscler Rep. 2016;18:40.
10. Borst J, Berkhemer OA, Roos YB, et al. Value of computed tomographic perfusion-based patient selection for intra-arterial acute ischemic stroke treatment. Stroke. 2015;46:3375–82.
11. Albers GW, Goyal M, Jahan R, et al. Ischemic core and hypoperfusion volumes predict infarct size in SWIFT PRIME. Ann Neurol. 2016;79:76–89.
12. Menon BK, Sajobi TT, Zhang Y, et al. Analysis of workflow and time to treatment on Thrombectomy outcome in the endovascular treatment for small core and proximal occlusion ischemic stroke (ESCAPE) randomized, controlled trial. Circulation. 2016;133:2279–86.
13. Goyal M, Jadhav AP, Bonafe A, et al. Analysis of workflow and time to treatment and the effects on outcome in endovascular treatment of Acute ischemic stroke: results from the SWIFT PRIME randomized controlled trial. Radiology. 2016;279:888–97.
14. Saver JL, Goyal M, van der Lugt A, et al. Time to treatment with endovascular Thrombectomy and outcomes from ischemic stroke: a meta-analysis. JAMA. 2016;316:1279–88.
15. Lavine SD, Cockroft K, Hoh B, et al. Training guidelines for endovascular ischemic stroke intervention: an international multi-society consensus document. AJNR. 2016;37:E31–4.
16. Berkhemer OA, van den Berg LA, Fransen PS, et al. The effect of anesthetic management during intra-arterial therapy for acute stroke in MR CLEAN. Neurology. 2016;87:656–64.

9 Principles and Practical Application of Brain CT in Acute Ischemic Stroke

Abdulaziz S. Al Sultan, Muneer Eesa, and Bijoy K. Menon

Abstract

Stroke is a leading cause of mortality and morbidity worldwide. Available effective therapies rely on imaging for decision making. Recent advances in the field now enable physicians to select appropriate patients for acute ischemic stroke treatment. Computed tomography continues to be the standard imaging modality in acute ischemic stroke assessment in most centers worldwide. Six recently published randomized trials, showing strong benefit from endovascular treatment in acute ischemic stroke, have mostly used computed tomography for patient selection. In this chapter, we will discuss non-contrast computed tomography, computed tomography angiography, and computed tomography perfusion imaging in patients with acute ischemic stroke. The different diagnostic, therapeutic, and prognostic implications, as well as the advantages and disadvantages of these modalities, will also be discussed.

Since the 1970s, computed tomography (CT) has been the single most important imaging technique in the evaluation of acute ischemic stroke (AIS). In this chapter, non-contrast computed tomography (NCCT), computed tomography angiography (CTA), and computed tomography perfusion imaging (CTP) applications in AIS will be discussed. The correlating diagnostic, therapeutic, and prognostic implications will be reviewed for each modality.

A.S. Al Sultan • B.K. Menon (✉)
Department of Clinical Neurosciences, University of Calgary, Calgary, AB, Canada
e-mail: docbijoymenon@gmail.com

M. Eesa
Department of Radiology, University of Calgary, Calgary, AB, Canada

9.1 Non-contrast Computed Tomography

NCCT has been extensively studied in patients with AIS. Given that differentiating between AIS and hemorrhagic stroke on a clinical basis is difficult, and that NCCT is readily available

S.-H. Lee (ed.), *Stroke Revisited: Diagnosis and Treatment of Ischemic Stroke*, Stroke Revisited, DOI 10.1007/978-981-10-1424-6_9

in most medical centers, NCCT is the initial modality for assessment in patients with suspected AIS. After obtaining a focused history (including time of onset and neurologic symptoms) and clinical examination, ruling out intracranial hemorrhage with an NCCT is the next step. Extent of ischemia on the non-contrast CT helps improve the evaluation and management in patients with AIS. Extent of ischemia is assessed systematically using methods that are summarized below.

9.1.1 Alberta Stroke Program Early CT Score (ASPECTS)

Since its inception in 2000, ASPECTS has been widely accepted in many centers providing care for AIS patients, as well as being a criterion for patient enrollment in multiple seminal AIS clinical trials [1].

ASPECTS is a standardized quantitative CT score that divides the middle cerebral artery (MCA) territory into ten divisions, each having one point. A score of 10/10 infers a normal MCA territory CT scan, whereas a 0/10 reflects a diffuse involvement of the ten regions of MCA territory. A point is lost for each region that displays early ischemic change (EIC). Originally, EIC was defined as either parenchymal hypoattenuation or focal swelling. Parenchymal hypoattenuation can be either in the form of lack of gray–white differentiation or reduced density of brain tissue in contrast to corresponding lesion in the contralateral hemisphere. This is in distinction to "focal swelling" that can be seen in the form of sulcal effacement resulting in narrowing of the adjacent cerebrospinal fluid spaces. However, because cortical focal swelling can be representative of penumbral tissue rather than infarction, detection of parenchymal hypoattenuation is a must when calculating ASPECTS.

For scoring ASPECTS, the MCA territory is divided into seven ganglionic level regions (caudate, internal capsule, insula, and lentiform nucleus, M1–3) and three supraganglionic level regions (M4–6) (Fig. 9.1a). Smaller regions of the brain (caudate, internal capsule, insula, and lentiform nucleus) are given equal weight as larger cortical areas (M1–6). Early ischemic changes should be visible on at least two adjacent cuts to ensure that the region is truly involved rather than being falsely positive due to a phenomenon called partial-volume effect. An example of partial-volume effects resulting in false positive detection of early ischemic changes is when there is associated chronic infarct. Head tilt, motion artifact, and bone artifacts can also lead to misinterpretation of early ischemic changes resulting in falsely low ASPECT scores.

Another method for assessing EIC was assessing whether >1/3 of the MCA territory was involved or not. The European Cooperative Acute Stroke Study (ECASS-1) used "one-third" of MCA distribution as patient selection criteria. This trial showed that in patients with NCCT hypoattenuation affecting one-third or less of the MCA distribution, administration of intravenous alteplase resulted in patients achieving good outcome at 90 days (odds ratio [OR] 3.43; 95% confidence interval [CI] 1.61–7.33). This was in contrast to patients with hypoattenuation more than one-third of the MCA distribution who did not achieve statistically significant good outcomes when compared to patients who did not receive intravenous alteplase (OR 1.27; 95% CI 0.82–1.95). Of note, however, estimating EIC extent using the one-third rule had modest to poor reliability (κ-value of 0.39; 95% CI 0.29–0.49).

9.1.2 Posterior Circulation Alberta Stroke Program Early CT Score (pc-ASPECTS)

The ASPECTS was developed for anterior circulation ischemic strokes. A posterior circulation ASPECTS was developed in 2007 for posterior circulation ischemic strokes on CT angiography-source images. This choice of modality was

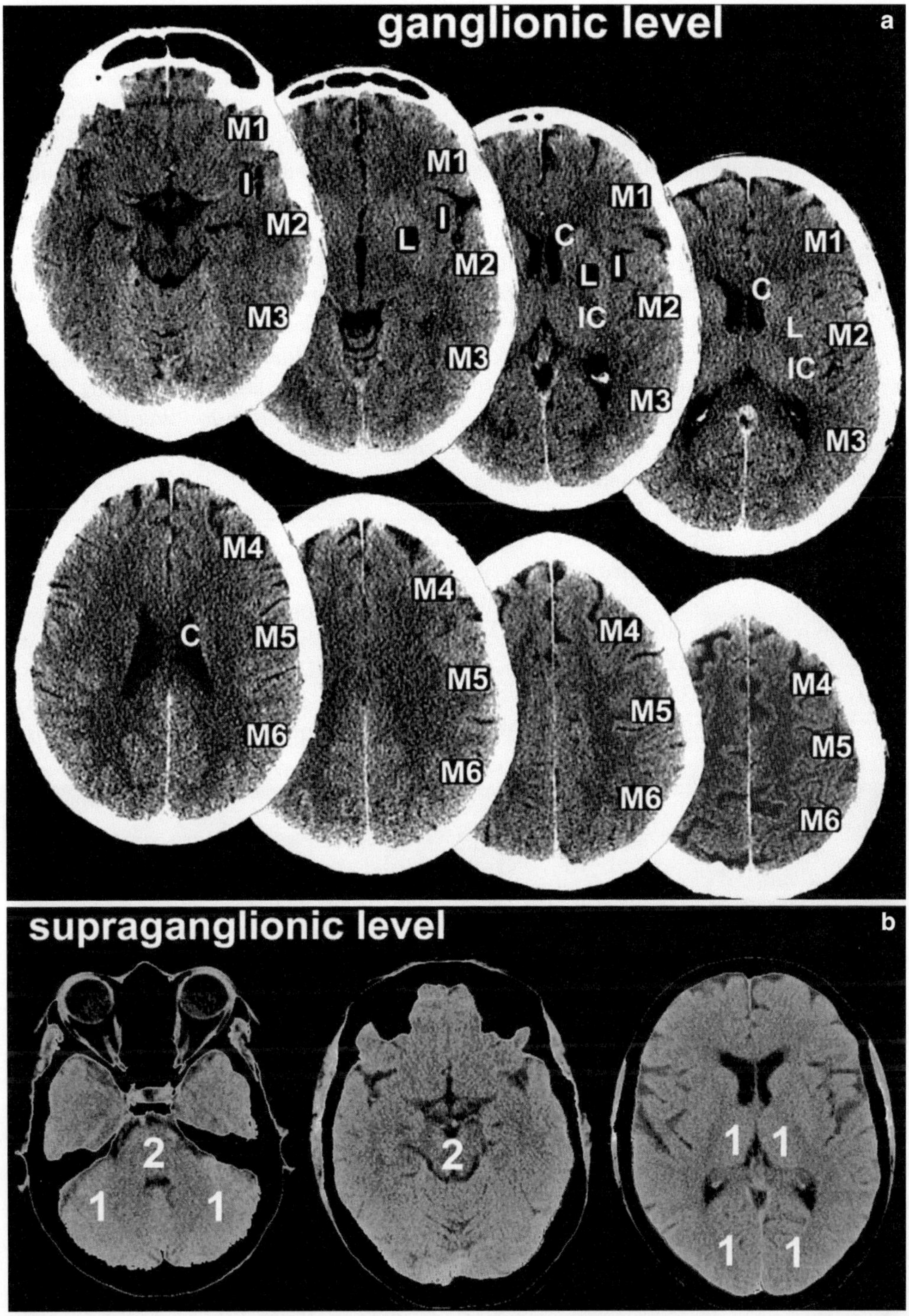

Fig. 9.1 ASPECT scoring system. The middle cerebral artery territory is divided into seven ganglionic level regions (caudate, internal capsule, insula, and lentiform nucleus, M1–3) and three supraganglionic level regions (M4–6) (**a**). For posterior circulation stroke, two points each are allocated to midbrain and pons, and one point is allocated to the thalamus, posterior cerebral artery (PCA) territory, and cerebellar hemisphere on each side (**b**). ASPECTS indicates Alberta stroke program early CT score

because non-contrast CT was not sensitive enough to detect EIC in brain parenchyma supplied by the posterior circulation. Similar to ASPECTS, pc-ASPECTS has a total of ten points. Two points each are allocated to midbrain and pons, and one point is allocated to the thalamus, posterior cerebral artery (PCA) territory, and cerebellar hemisphere on each side (Fig. 9.1b). Dichotomizing pc-ASPECTS at >7 vs <7 was able to predict patients who had a favorable functional outcome, using CTA-source images [2].

9.1.2.1 Hyperdense Artery Sign

In about a third of intraluminal MCA thrombus NCCT scans, a hyperdense MCA sign (HDMCAS) can be seen. In patients with higher hematocrit levels, dense MCA might be seen even within normal vessels; therefore, comparison of both MCAs is crucial. MCA "dot" sign can be identified in the Sylvian fissure affecting the M2/M3 branches of the MCA there (Fig. 9.2a). HDMCAS and MCA "dot" sign are relatively insensitive, with sensitivity of around 50% and 40%, respectively. However, they are both specific with their specificities reported to be 95% and 100%, respectively. Thin slice non-contrast CT scans (slice thickness <2.5 mm) in comparison have higher sensitivity and specificity for detecting intraluminal thrombus than non-contrast CT scans with average slice thickness >2.5 mm.

Of note, the hyperdense artery sign can be detected in the ICA, basilar artery, vertebral artery, and the posterior cerebral artery. The ability of thin slice non-contrast CT to detect proximal intraluminal thrombi with high sensitivity and specificity makes this imaging modality an important tool when deciding if a patient should be triaged for endovascular therapy [3].

9.2 CTA

Six recent randomized controlled trials (MR CLEAN, ESCAPE, Extend-IA, SWIFT-PRIME, REVASCAT, and THRACE) have shown that endovascular thrombectomy (with or without intravenous tPA) is superior to cur-

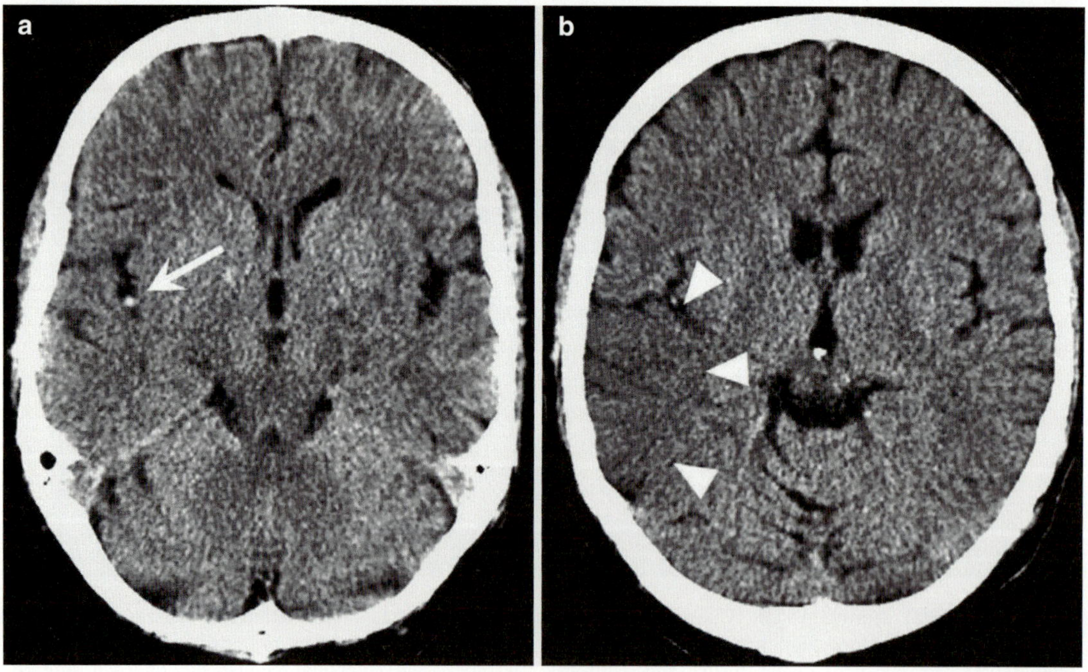

Fig. 9.2 Hyperdense MCA sign. Hyperdense MCA sign or MCA "dot" sign can be identified in the Sylvian fissure (*white arrow in* **a**) affecting the territory of M2/M3 branches of the MCA (*arrowheads in* **b**). MCA indicates middle cerebral artery

rent medical treatment [4, 5]. All of these trials used vascular imaging to determine patients' eligibility, with the majority undergoing CTA [6]. The CTA can be used to assess the following characteristics.

9.2.1 Intravascular Thrombus

Vascular imaging with CTA (or MRA) is the gold standard in detecting intravascular thrombi. The presence, extent, and location of the thrombi have diagnostic, therapeutic, and prognostic implications in almost every patient with AIS. Detecting the presence of an intravascular thrombus is the first step in assessing an AIS patient with a CTA. Patients with intravascular thrombi visualized on CTA have more severe clinical presentation (higher NIHSS). They are also more likely to benefit with thrombolysis or thrombectomy. The absence of intracranial thrombus on a CTA head however does not rule out ischemia [7].

A proximal thrombus, affecting the internal carotid artery (ICA), or the first segment of the MCA (M1), has a lower rate of recanalization with intravenous tPA in contrast to a more distal thrombus. These patients with proximal thrombi are more likely to benefit from endovascular thrombectomy (EVT). A recent meta-analysis shows that EVT is efficacious in patients with proximal intracranial occlusions when an arterial puncture is initiated within 7.3 h from onset of symptoms [8].

The length of the thrombus on CTA is an independent predictor of recanalization following tPA treatment. Thrombi >15 mm in length are less likely to reanalyze early with intravenous tPA in comparison to shorter thrombi. Length or extent of the clot can be measured semiquantitatively using the clot burden score (CBS). Similar to ASPECTS, the CBS is a 10-point scoring system with a score of 10 indicating absence of thrombi from ICA, M1, M2, and anterior cerebral artery (ACA). CBS of 0 would indicate a thrombus extending from involving all the aforementioned vessels (Fig. 9.3a). Patients with low CBS are less likely to benefit with intravenous tPA and therefore are better treated with EVT [9]. Intracranial thrombi that are porous (permeable) are more likely to dissolve early with intravenous tPA. Permeability of the thrombus can be assessed on CTA by looking

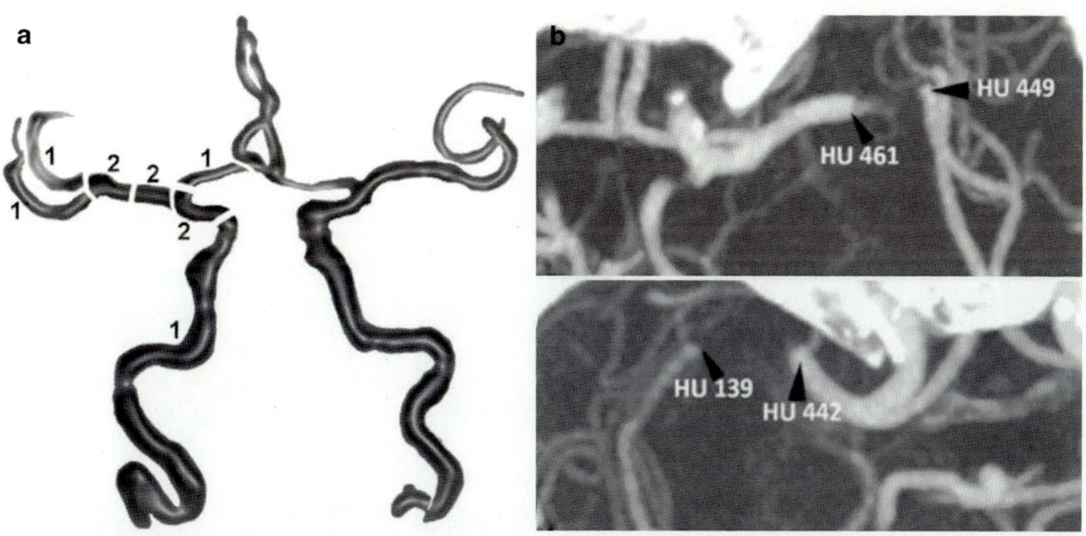

Fig. 9.3 Assessment of clot burden. The clot burden score is a 10-point scoring system with a score of 10 indicating absence of thrombi from ICA, M1, M2, and anterior cerebral artery (ACA) and a score of 0 indicating a thrombus extending from involving all the aforementioned vessels (**a**). Permeability of the thrombus can be assessed on CTA by looking for the presence of contrastation through the thrombus (**b**). *ICA* indicates internal carotid artery, *CTA* computed tomography angiography, *HU* Hounsfield unit

for the presence of contrastation through the thrombus. A helpful technique to assess permeable thrombi is shown in Fig. 9.3b [10].

9.2.2 Collateral Status

Collaterals supply the brain parenchyma through smaller arteriolar connections from the pial blood supply (leptomeningeal) or through larger arteriolar/arterial connections within the circle of Willis (Willisian) to the blood vessels supplying the brain. These collaterals provide retrograde filling to the blood vessels distal to the occluded segment of the intracranial artery. There is sufficient evidence that the presence of good collateral supply is associated with better clinical and radiological outcomes in AIS. Collateral imaging was used for patient selection in the ESCAPE trial; patients with poor collaterals on CTA were excluded (Fig. 9.4a) [11].

A recently developed technique for measuring collaterals is multiphase CTA (Fig. 9.4b). This technique has three distinct acquisition phases, using a multi-detector CT scanner and a single contrast bolus injection. The first phase starts from the aortic arch to the vertex, at 0.625 mm slice thickness, representing the peak arterial phase. The second and third phases scan the head from the skull base to the vertex, with 4-s delay per phase. The average total radiation dose using multiphase CTA with three phases in our center is 8.1 mSv for the three phases, which is less than the total radiation dose for a single-phase CTA in other established centers (8.2 mSv). This imaging protocol was used in ESCAPE trial. The technique of multiphase CTA avoids mislabelling of collateral status that is seen often with single-phase CTA. It is also more reliable than single-phase CTA in measuring collaterals. Other advantages include an ability to detect distal occlusions and to measure length/extent of intracranial thrombi more precisely [12].

Multiple scoring systems have been described for leptomeningeal collateral supply in AIS. Tan et al. described a collateral score with 0 reflecting the complete absence of collaterals and 3 reflecting the presence of collaterals with 100% filling. This score correlated well with clinical and radiological outcome. In patients with higher collateral scores, the clinical outcome was better, and the infarct volume was smaller in comparison to patients with lower collateral scores. Another way to assess collaterals that we use is shown in Fig. 9.4; this scor-

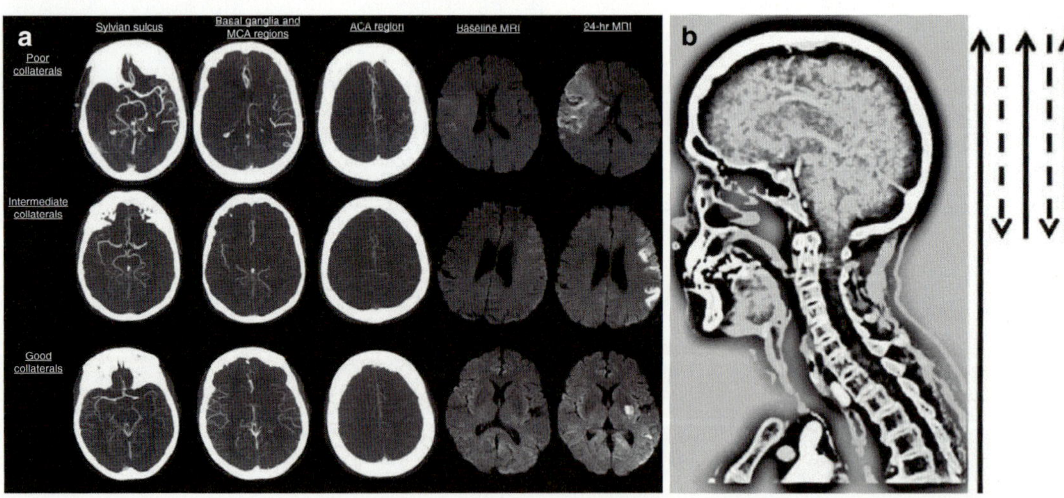

Fig. 9.4 Collateral status and neurological outcome. Patients who have good leptomeningeal collateral supply measured from baseline brain CT angiography had lower 3-month mRS and smaller final infarct volume size (**a**). Multiphase CT angiography image, with each phase represented by an arrow (**b**). The first phase (*long solid arrow*) is conventional arch-to-vertex CT angiography. The next two phases (*short solid arrows*) are sequential skull base-to-vertex acquisitions performed in the mid-venous and late venous phases. *Dashed arrows* indicate movement of the scanner in between image acquisitions. CT indicates computed tomography

ing scale has been shown to correlate well with clinical and radiological outcomes, with patients who have good collateral supply having lower 3-month mRS and smaller infarct volume size [13]. Hypo-contrastation on CTA-source image (CTA-SI) is associated with cerebral blood flow reduction. An issue with CTA-SI however is that timing of scan acquisition can result in the CTA-SI being either arterial weighted (blood flow weighted) or venous weighted (blood volume weighted). Thus, its utility in acute ischemic stroke has reduced over the past years [14].

9.3 CTP

A very important question to be answered in an almost every NCCT/CTA AIS evaluation is whether the EIC is more consistent with, irreversible, infarction core, or might rather be reflective of, a potentially salvageable, ischemic penumbra. CTP addresses these two critical issues. Despite its availability since the 1980s, CTP is a relatively recent addition to the arsenal of imaging techniques available for AIS assessment, due to significant improvements in speed of acquisition and processing of images. CTP is able to identify AIS patients with large ischemic penumbra, and smaller infarcted core, thus identifying patients likely to benefit from revascularization therapies. Other applications of CTP in ischemic stroke include assessment of post-intravenous tPA hemorrhagic transformation, as well as evaluation of ischemia after arterial vasospasm following subarachnoid hemorrhage.

Following the administration of iodinated contrast, multiple CT images obtained during the time of first pass of contrast are used to derive information on kinetics of the contrast. Mathematical algorithms like deconvolution are used to obtain estimates of cerebral blood flow, cerebral blood volume, and blood flow transit time functions like Tmax or mean transit time [15]. Target perfusion mismatch is then defined using thresholds for ischemic core and for penumbra. However, these thresholds might differ depending on CTP processing. We encourage readers to interact with their CTP vendor and use specific thresholds that are recommended for their specific CTP processing algorithms (Fig. 9.5).

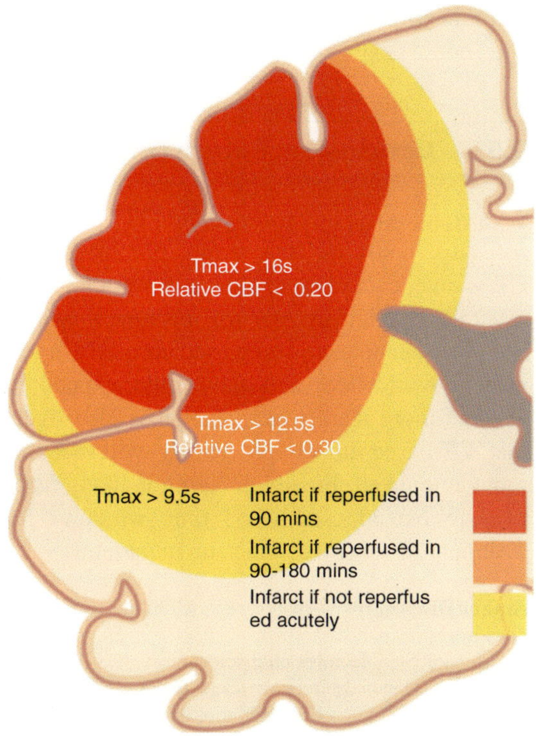

Fig. 9.5 Hypothetical model for time-based computed tomography perfusion thresholds for identifying final infarct volume. Optimal CTP parameter thresholds exist for identifying brain tissue that will likely infarct at different times from imaging if efficient reperfusion is not achieved. CTP indicates computed tomography perfusion imaging; CBF, cerebral blood flow; Tmax, time-to-maximum

9.4 Limitations of NCCT, CTA, and CTP

All the computed tomography modalities discussed in this chapter have some radiation risk. However, the radiation dose of a standard NCCT and CTA protocol for the assessment of AIS is less than that of a CTA chest or abdomen. Another limitation of CTA/CTP is the use of iodinated contrast agents, which historically have been associated with the development of "contrast-induced nephropathy." Nevertheless, a propensity score-matched study, involving 12,508 patients who had NCCT or contrast-enhanced computed tomography from Mayo Clinic, showed that acute kidney injury is, in fact, independent of exposure to contrast. In our opinion, therefore, a CT-based protocol for acute ischemic stroke has the advantage of speed of acquisition and low costs and has very low risk of radiation and contrast exposure.

9.5 Conclusion: Future Direction

As technological advances in the field involving software, hardware, tele-stroke platforms, and CT scanners continue to evolve, faster and more accurate imaging in AIS will become possible. Portable scanners are being used currently in few centers worldwide, and this could expand to become more readily available. It is also likely that CT-based image processing will become more automated. Finally, imaging is likely to be used to extend established time windows for treatment of acute ischemic stroke patients.

Author Disclosures Abdulaziz S. Al Sultan declares no disclosures.

Muneer Eesa declares no disclosures.

Bijoy K Menon declares membership of the Steering and Executive Committee; ESCAPE trial that received support from Covidien; Site Principal Investigator; SOCRATES Trial, sponsored by AstraZeneca; honoraria from Penumbra Incorporated; a provisional patent 62/086,077 for triaging systems in ischemic stroke; research funding from CIHR; Heart and Stroke Foundation of Canada; Alberta Innovates Health Solutions; Hotchkiss Brain Institute; the Faculty of Medicine, University of Calgary; and salary support from CIHR. In addition, he holds the current Heart and Stroke Foundation/University of Calgary Professorship in Stroke Imaging and receives salary support through the CIHR New Investigator Award.

Suggestions from Clinical Practice Guidelines Non-enhanced brain computed tomography (NECT) should be performed for initial and differential diagnosis of stroke before initiating any specific therapy. Hypointensity lesion on NECT as early ischemic changes may increase the risk of hemorrhagic transformation after intravenous fibrinolysis, and if the hypointensity involves more than one-third of the middle cerebral artery territory, intravenous fibrinolysis might be better to be avoided. Noninvasive vascular study such as computed tomography angiography or magnetic resonance angiography is very informative in emergency setting, but this study should not delay emergency treatment.

References

1. Menon BK, Puetz V, Kochar P, et al. ASPECTS and other neuroimaging scores in the triage and prediction of outcome in acute stroke patients. Neuroimaging Clin N Am. 2011;21:407–23.
2. Puetz V, Sylaja PN, Coutts SB, et al. Extent of hypoattenuation on CT angiography source images predicts functional outcome in patients with basilar artery occlusion. Stroke. 2008;39:2485–90.
3. Shobha N, Bal S, Boyko M, et al. Measurement of length of hyperdense MCA sign in acute ischemic stroke predicts disappearance after IV tPA. J Neuroimaging. 2014;24:7–10.
4. Bracard S, Ducrocq X, Mas JL, et al. Mechanical thrombectomy after intravenous alteplase versus alteplase alone after stroke (THRACE): a randomised controlled trial. Lancet Neurol. 2016;15:1138–47.
5. Goyal M, Menon BK, van Zwam WH, et al. Endovascular thrombectomy after large-vessel ischaemic stroke: a meta-analysis of individual patient data from five randomised trials. Lancet. 2016;387:1723–31.
6. Holodinsky JK, Yu AY, Assis ZA, et al. History, evolution, and importance of emergency endovascular treatment of acute ischemic stroke. Curr Neurol Neurosci Rep. 2016;16:42.
7. Qazi E, Al-Ajlan FS, Najm M, et al. The role of vascular imaging in the initial assessment of patients with acute ischemic stroke. Curr Neurol Neurosci Rep. 2016;16:32.
8. Saver JL, Goyal M, van der Lugt A, et al. Time to treatment with endovascular thrombectomy and outcomes from ischemic stroke: a meta-analysis. JAMA. 2016;316:1279–88.
9. Menon BK, Demchuk AM. Computed tomography angiography in the assessment of patients with stroke/TIA. Neurohospitalist. 2011;1:187–99.
10. Eswaradass P, Appireddy R, Evans J, et al. Imaging in acute stroke. Expert Rev Cardiovasc Ther. 2016;14:963–75.
11. Demchuk AM, Menon BK, Goyal M. Comparing vessel imaging: noncontrast computed tomography/computed tomographic angiography should be the new minimum standard in acute disabling stroke. Stroke. 2016;47:273–81.
12. Menon BK, d'Esterre CD, Qazi EM, et al. Multiphase CT angiography: a new tool for the imaging triage of patients with acute ischemic stroke. Radiology. 2015;275:510–20.
13. Menon BK, Qazi E, Nambiar V, et al. Differential effect of baseline computed tomographic angiography collaterals on clinical outcome in patients enrolled in the interventional management of stroke III trial. Stroke. 2015;46:1239–44.
14. Bal S, Bhatia R, Menon BK, et al. Time dependence of reliability of noncontrast computed tomography in comparison to computed tomography angiography source image in acute ischemic stroke. Int J Stroke. 2015;10:55–60.
15. d'Esterre CD, Boesen ME, Ahn SH, et al. Time-dependent computed tomographic perfusion thresholds for patients with acute ischemic stroke. Stroke. 2015;46:3390–7.

10 Principles and Practical Application of Brain MRI in Acute Ischemic Stroke

Bum Joon Kim

Abstract

Various pathomechanisms can cause acute ischemic stroke, and the treatment strategy differs according to the stroke mechanism. Therefore, rapid and accurate diagnosis of ischemic stroke is important. Furthermore, in the hyperacute stage, selecting appropriate patients who may benefit from reperfusion therapy is important. Despite several practical issues, multimodal MRI is useful for accurate diagnosis of acute ischemic stroke, for the evaluation of risks and benefits of reperfusion therapy, and finally for patient selection who may benefit from each treatment. The high sensitivity and specificity of diffusion-weighted image (DWI) helps in distinguishing acute ischemic stroke from stroke mimics. Furthermore, the lesion pattern on DWI reflects the underlying pathomechanism. The lesion mismatch between perfusion-weighted image (PWI) and DWI is thought to represent the potential salvageable tissue by reperfusion therapy. Signal changes of fluid-attenuated inversion recovery (FLAIR) image within DWI lesions may be a surrogate marker of tissue clock reflecting infarction age and might indicate the risk of hemorrhage after reperfusion treatment. Clot sign on gradient echo (GRE) image may reflect the nature of clot, and the location, length, and morphology of clot on GRE may provide predictive information on recanalization. Understanding the clinical implication of various findings of each sequences of multimodal MRI and comprehensively incorporating them into therapeutic decision-making may be a reasonable approach for expanding the indication of reperfusion treatment for acute ischemic stroke patients.

Rapid initial assessment and correct diagnosis of acute ischemic stroke are crucial. Though the diagnosis of stroke largely depends on the clinical presentation, imaging is useful for confirming the presence and the exact location of

B.J. Kim, M.D., Ph.D.
Department of Neurology, Kyung Hee University Hospital, Kyung Hee University College of Medicine, Seoul, South Korea
e-mail: medicj80@hanmail.net

S.-H. Lee (ed.), *Stroke Revisited: Diagnosis and Treatment of Ischemic Stroke*, Stroke Revisited, DOI 10.1007/978-981-10-1424-6_10

ischemic lesion, diagnosis of the underlying pathomechanism, prediction of the short- and long-term prognosis, and determination of the treatment strategy. Especially, multimodal magnetic resonance image (MRI) consists of various imaging sequences which are clinically valuable by each and by matched sequences. Multimodal MRI includes diffusion-weighted image (DWI), fluid-attenuated inversion recovery (FLAIR) image, gradient echo (GRE) image or susceptibility-weighted image (SWI), perfusion-weighted image (PWI), and MR angiography [1]. Advanced image such as high-resolution MRI (HR-MRI) gives additional information of the vessel wall pathology itself, which cannot be obtained by conventional MR angiography. The widely used mismatch concepts are PWI-DWI mismatch and the DWI-FLAIR mismatch.

Treatment strategy of stroke should not be determined based on information from a single sequence. Instead, the clinical significance of findings from each sequences of multimodal MRI must be fully understood, and the information from various sequences should be comprehensively considered when determining the treatment strategy of ischemic stroke [2]. This chapter shows what we have to look at from each sequences of multimodal MRI, and the usefulness of advance MRI techniques, in acute ischemic stroke patients.

10.1 Diffusion-Weighted Image: Lesion Pattern and Stroke Mechanism

DWI uses the Brownian motion of water molecules to generate contrast in MRI. Acute ischemic lesion appears as a hyperintense area on DWI and a hypointense on the corresponding area at apparent diffusion coefficient (ADC) map. This change occurs even within 3 min from the onset of ischemic stroke. At the subacute stage, ADC value continuously rises and becomes hyperintense after 2 weeks of stroke onset. DWI remains hyperintense due to the T2 shine-through effect. Therefore, ADC map is useful determining whether the lesions are in a single or multiple stages. Cerebral infarctions with multistage lesions have a higher chance to recur and may need more aggressive treatments. The accuracy in identifying ischemic lesions by DWI is high (88–100% sensitivity and 95–100% specificity). Therefore DWI is useful when the diagnosis is uncertain, in cases with stroke mimics.

Furthermore, small ischemic lesions at the cortex or posterior circulation, which are hardly visible by computed tomography (CT) at acute stage, can be easily detected by DWI. However, still in some cases with small brain stem infarction, the ischemic lesion can be initially negative on DWI, and follow-up DWI with a thin section can enhance the detection rate of those small brain stem lesions.

The treatment strategy of ischemic stroke highly depends on the mechanism of stroke. The characteristic ischemic lesion topography on DWI is useful for determining the mechanism of ischemic stroke. Several topographical types are representative of specific stroke mechanisms (Fig. 10.1) [3]:

- Multiple small scattered lesions in a single vascular territory: large artery atherosclerosis
  - Multiple small scattered cortical lesions only: extracranial artery disease
  - Perforator infarction in addition to multiple pial or border zone infarction: intracranial artery disease
- Single small subcortical infarction: small vessel occlusion
- Multiple territorial infarction: cardioembolic stroke or aortic arch disease
- Single large cortico-subcortical lesion: cardioembolic stroke

Specific lesion patterns are prone for a specific mechanism of stroke. For example, aortic arch embolism has a higher propensity of causing left hemisphere stroke, whereas cardioembolic stroke demonstrates a higher propensity to be located at the right hemisphere. Embolic stroke associated with patent foramen ovale (PFO) is dominantly found from the posterior circulation territory, which reflects the increased blood flow through the posterior circulation provoked by Valsalva

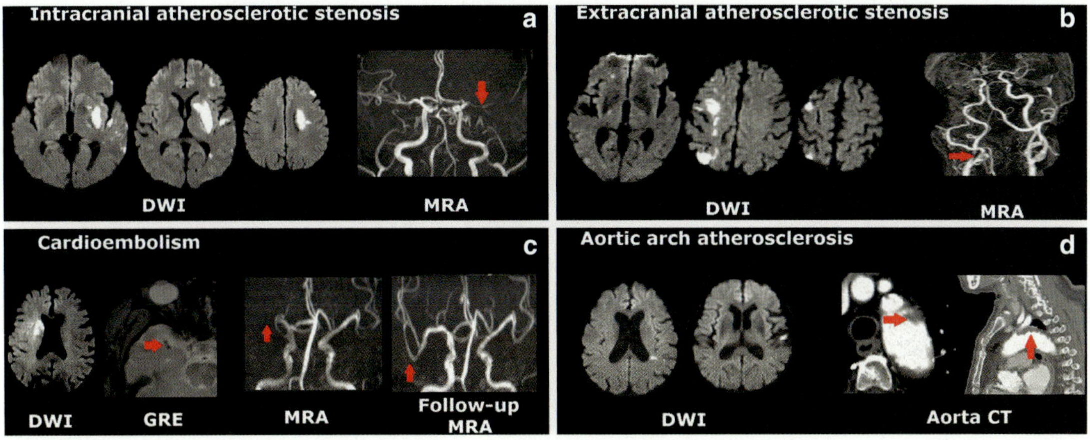

Fig. 10.1 Diffusion-weighted image lesion pattern according to stroke mechanism. Intracranial atherosclerotic stenosis (**a**), extracranial atherosclerotic stenosis (**b**), cardioembolism (**c**), and aortic arch atherosclerosis (**d**). Reproduced by permission of Journal of Stroke (Kim BJ, et al. J Stroke. 2014;16:131–45)

maneuver, which also increases the right-to-left shunt, simultaneously (paradoxical embolism) [4].

The volume of initial DWI lesion highly predicts the functional outcome of ischemic stroke. DWI volume less than 30–40 ml was associated with good outcome at 90 days after stroke. Benefit from intravenous thrombolysis was seen only with DWI lesions up to 25 ml. However, DWI >70 ml also demonstrated benefit from intravenous thrombolysis when the artery was recanalized. DWI lesion volume >100 ml is used as an indicator of malignant profile which predicts poor outcome.

10.2 Perfusion-Weighted Image: Imaging the Penumbra

Evaluation for the salvageable tissue is critical, selecting patients for reperfusion therapy in hyperacute stage of stroke. After a cerebral blood vessel is occluded, the core of the area develops infarction rapidly (ischemic core). However, though the neuronal function of the surrounding part is suspended, minimal blood flow supplied by collateral circulations maintains the viability of neurons. When the blood supply is restored, the neuronal activity of this area may be recovered. This conceptual area is named "penumbra," and when the difference between ischemic core and penumbra is large, it is regarded that the salvageable tissue is large, and the benefit of treatment can be large.

The perfusion status of the brain can be evaluated semiquantitatively by the PWI. The passage of contrast alters the local magnetic field and the signal intensity decreases rapidly in the surrounding brain tissue, due to the paramagnetic effect of the contrast. Echo-planar image technique is used to measure the signal intensity every second and voxel by voxel during the first 1 min after the injection of contrast. Finally, the time-concentration curve can be obtained from each voxel and the curve can be deconvolved by the arterial input function. The deconvolved curve is used to measure various parameters such as cerebral blood flow (CBF), cerebral blood volume (CBV), mean transit time (MTT), time to peak (TTP), and Tmax (Fig. 10.2):

- CBF: Blood supply in a given time period to the brain tissue. CBF is usually taken as the curve height at Tmax of the deconvolved curve. CBF most directly represents the final viability of the infarcted tissue.
- CBV: Whole blood quantity within the target area. CBV is presented as the area under the deconvolved curve. Initially, CBV increases by the dilation of blood vessels to maintain CBF in the infarcted tissue, but which decreases as the infarction evolves.

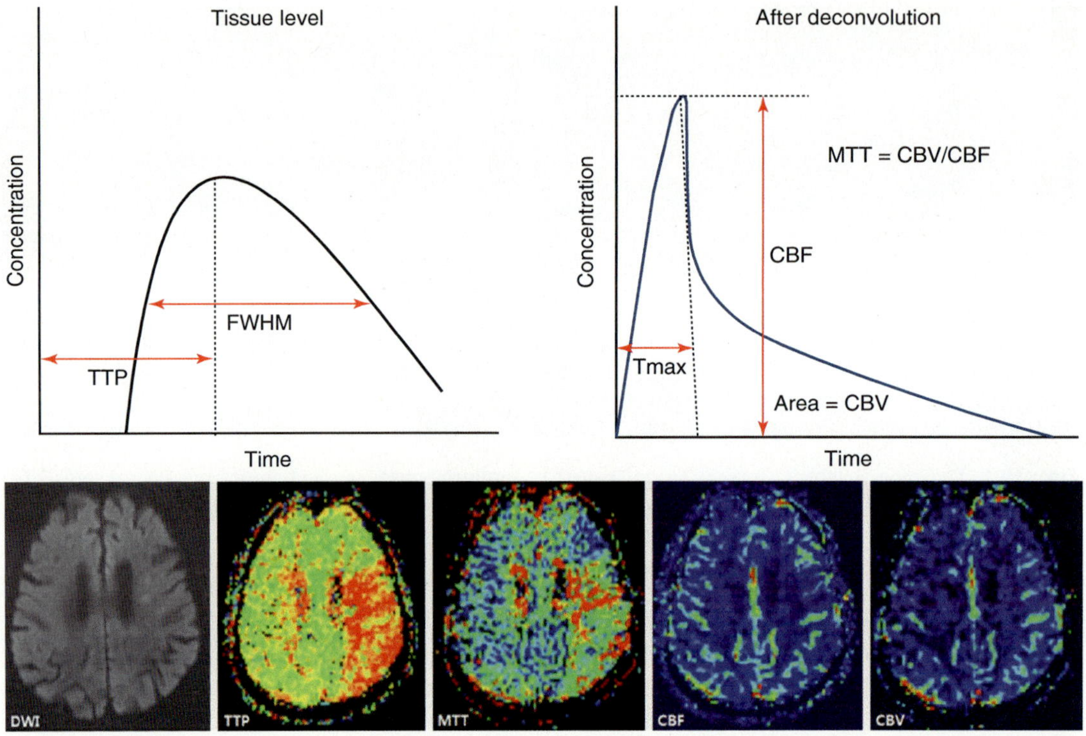

Fig. 10.2 Time-concentration curve at tissue level and after deconvolution. Various perfusion parameter maps are shown (*TTP* time to peak, *MTT* mean transit time, *CBF* cerebral blood flow, *CBV* cerebral blood volume). Reproduced by permission of Journal of Stroke (Kim BJ, et al. J Stroke. 2014;16:131–45)

- MTT: Average time required for the blood to enter the cerebral artery and maintain inside the tissue. MTT can be calculated by the following formula: [MTT = CBV/CBF]. MTT demonstrates the widest range of perfusion deficit and, therefore, may overestimate the true penumbra.
- Tmax: Time needed for the tissue residue function to reach maximum. Tmax is regarded as the most appropriate perfusion parameter representing the penumbra.

Though the optimal cutoff value of Tmax is still under debates, Tmax >6 s delay is most widely used to define the penumbra. PWI lesion visually exceeding 1.2–1.8 times of DWI lesion is considered as PWI-DWI mismatch positive. Patients with PWI-DWI mismatch demonstrated a more favorable outcome after thrombolysis than those without. However, using PWI-DWI mismatch solely in patient selection for thrombolysis failed to demonstrate a beneficial effect [5].

10.3 Gradient Echo or Susceptibility-Weighted Image: Microbleed and Clot Imaging

Cerebral microbleeds (CMBs) are small (2–10 mm) hypointense lesions observed from GRE or SWI, which are most often located at the deep structures (deep CMBs; Fig. 10.3a) or at the cortico-subcortical junctions (lobar CMBs; Fig. 10.3b). Deep CMBs have been closely linked to traditional vascular risk factors similar to small vessel disease (age and hypertension), whereas multiple lobar CMBs have been shown to be related to cerebral amyloid angiopathy or other degenerative diseases [6]. These conditions are bleeding prone, and large numbers of CMBs are associated with poor outcome of stroke. The risk of ICH after intravenous thrombolysis increases with the number of CMB in a dose-response relationship manner. The risk of ICH is higher in cases with lobar CMBs. But yet, it is not

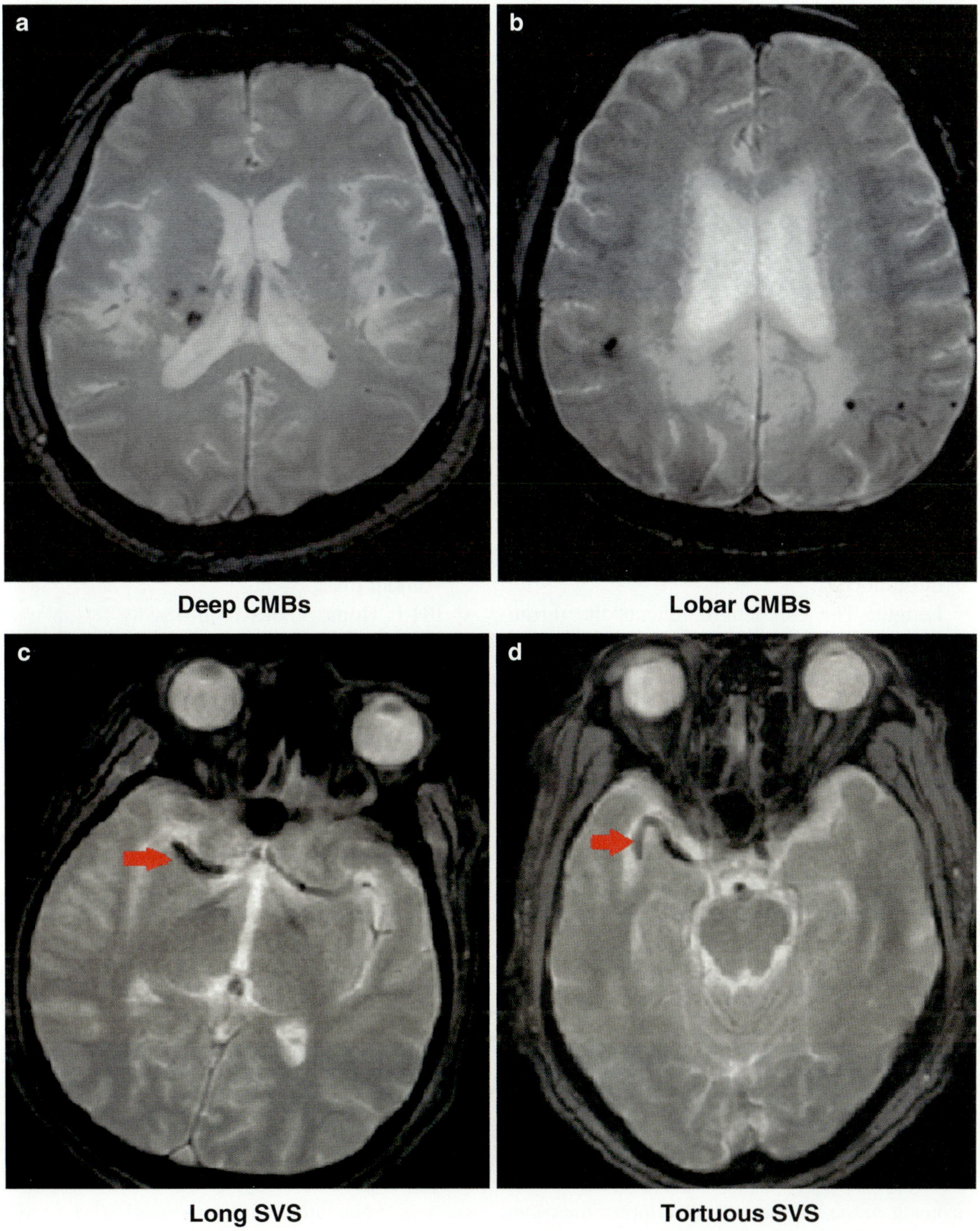

Fig. 10.3 Image findings from gradient echo. Deep cerebral microbleeds (**a**), lobar cerebral microbleeds (**b**), long susceptible vessel sign (**c**), and tortuous susceptible vessel sign (**d**). Reproduced by permission of Journal of Stroke (Kim BJ, et al. J Stroke. 2014;16:131–45)

conclusive weather CMBs should influence the decision-making in thrombolysis.

Ferromagnetic objects, such as red blood cells, distort the ambient field causing magnetic susceptibility artifacts. These artifacts enhance the detection of red blood cell-rich red thrombi clots, which are more common in cardioembolic strokes. Well-organized long-standing platelet-rich white thrombi are more resistant to thrombolytic therapy than fresh, fibrin-rich red thrombi. Therefore, susceptible vessel sign (SVS) itself may predict a higher possibility of recanalization. Several other factors of the SVS should be considered predicting the recanalization:

- Location: The recanalization rate by intravenous thrombolysis varies according to the occlusion site. Similarly, the location of SVS also matters; SVS of M1 is a strong predictor of recanalization failure after intravenous thrombolysis.
- Length: The clot length reflects the thrombotic burden of the clot. MCA occlusion with a SVS length >8 mm may have nearly no potential to be recanalized by intravenous thrombolysis (Fig. 10.3c).
- Morphology: Irregular or tortuous SVS decrease the possibility of successful thrombectomies in the M1 occlusion (Fig. 10.3d).

10.4 Evaluation for Risk of Hemorrhagic Transformation

Hemorrhagic transformation (HT) occurs after acute ischemic stroke and negatively affects the clinical outcome of stroke patients. The incidence of spontaneous HT occurs in one-third of patients with ischemic stroke. The increased permeability of the infarcted blood-brain barrier makes it prone for the extravasation of the blood component, especially when it is exposed to the restored blood flow. Disruption of the blood-brain barrier has been proposed to precede HT [7]. High initial severity, delayed treatment time, high blood pressure, large infarct core, and early ischemic sign on CT were factors associated with HT after thrombolysis.

MRI is also useful predicting HT after thrombolysis. A low ADC value, very low or absent apparent CBV or CBF (which demonstrates severe ischemic damage), large DWI lesion, and FLAIR hyperintensity within the DWI lesion (tissue clock) were associated with high chance of symptomatic HT. Considering the pathomechanism of HT, imaging directly indicating blood-brain barrier disruption may predict HT: (1) gadolinium enhancement of the CSF space on FLAIR image, (2) parenchymal enhancement of postcontrast T1-weighted image, and (3) direct permeability [8] image derived from PWI. HT can be classified as hemorrhagic infarction (HI: types I and II) and parenchymal hematoma (PH: types I and II) based on CT findings:

- HI-I: Isolated petechial staining of infarcted tissue without mass effect
- HI-II: Confluent petechiae in infarcted tissue without mass effect
- PH-I: Homogenous high-density lesion with minimal mass effect occupying less than 30% of the infarcted area
- PH-II: Lesion occupying more than 30% of the infarcted area with definite mass effect

10.5 FLAIR: Leukoaraiosis and Tissue Clock

FLAIR image is obtained by an inversion recovery technique that nulls fluids and suppresses the cerebrospinal fluid signals and thereby enhances the detection of cortical lesions. Furthermore, FLAIR image also demonstrates the burden of old subcortical white matter lesions (leukoaraiosis). Several scales are developed to present the burden of periventricular white matter and deep white matter changes, quantitatively, and severe leukoaraiosis was associated with increased ICH or HT after thrombolysis. However, as the net benefit of thrombolysis was persistent regardless to the presence of leukoaraiosis, there is no evidence to avoid thrombolysis in these patients.

The onset of stroke is very important regarding that reperfusion treatments are limited by time. The signal intensity of FLAIR image increases with a rise of water content inside the infarcted tissue caused by the disruption of blood-brain barrier (vasogenic edema). Therefore, DWI-FLAIR mismatch, a lesion visible on DWI but not FLAIR, reflects the lesion age (tissue clock) and can be helpful for the determination of thrombolysis in unclear-onset stroke patients (Fig. 10.4). DWI-FLAIR mismatch lesions are likely to be within the therapeutic time window for thrombolysis (specificity,

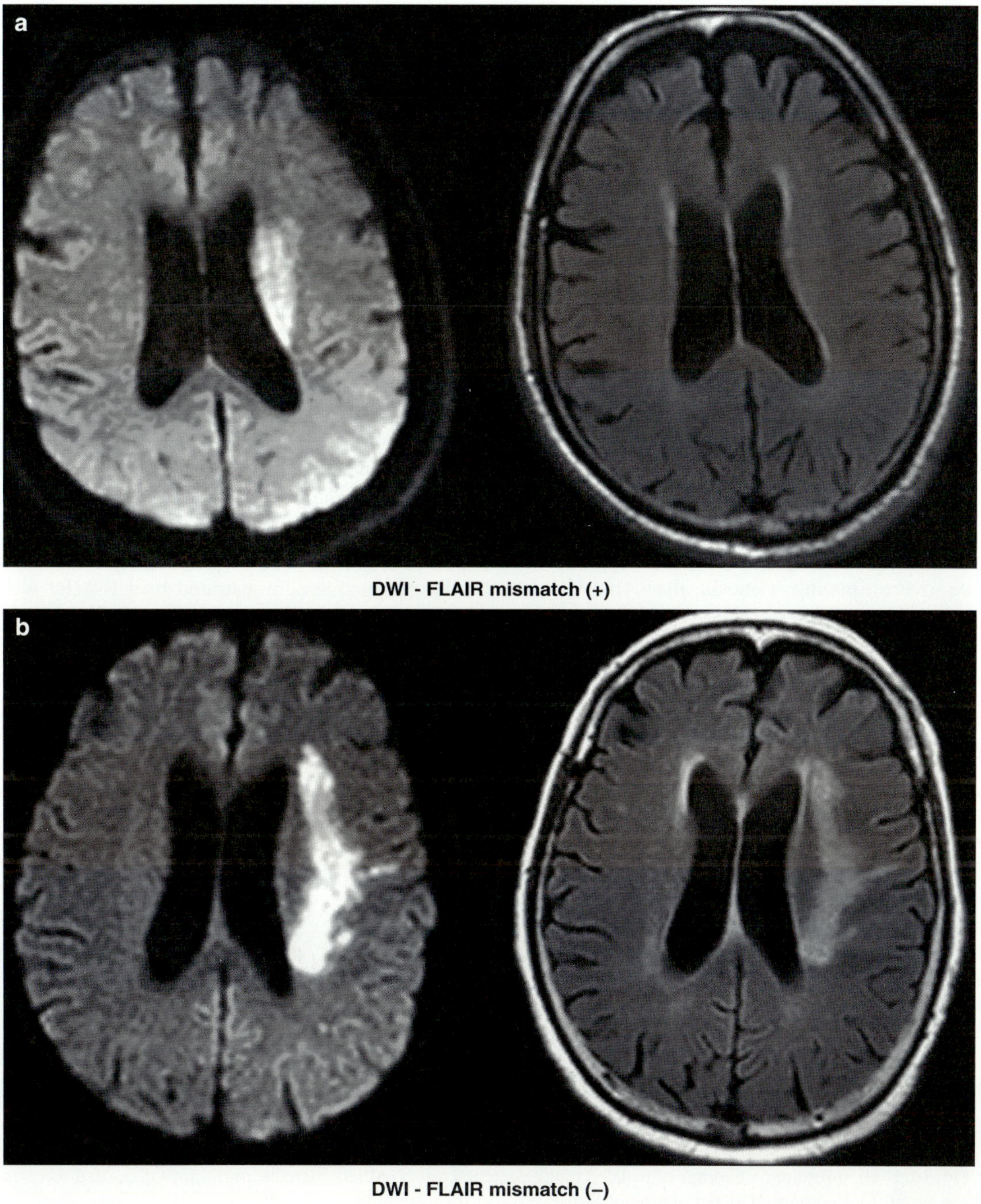

Fig. 10.4 DWI-FLAIR mismatch. Positive (**a**) and negative (**b**) cases. Reproduced by permission of Journal of Stroke (Kim BJ, et al. J Stroke. 2014;16:131–45)

93%, and positive predictive value, 94%). Finally some clinical trials using DWI-FLAIR mismatch for the selection of patients in unclear-onset stroke demonstrated promising results. However, potential confounders such as age and lesion volume affect the FLAIR change, and issues stemming from inter-rater reliability are still a problem to be solved.

10.6 MR Angiography: Site and Severity of the Steno-Occlusive Lesion

MR angiography is a set of vascular imaging techniques capable of depicting the extracranial (contrast-enhanced MR angiography; CE) and intracranial arteries (time-of-flight MR angiography; TOF). TOF MR angiography uses repeated radio frequency to saturate stationary tissue which shows relatively low signal. By contrast, flowing blood in cerebral arteries has relatively increased signal as it continuously carries unsaturated spins into the imaging volume. Therefore, TOF MR angiography is flow dependent and can be overestimating stenosis than the CE MR angiography.

MR angiography gives information about the site and severity of steno-occlusive lesion. Usually, stenosis more than 50% is regarded as a significant stenosis. Significant stenosis at the corresponding artery can cause stroke by artery-to-artery embolization, local branch occlusion of the perforators, perfusion deficits, and combination of these pathomechanisms. Furthermore, stenosis less than 50% can also cause stroke in the intracranial arteries by obliterating the orifice of perforators (small vessel occlusion; branch atheromatous disease).

The recanalization rate after intravenous thrombolysis highly depends on the site of occlusion; the rate of recanalization is low in ICA or M1 occlusion. Therefore, additional intra-arterial approach may be highly considered in those cases from the beginning of treatment. Considering intra-arterial thrombectomy, the technical difficulty and risk of complication during the approach inside the vasculature can be affected by the atherosclerosis burden and tortuosity of proximal vessels. Therefore, MR angiography may help planning intra-arterial treatment.

10.7 High-Resolution Vessel Wall MRI: Vessel Wall Pathology

Conventional MR angiography only demonstrates the lumen of cerebral vessels. However, HR-MRI may give additional information of the vessel wall pathology. The character of atherosclerotic plaque demonstrated by HR-MRI well correlated with the pathologic specimen (MRI-histologic correlation), and therefore, vulnerable plaques can be identified by HR-MRI. Especially, HR-MRI is useful detecting the pathomechanism of stenosis in intracranial cerebral arteries. The imaging characteristics of various mechanisms underlying intracranial stenosis are as follows (Fig. 10.5) [9]:

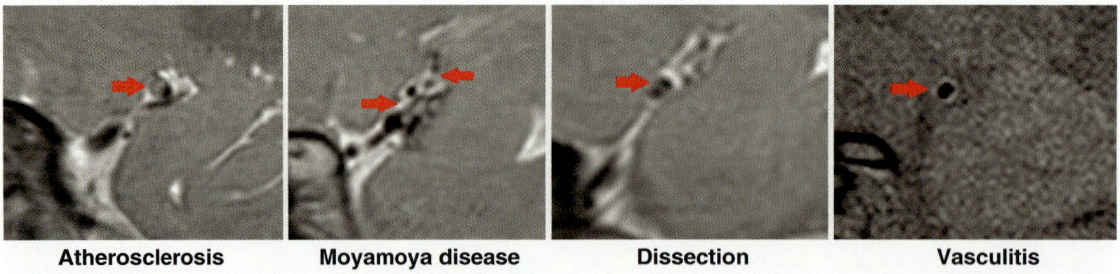

Fig. 10.5 High-resolution findings of isolated middle cerebral artery. Atherosclerosis, moyamoya disease, dissection, and vasculitis. Reproduced by permission of Stroke [9]

- Atherosclerosis: Eccentric, irregular wall thickening; gadolinium enhancement of the plaque may reflect the instability of plaque.
- Moyamoya disease: Concentric narrowing of the vessel lumen without an eccentric wall thickening or a plaque; extensive development of basal collateral vessels.
- Dissection: Dissecting flap or eccentric wall thickening associated with T1 bright wall components (intramural hematoma).
- Vasculitis: Smooth circumferential concentric wall thickening with diffuse gadolinium enhancement of the inflamed wall.

Furthermore, HR-MRI also demonstrated early atherosclerotic changes (small atherosclerotic plaques) which were not observed from the conventional MR angiography. The characteristics of patients with small plaques observed from HR-MRI (but normal MR angiography) were more similar to those with large artery atherosclerosis.

Conclusion

Multimodal MRI reveals various useful parameters for determining the treatment strategy of acute stroke. Multimodal MRI gives advantage when the diagnosis, the underlying stroke mechanism, and the onset of stroke are uncertain. Furthermore, multimodal MRI helps evaluating the risk and benefit of reperfusion therapy. In spite of these benefits, several practical issues exist limiting the use of MRI in the acute stage of cerebral infarction. One of them are the long scan time in comparison with CT. Recently multimodal MRI using echo-planar FLAIR and GRE image is under investigation to solve this issue. However, still depending on a single or a few parameters should be avoided in selecting appropriate patients for thrombolytic therapy. Instead, understanding and comprehensively combining the information from each MRI sequence (i.e., DWI, FLAIR, GRE, and PWI) and using various mismatch parameters (DWI-FLAIR mismatch and/or PWI-DWI mismatch) may be more helpful in establishing an indication of MRI-based thrombolysis (Fig. 10.6).

Suggestions from Clinical Practice Guidelines Diffusion-weighted imaging (DWI) visualizes infarct lesion by cytotoxic edema very accurately. When perfusion imaging by computed tomography or magnetic resonance imaging is analyzed with DWI, infarct core and penumbra may be estimated at that time, which can be used for selection of eligible patients for intravenous fibrinolysis and/or mechanical thrombectomy. With this information, causes, pathophysiology, lesion extent, and recanalization status can be obtained. However, these techniques are not mandatory in emergency setting for now because of possible neglect or delay in emergency care. Smart application is critical in individual patients.

Sequence	Basic principles	Clinical implications
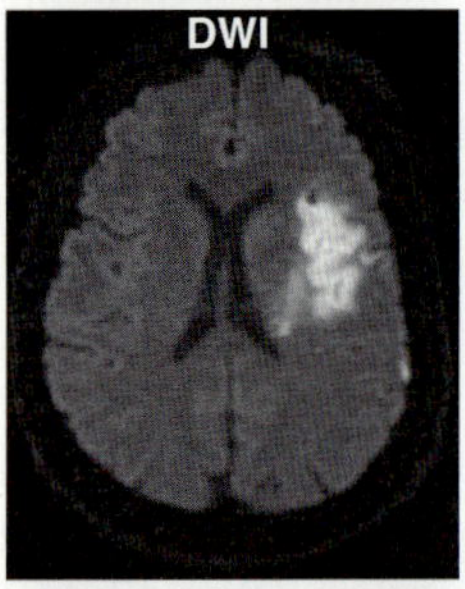	Represents area with cytotoxic edema.	• Appears rapidly after ischemic insult. • High specificity and sensitivity of detecting ischemia. • The mechanism of stroke affects the lesion pattern.
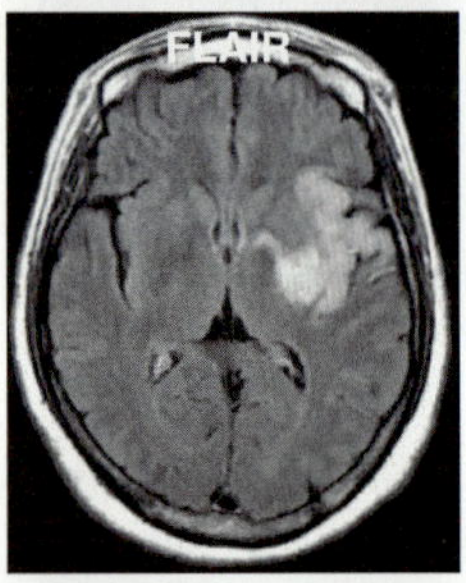	Represents the area with vasogenic edema	• Demonstrate the time from stroke onset (lesion age; DWI-FLAIR mismatch) • Visible lesion increases the risk of hemorrhage after reperfusion therapy. • Helpful evaluating the burden of old white matter ischemic change.
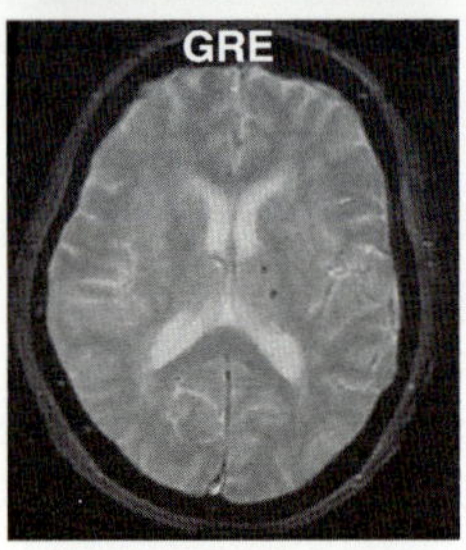	Susceptibility artifact enhances the detection of ferromagnetic material (i.e. blood).	• Sensitive to detect hemorrhagic infarction or hemorrhagic transformation. • Detects Cerebral microbleeds • Susceptible vessel sign is associated with red-blood cell rich clot, usually cardioembolism.
PWI 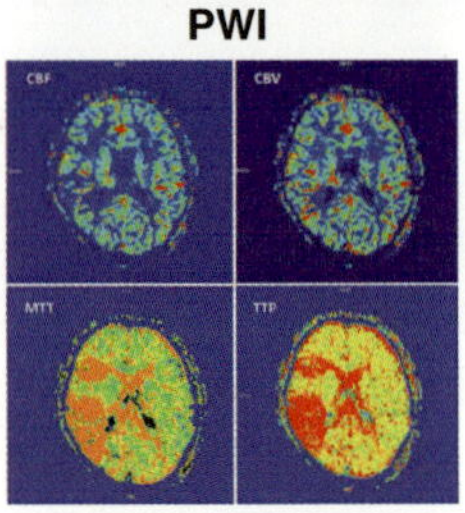	Represents the area with perfusion defect	Represents the penumbra and the potential benefit of recanalization (PWI-DWI mismatch)
MRA 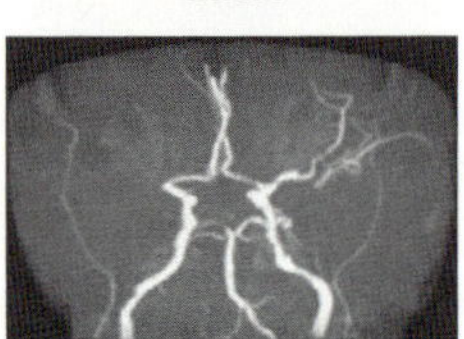	Represents the site and severity of stenosis	• Essential for determining the stroke mechanism. • Gives additional information of the possibility of recanalization after thrombolysis.

Fig. 10.6 Basic principles and clinical implications of multimodal MRI (*DWI* diffusion-weighted image, *FLAIR* fluid-attenuated inversion recovery image, *GRE* gradient echo image, *PWI* perfusion-weighted image, *MRA* magnetic resonance angiography, *CT* computed tomography)

References

1. Baird AE, Warach S. Magnetic resonance imaging of acute stroke. J Cereb Blood Flow Metab. 1998;18:583–609.
2. Campbell BC, Tu HT, Christensen S, et al. Assessing response to stroke thrombolysis: validation of 24-hour multimodal magnetic resonance imaging. Arch Neurol. 2012;69:46–50.
3. Kang DW, Chalela JA, Ezzeddine MA, et al. Association of ischemic lesion patterns on early diffusion-weighted imaging with toast stroke subtypes. Arch Neurol. 2003;60:1730–4.
4. Kim BJ, Sohn H, Sun BJ, et al. Imaging characteristics of ischemic strokes related to patent foramen ovale. Stroke. 2013;44:3350–6.
5. Nagakane Y, Christensen S, Ogata T, et al. Moving beyond a single perfusion threshold to define penumbra: a novel probabilistic mismatch definition. Stroke. 2012;43:1548–55.
6. Song TJ, Kim J, Song D, et al. Association of cerebral microbleeds with mortality in stroke patients having atrial fibrillation. Neurology. 2014;83:1308–15.
7. Khatri R, McKinney AM, Swenson B, et al. Blood-brain barrier, reperfusion injury, and hemorrhagic transformation in acute ischemic stroke. Neurology. 2012;79:S52–7.
8. Bang OY, Buck BH, Saver JL, et al. Prediction of hemorrhagic transformation after recanalization therapy using T2*-permeability magnetic resonance imaging. Ann Neurol. 2007;62:170–6.
9. Ahn SH, Lee J, Kim YJ, et al. Isolated MCA disease in patients without significant atherosclerotic risk factors: a high-resolution magnetic resonance imaging study. Stroke. 2015;46:697–703.

11 Identification of Stroke Mechanism: Stroke Classification

Seung-Hoon Lee

Abstract

In this chapter, the subtypes of stroke will be introduced to the readers. The classification of stroke into subtypes is not only for listing the causes of stroke through an academic approach but also helps in identifying the physiological behavior of stroke, which will help the physicians apply the optimal therapy to the patient, with a view to improving the prognosis of the patients. The most commonly used classification systems are the Oxfordshire Community Stroke Project (OCSP) classification system and the Trial of ORG 10172 in Acute Stroke Treatment (TOAST) classification system. Here, the readers will be introduced to both these classification systems and will be allowed to have a glimpse into their strengths and weaknesses.

If a patient who is suspected of having a stroke arrives at the emergency room, the first thing that must be done is to check the history of the patient, followed by the conduct of neurological tests, and the provision of immediate emergency care. A brain computed tomography (CT) scan should be performed as soon as possible to determine whether the patient is having an ischemic stroke or a hemorrhagic stroke, and if the criteria are met, intravenous thrombolysis or intra-arterial thrombectomy should be performed. During this process, if the patient has an ischemic stroke, the subtype of the stroke has to be identified based on the information gathered so far from the diagnosis process. There are limited information available in the initial stage of the treatment, and as such, it may be difficult to identify the correct stroke subtype. This notwithstanding, it is important for the physician to do his or her best to diagnose the stroke subtype. It is an appropriate treatment approach to change the subtype diagnosis as more information becomes available because the disease behavior differs by stroke subtype, making it appropriate to consider the stroke subtypes as totally different diseases. This may significantly change the prognosis of the stroke in the future, and the medical and surgical

S.-H. Lee, M.D., Ph.D., F.A.H.A.
Department of Neurology, Seoul National University Hospital, 101 Daehak-ro, Jongno-gu, Seoul 03080, South Korea
e-mail: sb0516@snu.ac.kr

S.-H. Lee (ed.), *Stroke Revisited: Diagnosis and Treatment of Ischemic Stroke*, Stroke Revisited, DOI 10.1007/978-981-10-1424-6_11

treatment to prevent recurrence may also differ significantly. Incidence rates of early neurological deterioration may even differ according to their stroke subtypes. Therefore, it is more helpful for the patient to identify the stroke subtype as early as possible. The recent progress in the brain magnetic resonance imaging (MRI) technology allows the blood flow in the brain and the process of brain stroke to be observed almost in real time. In addition, various kinds of multidimensional tests including hematological or imaging methods can be performed to find out the embolic source. With this, it has now become possible to diagnose the stroke subtype earlier than before and to provide a more personalized secondary preventive treatment to stroke patients.

11.1 Classification Methods of Ischemic Stroke

The purpose of classifying strokes is to make a decision regarding the basic direction of treatments to be provided to the patient. Such classification is used to describe the characteristics of the patient's stroke. In spite of the recent progress in the diagnostic test technologies, it is still true that the causes of stroke are not identified in 25–40% of the patients and is dependent upon the quality, completeness, and timing of the tests performed. As such, a stroke with an unrevealed cause is called "cryptogenic stroke." When classifying stroke, certain overlapping risk factors need to be considered, making it difficult to determine which of the two or more subtypes is correct. For example, in the case of a patient who has severe carotid artery stenosis and atrial fibrillation (AF), it is difficult to determine which of the two conditions arouses the present stroke.

The classification of strokes is based on the unified and standardized systems of classification, both in the academic and clinical domains. This is a result of decades of endeavors. The classification of the disease is not standardized across the world, however, due to the differences in the healthcare system and environment of countries. The United Kingdom (UK) and some British Commonwealth countries use the Oxfordshire Community Stroke Project (OCSP) classification system [1], while others use the Trial of ORG 10172 in Acute Stroke Treatment (TOAST) classification system [2], sometimes with minor modifications. These two subjects will be covered briefly herein.

11.1.1 Oxfordshire Community Stroke Project (OCSP) Classification System

OCSP classification was originally suggested to confirm the characteristics of the subjects in an epidemiological study in Oxfordshire, UK [1]. At that time, the researchers had to comply with their classification methods that were allowed under the UK's public healthcare system. All stroke patients were treated by primary care physicians in UK. Physical examination and CT were the diagnostic methods for stroke patients, but they had no other method to diagnose relevant problems in the cerebral vessels. For this reason, the researchers of OCSP chose to classify stroke patients only using physical examinations, based on the location and size of the ischemic stroke (Table 11.1). As the size and location of the stroke are not determined by the cause of the stroke, the analysis of the cause of stroke under this system is too difficult. A patient whose stroke is classified as lacunar stroke can still be having an embolic stroke. In contrast, this system is very easy to use in classifying stroke patients, and registration of the patient is rarely missed with a higher level of interobserver reliability. Because the prognosis of the patient is determined by the initial severity of the stroke, the estimation of the prognosis is relatively correct considering that the cause of the stroke is not known [3].

11.1.2 Trial of ORG 10172 in Acute Stroke Treatment (TOAST) Classification System

The earliest stroke classification system was the Stroke Data Bank Subtype Classification system

Table 11.1 OSCP classification

Type of infarct	Diagnosis
Cerebral infarction	If a CT scan performed within 28 days of symptom onset shows an area of low attenuation, no relevant abnormality, or an area of irregular high attenuation within a larger area of low attenuation (i.e., an area of hemorrhagic infarction) or if a necropsy examination shows an area of cerebral infarction (pale or hemorrhagic) in a region compatible with the clinical signs and symptoms
Lacunar infarct (LACI)	One of the four classic clinical lacunar syndromes. Patients with faciobrachial or brachiocrural deficits are included, but more restricted deficits are not
Total anterior circulation infarct (TACI)	Combination of new higher cerebral dysfunction (e.g., dysphasia, dyscalculia, visuospatial disorders), homonymous visual field defect, and ipsilateral motor and/or sensory deficit of at least two areas of the face, arm, and leg. If the conscious level is impaired and formal testing of higher cerebral function or the visual fields is not possible, a deficit is assumed
Partial anterior circulation infarct (PACI)	Only two of the three components of the TACI syndrome, with higher dysfunction alone, or with a motor/sensory deficit more restricted than those classified as LACI (e.g., confined to one limb, or to the face and hand but not the whole arm)
Posterior circulation infarcts (POCIs)	Any of the following: ipsilateral cranial nerve palsy with contralateral motor and/or sensory deficit, bilateral motor and/or sensory deficit, disorder of conjugate eye movement, cerebellar dysfunction without ipsilateral long-tract deficit (i.e., ataxic hemiparesis), or isolated homonymous visual field defect

OCSP Oxfordshire Community Stroke Project

[4]. It was composed of five classes developed when the National Institute of Neurological Disorders and Stroke (NINDS) established the Stroke Data Bank for the first time. These classes were brain hemorrhage, brain infarction (atherothrombotic and tandem arterial pathological abnormalities), cardioembolic stroke, lacunar stroke, and stroke from rare causes or with an undetermined etiology. Since 1993, almost all the clinical researchers in the world have been using the classification system suggested by the TOAST clinical researchers [2]. This classification method was originally intended to be used for comparing and analyzing the effect of danaparoid among the different subtypes of stroke. The basic principle of classification in this method was not significantly different from that of the Stroke Data Bank Subtype Classification system. The TOAST researchers originally divided stroke cases into eleven groups and then narrowed these down to five (Table 11.2). This classification method has the highest internal validity when the planned algorithms are followed strictly. Possible errors in classification are mostly corrected by discussion and agreement between specialized researchers. In the case of the lacunar stroke, however, which is defined by the clinical conditions and size of the stroke, there is still a risk of misclassification, where large-artery atherosclerosis (LAA) is mistaken as small-vessel occlusion (SVO) if there is an atherosclerotic artery that is too tiny to be spotted and clearly seen on MRI. As the definition of LAA includes 50% or more stenosis in the relevant arteries, it is still possible that a patient who is certain to have LAA can be classified with an undetermined etiology. It is also true that depending on the level of experience of the physician, the stroke cause may still be undetermined even if one of the candidate causes looks more promising. In this classification method, the ratio of undetermined causes is overestimated. Furthermore, while the cardioembolic stroke causes are classified into high- and medium-risk factors, patent foramen ovale (PFO), which has a high prevalence rate among normal individuals, is also a medium-risk factor. PFO may not be counted as cardioembolic causes and may be included in some cases. Accordingly, many researchers modify the TOAST classification system to suit their purposes. As there is no single modified version of this classification that is widely supported, however, it would suffice for the readers to understand the concept of the TOAST system clearly.

Table 11.2 TOAST classification

Type of infarct	Diagnosis
Large-artery atherosclerosis	Clinical evidence of cortical, subcortical, brain stem, or cerebellar dysfunction with more than 50% lesion or occlusion in an extracranial or intracranial vessel in the distribution of an infarct larger than 1.5 cm by CT or MRI. This diagnosis cannot be made if arterial studies show no evidence of pathology or if there is reasonable suggestion by history or studies that another mechanism is possible
Cardioembolism (high risk/medium risk)	Clinical evidence of cortical, subcortical, brain stem, or cerebellar dysfunction with a lesion size larger than 1.5 cm on CT or MRI and the presence of at least one high-risk (e.g., atrial fibrillation or mechanical heart valve) or medium-risk (e.g., lone atrial fibrillation or patent foramen ovale) cardiac pathology on diagnostic studies (electrocardiogram, rhythm strip, 24-h cardiac monitoring, transthoracic, or transesophageal echocardiography). Evidence of transient ischemic attacks or strokes in more than one vascular territory or of systemic emboli supports the diagnosis. Finally, other categories (large artery, small artery) must be excluded
Small-vessel occlusion (lacunar)	A lacunar syndrome (pure motor, sensorimotor, pure sensory, ataxia hemiparesis, dysarthria-clumsy hand) with normal CT or MRI or a lesion smaller than 1.5 cm on CT or MRI in the territories supplied by small-vessel penetrators. Large-artery and cardiac sources must be excluded
Stroke of other determined etiology	Stroke caused by nonatherosclerotic vasculopathies, hypercoaguable states, or hematologic disorders and other rare causes of stroke after diagnostic testing. Other categories must be excluded
Stroke of undetermined etiology (cryptogenic)	This diagnosis is made if two or more etiologies of stroke are possible, a complete evaluation reveals no possible source, or the patient had an incomplete evaluation

TOAST Trial of ORG 10,172 in Acute Stroke Treatment

11.2 Stroke Cases Classified Using the TOAST Classification System

To understand the classification and behavior of stroke, thrombosis, the main reason for the occlusion of the blood vessels, must first be understood. Thrombosis is the final product of the blood coagulation process and mainly consists of two parts: the platelet plugs and the fibrin meshwork. Normally, the conditions leading to the generation of thrombosis are collectively known as "Virchow's triad," which are (1) damages to the endothelial cells, trauma or arthrosclerosis; (2) abnormal blood flow, loss of laminar flow due to the delay of the flow in the veins or the turbulences in the arteries; and (3) hypercoagulability [5]. The thrombi can be classified into white thrombi, mostly composed of platelet plugs; red thrombi, mainly composed of red blood cells; and mixed thrombi, mixtures of the two. In stroke, all the three types of thrombi occur and are based on the type of thrombus that contributed most to the condition; the initial progress, the effectiveness of the treatment during the acute phase, and the treatment approaches for prognosis and secondary prevention are likely to be different. It is critical to identify the mechanism of thrombosis as well as relevant risk factors for the proper diagnosis and treatment of a stroke patient.

11.2.1 LAA

First, let me introduce the concept of the term large artery. This term is not basically used in the traditional anatomy, and it is not appropriate to understand it to be different from the small vessels based on the vascular histology. There are no clear definitions on the terms, but I suggest the following working definition: a blood vessel stemming from the vessels traveling toward the brain (aorta, brachiocephalic trunk, and common carotid artery) to those running the subarachnoid space in the brain. For more information, kindly refer to "Pathophysiology of Stroke," to be published as one of the *Stroke Revisited* series by the publisher, Springer Nature Inc.

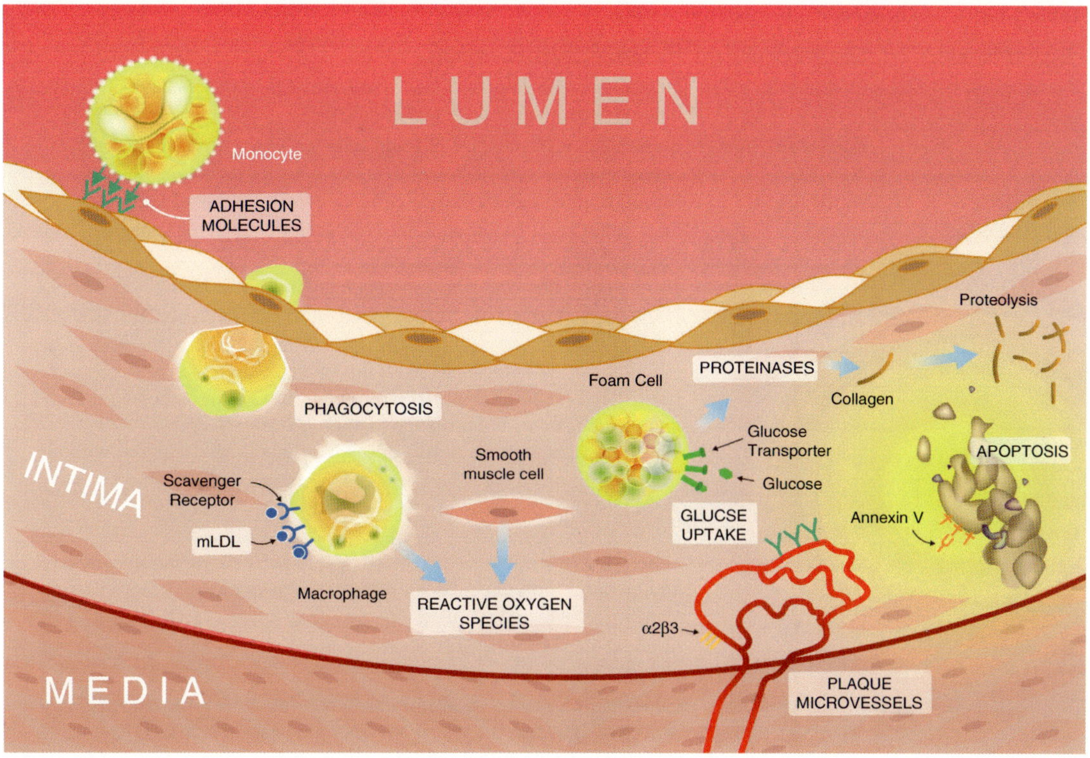

Fig. 11.1 Progression of atherosclerotic lesion (shown as time sequence from left to right)

The most important etiology of stroke among the vascular diseases in large arteries is atherosclerosis. Atherosclerosis is a chronic inflammatory disease mainly caused by the lipid on the walls of the artery due to innate and adaptive immunity. At first, it accompanies a functional disorder of the endothelial cells while the wall is exposed to an excessive amount of low-density lipoprotein (LDL), causing the LDL to pile up inside the intima (Fig. 11.1). With continued exposure to vascular risk factors (e.g., hypertension, diabetes, smoking, infection, stress, etc.), the damages to the endothelial cells are aggravated, and these damaged cells cause more LDL particles to be accumulated on the extracellular matrix. As a result, this area suffers the most from free radicals and cytokines. The modified LDL activates various inflammatory reactions. The main mechanism is the infiltration of the monocyte cells, which plays the most profound role in innate immunity. Monocytes come inside and reach the subendothelial areas to be differentiated into macrophages by the macrophage colony-stimulating factors. Macrophages accept the modified LDLs easily and develop pattern recognition receptors on the surface. Then it becomes lipid-containing macrophages and finally foam cells. The accumulation of foam cells leads to a disease in the arterial system through the movement of the vascular smooth muscle cells and the formation of a fibrous cap. Vascular status like this is called is "atherosclerotic plaques." The atherosclerotic plaques proceed to develop into thrombosis, which is the cause of LAA-related stroke.

Stable atherosclerotic plaques rarely result in stroke. Unstable or vulnerable plaques are the cause of LAA-related stroke. Most of these observations have originated from the coronary artery study reports. The World Health Organization (WHO) classified atherosclerotic plaques for the first time in 1958 [6]. Four classes were identified: fatty streak, atheroma, fibrous plaque, and complicated lesion. In the mid-1990s, the

Table 11.3 Classification of atherosclerotic lesion

Type of lesion	Subtype of lesion	Morphological description
Nonatherosclerotic intimal lesions	Intimal thickening	Natural accumulation of smooth muscle cells in the absence of lipid, macrophage foam cells, and thrombosis
	Intimal xanthoma	Superficial accumulation of foam cells without a necrotic core, fibrous cap, or thrombosis
Progressive atherosclerotic lesions	Pathological intimal thickening	Plaque rich in smooth muscle cells, with hyaluronan and proteoglycan matrix and focal accumulation of extracellular lipid. Absence of thrombosis
	Fibroatheroma	During early necrosis: focal macrophage infiltration into areas of lipid pools with an overlying fibrous cap. During late necrosis: loss of matrix and extensive cellular debris with an overlying fibrous cap. With or without calcification. Absence of thrombosis
	Intraplaque hemorrhage or plaque fissure	Large necrotic core (size >10% of plaque area) with hemorrhage and plaque area shows the presence of angiogenesis. Necrotic core communicates with the lumen through a fissure. Minimal tear without obvious thrombus
	Thin-cap fibroatheroma	A thin, fibrous cap (<65 μm) infiltrated by macrophages and lymphocytes, with rare or no smooth muscle cells and relatively large underlying necrotic core (>10% of plaque area). Intraplaque hemorrhage and/or fibrin might be present. Absence of thrombosis
Lesions with acute thrombi	Plaque rupture	Thin-cap fibroatheroma with cap disruption. Thrombosis is present and might or might not be occlusive. The luminal thrombus communicates with the underlying necrotic core
	Plaque erosion	Can occur on pathological intimal thickening or on a fibroatheroma. Thrombosis is present and might or might not be occlusive. No communication of the thrombus with the necrotic core
	Calcified nodule	Eruptive (shedding) of calcified nodule with an underlying fibrocalcific plaque with minimal or no necrosis. Thrombosis is usually not occlusive
Healed lesions	Healed plaque rupture, erosion, or calcified nodule	Healed lesion composed of smooth muscle cells, proteoglycans, and collagen type III with or without underlying disrupted fibrous cap, necrotic core, or nodular calcification. Lesions can contain large areas of calcification with few inflammatory cells and have a small or no necrotic core. The fibrotic or fibrocalcific collagen-rich plaque is associated with significant luminal stenosis. Absence of thrombosis

Reproduced by permission of Nature Reviews Cardiology [8]

American Heart Association (AHA) recommendeds new classification criteria for atherosclerotic plaque (Table 11.3; Fig. 11.2) [7, 8]. This classification was followed by recommendations from several researchers who found out that plaque erosion could result in coronary thrombosis, which further refined the classification system. Currently, the pathological classification of coronary artery atherosclerosis is based on this system, and the classification of atherosclerotic plaque on the cerebral artery is yet to be suggested. With minor differences in vascular histology among the organs, cerebral atherosclerotic process is not likely to be different from coronary atherosclerosis. Therefore, it is appropriate to understand ischemic stroke due to LAA from the classification system of coronary atherosclerosis. As the classification states, atherosclerotic plaques, which result in thrombosis, consist in plaque rupture, plaque erosion, and calcified nodules. Such lesions stimulate and activate platelets, and this marks the beginning of thrombosis. Later, due to the activated platelets, the platelets adhere to the atherosclerotic lesion and aggregate to form primary plugs. Due to the activation of clotting factors, the primary plugs condensate by fibrin meshwork, which completes the process of generating thrombosis. In this way, the thrombi that originate from a stroke caused by LAA are mainly white thrombi, while the thrombi

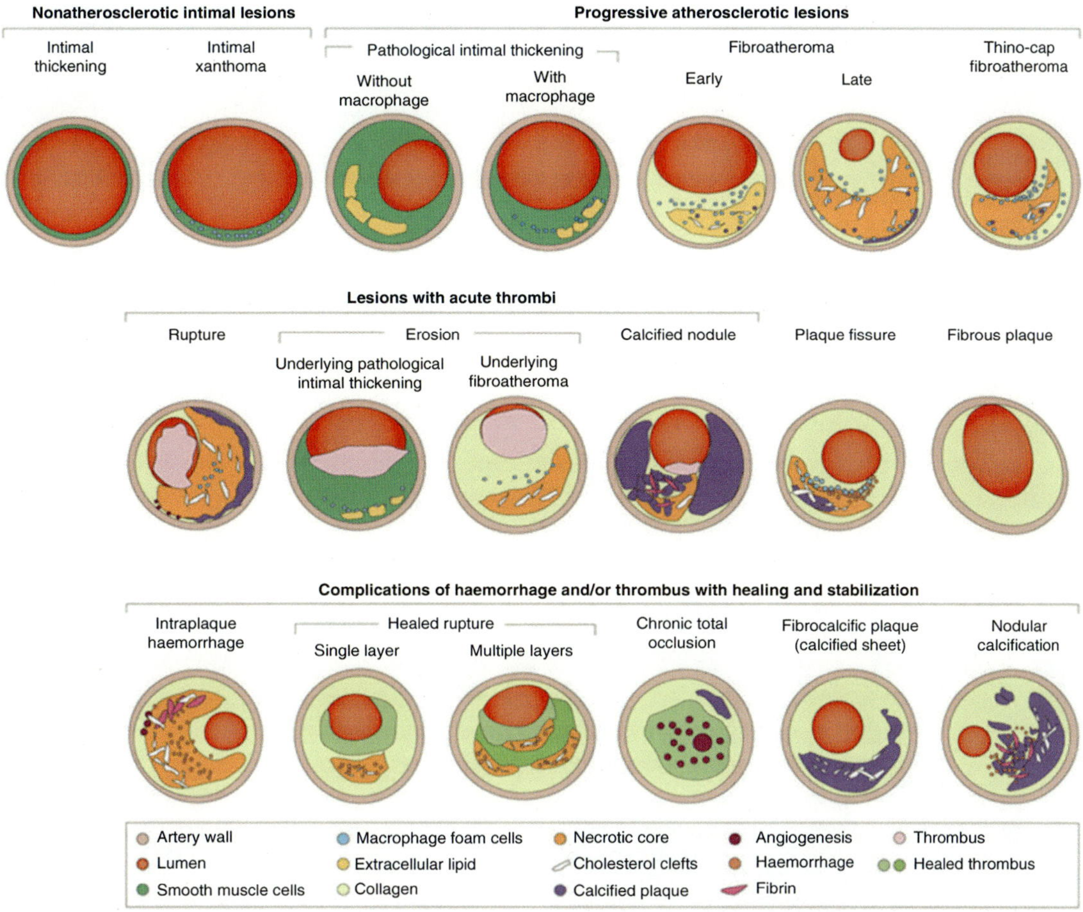

Fig. 11.2 Human coronary lesion morphologies categorized as nonatherosclerotic intimal lesions, progressive atherosclerotic lesions, lesions with acute thrombi, and complications of hemorrhage and/or thrombus with healing and stabilization. Reproduced by permission of Nature Reviews Cardiology [8]

generated from CE are basically red thrombi. Atherosclerotic plaque, which functions as the cause of thrombosis, is mostly attributable to plaque rupture, followed by plaque erosion and calcified nodule. These are the incidences in the coronary events, and it is yet to be confirmed if the incidences will be reproduce in the LAA-related stroke.

Briefly speaking, atherosclerosis, which may have been growing for years or even decades, develops into acute thrombosis due to a certain trigger, such as acute rupture. LAA-related stroke is divided into two kinds, depending on how the thrombi block the vessels. First one is in situ thrombosis, which blocks the cerebral vessel at the atherosclerotic lesion inducing thrombosis. In this case, ischemic infarction is likely to occur in the whole territory of the relevant blood vessel, but the size of the lesion may differ depending on the collateral circulation. The other one is artery-to-artery embolism: the thrombi, which are generated from the atherosclerotic lesion, crumble off and migrate to the distal vessels because of arterial pressure. In this case, stroke may involve a part of the vascular territory of the relevant artery, and the patient's symptoms are likely to be less severe. However, the atherosclerotic plaque from where the thrombi originated is still present, and a recurrent thromboembolism may cause a stroke recurrence or early neurological deterioration during the hospital

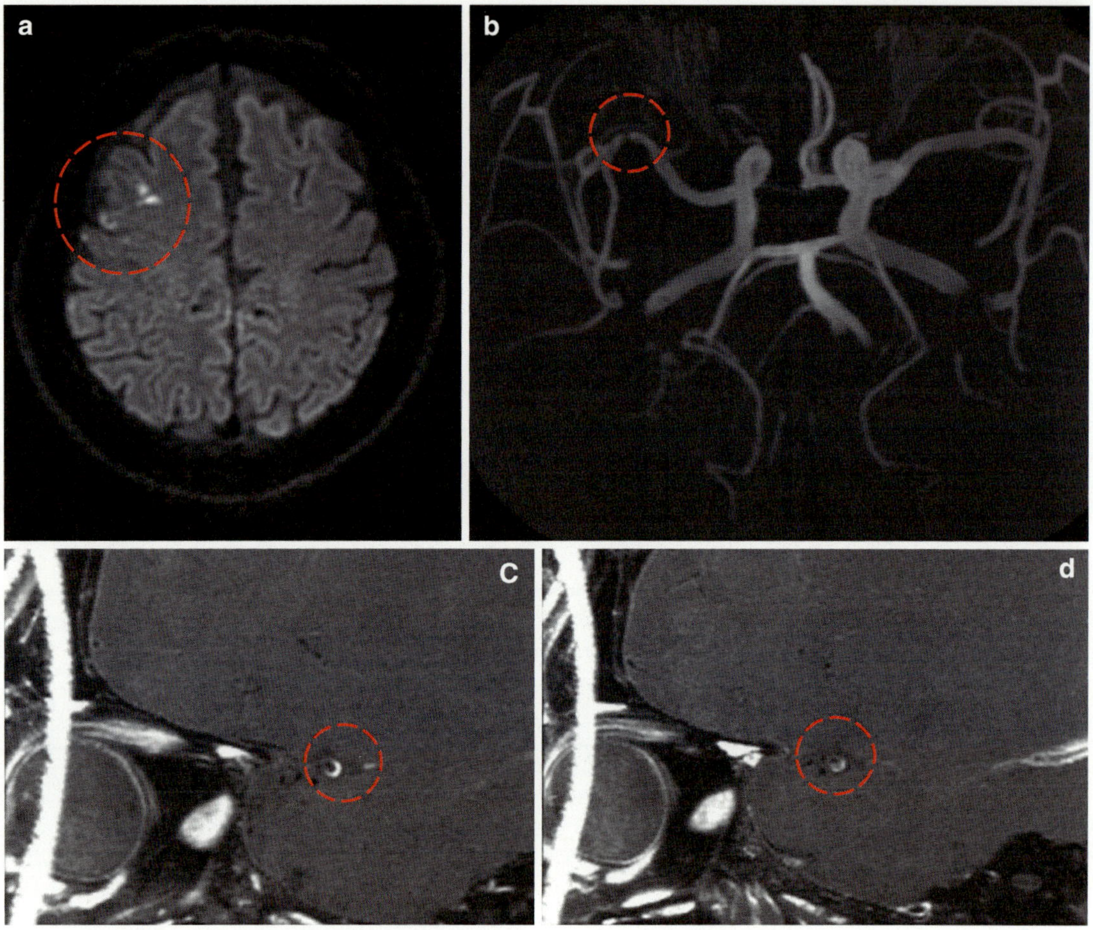

Fig. 11.3 A case of stroke caused by large-artery atherosclerosis. (**a**) New infarct lesions (*a dash-dot red circle*) were identified in diffusion-weighted imaging. (**b**) The patient had severe stenosis in the right middle cerebral artery lesions (*a dash-dot red circle*). (**c** and **d**) A vulnerable plaque with contrast enhancement was identified in the high-resolution magnetic resonance imaging (*dash-dot red circles*)

admission. In the TOAST classification, to decide that the stroke is caused by LAA, there must be a stenotic lesion on a vessel corresponding to LAA, and further, the stenosis degree should be at least 50% (Fig. 11.3). These criteria are under debate, but it does not change the fact that there is a need to find a stenotic lesion on the artery. Either magnetic resonance (MR) angiography or CT angiography may visualize the atherosclerotic lesion. The conventional angiography or digital-subtraction angiography (DSA) might be an option, but because of relatively frequent complications from the test, this test must be considered for patients with indications of carotid endarterectomy or carotid angioplasty with stenting. Carotid duplex ultrasonography and transcranial Doppler test are not usually counted as basic tests and are used as secondary confirmation methods. In the current status, it would be better that LAA is diagnosed via MR angiography or CT angiography.

11.2.2 SVO

In SVO, the mechanism of occlusion is quite different from that of LAA-related stroke. LAA-related stroke is basically caused by white thrombi related to activation of platelets, but the contribution of platelets is not major in SVO-related stroke. The mechanism of SVO was fully understood and mainly attributed to Dr. Miller Fisher's studies. Dr. Fisher, who analyzed lacunar strokes with numerous studies using serial sections of rodent brains, reached the conclusion that most of the lacunar strokes were caused by the occlusion of penetrating arteries and that the diameter of these arteries was in most cases within 225 μm [9]. Lacunar infarctions occurring in the 300 μm or higher diameter vessels were very rare. He guessed that it might be because of the lower possibility of collateral circulation in the vessels with a diameter less than 300 μm. In these vessels, occlusion occurs due to a mechanical blockage on the blood vessels by the degenerated vascular cells that form the wall of the blood vessels mostly denatured into "lipohyalinosis" (Fig. 11.4) [10]. That is, it occurs when the denatured vessel wall itself suddenly blocks the blood flow, and infarction caused by a thrombus, as in large-artery atherosclerosis, very rarely occurs. The SVO in the TOAST classification, however, basically means small-artery occlusion. Venous infarction is not included in the TOAST classification system, and it is included in the "other determined" category. Small-artery occlusion would be better in this context, which is one of the minor shortfalls of the TOAST classification system.

Among the lacunar strokes, around 50% are caused by occlusions originating from the thrombi in the blood vessels with a 300 μm or higher diameter, and the rest are caused by the atherosclerotic plaque itself, micro-stripping, plugging, etc., according to the reports. Arteriolosclerosis that is a cause of thrombus is located in the proximal penetrating artery in many cases, and this pathological finding is called "microatheroma." In particular, microatheroma occurring in the site branching from the great vessel is also called junctional atheroma, and in this case, the penetrating artery from which the thrombus that occurred here branches out is often completely closed. The definition of lacunar stroke is ambiguous in clinical setting. Traditionally, it is the occlusion of the penetrating artery that is called lacunar infarction, but it is difficult to tell them apart in the clinical settings without a pathologic information. Then, at the clinical settings in recent years, a less than 1.5 or 2 cm cerebral infarction that occurred deep inside as shown on the diffusion-weighted MRI is defined

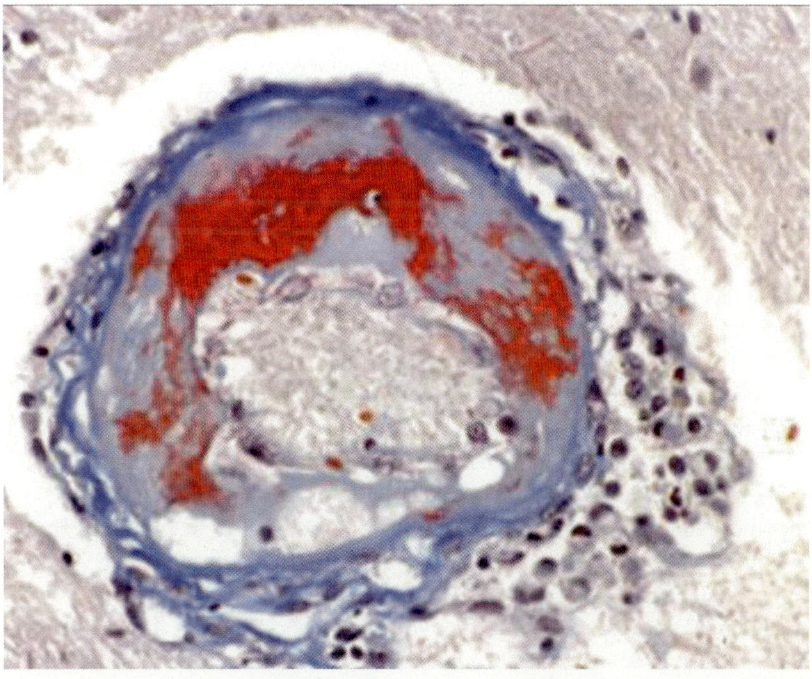

Fig. 11.4 Pathological features of lipohyalinosis. Reproduced by permission of Lancet Neurology [10]

Table 11.4 Lacunar syndromes

Syndrome	Lesion localization	Vessels involved
Pure motor stroke	Posterior limb of internal capsule Corona radiata Ventral pons Cerebral peduncle	Lenticulostriate perforators, anterior choroidal artery, perforators from basilar artery, or perforators from posterior cerebral artery
Pure sensory stroke	Ventroposterolateral (VPL) nucleus of thalamus	Perforators from thalamogeniculate artery
Sensorimotor stroke	Thalamocapsular area: posterior limb of internal capsule and VPL nucleus of thalamus	Lenticulostriate perforators, anterior choroidal artery, or perforators from thalamogeniculate artery
Dysarthria-clumsy hand syndrome	Same as pure motor stroke	Same as pure motor stroke
Ataxic hemiparesis	Same as pure motor stroke	Same as pure motor stroke

as lacunar infarction for classification. In this case, however, as even cerebral infarction with a hemodynamic cause or cerebral infarction caused by embolism meets this definition, misclassification is common. In most cases, it would be most reasonable if lacunar infarction would be considered to be caused by mechanical occlusion due to the blood vessels denatured into lipohyalinosis.

The stroke due to SVO is caused by the occlusion of a single perforating artery. Therefore, in many cases, they are found in the deeper areas, such as the internal border zone. As stated above, junctional atheroma or branch atheromatous diseases (which in fact belong to the LAA category) are not easy to be differentiated. Instead of the old name "lacunar infarction," some argued that they deserved a new name such as small deep infarction. Even if it is a misnomer, however, the name has been widely used for such a long time, and changing the status quo does not matter for now. It is more important to understand the difference between the meaning of lacunar infarction and its actual pathological characteristics.

The strokes caused by SVO cause a very small ischemic lesion, and the number of symptoms is not more than one or two. No matter how numerous they may be, they rarely go over three at a time. Acute cognitive decline is very rare as well. Lacunar syndromes are classified by citing its characteristics determined through clinicopathologic studies (Table 11.4). It is useful for communication between physicians and paramedical persons, but with the advances in stroke lesion pattern analysis through MRI, it would not be of much clinical importance. Moreover, lacunar syndromes are not always caused by SVO. Many patients with lacunar syndromes show LAA, cardioembolism (CE), or other determined causes of strokes, even small intracerebral hemorrhages. The OCSP classification system, which classifies patients based on physical symptoms and signs, may be exposed to critical errors, especially in lacunar stroke.

Symptoms are mild and the prognosis is very favorable in patients with SVO stroke. A lot of cases is likely to be fully recovered even without medical treatments. If the initial treatment is not properly done, however, the case might be worsened during the early phase. It would require a specific strategy to prevent a recurrence in different but graver forms of vascular events.

11.2.3 Cardioembolism (CE)

CE accounts for about 25% of all strokes. In most cases, LAA, SVO, and CE happen in similar proportions, each accounting for around 25% of the overall cases. The remaining 25% consist of strokes with undetermined or other determined

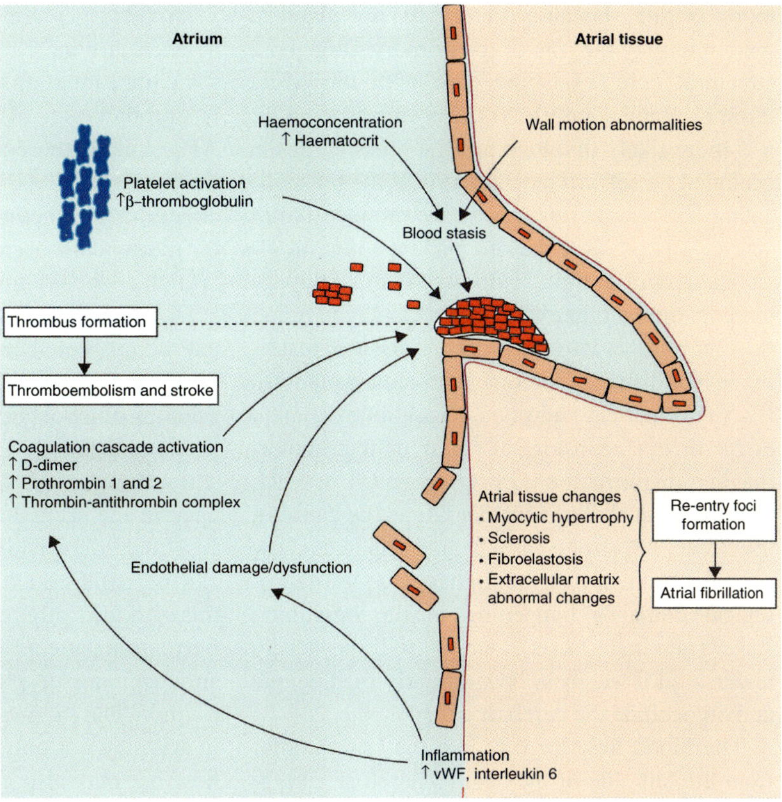

Fig. 11.5 Mechanism of thrombogenesis in atrial fibrillation. Reproduced by permission of Lancet Neurology [11]

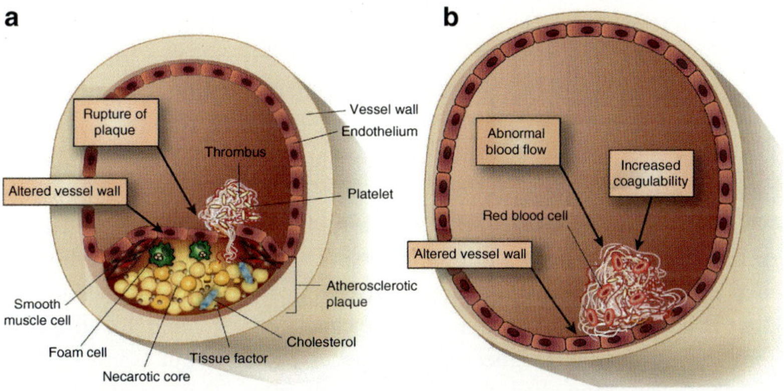

Fig. 11.6 White thrombus versus red thrombus. (**a**) White thrombus produced by platelet activation after plaque rupture. (**b**) Red thrombus formation by clotting factor activation. Reproduced by permission of Nature [12]

causes. CE is the type of stroke that occurs in patients with cardiac diseases with an obscured blood flow (i.e., acute myocardial infarction, left ventricular [LV] aneurysms, cardiomyopathies and myocarditis, valve disease and/or prosthesis, and AF) (Fig. 11.5) [11]. The activation of platelets and the resultant white thrombi are the main causes of LAA-related strokes. In strokes caused by CE, however, the clotting factor rather than the activation of platelets plays a more critical role. Stagnation of blood flow makes red blood cells form a passive, temporary core. Then, various physical and chemical stimuli activate the clotting factor cascade. The final product of this process, the fibrin meshwork, forms red thrombi (Fig. 11.6) [12]. The red thrombi mainly consist of red blood cells held together with fibrin, in which platelets are rarely discovered. They are more fragile, because there are no platelets therein to play the role of the primary plug and a structural core, as is the case with the white thrombi. Immediately after the occurrence of CE, it is more likely that high arterial pressure to the occluded vessel will recanalyze it. If the recanalization happens before any tissue damage is not severe, it is possible that the patient's neurological status will abruptly improve. If this happens too late, on the other hand, the recanalized blood flow may travel into the ischemic tissues, resulting in hemorrhage (hemorrhagic transformation). If a stroke patient shows an abrupt improvement of his or her neurological status or if a hemorrhagic transformation is observed on CT or MRI, the physician should consider CE as the cause of the stroke. CE stroke has a characteristic to show a greater tendency of the highest level of neurological damages happening in the beginning stage (maximal onset), which will be easily understood if we guess how abruptly cardiogenic emboli occlude the cerebral vessel.

The blood flow directly into the brain comes from the left side of the heart. Therefore, except for the diseases leading to a right-to-left (R–L) shunt, the heart diseases that create thrombi in the LV and left atrium (LA) are the main causes of CE. The heart diseases that generate thrombi in the LV mainly occur at the LV apex, but if the patient has an LV aneurysm or acute myocardial infarction, the chance that the thrombi may be generated from the LV is also high. This is because with myocardial infarction, dyskinesia (akinesia or hypokinesia) on the wall of the heart in the LV may result in a serious obstruction of the blood flow. In acute myocardial infarction, the chance of thrombus formation is highest after the occurrence of the disease, and then the possibility sharply decreases over time. However, the proportion of the strokes caused by acute myocardial infarction is by far surpassed by those caused by old myocardial infarction. This is because of the higher morbidity rate of old myocardial infarction, which contributes to the higher frequency of occurrence while the chance of forming thrombi is still lower. Likewise, with AF, the chance of thrombus formation is not as high as with the others, but due to the higher morbidity rate of the elderly population, it is known as the most frequent cause of CE.

Appendages are the pocket-like attachments to each atrium. The left atrial appendage has a structure extending to the narrow entrance, and it is a probable site of blood stasis. If the history of AF is longer, there are bound to be changes with the structures and tissues on the left atrium. Such changes are sometimes linked with the frequency of thrombosis occurrence. The change, called "rough endocardium," refers to a finding of wrinkled appearance caused by edema and is characterized by peeled endothelial cells, so that fibrin or thrombi may be easily generated. Besides, findings of myocytic hypertrophy or necrosis and a mononuclear cell infiltrate, etc. are observed. The phenomenon where it is difficult to come back to the normal atrial rhythm even after successful cardioversion in atrial fibrillation patients can be explained by pathological findings like this. Additionally, due to these findings, atrial fibrillation patients are highly likely to require an anticoagulant despite the return to the normal rhythm. The failure of contraction of the atrium in AF may not only delay or obstruct the blood flow but may also aggravate the situation as the left atrium may be enlarged progressively. Such condition is further aggravated by mitral stenosis. The expansion of the left atrium increases the chance of the occurrence of thrombosis and stroke. This has been confirmed by other studies, where the sizes of the left atrium were standardized in accordance with the physical dimensions. The blood flow stasis in the left atrium or left atrium appendage is confirmed via transesophageal echocardiography (TEE) through spontaneous echo contrast (SEC). This SEC may be related to stroke occurrence. It is known that about 1/3 of the SEC persists after an AF returns to a normal rhythm, which necessitates continued anticoagulation treatment.

11.2.4 Other Determined (OD) Causes

This category does not refer to the category of strokes that occur in accordance with certain definitions. Literally, it means that the stroke has not been classified as it is rare, while the direct cause of a particular stroke case has been identified. It is important not to confuse this category with the "undetermined" category as OD includes only those with clearly known causes. Therefore, if the cause of a particular stroke is known but it is not included in the LAA, SVO, or CE categories, it is classified as an OD. This particular category is a collection of a variety of causes of strokes. Their prevalence and distribution, while being scarce, differ among countries and races. As such, the distribution within countries and races is expected to be significantly different. For example, moyamoya disease is a very important cause of stroke in Asia but is extremely rare in Western countries, while the opposite is true for carotid artery dissection. Due to population aging, the frequency of cancer-related stroke is increasing sharply. In addition, a number of genetic factors have been confirmed. For the strokes that correspond to this definition, please refer to Sect. 8.3, where they are discussed in detail.

11.2.5 Undetermined (UD) Causes

The strokes belonging to this category have not been clearly explained in terms of their causes. This category is divided into two types: that with a cryptogenic source and that with two or more sources. In strokes with a cryptogenic source, the cause of the stroke is not definitely identified. While the patient has a territorial infarction, there is no LAA in the vessel, and the patient does not have a CE source, and this case belongs to UD category. The case where multiple embolic infarction occurs but CE or a systemic embolic source is not found is a common example of UD stroke. If a patient has stenosis that is not high enough to satisfy the definitions of LAA, how do you classify this case? In the TOAST classification system, the criterion for LAA is 50% or more vessel stenosis. If the relevant vascular stenosis is found below such threshold on MR or CT angiography (e.g., 30% M1 stenosis), we have to classify the case into the UD category. While the grade of stenosis itself is important, however, it is understood that the unstable or vulnerable plaque, which causes thrombosis, is more common in 50% or lower stenosis. Would it not be reasonable to classify this case as an LAA patient? This weakness in the TOAST system explains why many of the studies do not use the definition of 50% stenosis as it is. The 50% threshold was only an arbitrary consensus among the TOAST researchers, and moreover, there were no conditions specifying the type of imaging. Thus, the current consensus is that it would be reasonable to classify the patient as an LAA patient if there is a stenosis, even if it is as low as 10%, which could lead to LAA-related stroke. This strategy is not without problems, however, because the level of the diagnostic tests given to identify the cause of the stroke differs across countries. In addition, the MRI technology is advancing at a fast pace, and as such, it is not possible to set a high-resolution MRI with 3.0 T or higher as the norm. It would be appropriate to have an experienced stroke team and to share and communicate their own classification system.

If a patient has multiple embolic infarctions with no cardioembolic source, the patient is classified as having stroke with a cryptogenic source. During the hospitalization period, the patient goes through 24-h Holter monitoring, but if the patient shows AF in ECG 6 months after discharge, what category should the initial stroke be classified into? In principle, it may be classified as a stroke with a cryptogenic source, but we are likely to guess that the original stroke was caused by CE. The cause of the stroke might have been paroxysmal AF, which was not discovered during the hospitalization period. When paroxysmal AF is to be discovered long after discharge, it would be reasonable to consider anticoagulation.

Here is another example. A patient visits the hospital with multiple embolic infarctions, but no one is sure about the cause. One year after discharge, however, the patient receives a lupus anticoagulant test from another department. The result is positive, and in the follow-up test after 12 weeks, the result is again positive. This patient has antiphospholipid syndrome, but during the hospitalization period, the patient was not tested for it. Perhaps the patient had a stroke caused by antiphospholipid syndrome and should have been classified as an OD patient. If so, what level of diagnostic tests should be considered to be performed while the patient is admitted to a hospital? This is a question without a clear answer and that is significantly affected by the healthcare insurance issues of each country. The chance of finding the real cause will be higher, however, if the physician finds some clues and pursuits undiscovered causes enthusiastically.

As for strokes with two or more sources, if a patient have 60% stenosis in a carotid artery and AF at the same time, the typical classification will be stroke with two or more sources. What should be done, however, if the patient has 60% stenosis in the carotid artery and also has PFO? PFO, according to the TOAST classification, is a medium-risk cardioembolic source, but after many studies, the PFO morbidity rate among normal elderly adults was found to be as high as 20–30%. If all PFOs will be taken as cardioembolic sources, too many patients will be classified as having had a stroke with two or more sources. It is not that PFO should be removed from the list of CE sources, however, as it is still true that there are patients who suffer strokes caused by it. In the end, it is clear that not a single classification regime should be accepted as it is. The intuition and experience of the stroke neurologists who observe the patients in person remain important.

Conclusion

In this chapter, the history of the existing major stroke classification systems was examined, and a closer look was made into several classification regimes commonly used today. Currently, most of the studies use the OCSP or TOAST classification system, but the OCSP system has the critical weakness of not being able to identify the cause of stroke. The TOAST classification system, on the other hand, was developed in 1993 and has been used ever since, for more than two decades. Even today, this system is widely used. As was discussed earlier, however, the use of this system may pose problems as it may involve critical flaws and as there are too many loopholes in the system. What is most important is to understand why there is a need to classify the stroke of the patient to begin with. If the purpose of the classification is to find out the severity distribution of the patient, even the OCSP system will provide a good deal of information, but if the purpose of the classification is to find the optimal therapy and to provide the highest level of preventive effect after hospital discharge, the TOAST classification system may well serve such purpose, but there is a need to customize it based on the accumulated experience of the center.

Suggestions from Current Clinical Practice Guidelines Not applicable to this chapter.

References

1. Bamford J, Sandercock PA, Dennis MS, et al. Classification and natural history of clinically identifiable subtypes of brain infarction. Lancet. 1991;337:1521–6.
2. Adams HP, Bendixen BH, Kappelle LJ, et al. Classification of subtype of acute ischemic stroke: definitions for use in a multicenter clinical trial. Stroke. 1993;24:35–41.
3. Amarenco P, Bogousslavsky J, Caplan LR, et al. Classification of stroke subtypes. Cerebrovasc Dis. 2009;27:493–501.
4. Sacco RL, Ellenberg JH, Mohr JP, et al. Infarcts of undetermined cause: the NINCDS Stroke Data Bank. Ann Neurol. 1989;25:382–90.
5. Anning ST. The historical aspects of venous thrombosis. Med Hist. 1957;1:28–37.
6. Classification of atherosclerotic lesions; report of a study group. World Health Organ Tech Rep Ser. 1958;57:1–20.
7. Stary HC, Chandler AB, Dinsmore RE, et al. A definition of advanced types of atherosclerotic lesions and a histological classification of atherosclerosis. A report from the Committee on Vascular Lesions of the Council on Arteriosclerosis, American Heart Association. Arterioscler Thromb Vasc Biol. 1995;15:1512–31.
8. Yahagi K, Kolodgie FD, Otsuka F, et al. Pathophysiology of native coronary, vein graft, and in-stent atherosclerosis. Nat Rev Cardiol. 2016;13:79–98.
9. Fisher CM. Lacunar strokes and infarcts: a review. Neurology. 1982;32:871–6.
10. Pantoni L. Cerebral small vessel disease: from pathogenesis and clinical characteristics to therapeutic challenges. Lancet Neurol. 2010;9:689–701.
11. Watson T, Shantsila E, Lip GY. Mechanisms of thrombogenesis in atrial fibrillation: Virchow's triad revisited. Lancet. 2009;373:155–66.
12. Mackman N. Triggers, targets and treatments for thrombosis. Nature. 2008;451:914–8.

Selections of Antithrombotic Agents During Acute Stage

12

Tomohisa Nezu, Naohisa Hosomi, and Masayasu Matsumoto

Abstract

There are two major classes of antithrombotic agents that can be used in acute stroke settings, namely, antiplatelet agents and anticoagulant agents. Aspirin is recommended to use as soon as possible (within 48 h after stroke onset) for acute ischemic stroke patients. Recently, short-term dual antiplatelet therapy (aspirin plus clopidogrel) has been indicated to be safe and superior to aspirin in acute ischemic stroke patients in China. However, the dual antiplatelet therapy with aspirin and clopidogrel is not recommended as stroke prevention for the long term. Early anticoagulation occasionally might be used for certain stroke patients, although it is not recommended in general. Oral anticoagulation is recommended for secondary stroke prevention in patients with cardioembolic stroke. However, the initial timing of anticoagulation in acute stroke setting in cardioembolic stroke patients remains unclear. Further prospective studies to evaluate the safety, efficacy, optimal term, or optimal selections of antithrombotic agents will be needed for the acute ischemic stroke patients, considering the etiology of stroke. Physicians should consider the etiology of stroke (at least, cardioembolic stroke or non-cardioembolic stroke) to select the antithrombotic agents.

There are two major classes of antithrombotic agents that can be used in acute stroke settings, namely, antiplatelet agents and anticoagulant agents. In general, aspirin, which is one of the antiplatelet agents, is widely used and recommended to use early (within 48 h) for acute ischemic stroke patients [1, 2]. Recently, short-term dual antiplatelet therapy (aspirin plus clopidogrel) in acute stroke settings has been thought to be more effective as secondary prevention of stroke or transient ischemic attack (TIA) without increasing risk of hemorrhagic stroke and major bleeding events [3]. Early anticoagulation

T. Nezu, M.D., Ph.D. (✉) • N. Hosomi, M.D., Ph.D.
Department of Clinical Neuroscience and Therapeutics, Hiroshima University Graduate School of Biomedical & Health Sciences,
1-2-3 Kasumi, Minami-ku, Hiroshima, Hiroshima 734-8551, Japan
e-mail: tomonezu@hiroshima-u.ac.jp

M. Matsumoto, M.D., Ph.D.
Department of Clinical Neuroscience and Therapeutics, Hiroshima University Graduate School of Biomedical & Health Sciences,
1-2-3 Kasumi, Minami-ku, Hiroshima, Hiroshima 734-8551, Japan

Japan Community Healthcare Organization (JCHO), Hoshigaoka Medical Center, Hirakata, Japan

S.-H. Lee (ed.), *Stroke Revisited: Diagnosis and Treatment of Ischemic Stroke*, Stroke Revisited, DOI 10.1007/978-981-10-1424-6_12

therapy is generally not recommended because there is an increased risk of bleeding complications [1, 2]. However, several clinical trials did not evaluate the stroke subtype. To select antithrombotic agents in acute stroke settings, physicians should also consider the etiology of stroke. Anticoagulation occasionally might be used for certain stroke patients such as cardioembolic stroke, large artery atherosclerosis, and cerebral artery dissection.

In this chapter, we described the type or efficacy of antiplatelet therapy for acute ischemic stroke patients based on several large clinical trials. In addition, we mentioned the potential use of anticoagulation in acute stroke settings according to stroke subtype, although there was a lack of evidence. Antithrombotic therapy related to thrombolytic therapy, mechanical thrombectomy, or carotid artery stent is not included in this chapter. In general, antithrombotic therapy should not be given for the first 24 h if the patients were treated with intravenous tissue plasminogen activator.

12.1 Antiplatelet Agents

12.1.1 Aspirin

Aspirin, an inhibitor of cyclooxygenase hence preventing thromboxane A2 synthesis, is an old medicine and most extensively used for the treatment of acute ischemic stroke. Two large studies, the International Stroke Trial (IST) and the Chinese Acute Stroke Trial (CAST), showed the benefit of aspirin for acute ischemic stroke patients in 1997 [4, 5]. The IST enrolled 19,435 patients with suspected acute ischemic stroke, who were randomized of aspirin, subcutaneous heparin, both, or neither. The patients allocated to aspirin (300 mg daily) within 48 h of stroke onset had significantly fewer recurrent ischemic strokes within 14 days with no significant excess of hemorrhagic strokes. In addition, the reduction in combined outcome of death or nonfatal recurrent stroke at 6 months with aspirin was significant. The CAST was a randomized, placebo-controlled trial of the effects of aspirin treatment (160 mg daily) started within 48 h of the onset of suspected acute ischemic stroke ($n = 21{,}106$). The patients allocated to aspirin had a 14% relative risk reduction in mortality at 4 weeks after stroke onset. A recent systematic review assessed the efficacy and safety of immediate oral antiplatelet therapy in acute stroke settings [6]. Those results were based on eight trials involving over 40,000 participants, but the 98% of the data came from IST and CAST trials. The investigators concluded that antiplatelet therapy with aspirin 160–300 mg daily and started within 48 h of onset of presumed ischemic stroke reduced the risk of early recurrent ischemic stroke without a major risk of early hemorrhagic complications and improved long-term outcomes. Recent guidelines (the American College of Chest Physicians and the American Heart Association/American Stroke Association) also recommended that aspirin should be started as early as possible after the diagnosis of ischemic stroke [1, 2]. Evidence of aspirin trial shows a necessity of antiplatelet therapy for preventing acute recurrence in non-cardioembolic stroke.

12.1.2 Clopidogrel

Clopidogrel is a platelet ADP receptor antagonist (P2Y12 inhibitors) that has been tested for secondary stroke prevention in several trials. However, there has been limited evidence with the use of clopidogrel alone in acute stroke settings. Initiation of treatment with clopidogrel in a daily dose of 75 mg does not produce maximal inhibition of platelet aggregation. Therefore clopidogrel loading dose (300–600 mg) or the combination of aspirin and clopidogrel might be used in acute ischemic stroke patients similar to patients with acute myocardial infarction. Although the dual antiplatelet agents are the standard use for acute coronary syndrome, several large trials have failed to show the efficacy and safety of combination of aspirin and clopidogrel in long-term secondary stroke prevention [7, 8]. In the acute stroke settings, the Fast Assessment of Stroke and TIA to prevent Early Recurrence

(FASTER) trial was conducted in 392 acute ischemic stroke patients within 24 h of stroke onset randomly assigned to either aspirin plus clopidogrel (300 mg loading dose, then 75 mg daily) or aspirin alone [9]. Although the FASTER trial failed to show significant reduction in the primary outcome of combined ischemic and hemorrhagic stroke at 90 days after stroke onset, the trial was limited by small sample size. On the other hand, the CLAIR (clopidogrel plus aspirin versus aspirin alone for reducing embolization in patients with acute symptomatic cerebral or carotid artery stenosis) [10] and the CARESS (Clopidogrel and Aspirin for Reduction of Emboli in Symptomatic Carotid Stenosis) [11] trials which included acute ischemic stroke patients with large artery stenosis showed that dual antiplatelet therapy was more effective in reducing cerebral embolization than monotherapy (aspirin alone).

Recently, the Clopidogrel in High-Risk Patients with Acute Nondisabling Cerebrovascular Events (CHANCE) trial was conducted to test the effect of early dual antiplatelet treatment for the prevention of secondary stroke within the first 90 days following a qualifying transient ischemic attack (TIA) or minor stroke [12]. The CHANCE was a large, randomized, double-blind, placebo-controlled trial, and a total 5170 patients within 24 h were recruited in China. The trial showed that early initiation and short-term use of dual antiplatelet therapy (clopidogrel 300 mg loading dose, then 75 mg daily for 90 days, plus aspirin 75 mg daily for the first 21 days) had a significant reduction in all stroke recurrence at 90 days compared with the placebo plus aspirin (75 mg daily for 90 days). In addition, there was no difference in the rate of moderate or severe hemorrhages between patients with dual antiplatelet therapy and those with aspirin alone. More recently, the Combination of Clopidogrel and Aspirin for Prevention of Early Recurrence in Acute Atherothrombotic Stroke (COMPRESS) trial was conducted in 358 acute ischemic stroke patients of presumed large artery atherosclerosis origin within 48 h of onset to clopidogrel (75 mg daily without loading dose) plus aspirin (300 mg loading, then 100 mg daily) or to aspirin alone (300 mg loading, then 100 mg daily) for 30 days [13]. However, the dual antiplatelet therapy was not superior to aspirin alone for preventing new ischemic lesions and clinical vascular events at 30 days after stroke onset. Those negative results might be due to the timing of randomization, the absence of loading dose, and the small sample size, compared to the CHANCE trial. Although the CHANCE trial provided the strong evidence that the short-term intervention of dual antiplatelet therapy (clopidogrel plus aspirin) could significantly reduce the risk of stroke recurrence, the results of the CHANCE trial are not applied to the other acute ischemic stroke patients, such as Western populations. The inclusion criteria also selected for patients with minor stroke, defined as a National Institutes of Health Stroke Scale (NIHSS) score of 3 or less at the time of randomization. Further studies whether short-term dual antiplatelet therapy is safe and superior to aspirin alone in other racial populations including moderate or severe stroke will be needed. Of note, lack of evidence in comparison of clopidogrel alone with aspirin alone for reducing early stroke recurrence, there is still a possibility that the similar results with the CHANCE trial can be obtained with clopidogrel alone.

Clopidogrel is a prodrug activated by several enzymes including CYP2C19, and functional genetic variations in CYP genes are thought to affect the effectiveness of platelet inhibition in patients with clopidogrel. The subanalysis of 2933 patients in the CHANCE trial showed the other important interpretations for the association between CYP2C19 genetic variants and clinical outcomes of clopidogrel-treated patients with acute ischemic stroke [14]. In the results, the use of clopidogrel plus aspirin compared with aspirin alone reduced the risk of a new stroke in the subgroup of patients who were not carriers of the CYP2C19 loss-of-function alleles ($n = 1207$), but did not in carriers of the loss-of-function alleles (*2, *3) ($n = 1726$). These findings might support a role of CYP2C19 genotype in the efficacy of clopidogrel. A promising antiplatelet agent and new P2Y inhibitors (prasugrel, cangrelor, ticagrelor, and elinogrel) have a faster onset of platelet inhibition and less variability of response compared with clopidogrel. New P2Y inhibitors decrease mortality after percutaneous intervention for the patients with acute coronary syndrome [15]. However, there was few evidence to evaluate the efficacy and safety of new P2Y inhibitors for the acute ischemic stroke patients. The Acute Stroke or Transient Ischemic Attack Treated with Aspirin or Ticagrelor and Patient Outcomes (SOCRATES) trial was designed to compare ticagrelor with aspirin with regard to their effectiveness for the prevention of major vascular events over a period of 90 days in acute stroke settings [16]. In the SOCRATES trial, total 13,199 patients who had a high-risk TIA or acute ischemic stroke patients with a NIHSS score of 5 or less were enrolled. In the results, ticagrelor was not found to be superior to aspirin in reducing the rate of stroke, myocardial infarction, or death at 90 days. Further studies whether other P2Y inhibitors (monotherapy) or the combination of ticagrelor and aspirin (dual therapy) are superior to aspirin alone in acute ischemic stroke settings will be needed.

12.1.3 Dipyridamole or Cilostazol

Dipyridamole inhibits phosphodiesterase (PDE) and augments prostacyclin-related platelet aggregation inhibition. Several large clinical trials indicated that the combination therapy dipyridamole and aspirin was at least as effective as aspirin alone for secondary stroke prevention [17, 18]. However, the combination therapy (dipyridamole plus aspirin) was shown to be less well tolerated than aspirin alone, because the patients with dipyridamole sometimes have headache. In the acute stroke settings, there was scarce evidence for use of dipyridamole. The early treatment with aspirin plus extended-release dipyridamole for transient ischemic attack or ischemic stroke within 24 h of symptom onset (EARLY) trial was conducted to compare outcome between patients with aspirin plus extended-release dipyridamole twice daily and those with aspirin monotherapy for 7 days [19]. After 7 days, all patients received open-label aspirin plus extended-release dipyridamole. Total 539 patients were recruited in the EARLY trial. In the results, there was no significant difference in the functional good outcome defined as a modified Rankin Scale score of 0–1, vascular events, and mortality at 90 days between patients with aspirin plus extended-release dipyridamole and those with aspirin.

Cilostazol, which is one of a PDE inhibitor, also has been shown to be effective in the secondary prevention of stroke. The second Cilostazol Stroke Prevention Study (CSPS 2) was conducted to establish non-inferiority of cilostazol versus aspirin for prevention of stroke and to compare the efficacy and safety of cilostazol and aspirin in patients with non-cardioembolic stroke [20]. Total 2757 patients who had had a cerebral infarction within the previous 26 weeks were enrolled. In the results, the incidence of stroke recurrence was lower in patients receiving cilostazol than in those receiving aspirin. Several clinical trials were conducted to confirm whether combination antiplatelet therapy with cilostazol could be useful for the acute ischemic stroke patients, especially with intracranial branch atheromatous disease or intracranial atherosclerotic stenosis [21–23]. The Trial of Cilostazol in Symptomatic Intracranial Arterial Stenosis (TOSS) showed that cilostazol plus aspirin was superior to aspirin alone in preventing the progression of symptomatic intracranial atherosclerotic stenosis [23]. However, it remains unclear whether cilostazol could be effective for prevention of stroke in acute stoke settings.

12.2 Anticoagulant Agents

Anticoagulation with heparin or low molecular weight heparin within 48 h of ischemic stroke onset was associated with a higher mortality and worse outcomes compared with aspirin [24]. Therefore, several guidelines described that early administration of anticoagulation was not recommended for the treatment of patients with acute ischemic stroke [1, 2]. On the other hand, Japanese guidelines described that the use of heparin can be considered for acute ischemic stroke within 48 h after stroke onset, although adequate scientific evidence was lacking [25].

Most clinical trials have not evaluated the initial dose and initial timing of anticoagulation, considering the infarct size or the stroke subtype. Considering those factors, early anticoagulant therapy occasionally might be useful for certain stroke patients such as cardioembolic stroke, large artery atherosclerosis, and cerebral artery dissection.

12.2.1 Cardioembolic Stroke

Oral anticoagulation is recommended for secondary stroke prevention in patients with atrial fibrillation (AF) and other high-risk cardioembolic source. However, the initial timing of anticoagulation after stroke onset remains unclear. The timing of administration might be dependent on the size of the infarct, which is presumed to associate with the risk of hemorrhagic transformation. Although a 2007 meta-analysis showed no net benefit of early anticoagulant therapy (within 48 h after stroke onset) over antiplatelet therapy in patients with cardioembolic stroke [26], some patients at high risk of early stroke recurrence (e.g., intracardiac thrombus or mechanical heart valve) were not included in most clinical trials. Early anticoagulant therapy could be considered in those patients when the risk of hemorrhagic complications is low (e.g., small brain infarct or TIA).

Recent several large studies have shown that direct oral anticoagulants (DOACs) are at least equivalent to warfarin for reducing ischemic stroke and superior to warfarin for reducing intracranial hemorrhage among patients with nonvalvular AF (NVAF) [27–30]. However, limited evidence existed for the effectiveness of DOACs for the secondary prevention of ischemic stroke patients with NVAF in acute stroke settings, because those studies found that DOACs could not be started within 7–14 days of a stroke onset. In Japan, the prospective, multicenter, observational Stroke Acute Management with Urgent Risk-factor Assessment and Improvement (SAMURAI)-NVAF Study was conducted to elucidate real-world risks and benefits of anticoagulation including DOAC use, mostly initiated early after stroke or TIA onset [31]. In the results, both warfarin and DOACs were initiated within 4 days after stroke or TIA onset in the majority of cases. Intracranial hemorrhage within 3 months after stroke onset occurred in only 0.23% of the present DOACs users, and its relative risk was only 17% of that in warfarin users. Therefore, DOAC might be relatively safe for acute stroke patients.

12.2.2 Large Artery Atherosclerosis

The Trial of Org 10172 in Acute Stroke Treatment (TOAST) trial evaluated the efficacy of the low molecular weight heparinoid (danaparoid) administered as an intravenous bolus within 24 h of stroke onset and continued for 7 days in 1281 patients with acute ischemic stroke [32]. Subgroup analysis of that trial showed a higher rate of favorable outcomes at 3 months in patients treated with danaparoid who had a large artery atherosclerotic stroke (68 vs 55% with placebo, $P = 0.04$). The FISS-tris trial evaluated the low molecular weight heparin (nadroparin) versus aspirin within 48 h after stroke onset for Asian acute stroke patients with large artery occlusive disease [33]. Although the proportion of patients with good outcomes (defined by a Barthel Index ≥85) at 6 months were not significantly different, there was a significant benefit to low molecular weight heparin in a prespecified secondary outcomes (defined by a modified Rankin Scale score of 0–1).

Japanese guidelines recommended argatroban, a selective thrombin inhibitor developed in Japan, for acute ischemic stroke within 48 h after non-cardioembolic stroke onset and with a maximum diameter of ≥1.5 cm based on several randomized clinical trials in Japan [25]. However, recent retrospective study showed that argatroban might not have an added benefit on functional outcomes at discharge in patients with atherothrombotic stroke compared to controls after propensity score matching [34]. On the other hand, previous retrospective study found that argatroban might be useful on cardioembolic stroke, increasing the improvement of recovery of stroke severity without increasing the risk of hemorrhage [35], although Japanese guidelines showed that argatroban was thought to be contraindicated in cardioembolic stroke patients. Additional prospective clinical trials whether argatroban could be effective in acute ischemic stroke patients (large artery atherosclerosis or cardioembolic stroke) will be needed.

12.2.3 Cerebral Artery Dissection

There is no evidence for superiority of anticoagulation or antiplatelet therapy in prevention of stoke after cerebral artery dissection. The Cervical Artery Dissection In Stroke Study (CADISS) was established to compare the effectiveness of antiplatelet use with anticoagulant use for the prevention of recurrent stroke in patients with carotid and vertebral artery dissection [36]. The total 250 patients were recruited, and the primary endpoint was set for the ipsilateral stroke or death within 3 months. In results, stroke or death occurred in three (2%) of 126 patients with antiplatelet use versus one (1%) of 124 patients with anticoagulant use. Early recurrences are very rare in ischemic stroke patients with cerebral artery dissection. Therefore, the antithrombotic treatments in ischemic stroke patients with cerebral artery dissection remain unknown. The clinical trials to clarify the optimal antithrombotic medications for secondary prevention among patients with cerebral artery dissection will need a very large sample size. The details of management for the acute ischemic stroke patients with cerebral artery dissection are described in the other chapter.

12.3 Approach to Antithrombotic Therapy for Acute Ischemic Stroke Patients

The approaches to antithrombotic therapy are summarized for acute ischemic stroke patients with non-cardioembolism in Fig. 12.1 and for those with cardioembolism in Fig. 12.2. These algorithms are excepted about the management of thrombolysis (including intravenous tissue plasminogen activator), mechanical thrombectomy, carotid endarterectomy, and carotid artery stent. The details of long-term antithrombotic therapy for the secondary prevention in patients with other etiologies are described in the other

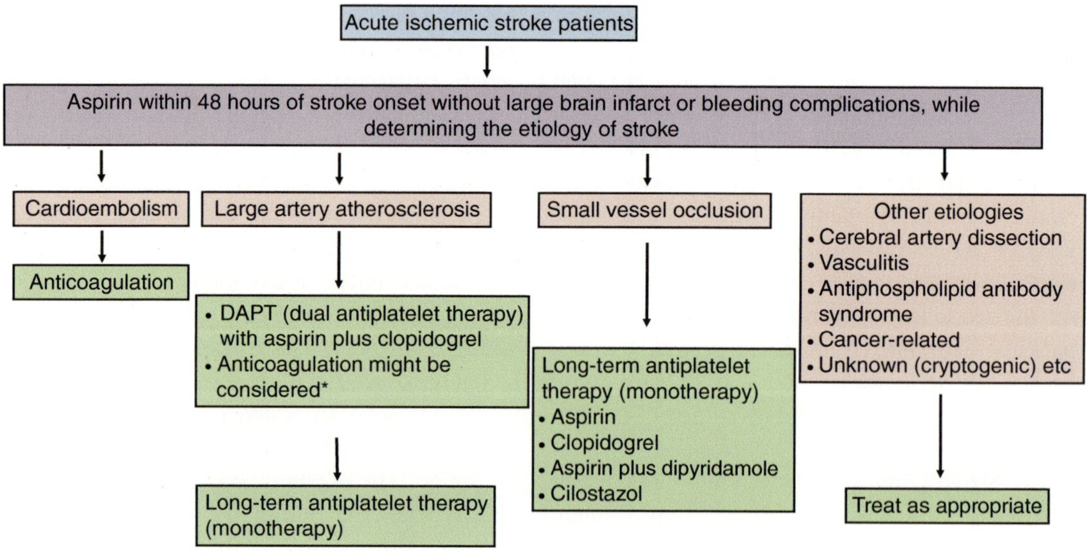

Fig. 12.1 The approach to antithrombotic therapy for acute ischemic stroke patients with non-cardioembolic stroke. * Several guidelines suggest that early anticoagulation is not recommended

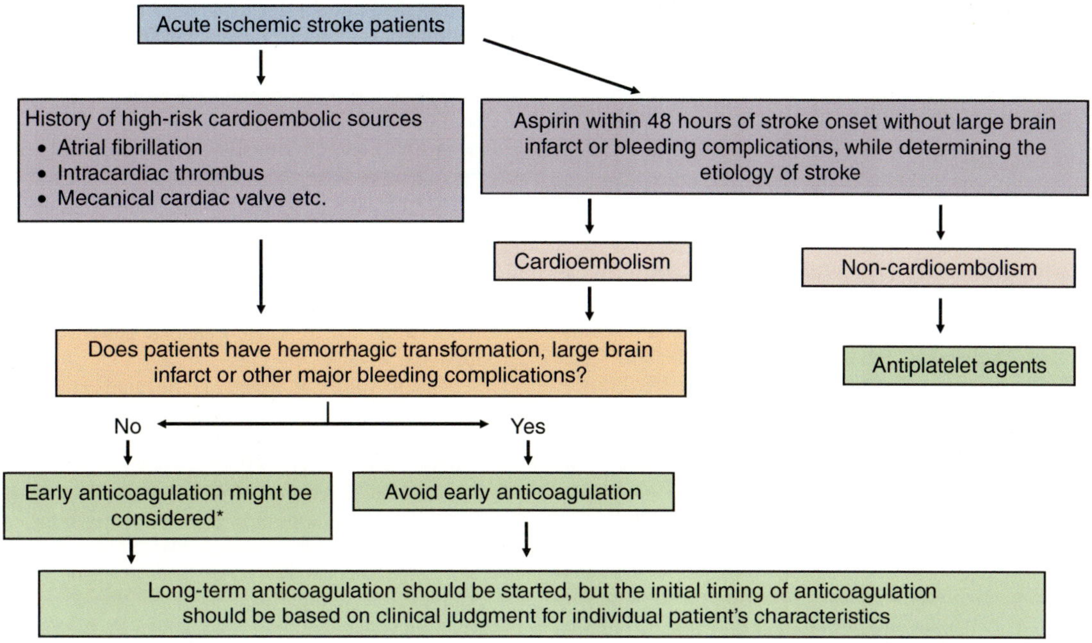

Fig. 12.2 The approach to antithrombotic therapy for acute ischemic stroke patients with cardioembolic stroke. * Several guidelines suggest that early anticoagulation is not recommended

chapter. Although several guidelines suggested that early anticoagulation therapy in acute stroke setting was not recommended, we described that anticoagulation might be considered in the patients with large artery atherosclerosis or cardioembolic stroke in those algorithms based on Japanese guidelines [1, 2, 25]. We did not mention the selections of antithrombotic agents for patients with progressing stoke in this algorithm. Although the results of the CHANCE trial might support the early and short-term dual antiplatelet therapy that could be beneficial for the patients with progressing stroke, the optimal selection of antithrombotic therapy remains unclear.

Conclusions

Aspirin is recommended to use as soon as possible for acute ischemic stroke patients. The CHANCE trial provided the additional evidence that short-term dual antiplatelet therapy (aspirin plus clopidogrel) was safe and superior to aspirin alone in acute ischemic stroke patients. The Platelet-Oriented Inhibition in New TIA and Minor Ischemic Stroke (POINT) trial is currently enrolling North American patients with inclusion or exclusion criteria similar to CHANCE trial. In addition, the Triple Antiplatelets for Reducing Dependency after Ischemic Stroke (TARDIS) trial which is comparing the safety of triple antiplatelet therapy (combined aspirin, clopidogrel, and dipyridamole) versus guideline therapy (aspirin and dipyridamole or clopidogrel alone) in 4100 patients with acute stroke or TIA is ongoing. A conclusive determination of the usefulness of the aggressive short-term combination of antithrombotic agents for the secondary prevention of ischemic stroke in acute stroke settings awaits several large randomized trials.

Suggestions from Clinical Practice Guidelines Aspirin should be administered orally as early as possible after diagnosis of acute ischemic stroke. Initial aspirin dose depends on various situations and is 160–325 mg per day in most countries. Clopidogrel might be effective, but not fully evaluated in acute stroke setting.

Usefulness of urgent anticoagulation is not proven in any cases. However, use of clopidogrel or urgent anticoagulation should be based on individual situations.

References

1. Lansberg MG, O'Donnell MJ, Khatri P, et al. Antithrombotic and thrombolytic therapy for ischemic stroke: Antithrombotic Therapy and Prevention of Thrombosis, 9th ed: American College of Chest Physicians Evidence-Based Clinical Practice Guidelines. Chest. 2012;141:e601S–36S.
2. Jauch EC, Saver JL, Adams HP, et al. Guidelines for the early management of patients with acute ischemic stroke: a guideline for healthcare professionals from the American Heart Association/American Stroke Association. Stroke. 2013;44:870–947.
3. Zhang Q, Wang C, Zheng M, et al. Aspirin plus clopidogrel as secondary prevention after stroke or transient ischemic attack: a systematic review and meta-analysis. Cerebrovasc Dis. 2015;39:13–22.
4. The International Stroke Trial (IST): a randomised trial of aspirin, subcutaneous heparin, both, or neither among 19435 patients with acute ischaemic stroke. International Stroke Trial Collaborative Group. Lancet. 1997;349:1569–81.
5. CAST: randomised placebo-controlled trial of early aspirin use in 20,000 patients with acute ischaemic stroke. CAST (Chinese Acute Stroke Trial) Collaborative Group. Lancet. 1997;349:1641–9.
6. Sandercock PA, Counsell C, Tseng MC, et al. Oral antiplatelet therapy for acute ischaemic stroke. Cochrane Database Syst Rev. 2014;(3):CD000029.
7. Diener HC, Bogousslavsky J, Brass LM, et al. Aspirin and clopidogrel compared with clopidogrel alone after recent ischaemic stroke or transient ischaemic attack in high-risk patients (MATCH): randomised, double-blind, placebo-controlled trial. Lancet. 2004;364:331–7.
8. Benavente OR, Hart RG, McClure LA, et al. Effects of clopidogrel added to aspirin in patients with recent lacunar stroke. N Engl J Med. 2012;367:817–25.
9. Kennedy J, Hill MD, Ryckborst KJ, et al. Fast assessment of stroke and transient ischaemic attack to prevent early recurrence (FASTER): a randomised controlled pilot trial. Lancet Neurol. 2007;6:961–9.
10. Wong KS, Chen C, Fu J, et al. Clopidogrel plus aspirin versus aspirin alone for reducing embolisation in patients with acute symptomatic cerebral or carotid artery stenosis (CLAIR study): a randomised, open-label, blinded-endpoint trial. Lancet Neurol. 2010;9:489–97.
11. Markus HS, Droste DW, Kaps M, et al. Dual antiplatelet therapy with clopidogrel and aspirin in symptomatic carotid stenosis evaluated using doppler embolic signal detection: the Clopidogrel and Aspirin for Reduction of Emboli in Symptomatic Carotid Stenosis (CARESS) trial. Circulation. 2005;111:2233–40.
12. Wang Y, Zhao X, Liu L, et al. Clopidogrel with aspirin in acute minor stroke or transient ischemic attack. N Engl J Med. 2013;369:11–9.
13. Hong KS, Lee SH, Kim EG, et al. Recurrent ischemic lesions after acute atherothrombotic stroke: clopidogrel plus aspirin versus aspirin alone. Stroke. 2016;47:2323–30.
14. Wang Y, Zhao X, Lin J, et al. Association between CYP2C19 loss-of-function allele status and efficacy of clopidogrel for risk reduction among patients with minor stroke or transient ischemic attack. JAMA. 2016;316:70–8.
15. Bellemain-Appaix A, Brieger D, Beygui F, et al. New P2Y12 inhibitors versus clopidogrel in percutaneous coronary intervention: a meta-analysis. J Am Coll Cardiol. 2010;56:1542–51.
16. Johnston SC, Amarenco P, Albers GW, et al. Ticagrelor versus aspirin in acute stroke or transient ischemic attack. N Engl J Med. 2016;375:35–43.
17. Sacco RL, Diener HC, Yusuf S, et al. Aspirin and extended-release dipyridamole versus clopidogrel for recurrent stroke. N Engl J Med. 2008;359:1238–51.
18. Halkes PH, van Gijn J, Kappelle LJ, et al. Aspirin plus dipyridamole versus aspirin alone after cerebral ischaemia of arterial origin (ESPRIT): randomised controlled trial. Lancet. 2006;367:1665–73.
19. Dengler R, Diener HC, Schwartz A, et al. Early treatment with aspirin plus extended-release dipyridamole for transient ischaemic attack or ischaemic stroke within 24 h of symptom onset (EARLY trial): a randomised, open-label, blinded-endpoint trial. Lancet Neurol. 2010;9:159–66.
20. Shinohara Y, Katayama Y, Uchiyama S, et al. Cilostazol for prevention of secondary stroke (CSPS 2): an aspirin-controlled, double-blind, randomised non-inferiority trial. Lancet Neurol. 2010;9:959–68.
21. Shimizu H, Tominaga T, Ogawa A, et al. Cilostazol for the prevention of acute progressing stroke: a multicenter, randomized controlled trial. J Stroke Cerebrovasc Dis. 2013;22:449–56.
22. Teruo K, Tucker A, Sugimura T, et al. Ultra-early combination antiplatelet therapy with cilostazol for the prevention of branch atheromatous disease: a multicenter prospective study. Cerebrovasc Dis Extra. 2016;6:84–95.
23. Kwon SU, Cho YJ, Koo JS, et al. Cilostazol prevents the progression of the symptomatic intracranial arterial stenosis: the multicenter double-blind placebo-controlled trial of cilostazol in symptomatic intracranial arterial stenosis. Stroke. 2005;36:782–6.
24. Berge E, Sandercock P. Anticoagulants versus antiplatelet agents for acute ischaemic stroke. Cochrane Database Syst Rev. 2002;(4):CD003242.
25. Kern R, Nagayama M, Toyoda K, et al. Comparison of the European and Japanese guidelines for the management of ischemic stroke. Cerebrovasc Dis. 2013;35:402–18.

26. Paciaroni M, Agnelli G, Micheli S, et al. Efficacy and safety of anticoagulant treatment in acute cardioembolic stroke: a meta-analysis of randomized controlled trials. Stroke. 2007;38:423–30.
27. Patel MR, Mahaffey KW, Garg J, et al. Rivaroxaban versus warfarin in nonvalvular atrial fibrillation. N Engl J Med. 2011;365:883–91.
28. Connolly SJ, Ezekowitz MD, Yusuf S, et al. Dabigatran versus warfarin in patients with atrial fibrillation. N Engl J Med. 2009;361:1139–51.
29. Granger CB, Alexander JH, McMurray JJ, et al. Apixaban versus warfarin in patients with atrial fibrillation. N Engl J Med. 2011;365:981–92.
30. Giugliano RP, Ruff CT, Braunwald E, et al. Edoxaban versus warfarin in patients with atrial fibrillation. N Engl J Med. 2013;369:2093–104.
31. Arihiro S, Todo K, Koga M, et al. Three-month risk-benefit profile of anticoagulation after stroke with atrial fibrillation: the SAMURAI-Nonvalvular Atrial Fibrillation (NVAF) study. Int J Stroke. 2016;11:565–74.
32. Low molecular weight heparinoid, ORG 10172 (danaparoid), and outcome after acute ischemic stroke: a randomized controlled trial. The Publications Committee for the Trial of ORG 10172 in Acute Stroke Treatment (TOAST) Investigators. JAMA. 1998;279:1265–72.
33. Wong KS, Chen C, Ng PW, et al. Low-molecular-weight heparin compared with aspirin for the treatment of acute ischaemic stroke in Asian patients with large artery occlusive disease: a randomised study. Lancet Neurol. 2007;6:407–13.
34. Wada T, Yasunaga H, Horiguchi H, et al. Outcomes of argatroban treatment in patients with atherothrombotic stroke: observational nationwide study in Japan. Stroke. 2016;47:471–6.
35. Hosomi N, Naya T, Kohno M, et al. Efficacy of anticoagulant treatment with argatroban on cardioembolic stroke. J Neurol. 2007;254:605–12.
36. Markus HS, Hayter E, Levi C, et al. Antiplatelet treatment compared with anticoagulation treatment for cervical artery dissection (CADISS): a randomised trial. Lancet Neurol. 2015;14:361–7.

Ischaemic Stroke: Indication and Techniques of Decompressive Surgery

13

Stephen Honeybul

Abstract

There continues to be a considerable amount of interest in the use of decompressive hemicraniectomy in the context of "malignant" middle cerebral artery infarction. There is now a significant amount of evidence that is a lifesaving intervention; however it is by no means restorative, and many patients will survive but remain dependent, especially those patients over 60 years of age. The degree to which that outcome is acceptable to any one individual is difficult to determine, especially in the time-constrained context of acute stroke. However, it is important to consider the issues of appropriate patient selection in order to avoid exposing patients to an outcome that they might previously perceived to be unacceptable. For those patients on whom surgery is considered beneficial, there remain some issues regarding timing of surgical decompression and complications of the initial decompression and subsequent reconstructive cranioplasty.

There continues to be a considerable amount of interest in the use of decompressive hemicraniectomy in the context of "malignant" middle cerebral artery infarction. Despite advances in endovascular management that have the potential to reverse or significantly reduce the neurological deficit, the time-dependent nature of these interventions means that there will always be patients who either present outside the therapeutic window or for whom endovascular therapy fails. Approximately 1–10% of these patients will develop life-threatening cerebral oedema, and the prognosis for these patients is poor with a fatality rate in the region of 80%. In these circumstances, consideration may be given to decompressive hemicraniectomy as a lifesaving intervention (Fig. 13.1). The procedure itself is technically straightforward and involves temporarily removing a large segment of the calvarium on the same side of the stroke in order to provide extra

S. Honeybul
Department of Neurosurgery, Sir Charles Gairdner Hospital and Royal Perth Hospital, Nedlands, WA, Australia

Department of Neurosurgery, Royal Perth Hospital, Perth, WA, Australia
e-mail: stephen.honeybul@health.wa.gov.au

S.-H. Lee (ed.), *Stroke Revisited: Diagnosis and Treatment of Ischemic Stroke*, Stroke Revisited, DOI 10.1007/978-981-10-1424-6_13

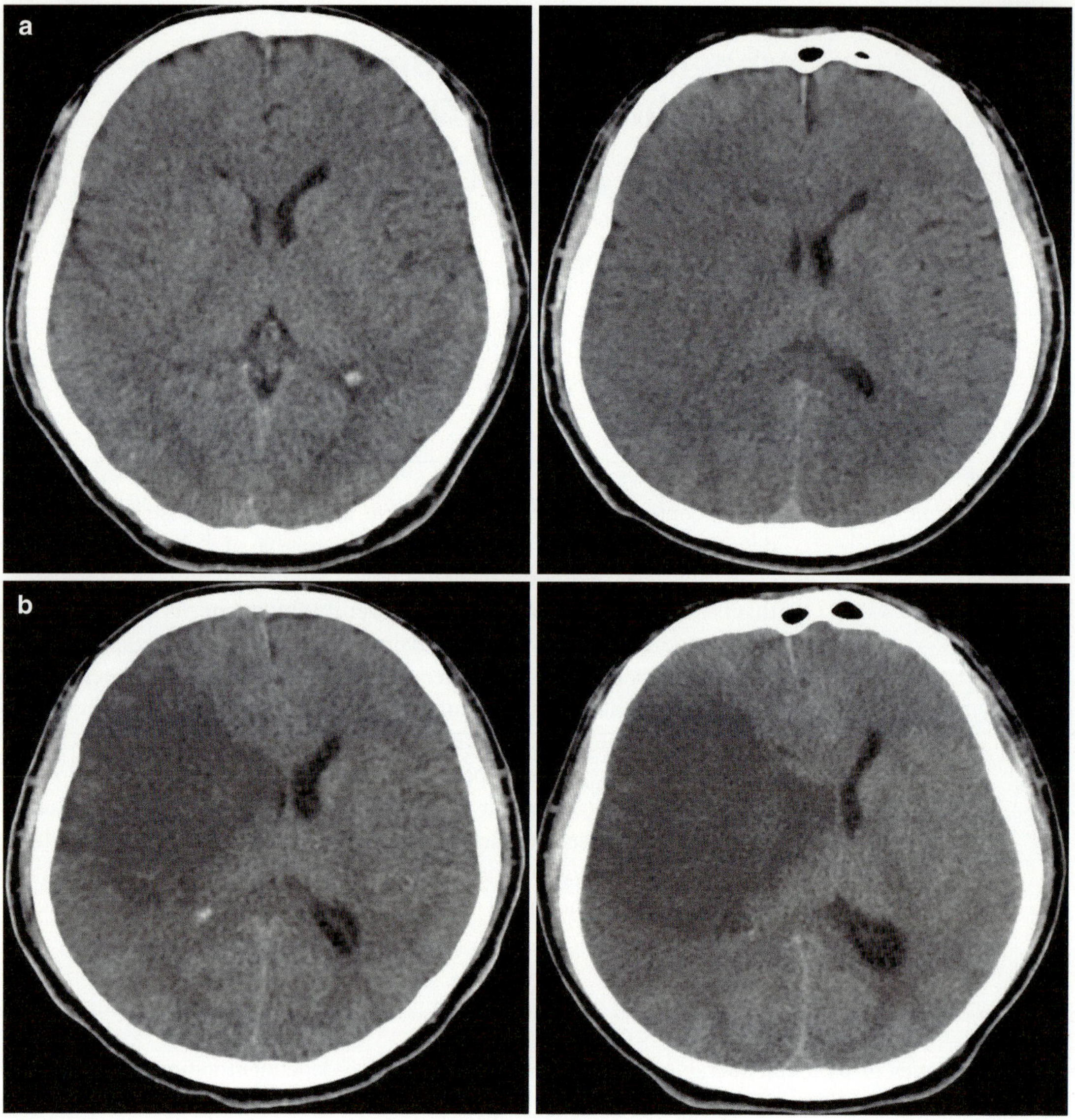

Fig. 13.1 A case of malignant middle cerebral infarction. (**a**) Development of malignant middle cerebral infarction in a 40-year-old adult male. Presented with acute left hemiparesis. *Left*. Initial presentation. Early global cerebral swelling with preservation of grey/white interface and minimal sulcal effacement. *Right*. Eight hours. Following failure of endovascular therapy, there is now a large right middle cerebral artery infarct with effacement of cerebral sulci, effacement of the lateral ventricle and midline shift. (**b**) Temporal evolution of the "malignant" middle cerebral artery infarct. *Left*. Thirty-eight hours. Progressive midline shift with involvement of the basal ganglia. *Right*. Forty-eight hours. Clinical deterioration and prior to surgical decompression. Further progression with involvement of middle cerebral artery territory and basal ganglia

space into which the ischaemic brain can expand. The rationale is that death due to tonsillar herniation is prevented and cerebral perfusion is improved such that damage due to secondary insults may be reduced.

The procedure was first described in 1894 by Annandale and thereafter by Kocher in 1901. Its use gained popularity in the early 1970s predominantly in the setting of severe traumatic brain injury (TBI). However, the combination of poor clinical outcomes and experimental studies suggesting that decompression may actually worsen cerebral oedema led to the procedure being almost abandoned. Throughout the 1980s there was a resurgence in interest, and an increasing number of retrospective studies described the use of the procedure not only following severe TBI and stroke but also in the context of subarachnoid haemorrhage, severe intracranial infection and dural sinus thrombosis [1].

Overall there appeared to be a considerable amount of evidence that decompressive surgery could reduce mortality; however evidence that surgical intervention improved clinical outcome was less forthcoming. Certainly in the context of stroke, surgical intervention will not reverse the ischaemic deficit that precipitated the cerebral swelling, and the concern amongst clinicians was that any reduction in mortality came at the expense of an unacceptable increase in the number of survivors with severe disability and dependency. In order to address this issue, a number of prospective randomised controlled trials were conducted.

13.1 Current Evidence for Clinical Efficacy of Decompressive Hemicraniectomy in Stroke

13.1.1 The European Stroke Trials: Patients Under 60 Years of Age

In the early 2000s, three trials were independently conducted in Europe which compared decompressive hemicraniectomy with standard medical therapy within 48 h of presentation for patients under 60 years of age who developed clinical deterioration following middle cerebral artery infarction. The DECIMAL and DESTINY trials were interrupted early because of slow recruitment and a significant difference in mortality between the treatment groups favouring surgery [2, 3]. The HAMLET trial was stopped because it was thought that it would be highly unlikely that a statistically significant difference would be seen for the primary neurological outcome measure which was defined as good (modified Rankin Score [mRS] 0–3) or poor (mRS 4–6) [4].

Table 13.1 Results of the randomised controlled trials [4, 5]

mRS	Hemicraniectomy	Conservative
Pooled analysis of the European stroke trials		
	n = 51 patients (%)	*n* = 42 patients (%)
6	11 pts (22%)	30 pts (71%)
5	2 pts (4%)	2 pts (5%)
4	16 pts (31%)	1 pt (2%)
3	15 pts (29%)	8 pts (19%)
2	7 pts (14%)	1 pt (2%)
DESTINY II trial		
	n = 49 patients (%)	*n* = 63 patients (%)
6	16 pts (33%)	44 pts (70%)
5	14 pts (28%)	8 pts (13%)
4	16 pts (32%)	9 pts (15%)
3	3 pts (7%)	2 pts (3%)
2	0	0

What each trial independently demonstrated was that survival was improved in those patients who were randomised to receive decompressive surgery. However each individual trial was insufficiently powered to determine whether there was an improvement in favourable outcome. Thereafter, a pooled analysis of the 93 patients involved in all three trials was performed, and this confirmed not only the significant reduction in mortality, but it was also concluded that there was an increase in the number of patients with a favourable outcome (Table 13.1).

On initial examination, this would appear to provide compelling evidence for the efficacy of surgical decompression for patients less than 60 years of age (as per the trial enrolment criteria); however, there were some issues that required clarification. In the first instance, in order to obtain this positive result, favourable outcome had to be redefined. Previously, in the stroke literature the mRS had been used to assess outcome, and this was usually dichotomised into favourable (mRS 0–3) or unfavourable (mRS 4–6). The implication being that the aim of surgery is to achieve an outcome which is felt to be acceptable to the person on whom the procedure is being performed. Notwithstanding some limitations of the mRS, the fundamental issue that denotes a favourable outcome is that a person has a degree of independence.

In the pooled analysis, favourable was reclassified such that it included patients with a mRS of 4. This would therefore include patients who cannot walk unaided and cannot look after their bodily needs which is an outcome that has been regarded as unfavourable for many years. Indeed, closer examination of the data confirms that the increase in survival came almost directly at the expense of an increase in the number of patients with a mRS of 4 [6]. Amongst the survivors who were randomised to receive standard medical care, 75% (9 of 12) had a mRS of 3 or less, an outcome previously defined as favourable. A similar favourable outcome was only achieved in the 55% of the patients treated surgically (22 of 40). It would seem that the most likely outcome following medical therapy is either death or a favourable outcome (mRS 0–3), whereas surgery considerably increases the risk of survival with a mRS of 4 [6].

13.1.2 The DESTINY II Trial: Patients Over 60 Years of Age

The DESTINY II trial investigated the use of decompressive hemicraniectomy in patients over 60 years of age. In a similar design to the previous European trials, patients were randomised within 48 h of presentation to either surgical decompression or standard medical therapy. The results of this study confirmed that surgical intervention significantly reduced mortality; however the conclusion that "hemicraniectomy increased survival without severe disability" requires clarification (Table 13.1).

Most of the survivors in the hemicraniectomy group were adjudged to be either a mRS of either 4 or 5 which would seem to confirm the results of the previous studies that an increase in survival comes at the expense of survival with dependency. However, the finding that 63% of the survivors in the hemicraniectomy group gave retrospective consent to treatment would appear to support ongoing use of the procedure in this age group because it is difficult to argue that it is not on a patient's best interest to have surgery if they are able to state that they are satisfied with their outcome and they would do the same again.

Yet closer examination of results shows that amongst the 27 survivors in the hemicraniectomy group, only 11 could adequately answer this question. The remaining 16 patients had to have a surrogate response from their next of kin because they themselves could not adequately answer the question because they had either severe aphasia or neuropsychological deficits. Given that only 7% (or three patients) achieved a mRS of 3, the remaining 24 patients had either mRS of 4 or 5. Assuming those patients with a mRS of 3 responded positively to the question regarding retrospective consent, amongst the remaining 24 patients, 16 patients could not walk without assistance, could not take care of their basic bodily needs and did have sufficient neurocognitive function such that they could answer a relatively simple question. Given what many informed commentators of sound mind would regard as an unacceptable outcome, these findings would encourage a reconsideration of the aforementioned conclusion [7].

Notwithstanding these observations, there is no doubt that the results of the trials provide good quality level 1 evidence on which to base clinical decision-making especially when considering patient selection and timing of surgery.

13.2 Patient Selection

When considering patient selection, age has always been an important factor because, generally, older patients have reduced brain plasticity, increased comorbidities and are less able to cope with the stress of surgical intervention and subsequent rehabilitation. However, in the light of the evidence currently available, the time may have come for a more nuanced approach to patient selection that seeks to explore an individual's healthcare preferences once they have lost competency.

The fundamental issue rests the acceptability or otherwise of survival with severe disability, and broadly speaking there will be three categories of healthcare preferences that require consideration. Firstly, there are those patients whose preferences are unknown; secondly, there are those patients who have expressed an opinion that survival is paramount even with severe disability; and finally, there are those patients who expressed a view that survival with disability would be unacceptable.

13.2.1 Patients with No Previously Documented or Expressed Healthcare Preferences

Realistically, in the emotionally charged atmosphere of an acute stroke, it would be very difficult to withhold therapy in a person under 60 years of age if there was at least some chance of survival with an acceptable level of disability, and the possibility of unacceptable dependency was acknowledged and accepted by those involved in making the decision. Treatment based on such reasoning can be justified even if the eventual outcome seems unacceptable to the injured party because risks and uncertainties are inevitable in all fields of medicine. It could also be argued given the alternative would be not to survive at all, a young person may quite reasonably be given the chance to "risk" survival with a mRS of 4 in the hope that they will either improve to achieve a mRS of 3 or learn to accept a level of disability that they might previously have deemed unacceptable.

For patients over 60 years of age, it must be acknowledged that there is only a very small chance that that person may achieve independence and there is a high chance that they may be left with very significant neurocognitive and neuropsychological deficits. Ideally, the acceptability or otherwise of this outcome for that particular individual must be fully explored prior to surgical intervention.

13.2.2 Survival Is Paramount

There is little doubt that certain individuals may feel that life is sacrosanct and worth preserving under any circumstances, and this may be based on certain religious, cultural or personal values. These individuals may also be willing to "run the risk" of survival with severe disability, in the hope that they may achieve a good functional outcome. They might also want the opportunity to adapt and learn to live with a level of disability that they and many others, perhaps, might previously have thought to be unacceptable. Whilst these views may fall outside what is deemed acceptable to the majority, where possible, these views should be acknowledged and acted upon. For this group of patient's surgical intervention, following the development of "malignant" cerebral infarction is entirely reasonable.

13.2.3 Survival with Disability Is Unacceptable

The final group of patients will be those patients who have previously expressed a view (either previously voiced or documented) that they would not want to survive with severe disability. In these circumstances the surgeon cannot reasonably assume that they would be able to obtain consent for the operation and, if they did proceed, would have to justify acting on their own judgement against a properly considered assessment of the wishes of the patient.

It could of course be argued that competent individuals do not necessarily predict what they will later find acceptable or unacceptable as a quality of life, and this has been demonstrated when investigators have obtained "retrospective consent" amongst hemicraniectomy survivors. However, to add determinative weight to this as a variation of the consenting process would undermine one of the fundamental tents of modern medicine which requires informed consent to be obtained from competent individuals prior to medical intervention of any sort. Notwithstanding the limitations of making somewhat abstract statements such as "I would rather be dead than live with severe disability" if a person has previously made this assessment, it should be acted upon accordingly. Withholding surgical intervention is further justified by reviewing the results of the pooled analysis of the three European trials in which the most likely outcome following standard medical therapy is either death or survival with a mRS of 3 and thereby some degree of independence.

Overall there is unlikely to be a one-size-fits-all approach to the difficult problem of patient selection especially in the time-constrained circumstances of acute stroke. However, given the evidence available, it is clear that outcome cannot be dichotomised into life or death and these issues must be considered as early as possible following diagnosis of stroke ideally when the patient is relatively stable. This avoids the need for hasty decisions following a catastrophic deterioration where the ethical issues are either sidelined or not really considered at all.

Once the decision regarding surgical intervention has been made, the next issue that requires consideration is that of timing of surgical decompression.

13.3 Surgical Timing

It would seem to be reasonable to proceed with surgical decompression as soon as possible given that there is experiment evidence that early decompression can reduce secondary insults in the context of both traumatic brain injury and ischaemic stroke. However, there are two problems that arise when attempting to apply this concept to clinical practice. On the one hand, it would appear logical to decompress the brain before uncontrolled cerebral swelling leads to impaired perfusion and possibly worsening ischaemia. On the other hand, if early decompression is performed prior to the development of significant cerebral swelling, it may be that certain patients are submitted to surgery who would otherwise have been managed conservatively. Some clinical studies have reported a trend to reduced mortality and improved outcome when surgery was performed early prior to clinical deterioration [8]. Other studies have reported precisely the opposite, and this probably reflects an earlier intervention for a more rapid clinical deterioration and therefore more severe underlying disease [9].

The main problem is determining which patients will subsequently develop the more malignant brain oedema, and whilst there is no definitive predictive measure, a number of clinical and radiological features have been identified which can be combined with evidence gained from the clinical trials.

13.3.1 Clinical Parameters that Predict Malignant Progression

The National Institutes of Health Stroke Scale (NIHSS) provides a useful indication of stroke severity, and this may highlight those patients that are more likely to develop "malignant" infarction. Patients with a score of greater than 20 for dominant hemispheric involvement or greater than 15 for non-dominant hemispheric within 6 h of presentation are particularly at risk. Nausea, vomiting and hyperthermia are also suggestive of malignant progression. In addition, a number of biochemical markers such as hyperglycaemia, leukocytosis and S100B have been shown to have predictive value, but they are not commonly used in clinical practice. Interestingly the role of intracranial pressure (ICP) monitoring in these patients is limited as neurological deterioration can occur without an increase in the ICP.

13.3.2 Radiological Features that Predict Malignant Progression

The morphology of the stroke on either CT or MRI has been shown to have some predictive value. Early CT hypodensity of greater than 50% of the middle cerebral artery territory, involvement of anterior cerebral, posterior artery territory and basal ganglia (Fig. 13.1), midline shift as well as infarct volume of greater than 145 ml on diffusion-weighted MRI have all been shown to predict the development of malignant oedema.

13.3.3 Evidence from the Randomised Controlled Trials

The pooled analysis from the three prospective trials could not demonstrate any difference in functional outcome when comparing those patients treated in less than 24 h after symptom onset with those treated in 24–48 h, and it may be that the latter timeframe is more clinically realistic. The HAMLET study included patients who had been decompressed up to 96 h after symptom onset, and secondary outcome analysis showed that surgery within 48 h significantly reduced the probability of severe disability or death (mRS 5 or 6); however, surgery beyond 48 h provided no such benefit.

Overall, in the clinical setting, the issue of optimal timing remains somewhat unresolved. If surgery is performed too early, there may be a tendency to overtreat and include patients who may have been managed conservatively, and this issue requires further study. Certainly a 24–48 h time window would seem reasonable; however in some patients cerebral swelling can peak later than 48 h after symptom onset. Whilst benefit was not demonstrated by the HAMLET study, it must be noted that the numbers treated were relatively small, and it may be that there is a wider clinical window in which to select appropriate patients.

Table 13.2 Complications following decompressive hemicraniectomy

Complications following decompressive hemicraniectomy
• Postoperative subdural, extradural or subgaleal haematoma
• Cortical herniation
• Damage to herniated cortex
• Subdural/subgaleal effusion
– Managed conservatively
– Simple drainage
– Subdural peritoneal shunt
• Hydrocephalus
• Seizures
• Syndrome of the trephined (confirmed if symptoms were reversed following cranioplasty)
Complications following cranioplasty
• Sudden death following cranioplasty
• Postoperative subdural, extradural or subgaleal haematoma
• Infected cranioplasty (requiring removal of cranioplasty)
• Seizures
• Bone flap resorption
– Requiring replacement
– Clinically significant, not augmented
– Radiologically evident but not clinically significant

13.4 Surgical Considerations

In terms of the technical aspects of surgery, both the initial decompressive surgery and the subsequent reconstructive cranioplasty are technically straightforward; however it is becoming increasingly apparent that both procedures are associated with significant complications (Table 13.2). An exhaustive description is not really required as they are fairly standard neurosurgical procedures; however a brief overview will aim to emphasise complication avoidance.

13.4.1 Decompressive Hemicraniectomy

The aim of the initial hemicraniectomy procedure is to provide as wide and extensive decompression as possible. A question incision is used to exposure as much of the hemicranium as possible within the confines of patient positioning. If the craniotomy is too small, there will be an increased risk of herniation of the brain through the craniectomy, and this may lead to cortical injury. A scalp flap is reflected laterally, and whilst there are some minor variations in the manner in which the temporal muscle is dissected, it is usually easiest to reflect as a single myocutaneous flap. The craniectomy is then performed, and it is important that the bone edge is approximately 1 cm within the confines of the scalp incision. If the craniectomy margin extends beneath the skin incision, there is a risk of cortical injury when performing the cranioplasty because the dissection plan may be compromised. The dura is opened in either a cruciate fashion or circumferentially and a duroplasty performed with either pericranium or a proprietary dural substitute. These can be sutured in position, but it is probably not necessary to accomplish a watertight closure; indeed communication of the subdural space with the subgaleal space may help resorb some of the effusions that are commonly encountered postoperatively. These can have a fairly impressive appearance; however most can be managed conservatively. Following placement of a wound drain, the wound is closed in a routine fashion. Once the patient has recovered and the cerebral swelling has subsided, consideration must be given to cranial reconstruction.

13.4.2 Cranioplasty

A cranioplasty is important in terms of rehabilitation because it restores cerebral protection and cosmesis and, in certain patients, it can improve neurological function. In most institutions the material most commonly used is the patient's own bone because it is cheap, is biocompatible and obviously has the ideal contour. The procedure is technically straightforward; however, as with the initial craniectomy, the number of complications appears disproportionate to the level of technical complexity required to perform the procedure. Three of these require specific consideration given the significant impact that they have on patient outcome.

First, in 2011, three cases of massive uncontrolled cerebral swelling leading to death following an uneventful cranioplasty were reported in three young males who had survived following decompressive craniectomy for severe traumatic brain injury [10]. Within the same neurosurgical service in Western Australia, there were three further deaths following cranioplasty in patients who had had a decompressive hemicraniectomy for ischaemic stroke [11]. Overall, this brings the overall mortality rate to approximately 1% which is extraordinarily high for a relatively simple elective procedure. Until recently this was thought to be a very rare event; however there have since been a number of publications documenting this complication with an incidence ranging from 1 to 7%, and it may be that this phenomenon is merely under-reported. Indeed, a recent publication listed death following bone flap replacement on the outcome algorithm for patients who have had a decompressive craniectomy following ischaemic stroke [12]. The pathophysiology remains to be established; however, it has been suggested that it may be due to some sort of autoregulatory failure. This would mean that the cerebral vasculature is unable to respond adequately when the bone flap is replaced and there are rapid haemodynamic pressure changes such as may occur following application of a suction drain or following a seizure.

Whilst this has yet to be established, it would be difficult to attribute the massive and uncontrolled cerebral swelling to any other mechanism. Certainly within the neurosurgical service of Western Australia, there have been no further deaths following cranioplasty, and this may be because close attention is now given to seizure prophylaxis and cardiovascular stability in the immediate postoperative period and suction drains are not placed on high suction in order to prevent significant pressure differentials. If interest is maintained in the use of the decompressive craniectomy, wider reporting of this type of complication should be encouraged in order to determine not only which patients are most at risk of this devastating complication but also to develop appropriate management strategies.

Second, the reported incidence of cranioplasty infection ranges from 1–12% which is higher than for most elective neurosurgical procedures. A number of reasons have been suggested including skin colonisation whilst in hospital, immune compromise following trauma and the need for multiple operations. However, the results of a recent randomised controlled cranioplasty trial would seem to suggest that surgical technique may be a significant factor [13]. The trial compared outcome following cranioplasty with either autologous bone or primary titanium, and in order to limit confounding within and between both arms of the trial, all procedures were performed by a single senior neurosurgeon using a standardised surgical technique with strict adherence to asepsis. This resulted in no primary infections in the 64 patients in either arm of the trial, and the subsequent changes in management of cranioplasty patients were such that there have been no cranioplasty infections for the past 3 years within the two public hospitals in Western Australia in which cranial neurosurgery is undertaken.

The procedure is usually performed by relatively junior neurosurgical staff because it is perceived to be relatively simple. However, the reopening of previous incisions, the dissection of scarred tissue planes and the use of implants can lead to many instances where sterility may be compromised in inexperienced hands, and the results of the aforementioned trial seem to confirm this observation. Given the impact that further surgery to removal of the infected bone, prolonged antibiotic therapy and addition cranioplasty procedures can potentially have on patient outcome, it may be necessary to reconsider the involvement of senior clinicians when these procedures are being performed.

Third, the reported incidence of bone flap resorption varies between 3% and 12%, and whilst this may be a reflection of biological variability, it may also be a reflection of varying patterns of follow-up and clinical assessment. In addition there is no consensus as to what is clinically significant bone flap resorption. One working definition that has been proposed is that resorption is clinically significant when there has been bicortical loss of bone flap integrity [14]. The rationale for this definition is that once there has been resorption through both the inner and outer table of the bone flap, the protective capacity of the skull vault becomes compromised especially if the patient were to sustain a direct blow to the affected region (Fig. 13.2a). As such the cranioplasty would have failed to fulfil the criteria of restoring cranial protection. The results of the aforementioned trial found that primary titanium cranioplasty provided a better cosmetic and functional outcome and was cost neutral when compared with primary autologous cranioplasty. Although there were costs associated with the custom-made titanium plates, these costs were offset by the extra costs incurred by the operation and hospital stay costs associated with the increase in the number of patients that required secondary cranioplasty after their autologous cranioplasty had failed (Fig. 13.2b). It was also found that bone resorption appeared to be more common in young patients, and therefore in this group of patients, primary titanium cranioplasty should be seriously considered for skull vault reconstruction following decompressive hemicraniectomy.

Conclusion

The role of decompressive craniectomy in the context of "malignant" middle cerebral infarction continues to be refined. The technique of decompressive surgery is simply illustrated in Fig. 13.3, and surgical indications were summarised in Fig. 13.4. There is now little doubt that it is a lifesaving intervention, but it is by no means restorative, and many patients will survive with a level of disability that leaves them dependent. When considering surgical intervention in the time-constrained context of acute stroke, it is important that the ethical issues that arise are fully explored in order to prevent some individuals being exposed to an outcome that they might previously have thought to be unacceptable. More work is also required in this field in order to determine which patients are most likely to develop this "malignant" cerebral swelling so that timing of surgery can be refined and complications minimised.

Conflict of Interest None declared.

Funding None.

Suggestions from Clinical Practice Guidelines
In malignant hemispheric infarction, decompressive surgery is strongly recommended, but in real practice, conduction of the surgery depends on patients' age, valuations of achievable outcome states, etc. In terms of cerebellar infarction, impending brain stem compression can be treated by decompressive surgical evacuation.

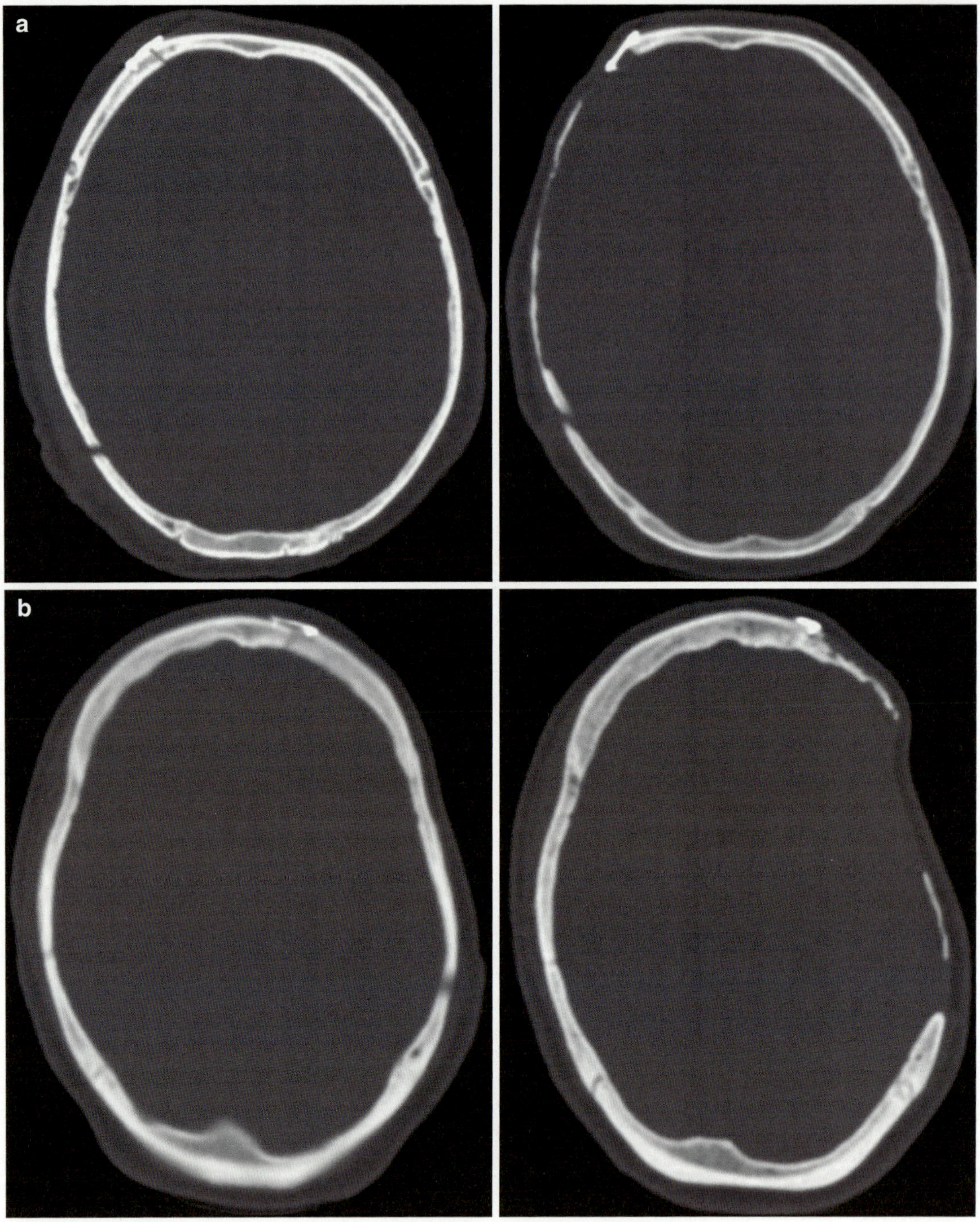

Fig. 13.2 Failure of autologous cranioplasty. (**a**) Partial failure of autologous cranioplasty. Axial CT bone windows. *Left*. Day 1 following cranioplasty showing good bone apposition. *Right*. Nine months following cranioplasty showing resorption through both inner and outer table anteriorly. Augmentation was recommended, but the patient declined. (**b**) Complete failure of autologous cranioplasty. Axial CT bone window. *Left*. Day 1 following autologous cranioplasty showing good bone apposition. *Right*. Six months following cranioplasty showing extensive resorption of bone flap despite evidence of fusion anteriorly. The patient had a titanium cranioplasty performed

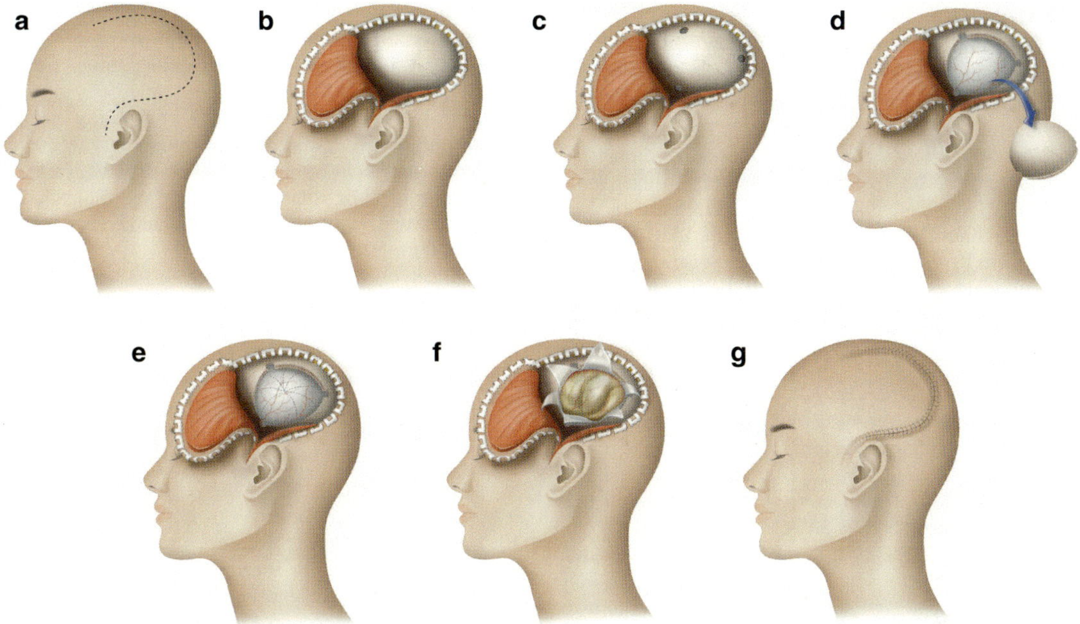

Fig. 13.3 Techniques of decompressive craniectomy. (**a**) Scalp incision: standard question mark skin incision is made from the zygoma to behind the ear. (**b**) Scalp reflection: muscle and soft tissue of scalp are dissected. The scalp flap is reflected anteriorly. (**c**) Creation of bone flap: at least three burr holes are made in the skull. The bone flap is created anteriorly-posteriorly. (**d**) Removal of bone flap: the residual temporal bone is cut by rongeur down to the floor of the middle cranial fossa for maximal decompression of brainstem after removing the bone flap. (**e**) Dural opening: performing the dura opening by multiple radial incisions for maximal cerebral decompression. (**f**) Resection of lesion: the ischaemic brain lesion can be resected. (**g**) Closing the incision: the scalp skin is closed with suture or staples

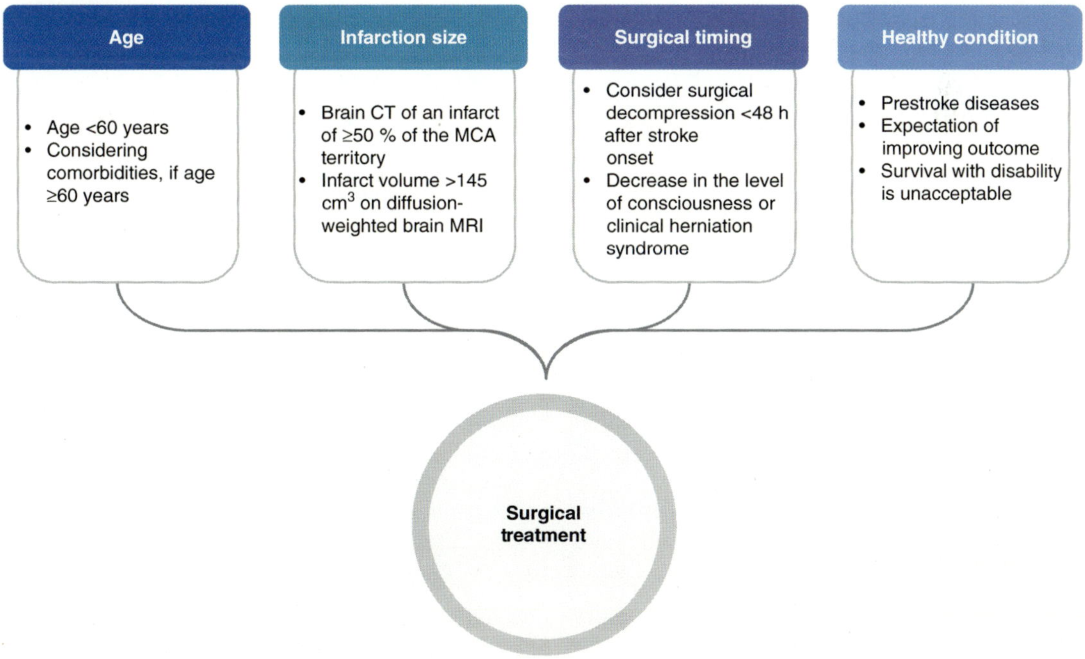

Fig. 13.4 A schematic diagram showing indications of decompressive surgery

References

1. Honeybul S, Ho KM. The current role of decompressive craniectomy in the management of neurological emergencies. Brain Inj. 2013;27:979–91.
2. Jüttler E, Schwab S, Schmiedek P, et al. Decompressive Surgery for the Treatment of Malignant Infarction of the Middle Cerebral Artery (DESTINY): a randomized, controlled trial. Stroke. 2007;38:2518–25.
3. Vahedi K, Vicaut E, Mateo J, et al. Sequential-design, multicenter, randomized, controlled trial of early decompressive craniectomy in malignant middle cerebral artery infarction (DECIMAL Trial). Stroke. 2007;38:2506–17.
4. Hofmeijer J, Kappelle LJ, Algra A, et al. Surgical decompression for space-occupying cerebral infarction (the Hemicraniectomy After Middle Cerebral Artery infarction with Life-threatening Edema Trial [HAMLET]): a multicentre, open, randomised trial. Lancet Neurol. 2009;8:326–33.
5. Vahedi K, Hofmeijer J, Juettler E, et al. Early decompressive surgery in malignant infarction of the middle cerebral artery: a pooled analysis of three randomised controlled trials. Lancet Neurol. 2007;6:215–22.
6. Jüttler E, Unterberg A, Woitzik J, et al. Hemicraniectomy in older patients with extensive middle-cerebral-artery stroke. N Engl J Med. 2014;370:1091–100.
7. Puetz V, Campos CR, Eliasziw M, et al. Assessing the benefits of hemicraniectomy: what is a favourable outcome? Lancet Neurol. 2007;6:580–1.
8. Honeybul S, Ho KM, Gillett G. Outcome following decompressive hemicraniectomy for malignant cerebral infarction: ethical considerations. Stroke. 2015;46:2695–8.
9. Mori K, Nakao Y, Yamamoto T, et al. Early external decompressive craniectomy with duroplasty improves functional recovery in patients with massive hemispheric embolic infarction: timing and indication of decompressive surgery for malignant cerebral infarction. Surg Neurol. 2004;62:420–9.
10. Kilincer C, Asil T, Utku U, et al. Factors affecting the outcome of decompressive craniectomy for large hemispheric infarctions: a prospective cohort study. Acta Neurochir. 2005;147:587–94.
11. Honeybul S. Sudden death following cranioplasty: a complication of decompressive craniectomy for head injury. Br J Neurosurg. 2011;25:343–5.
12. Honeybul S, Damodaran O, Lind CR, et al. Malignant cerebral swelling following cranioplasty. J Clin Neurosci. 2016;29:3–6.
13. Kelly AG, Holloway RG. Health state preferences and decision-making after malignant middle cerebral artery infarctions. Neurology. 2010;75:682–7.
14. Honeybul S, Morrison DA, Ho KM, et al. A randomized controlled trial comparing autologous cranioplasty with custom-made titanium cranioplasty. J Neurosurg. 2016;18:1–10.
15. Honeybul S, Ho KM. How "successful" is calvarial reconstruction using frozen autologous bone? Plast Reconstr Surg. 2012;130:1110–7.

14 Critical and Medical Management in Acute Stage of Ischemic Stroke

Sang-Bae Ko

Abstract

Patients with acute ischemic stroke may have different prognosis based on the ischemic lesion burden, the reperfusion status after thrombolytic therapy or endovascular thrombectomy. In addition, the quality of neurocritical care has a different effect on clinical outcome, according to the appropriateness of diagnosis and treatment of neurologic worsening. Here, we will mainly focus on general medical care, such as intravenous fluid therapy, glucose control, and hemodynamic optimization. In the latter part, we will briefly discuss the specific issues on neurocritical care in treating patients with large ischemic burden, especially on managing brain edema and elevated intracranial pressure.

14.1 General Medical Care

14.1.1 Fluid Therapy and Choice of Intravenous Fluid

The major purpose of fluid therapy in ischemic stroke patients is to maintain adequate intravascular blood volume, aiming at augmenting cardiac output to optimize cerebral perfusion. Except for patients with coexisting medical conditions such as congestive heart failure, most ischemic stroke patients are either euvolemic or hypovolemic at presentation. Moreover, when the patients have fever or dysphasia, they may indeed require enough hydration.

When choosing fluids for intravenous infusion, it remains unresolved whether crystalloids (e.g., normal saline or Ringer's lactate) or colloids (hydroxyethyl starch or albumin) are preferable. Electrolyte concentrations of commonly used fluids are described (Table 14.1). Normal saline (0.9%) is the most commonly used for fluid resuscitation. Normal saline is cheap and has been widely used in various conditions. On the other hand, it has higher chloride ion concentration (155 mEq/L) compared to physiologic concentration (98 ~ 110 mEq/L). Therefore, its excessive use may lead to unwanted hyperchloremic metabolic acidosis, which may have risk of

S.-B. Ko, M.D., Ph.D.
Department of Neurology, Seoul National University Hospital, 101 Daehak-ro, Jongno-gu, Seoul 110-744, South Korea
e-mail: sangbai1378@gmail.com

S.-H. Lee (ed.), *Stroke Revisited: Diagnosis and Treatment of Ischemic Stroke*, Stroke Revisited, DOI 10.1007/978-981-10-1424-6_14

Table 14.1 Chemical properties of commonly used fluid solutions

	Na (mEq/L)	Cl (mEg/L)	Osmolarity (mOsm/L)	Others (mEq/L)
Crystalloid				
Normal saline (0.9%)	155	155	310	
Ringer's lactate	130	109	273	Lactate (28), K (5.4)
Plasma-Lyte A	140	98	295	Acetate 27/gluconate 23/K(5)
Colloid				
4% albumin	148	128	250	
Hydroxyethyl starch (6%): Voluven	154	154	308	
Hydroxyethyl starch (6%): Volulyte	137	110	286	K (4), Mg (1.5), acetate (34)

renal impairment. By contrast, Ringer's lactate (Hartmann solution) or Plasma-Lyte A have lower chloride ions, close to physiologic concentration, and are called as "balanced" solutions. Even though Plasma-Lyte A is better in terms of electrolyte balance, it is more expensive than normal saline and did not show superiority to normal saline when used in patients with septic shock. In theory, colloids (albumin or hydroxyethyl starch [HES]) may have advantages over crystalloids in maintaining intravascular volume, because higher percentage of infused colloids remain in the intravascular compartment compared to crystalloids. However, even in patients with septic shock or hemorrhagic shock who require large amount of fluid therapy than ischemic stroke, colloids infusion did not show clinical benefit. To the contrary, prolonged use of HES (Voluven or Volulyte) did actually lead to more renal complications requiring renal replacement therapy. In the recent Cochrane review, focusing on the effect of fluid therapy in patients with stroke, intravascular fluid therapy to induce hemodilution did not show either short-term (up to 28 days) or long-term (3–6 months) mortality benefit [1]. Functional outcomes (measured by modified Rankin Scale of 3–6) were also not different. More specifically, crystalloids and colloids did not show any difference in terms of mortality and the risk of brain edema. However, colloids therapy had 2.3 times higher risk of pulmonary edema due to volume overload. In ALIAS-2 trial, which infused albumin for neuroprotection, a higher percentage of patients in the albumin group had pulmonary edema compared to placebo. Taken together, intravascular fluid therapy can be used in patients with acute stroke. However, its net clinical benefit has not been validated yet. Moreover, colloids have higher risk of pulmonary edema.

14.1.2 Blood Pressure Control

14.1.2.1 Pathophysiology of Elevated Blood Pressure in Acute Ischemic Stroke

Elevated blood pressure is common in acute phase, and approximately 60% of patients have systolic blood pressure greater than 140 mmHg on presentation. The percentage is even higher when the patients have a history of hypertension. The suggested mechanisms of blood pressure surges are partly explained by an increase in plasma catecholamine, anxiety, and noxious stimuli including severe pain or bladder distention. In addition, an increase in intracranial pressure often leads to additional blood pressure elevation in severe stroke (Cushing phenomenon). Regardless of its cause, acute blood pressure elevation is associated with poor neurologic outcome.

14.1.2.2 Cerebral Autoregulation and Optimal Blood Pressure

Cerebral autoregulation means cerebral blood flow is maintained in a constant level despite the changes in blood pressure (more correctly cerebral perfusion pressure, which is defined as mean arterial pressure minus intracranial pressure) (Fig. 14.1). In cases with intact autoregulation, an

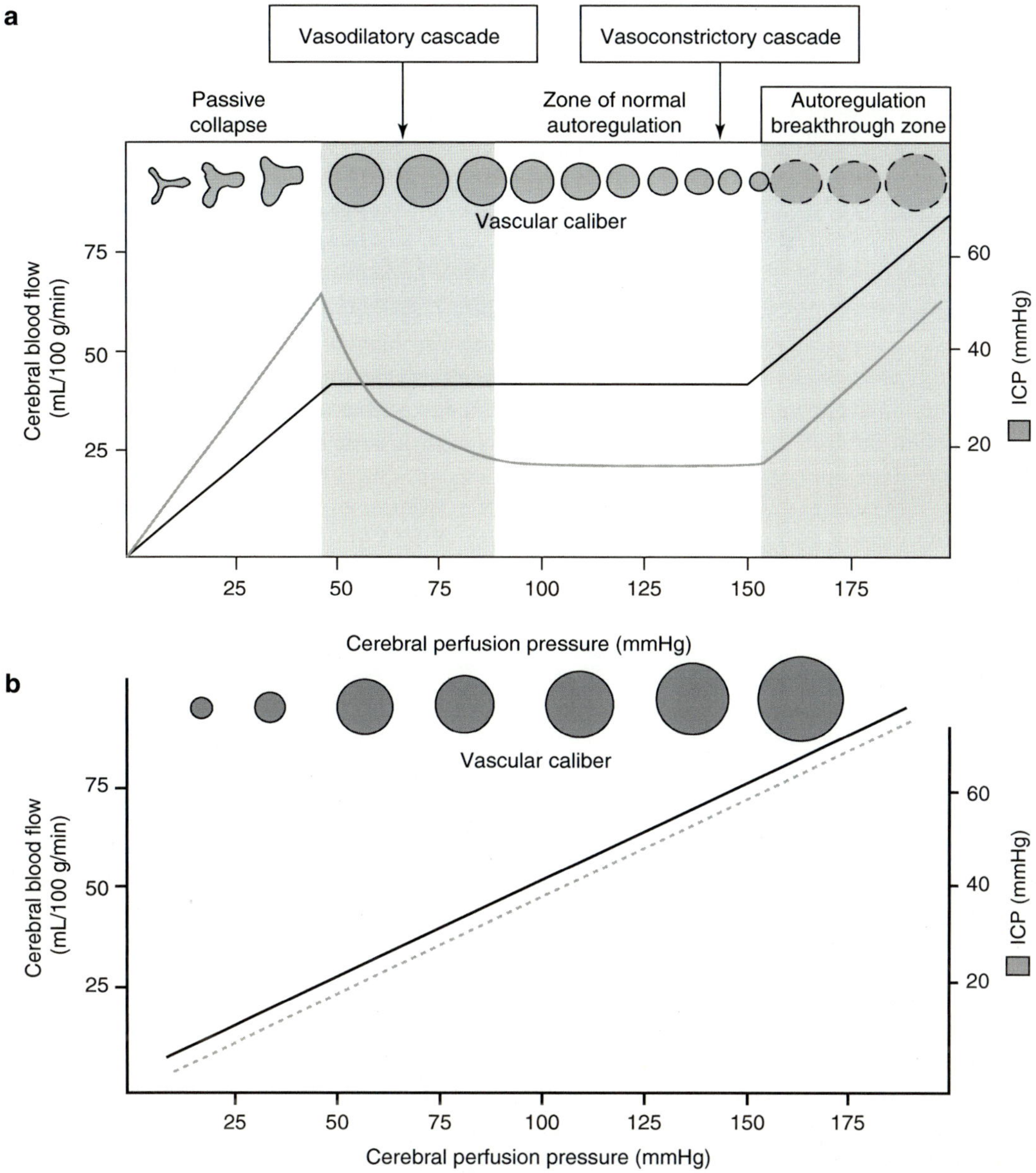

Fig. 14.1 Relationship among the cerebral hemodynamic parameters. In patients with intact cerebral autoregulation, constant cerebral blood flow is maintained within autoregulating ranges of blood pressure. When blood pressure drops, cerebral blood vessels dilate to maintain constant blood flow, in which paradoxically increases intracranial pressure (**a**). In patients with disturbed cerebral autoregulation, the caliber of blood vessel is passively dependent on perfusion pressure. Therefore, cerebral blood flow and intracranial pressure are directly affected by mean artery pressure (**b**). Reproduced by permission of Journal of Stroke [2]

increase in blood pressure leads to vasoconstriction which increases vascular resistance and maintains constant cerebral blood flow. By contrast, progressive drop in blood pressure induces vasodilation which decreases vascular resistance and helps with constant blood flow [2]. In patients with acute ischemic stroke, cerebral autoregulation is often disturbed. With disturbed autoregulation, cerebral blood flow is more directly dependent on blood pressure, and a decrease in blood pressure may lead to concomitant decrease in cerebral blood flow, which may aggravate perfusion deficit in the penumbra area. The status of autoregulation on each patient can be identified using correlation analysis between continuous blood pressure and intracranial pressure (pressure reactivity index, PRx) or cerebral blood flow (flow reactivity index, FRx). If patients' autoregulation status is not known, abrupt drop in blood pressure should be avoided not to aggravate perfusion deficit just in case the patient have disturbed autoregulation. In a healthy person, within the ranges of mean arterial pressure between 60 mmHg and 150 mmHg, cerebral blood flow remained constant based on with autoregulation physiology.

14.1.2.3 Management of Blood Pressure Elevation

Patients who are treated with intravenous tissue plasminogen activator (t-PA) therapy, blood pressure should be controlled under 180/105 mmHg. In general, there is no sweet spot for pressure in treating patients with acute ischemic stroke. Based on American Stroke Association guidelines, it is reasonable to start using blood pressure-lowering drugs from 220 to 120 mmHg, which is 150 mm Hg in terms of mean arterial pressure. Blood pressure above this level can be in the autoregulatory breakthough zone, which requires lowering blood pressure.

Most commonly used blood pressure-lowering drugs are intravenous injections including labetalol (10–20 mg bolus) or nicardipine (infusion at a rate of 3–5 mg/h or bolus injection of 1–2 mg based on pressure level). In refractory cases, nitroprusside injection may be tried, but it has rarely been used in stroke patients because nitroprusside has an unpredictable effect on blood pressure and has rebound hypertension which may actually aggravate ICP surges.

14.1.2.4 Unsolved Issues in Blood Pressure Control in Acute Ischemic Stroke

When patients are treated with t-PA, blood pressure is strictly controlled under 180/105 mmHg because high blood pressure is associated with hemorrhagic transformation [3]. However, it is unknown whether more intensive blood pressure control is beneficial to the patients treated with t-PA or not. In ENCHANTED trial (part B), effectiveness of intensive blood pressure lowering (SBP 130–140 mmHg) were compared with standard treatment (SBP < 180 mmHg), which will be published in the near future [4]. Moreover, in patients with intra-arterial thrombectomy with complete recanalization, appropriate blood pressure level is not known. Those patients may not require high blood pressure to optimize perfusion and may need strict blood pressure control to prevent hemorrhagic transformation. This should be addressed in the upcoming clinical trials.

14.1.3 Glucose Control

Extreme blood glucose, either high or low, can be detrimental in patients with acute ischemic stroke. Hypoglycemia may present with stroke-mimicking symptom and should be rapidly corrected above 60 mg/dL, if identified. Hyperglycemia is associated with ischemic progression, hemorrhagic transformation, and poor neurologic outcome. In the acute phase, transient elevation of glucose is common, and it gradually decreases over time. Strict glucose control with insulin infusion is frequently associated with hypoglycemic episodes and did not translate into better clinical outcome. The optimal range of serum glucose is not known in acute ischemic stroke. However, currently recommended ranges of serum glucose are between 140 and 180 mg/dL [3].

Ideally, direct measurement of brain tissue glucose may have more direct information in each patient. However, invasive monitoring on metabolism is required such as microdialysis, which needs more study in patients with acute ischemic stroke. Low brain glucose has been identified as a critical factor for metabolic crisis in patients with severe brain injury [2]. Brain tissue glucose is affected in part by serum glucose and in part by cerebral perfusion pressure or cerebral blood flow (Fig. 14.2). In normal condition, brain glucose concentration is measured higher than 2 mmol/L, and brain/serum glucose ratio is regarded as more than 0.4. A decrease in brain glucose leads to brain tissue starvation with energy failure in patients with severe brain injury. Moreover, a decrease in brain/serum glucose ratio below 0.12, compared to a normal ratio of 0.4, has been considered as an independent risk factor for metabolic crisis.

14.1.4 Fever

Elevated body temperature is common in acute stroke and most frequently observed within 2 days after presentation. The etiologies of fever, including infectious and noninfectious origins, are very diverse and need to be differentiated appropriately. When infectious fever is suspected, sensitive antibiotics covering suspected pathogen should be initiated based on the presumed source of infection. On the other hand, patients with severe stroke often have elevated temperature without definite infection source. In this case, fever is often associated with herniation or mass effect.

Although fever is linked with poor neurologic outcome, active control of fever using cooling devices is not proven to be beneficial in acute stroke. However, extreme elevation of body temperature may aggravate brain swelling and infarc-

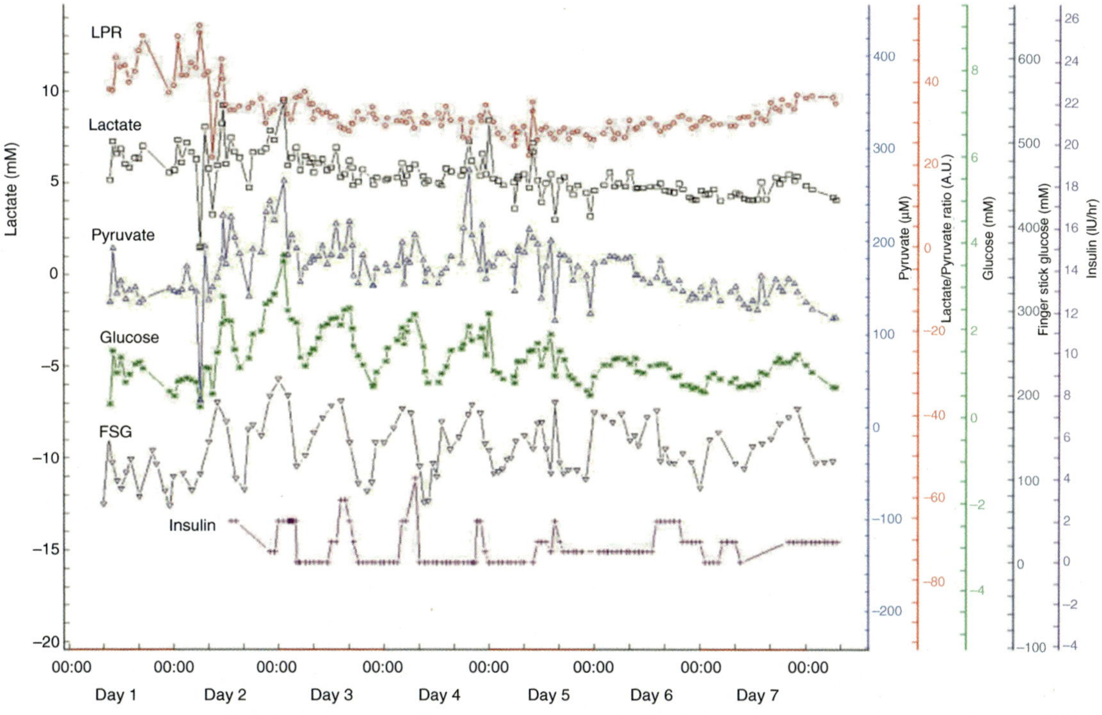

Fig. 14.2 Relationship between peripheral glucose and brain glucose in severe stroke patients. Brain tissue glucose, measured by microdialysis, fluctuates followed by systemic glucose level. When insulin infusion was given, a sudden drop of systemic glucose can lead to very low brain tissue glucose, which is associated with brain energy failure and metabolic crisis. *LPR* Lactate/pyruvate ratio, *FSG* fingerstick glucose, *AU* arbitrary unit, and *IU* international unit. Reproduced by permission of Journal of Stroke [2]

tion extension, it is reasonable to control fever with antipyretics or cooling methods. Although rare, paroxysmal sympathetic hyperactivity can be a cause of fever in patients with severe ischemic stroke [5].

14.2 Cardiac Evaluation and Control in Acute Stage

14.2.1 Embolic Source Evaluation

Investigation of potential embolic source is the most important diagnostic step in evaluating patients with acute ischemic stroke [6]. Evaluating methods include transthoracic echocardiography (TTE), transesophageal echocardiography (TTE), and heart rhythm monitoring (electrocardiogram or Holter monitoring). Current evidence suggests that even longer monitoring, up to several weeks using implantable loop recorder, may detect more atrial fibrillation in high-risk patients.

TTE is generally performed as a screening test to find cardiac embolic sources. Well known embolic sources are described in Table 14.2. If indicated TEE can be performed (Fig. 14.3). TEE is superior to TTE in identifying small embolic sources located in the posterior part, such as valve vegetation, left atrial appendage thrombus, patent foramen ovale, or aortic atheroma. However, TEE also has limitations; high intra and interrater variability, not always available at any time, may require patients' cooperation. Therefore, patients with severe stroke may not tolerate TEE due to poor cooperation. Cardiac multidetector CT (MDCT) has roles in identifying intra- or extracardiac embolic sources because MDCT has less interrater variability and has better visualization of aortic arch atheroma [7]. Therefore, those who cannot tolerate TEE, cardiac MDCT can be used as an alternative in evaluating intracardiac or extracardiac embolic sources.

Table 14.2 List of potential embolic sources

Sources with high embolic potential: intracardiac
Arrhythmia
Atrial fibrillation (valvular > non-valvular)
Atrial flutter
Sick sinus syndrome
Ischemic heart disease
Recent myocardial infarction (<1 month)
Chronic myocardial infarction with LV aneurysm
Akinetic/dyskinetic LV wall
Valvular heart disease
Mitral stenosis, aortic stenosis
Prosthetic valve
Intracardiac thrombus
LV or LA thrombus
Cardiomyopathy
Dilated cardiomyopathy with low ejection fraction
Cardiac tumors
Myxoma
Fibroelastoma
Other cardiac tumors
Intracardiac vegetations
Endocarditis
Sources with high embolic potential: extracardiac
Aortic atheroma
Complex aortic plaque (>4 mm, ulceration or mobile)
Sources with low embolic potential
Mitral valve prolapse
Patent foramen ovale
Spontaneous echogenic contrast
Mitral annular calcification
Atrial septal aneurysm
Lambl's excrescences

Stroke unit care with continuous ECG monitoring indeed increased the chances of detecting a new onset atrial fibrillation. The longer the duration of monitoring, the higher chance of finding an atrial fibrillation. In addition, the size of left atrium diameter, the frequency of left atrial premature complex, and cardiac diastolic dysfunctions are associated with the risk of cardiac embolic stroke.

14.2.2 Atrial Fibrillation and Rapid Ventricular Response

Previous trials showed that rhythm control is not superior to rate control in reducing mortality. However, meta-analysis suggested that rhythm control may be beneficial in young patients if

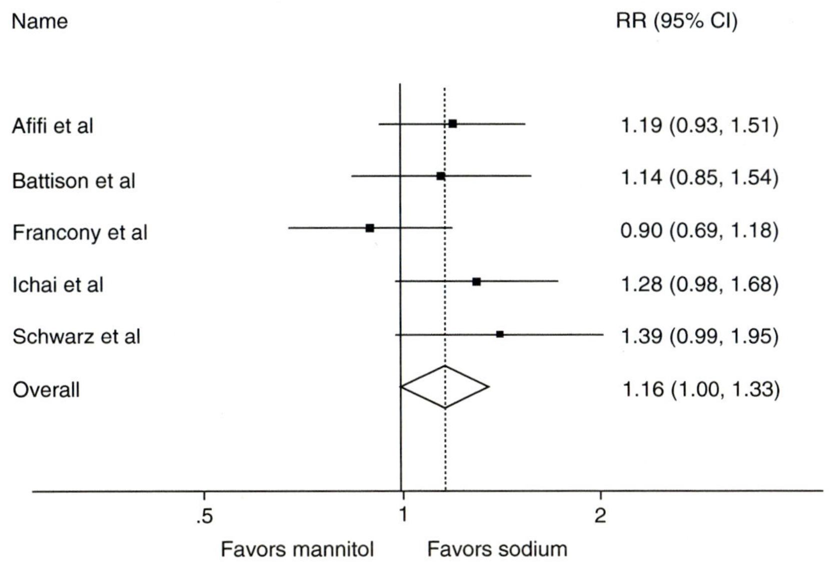

Fig. 14.3 Forest plot showing the relative risk of successful control of elevated intracranial pressure. Meta-analysis from randomized controlled trials showed that hypertonic saline more effectively decreased elevated intracranial pressure compared to mannitol. Source: Hypertonic saline versus mannitol for the treatment of elevated intracranial pressure: A meta-analysis of randomized clinical trials. Reproduced by permission of Critical Care Medicine [10]

maintained long enough. Rate control aims at limiting heart rate below 100 beats per minute; prolonged tachycardia may end up with tachycardia associated cardiomyopathy, which is reversible. In treating patients with acute phase, rapid ventricular response in atrial fibrillation is more frequently confronted condition. In mild cases, patients just feel palpitation, dizziness, or short breath. However, in severe cases, blood pressure drops with empty heart requiring immediate treatment. First-line drugs are intravenous beta-blockers or calcium channel blockers (diltiazem or verapamil) except in patients with known pre-excitation such as Wolff-Parkinson-White (WPW) syndromes. Doses and regimens are described in Table 14.3. Digoxin shows rate control effect via increasing vagal tones. Therefore, digoxin is very ineffective in reducing heart rate in majority of cases with rapid ventricular response because it is often triggered by an increased sympathetic tone, hyperthyroidism, or fever. In general, digoxin is considered in patients with hypertrophic cardiomyopathy, or WPW syndrome, only if patients have left ventricular dysfunction. Digoxin

Table 14.3 Frequently used drugs for controlling heart rate in atrial fibrillation

	Recommended regimen
Beta-blocker	
Propranolol	Bolus injection of 1.0 mg over 5 min then continuous infusion at a rate of 0.5 mg/min (maximum dose of 0.1 mg/kg)
Esomolol	Bolus injection of 0.5 mg/kg over 1 min followed by 0.05–0.1 mg/kg per min
Metoprolol	0.15 mg/kg (to a maximum dose of 10 mg)
Calcium channel blocker	
Diltrazem	Bolus injection of 0.2 mg/kg over 2 min. A second dose of 0.35 mg/kg over 2 min in 15 min after the first dose. Maintenance dose: 5–15 mg/h
Verapamil	Bolus injection of 0.075 mg/kg (to a maximum dose of 5 mg). A second bolus dose of 0.075 mg/kg (to a maximum dose of 5 mg) can be given 10 min after the first dose. A third dose of 0.15 mg/kg (to a maximum dose of 10 mg) can be injected 30 min after the second dose
Amiodarone	150 mg over 10 min, maintenance dose 1 mg min over 6 h then 0.5 mg/min
Digitalis	Intravenous loading: 8–12 mcg/kg, 50% initially then 1/4 the loading dose q6–8 h twice

should be avoided in patients with paroxysmal atrial fibrillation, because digoxin may aggravate the frequency of atrial fibrillation.

14.3 Neurocritical Care for Ischemic Stroke Patients

14.3.1 ICU Indication of Ischemic Stroke

The admission criteria to the neurological ICU may differ in each institution but usually admit patients with major organ dysfunction as well as severe brain damage. Therefore, acute stroke patients in the middle cerebral or basilar artery territory are good candidate for admission to the neurological ICU. In addition, any patients who require intensive neurological, hemodynamic monitoring, or need intensive respiratory care, are also a candidate for ICU care.

14.3.2 Malignant Middle Cerebral Artery Infarction

The majority of patients with large hemispheric infarction are admitted to the neurological ICU for monitoring of brain swelling. Patients with admission NIHSS >20 in the dominant hemisphere, or NIHSS >15 in the nondominant hemisphere, are likely to have large infarctions, requiring close observation for neurological worsening. Although there are no perfect clinical or radiological factors predicting malignant cerebral infarction, infarction volume > 80 cc within 6 h or infarct volume > 145 cc within 14 h have been suggested as an imaging risk factor for malignant infarction. Brain edema becomes evident within 24–36 h from onset, which peaks over the course of 72–96 h Therefore, most patients may deteriorate within 2–3 days from onset [8].

14.3.3 Brain Edema and Increased Intracranial Pressure

Patients with huge hemispheric infarction need frequent neurological assessment including consciousness level and pupillary light reflex. A progressive decline in level of consciousness is a strong predictor of worsening of brain edema. Ipsilateral or contralateral pupillary dysfunction, adduction palsy, or extensor posturing suggest downward herniation. Currently, more objective measurement of pupil size and light reflex are possible using automated pupilometer, which help with early decision making. It is still under debate whether patients with large hemispheric stroke require continuous intracranial pressure monitoring. Brain swelling does not always correlate with an increase in intracranial pressure. Therefore, it should be kept in mind that patient can deteriorate even with normal intracranial pressure.

14.3.4 Medical Management of Increased Intracranial Pressure

Medical management of intracranial pressure will also be discussed in Chap. 21. When ICP elevation is suspected, ICP care bundle should be initiated. Head elevation should be up to 30 degree with limiting head rotation to facilitate intracranial venous drainage. When considering osmotic agents, 20% mannitol (0.5 ~ 1 g/kg) is often used. The ICP lowering effect peaks within 30 min to 1 h after infusion and persist over 4 or 6 h. Prolonged use of mannitol often leads to renal insufficiency, mediated by dehydrating effect and direct toxic effect to renal tubules. To prevent renal deterioration, patients' intravascular volume status should be managed with euvolemic because the dehydrating effect of mannitol aggravates prerenal-type azotemia. In addition, direct toxic effect of mannitol is dependent on serum concentration of mannitol. However, direct measurement of blood mannitol concentration is not practically available except for research setting. Instead, osmolar gap (a difference between measured and calculated osmolarity) was used to estimate serum mannitol concentration. As mannitol concentration increases with repeated uses, serum-measured osmolarity increases. However, calculated osmolarity (2Na + BUN/2.8 + Glucose/18) does not have factors reflecting mannitol concentration.

Therefore, the osmolar gap shows fair correlation with mannitol concentration, and it is practically used to estimate serum mannitol concentration. With high osmolar gap above 50 or 60, mannitol should be withheld due to high chances of renal failure.

Hypertonic saline is a good alternative to mannitol. In a recent meta-analysis, hypertonic saline has shown more effectively to control intracranial pressure in the neurological ICU (Fig. 14.4) [9, 10]. A variety of concentration of hypertonic saline, from 3 to 23.4%, has been used in the practice. Among them, 11.7% (60 ml) or 23.4% (30 ml) are frequently used to control ICP surges. In a study using invasive multimodality monitoring, administration of osmotic agent (mannitol or hypertonic saline) reduced brain water content by 1.4% in 1 h after injection, proving its direct tissue drying effect in the peri-lesion area at risk of edema [11].

Other promising therapy to prevent brain edema is glyburide. Glyburide decreases brain edema through inhibition of nonselective channel composed of sulfonylurea receptor 1 (SUR1) and transient receptor potential cation channel subfamily M member 4 (TRPM4). In a recent randomized phase 2 clinical trial, intravenous glyburide was well tolerated and showed effect in controlling brain edema, measured by the midline shift on CT scan [12]. But it failed to change clinical outcomes. This needs to be validated on further clinical trials.

14.3.5 Decompressive Hemicraniectomy in Malignant MCA Infarction

The most effective method in controlling brain swelling in malignant MCA infarction is decompressive hemicraniectomy [8]. Hemicraniectomy was proven to reduce mortality by 50% (from 77 to 22%) in young patients (age < 60). In an additional trial, mortality benefit persisted even in older patients with age over 60. In this trial among elderly patients, the median age was 70 and confirmed that hemicraniectomy decreased mortality from 70 to 33%. However, the mortality benefit was small compared to younger patients.

Timing of decompressive hemicraniectomy is still debatable. Most surgical hemicraniectomy trial was performed within 24–48 h after onset.

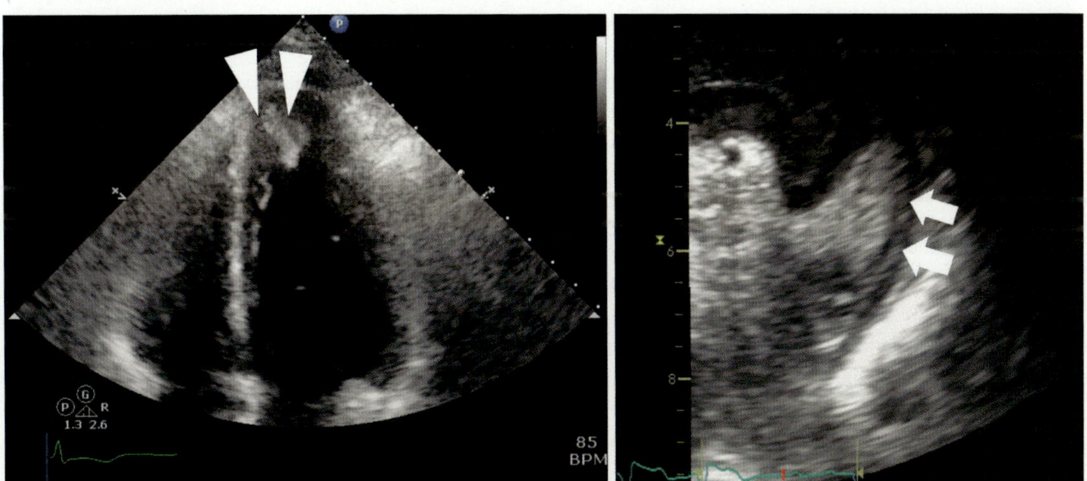

Fig. 14.4 Echocardiographic evaluation of cardiac embolic sources. A 56-year-old male patient was presented with multiple scattered embolic infarctions. Initial electrocardiogram was normal. Transthoracic echocardiogram showed mobile thrombus at the apex of left ventricle (2.5 cm × 1.8 cm, *panel A*, *arrowhead*), which disappeared after anticoagulation. A 62-year-old woman was presented with multiple recurrent stroke events. Transthoracic echocardiography was normal, but transesophageal echocardiogram showed thrombus in the left atrial appendage (*arrows*, *Panel B*)

Even though not all of the patients with malignant infarction have actual herniation, early surgery within 12 h may be more beneficial compared to delayed surgery 48–72 h after onset. Patients who waited for clinical deterioration then performed hemicraniectomy had worse clinical outcome. Therefore, early surgery may be better when indicated. The natural course and the effect of hemicraniectomy on functional outcome and mortality should be discussed with family members.

14.3.6 Targeted Temperature Management

Targeted temperature management (TTM) was proven to show benefit only in patients with out of hospital cardiac arrest (OHCA) with shockable rhythm such as ventricular fibrillation. Clinical trials of TTM on ischemic stroke are still undergoing. Brain cooling has neuroprotective effect and reduces ischemic reperfusion injury, which prompted its use in hyperacute stroke patients. In addition, hypothermia lowers metabolic rate in the brain, which leads to decrease in cerebral blood flow due to metabolism-flow coupling phenomenon, and ends up with decrease in cerebral blood volume and reduction in intracranial pressure. Therefore, TTM can be used in cases with severe brain edema with ICP crisis, if patients reject or cannot tolerate decompressive hemicraniectomy.

There are several cooling methods in the clinical practice, surface cooling with gel pad system (Arctic Sun) and intravascular cooling (InnerCool or CoolGarD). Intravascular cooling requires a new central line insertion via the femoral vein, which may somewhat delay initiating treatment. However, intravascular cooling is more effective in rapid cooling, and patients' body temperature deviates less from the target temperature. On the other hand, surface cooling is easier to apply and handle. The effect on neurologic outcome is similar, and any types of methods can be used based on user's experience.

Earlier phase 1 studies on TTM in hyperacute stroke showed that intravascular cooling after t-PA infusion was generally well tolerated but did increase the risk of pneumonia. In recent phase 2 study (ICTuS2), intravascular cooling right after administration of t-PA, targeting at 33 °C for 24 h and controlled rewarming for 12 h, did not improve clinical outcome (defined by mRS 0–1 on 90 days, 33% in hypothermia group vs. 38% in normothermia group). In this trial, intra-arterial thrombectomy was not allowed. As expected, more pneumonia event was observed in hypothermia group (19%) compared to normothermia (10.5%). The reasons of higher pneumonia rate are partly due to sedative, anti-shivering drug, or hypothermia itself. More safe regimens are needed to use TTM in clinical practice. Another European trial on an acute stroke patient (EuroHYP-1) is currently ongoing, and the effect of TTM on hyperacute stroke will be validated.

One randomized clinical trial was performed to evaluate the effect of TTM on brain swelling and functional outcome in patients with malignant MCA infarction who rejected or could not tolerate decompressive hemicraniectomy [13]. TTM was initiated targeting at 33–34 °C for 24 h and extended up to 72 h depending on physician's decision with slow-controlled rewarming at a rate of 0.1 °C/h. Patients with TTM had a trend for better functional outcome without changes in mortality. Therefore, TTM can be used as an alternative for surgery in patients who cannot tolerate or reject decompressive hemicraniectomy (Fig. 14.5).

14.3.7 Early Tracheostomy Versus Late Tracheostomy

Patients with severe stroke tend to be intubated for airway protection and respiratory care. Although Glasgow Coma Scale higher than 8 with eye score of 4 has high likelihood of successful extubation, patients who failed extubation more than twice will be considered for tracheostomy. Usual timing of decision on tracheostomy is around 14 days. In one randomized trial (SETPOINT trial) in stroke patients, early tracheostomy (<3 days) reduced the sedation needs compared to late tracheostomy (7–14 days).

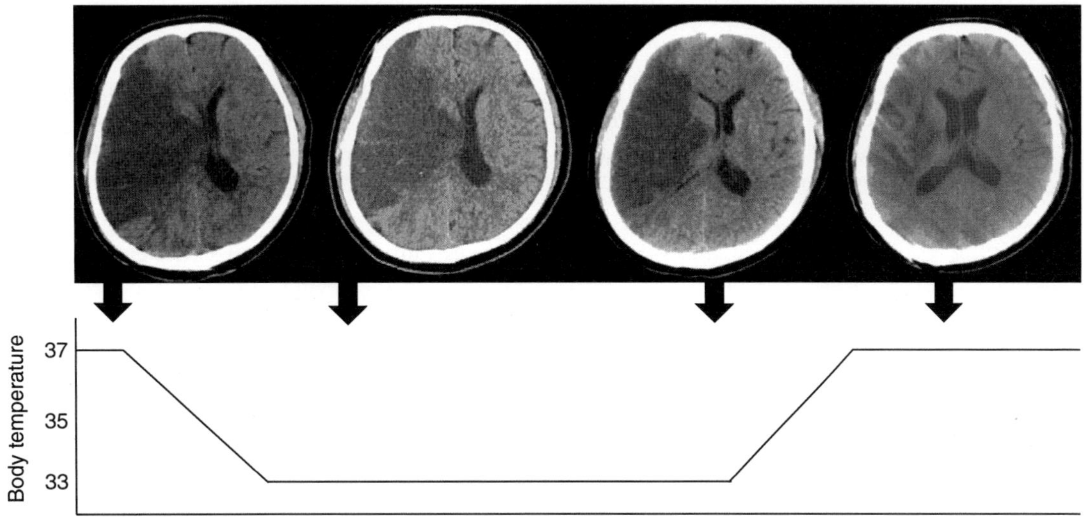

Fig. 14.5 The effect of targeted temperature management in patients with malignant middle cerebral artery infarction. A 55-year-old mala patient with atrial fibrillation presented with left side weakness. After successful intra-arterial thrombectomy with Solitaire stentriever, progressive brain swelling was identified on hospital day 1. Hemicraniectomy was planned, but hemodynamically unstable supraventricular tachycardia was developed without response to medication in the operating room. Surgery was canceled, and patient was treated with targeted temperature management at 33 degree. After initiation of hypothermia, midline shift was halted, and slow controlled rewarming was initiated on day 4. On day 10, follow up CT scan showed mass effect due to brain edema was subsided

14.3.8 Early Neurologic Deterioration After Ischemic Stroke

Early neurologic deterioration (END) is defined as an aggravation of neurologic deficit after initial stroke symptom. The frequency of END may differ based on definitions, but about 15–25% of acute stroke patients experiences END in the course of acute treatment. Generally, END is defined by an aggravation of the total NIHSS score of ≥2 points, the consciousness score of ≥1, or the motor score of ≥1. Causes of END are diverse but are reported to be associated with stroke recurrence, progression, or symptomatic hemorrhagic transformation. Risk factors of END are hypertriglyceridemia or hyperglycemia (metabolic factor), parent vessel severe stenosis (perfusion factor), and seizures.

END is associated with poor neurologic outcome. Therefore, close monitoring and early treatment of triggering factors is very important.

14.4 Prevention and Management of Stroke Complication

14.4.1 Aspiration Pneumonia and Ventilator-Associated Pneumonia

Aspiration pneumonia is one of the most common systemic complications after stroke. In general, approximately 20% of stroke patients may experience pneumonia in acute periods. Pneumonia is highly associated with poor outcome. However, there is no effective preventive method. Suggested risk factors are old age (>75 years), congestive heart failure, dysarthria, swallowing difficulty, and the use of proton pump inhibitors. Therefore, bedside swallowing evaluation is required to minimize aspiration pneumonia, especially in patients with these risk factors. In addition to these, a growing of evidence suggests that stroke itself induce transient immune depression, which is independently related with systemic infection and may lead to the development of pneumonia.

In order to minimize infection complication and to improve clinical outcome, a preventive treatment of antibiotics was tried but did not show clinical benefit in stroke patients. By contrast, head elevation (rather than flat position) and maintaining good oral hygiene are simple but important preventive maneuvers to minimize pneumonia risk in stroke patients. One single center randomized trial showed that routine use of gastrointestinal motility drug decreased the risk of aspiration pneumonia. Common clinical manifestations and laboratory markers in diagnosing pneumonia are new crackles, tachypnea (>25/min), desaturation (<90%), new onset cough, purulent sputum, pyrexia (>38 °C), leukocytosis (>11,000/mL), and elevated C-reactive protein (>25 mg/L). Therefore, daily pneumonia surveillance is required.

Appropriate choice of antibiotics requires the awareness of common pathogens in each treating unit. However, suggested empirical regimens include piperacillin-tazobactam, cefepime, ceftazidime, levofloxacin, carbapenem, or its combination. When methicillin resistance infection is highly suspected, vancomycin should be covered. After initiation of broad spectrum antibiotics, de-escalation of therapy is recommended based on the sputum or blood culture profiles. Usual duration of antibiotics coverage is 7 days but may be longer if isolated pathogens have drug resistance.

Suggestions from Clinical Practice Guidelines General medical care for stroke patients were illustrated in Fig. 14.6. Blood pressure control during acute stage has not been established, but systolic blood pressure more than 180 mm Hg might be better to be controlled. Hypoxia (oxygen saturation less than 94%) needs to be treated with supplementary oxygen supply. Electrocardiographic monitoring is needed to identify paroxysmal atrial fibrillation as a stroke cause or potential serious arrhythmias. Hyperthermia more than 38 °C is needed to be treated with antipyretic medications or surface cooling, and its source should be identified. Both hyperglycemia and hypoglycemia should be identified and immediately corrected. Patients with risk of herniations due to increased intracranial pressure are considered to be treated by measures to lower the intracranial pressure with/without close monitoring of intracranial pressure.

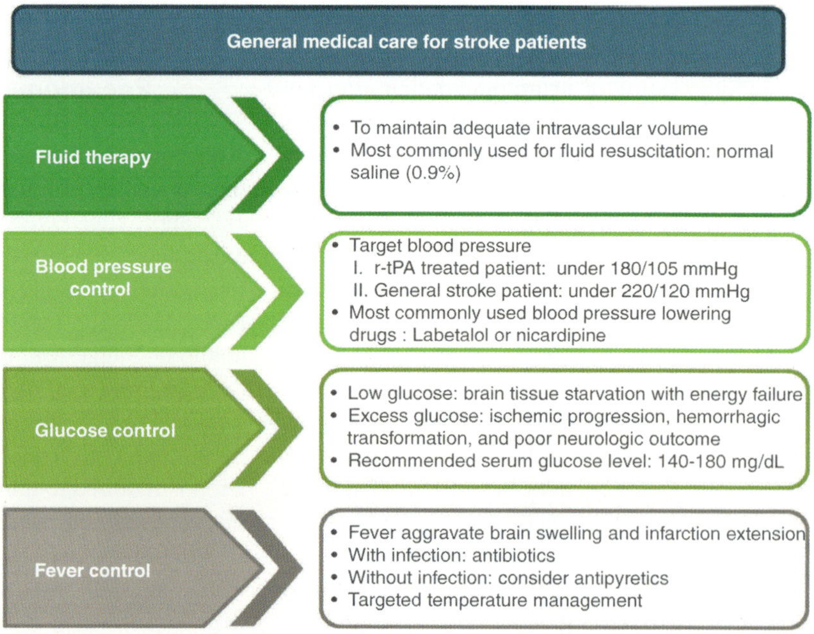

Fig. 14.6 General medical care for stroke patients

References

1. Visvanathan A, Dennis M, Whiteley W. Parenteral fluid regimens for improving functional outcome in people with acute stroke. Cochrane Database Syst Rev. 2015:CD011138.
2. Ko SB. Multimodality monitoring in the neurointensive care unit: a special perspective for patients with stroke. J Stroke. 2013;15:99–108.
3. Jauch EC, Saver JL, Adams HP Jr, et al. Guidelines for the early management of patients with acute ischemic stroke: a guideline for healthcare professionals from the American heart association/American stroke association. Stroke. 2013;44:870–947.
4. Huang Y, Sharma VK, Robinson T, et al. Rationale, design, and progress of the enhanced control of hypertension and thrombolysis stroke study (enchanted) trial: an international multicenter 2 × 2 quasi-factorial randomized controlled trial of low- vs. standard-dose rt-pa and early intensive vs. guideline-recommended blood pressure lowering in patients with acute ischaemic stroke eligible for thrombolysis treatment. Int J Stroke. 2015;10:778–88.
5. Meier K, Lee K. Neurogenic fever: review of pathophysiology, evaluation, and management. J Intensive Care Med. 2016;32(2):124–9. [Epub ahead of print]
6. Saric M, Armour AC, Arnaout MS, et al. Guidelines for the use of echocardiography in the evaluation of a cardiac source of embolism. J Am Soc Echocardiogr. 2016;29:1–42.
7. Ko SB, Choi SI, Chun EJ, et al. Role of cardiac multidetector computed tomography in acute ischemic stroke: a preliminary report. Cerebrovasc Dis. 2010;29:313–20.
8. Zha AM, Sari M, Torbey MT. Recommendations for management of large hemispheric infarction. Curr Opin Crit Care. 2015;21:91–8.
9. Marko NF. Hypertonic saline, not mannitol, should be considered gold-standard medical therapy for intracranial hypertension. Crit Care. 2012;16:113.
10. Kamel H, Navi BB, Nakagawa K, et al. Hypertonic saline versus mannitol for the treatment of elevated intracranial pressure: a meta-analysis of randomized clinical trials. Crit Care Med. 2011;39:554–9.
11. Ko SB, Choi HA, Parikh G, et al. Real time estimation of brain water content in comatose patients. Ann Neurol. 2012;72:344–50.
12. Sheth KN, Elm JJ, Molyneaux BJ, et al. Safety and efficacy of intravenous glyburide on brain swelling after large hemispheric infarction (games-rp): a randomised, double-blind, placebo-controlled phase 2 trial. Lancet Neurol. 2016;15:1160–9.
13. Su Y, Fan L, Zhang Y, et al. Improved neurological outcome with mild hypothermia in surviving patients with massive cerebral hemispheric infarction. Stroke. 2016;47:457–63.

Rehabilitation in Acute Stage

15

Byung-Mo Oh and Han Gil Seo

Abstract

The goal of rehabilitation for stroke victims in acute stage has been primarily focused on preventing immobility-related complications such as deep vein thrombosis, cardiopulmonary deconditioning, pressure ulcer, and joint contractures. Early mobilization is the first-line preventive strategy for most of these complications. Although many clinical guidelines for stroke management recommend starting mobilization as soon as patients are medically stabilized, the definition of mobilization remains unclear, and the supporting evidence has been insufficient. In the phase III A Very Early Rehabilitation Trial for Stroke (AVERT), mobilization started very early (<24 h after onset) showed worse outcome as compared to standard care. A lively controversy is currently underway on the phase III AVERT and its ramifications. In this review, the background rationale and ensuing debate regarding phase III AVERT will be summarized and appraised. In addition, a succinct review on the management strategy for swallowing difficulty will follow.

The ultimate goal of stroke rehabilitation is to maximize the victims' independence in their everyday lives by facilitating neurological as well as compensatory functional recovery. A goal-oriented, multidisciplinary team approach is also an indispensable quality of acute rehabilitation after stroke. The emphasis of rehabilitation service, however, can differ according to the stages after stroke. For instance, intensive multidisciplinary training program should be provided in order to achieve maximal functional recovery in the post-acute phase, whereas the prevention of complication should be the core element in the acute stage. Unfortunately, there have been conflicting rationales and consequent strategies on the acute-stage rehabilitation. More cautious groups advocate bed rest for the first couple of days after stroke in order to save the penumbra zone, while mobilization as early as within 24 h

B.-M. Oh, M.D., Ph.D. (✉) • H.G. Seo, M.D., M.S.
Department of Rehabilitation Medicine,
Seoul National University Hospital,
101 Daehak-ro Chongno-gu, Seoul 03080,
South Korea
e-mail: keepwiz@gmail.com

S.-H. Lee (ed.), *Stroke Revisited: Diagnosis and Treatment of Ischemic Stroke*,
Stroke Revisited, DOI 10.1007/978-981-10-1424-6_15

has been gaining more popularity lately. Serious debate still going on the timing, methods, intensity and frequency of acute-stage rehabilitation will be summarized and critically appraised in this review. In addition, recent advances in screening and management of swallowing difficulties will follow.

15.1 Common Settings of Inpatient Medical Care

The care settings where acute-stage rehabilitation services are provided vary greatly from country to country. In the United States, the median length of stay in the acute care hospital for patients with ischemic stroke is around 4 days [1]. Although combined acute-subacute stroke units (SUs) are associated with greater odds reduction for death or dependency as compared with general rehabilitation wards [2], SUs in acute care hospitals are getting more distinguished from post-acute rehabilitation facilities, which are driven primarily by nonmedical cause such as insurance reimbursement. Multidisciplinary rehabilitation service is, thus, not feasible in many acute settings. Although the medical and social influence of this radical cutdown in the length of stay for stroke survivors are worthy of in-depth discussion, it is out of the scope of the present article. Readers can refer to the recent guideline for practical details on this topic [1].

15.2 Early Mobilization

The results of phase III A Very Early Rehabilitation Trial for Stroke (AVERT) provoked a great debate about early mobilization. The ongoing discussion is focused on the detailed aspects of the results and is likely to result in substantial changes of the current clinical guidelines.

15.2.1 Definition

Mobilization, as a rehabilitation term, is used to describe out-of-bed interventions, such as sitting, standing, and walking, not just passively moving patients' limbs. Although many acute stroke guidelines recommend beginning active rehabilitation as early as possible, the ideal launch time of mobilization has not been described. The period of clinical interest may fall in the first 24–72 h after stroke [3]. Very early mobilization (VEM) is a rehabilitation strategy getting patients out of bed within 24 h of stroke onset. The questions on optimal intensity, frequency, and duration of early mobilization remain largely unanswered.

15.2.2 Background

Most stroke patients experience mobility problems caused by neurological deficits or combined medical conditions. Potential complications of immobility after stroke include deep venous thrombosis, urinary tract infection and retention, orthostatic hypotension, atelectasis, constipation, decubitus ulcer, depression, osteoporosis, and musculoskeletal deconditioning [4]. Early mobilization is the first-line preventive strategy for most of these complications.

Increased brain plasticity in an early phase of stroke also warrants initiation of rehabilitation as early as possible. It has been identified that waves of growth-promoting genes begin in the first day and peak at approximately 7 days after stroke, whereas growth-inhibitory molecules have a delayed induction reaching a peak several weeks after stroke [5]. When the enriched rehabilitation started 5, 14, and 30 days after focal ischemia in rats, the "day 5" group showed the greatest improvement in skilled forelimb reaching ability as well as general mobility [6]. With "day 30" initiation after stroke, enriched rehabilitation did not yield any benefit as compared to control group (social housing). The brain shows heightened plasticity to rehabilitation early after stroke but it is finite. It is generally believed that the optimal time window beyond which rehabilitation is less effective may exist. However, concern about exacerbated brain injury by too early initiation of therapy after stroke arose based on the results from animal studies [5]. A meta-analysis on training strategies in animal models of ischemic stroke has reported that training initiated between 1 and 5 days after stroke onset was more efficacious for infarct volume reduction and functional improvement than that initiated <1 day or >5 days after stroke onset [7].

Cerebral blood flow and blood pressure changes are other concerns of early mobilization during the acute phase of stroke. Although change of cerebral blood flow velocity depending on head position was controversial in stroke patients, it is expected that horizontal positioning may support newly established leptomeningeal or transcortical collateral channels [3]. This concern leads to Lausanne and SEVEL trials and ongoing HeadPoST (http://www.clinicaltrials.gov: NCT02162017). SEVEL trial was prematurely terminated because of slow enrollment rate ($n = 138$) and suggested no extreme effect of the early sitting within 1 calendar day after stroke onset in either direction of stroke outcome [8]. In addition, potential adverse effect of increased blood pressure by physical activity and postural hypotension has been considered in early mobilization after stroke.

15.2.3 Evidence

Before phase III AVERT, four small-sized trials on VEM within 24 h of acute stroke, including phase II AVERT, were completed [3]. No trial has demonstrated significant effect on complications, mortality, or global disability. Faster return to unassisted walking, improved functional recovery, and cost-effectiveness were also suggested from phase II AVERT. A meta-analysis on three randomized controlled trials ($n = 159$) reported nonsignificant functional improvement, but increased mortality with VEM compared with usual care [9].

Phase III AVERT is a single-blind, multicenter randomized controlled trial including 2104 stroke patients [10]. Patients with ischemic or hemorrhagic stroke, first or recurrent, were enrolled, and treatment with recombinant tissue plasminogen activator was allowed. Three crucial elements of VEM intervention were (1) beginning within 24 h of stroke onset; (2) focusing on sitting, standing, and walking (i.e., out-of-bed) activity; and (3) resulting in at least three additional out-of-bed sessions to usual care. The results demonstrated that VEM was associated with a reduction in the odds of favorable outcome at 3 months, defined as a modified Rankin scale score of 0–2. In subgroup analysis, patients with severe stroke and those with intracerebral hemorrhage showed reduced favorable outcome if treated with VEM. It is notable that VEM and usual care groups were mobilized after 18.5 h (median; IQR, 12.8–22.3) and 22.4 h (16.5–29.3), respectively. Considering that the median time to first mobilization in the standard care group was 30.8 h (23.0–39.9) in phase II AVERT, this finding indicates that the standard clinical practice on early mobilization after stroke has changed during the study period. Dose-response analysis demonstrated that increased daily frequency of out-of-bed sessions was associated with improved outcome at 3 months, whereas increased amount of mobilization reduced the odds of a good outcome [11]. Therefore, short and frequent mobilization may be beneficial early after acute stroke.

Although early mobilization has become a standard practice in acute stroke management, risk and benefit of VEM should be reevaluated carefully. Detailed review of current evidence is needed to draw clinical guidelines for early mobilization after stroke. At this point, individualized approach considering the patients' characteristics, such as stroke type and severity, and the amount and frequency of mobilization may be a proper strategy of early mobilization.

15.3 Swallowing Difficulty

15.3.1 Scope of the Problem

Although swallowing is a robust, patterned human movement normally starting in utero, its sensorimotor control involves the complex neural mechanisms over the sequential contraction and relaxation of dozens of small muscles. In this regard, it is no surprise that such a high prevalence (29–67%) of dysphagia—a difficulty with swallowing—exists among stroke victims in acute stage [12]. Clinical significance of dysphagia is far from trivial because severe dysphagia poses almost 11 times higher risk for aspiration

a

GUSS
(Gugging Swallowing Screen)

Name:________
Date:________
Time:________

1. Preliminary Investigation /Indirect Swallowing Test

	YES	*NO*
Vigilance *(The patient must be alert for at least for 15 minutes)*	1 ☐	0 ☐
Cough and/or throat clearing *(voluntary cough)* *(Patient should cough or clear his or her throat twice)*	1 ☐	0 ☐
Saliva Swallow: • Swallowing successful	1 ☐	0 ☐
• Drooling	0 ☐	1 ☐
• Voice change (hoarse, gurgly, coated, weak)	0 ☐	1 ☐
SUM:	(5)	
	1 - 4= Investigate further¹ 5= Continue with part 2	

2. Direct Swallowing Test (Material: Aqua bi, flat teaspoon, food thickener, bread)

In the following order:	1 →	2 →	3 →
	SEMISOLID*	LIQUID**	SOLID ***
DEGLUTITION:			
• Swallowing not possible	0 ☐	0 ☐	0 ☐
• Swallowing delayed (> 2 sec.) (Solid textures > 10 sec.)	1 ☐	1 ☐	1 ☐
• Swallowing successful	2 ☐	2 ☐	2 ☐
COUGH (involuntary): *(before, during or after swallowing - until 3 minutes later)*			
• Yes	0 ☐	0 ☐	0 ☐
• No	1 ☐	1 ☐	1 ☐
DROOLING:			
• Yes	0 ☐	0 ☐	0 ☐
• No	1 ☐	1 ☐	1 ☐
VOICE CHANGE: *(listen to the voice before and after swallowing - Patient should speak „O")*			
• Yes	0 ☐	0 ☐	0 ☐
• No	1 ☐	1 ☐	1 ☐
SUM:	(5)	(5)	(5)
	1 - 4= Investigate further¹ 5= Continue Liquid	1 - 4= Investigate further¹ 5= Continue Solid	1 - 4= Investigate further¹ 5= Normal

SUM: (Indirect Swallowing Test AND Direct Swallowing Test) ______ (20)

*	First administer ⅓ up to a half teaspoon Aqua bi with food thickener (pudding-like consistency). If there are no symptoms apply 3 to 5 teaspoons. Assess after the 5th spoonful.
**	3, 5, 10, 20 ml Aqua bi - if there are no symptoms continue with 50 ml Aqua bi (Daniels et al. 2000; Gottlieb et al. 1996) Assess and stop the investigation when one of the criteria is observed!
***	Clinical: dry bread; FEES: dry bread which is dipped in coloured liquid
¹	Use functional investigations such as Videofluoroscopic Evaluation of Swallowing (VFES), Fiberoptic Endoscopic Evalutation of Swallowing (FEES)

b

GUSS
(Gugging Swallowing Screen)
GUSS-EVALUATION

RESULTS		SEVERITY CODE	*RECOMMENDATIONS*
20	Semisolid / liquid and solid texture successful	Slight / No Dysphagia minimal risk of aspiration	• Normal Diet • Regular Liquids (First time under supervision of the SLT or a trained stroke nurse!)
15-19	Semisolid and liquid texture successful and Solid unsuccessful	Slight Dysphagia with a low risk of aspiration	• Dysphagia Diet (pureed and soft food) • Liquids very slowly – one sip at a time • Funcional swallowing assessments such as Fiberoptic Endoscopic Evaluation of Swallowing (FEES) or Videofluoroscopic Evaluation of Swallowing (VFES) • Refer to Speech and Language Therapist (SLT)
10-14	Semisolid swallow success sful and Liquids unsuccessful	Moderate dysphagia with a risk of aspiration	Dysphagia diet beginning with: • Semisolid textures such as baby food and additional parenteral feeding. • All liquids must be thickened! • Pills must be crushed and mixed with thick liquid. • No liquid medication! • Further functional swallowing assessments (FEES, VFES) • Refer to Speech and Language Therapist (SLT) *Supplementation with nasogastric tube or parenteral*
0-9	Preliminary investigation unsuccessful or Semisolid swallow unsuccessful	Severe dysphagia with a high risk of aspiration	• NPO (non per os = nothing by mouth) • Further functional swallowing assessment (FEES, VFES) • Refer to Speech and Language Therapist (SLT) *Supplementation with nasogastric tube or parenteral*

Fig. 15.1 The Gugging Swallowing Screen (GUSS). (**a**) Test form of GUSS. (**b**) Evaluation form of GUSS (Reproduced by permission of Stroke) [15]

pneumonia after stroke [13]. Videofluoroscopic swallowing study (VFSS) or modified barium swallow fluoroscopy is the gold standard for assessment of swallowing function. However, up to 27% of stroke survivors who have symptomatic dysphagia are reportedly "silent aspirators" [12], which require well-validated clinical screening tests.

15.3.2 Screening and Management of Swallowing Difficulty in the Acute Stage

In most cases, nasogastric (NG) tube is used as a first-line secure route of administration for medication and nutrition. Standardized screening tests are used to judge if the patient's swallowing function is safe enough for full oral feeding [14]. Screening tools validated in stroke include Oral Pharyngeal and Clinical Swallowing Examination, Bedside Aspiration Test, the Gugging Swallowing Screen (Fig 15.1), and the Toronto Bedside Swallowing Screening Test [14, 15]. If a patient fails a screening test or shows repetitive episodes of saliva aspiration, standardized instrumental assessment such as VFSS or fiber-optic endoscopic evaluation of swallowing (FEES) is warranted. Percutaneous or endoscopic gastrostomy is indicated for patients with persistent severe dysphagia. In most cases, rehabilitation using therapeutic exercise and compensatory maneuver lead to safe oral feeding within a couple of weeks.

Conclusion

Phase III AVERT trial posed a serious question on the safety of VEM in acute stroke, which demands revision of the current clinical guidelines. The bottom line is that current evidence does not support active out-of-bed mobilization within 24 h after the onset for all stroke patients. Individualized approach with gentle in-bed mobility for the first 24–48 h would be a reasonable alternative to reduce immobility-related complications as well as not to harm the penumbra zone.

Swallowing difficulty is one of the most common functional impairments after stroke. The purpose of initial use of enteral nutrition such as NG tube is to prevent serious complication such as aspiration pneumonia or asphyxia. Although swallowing difficulty is very common after stroke, ability to eat with safety and efficiency can be regained within a couple of weeks in most cases. Validated screening tools are readily available for early clinical decision making.

The ever-worsening brevity of stay in the specialized SUs in acute care hospitals offers a very narrow window of opportunity for comprehensive rehabilitation. More research will be required to delineate the optimal timing, intensity, frequency, and mode of exercise for the acute phase of stroke.

Suggestions from Clinical Practice Guidelines After admission to the center, the stroke patient should be assessed with regard to swallowing ability before eating, drinking, or taking oral medications using a structured, standardized dysphagia scoring system. If the patient has a significant dysphagia, a nasogastric tube (i.e., Levin tube) should be used to maintain hydration and nutrition.

References

1. Winstein CJ, Stein J, Arena R, et al. Guidelines for adult stroke rehabilitation and recovery: a guideline for healthcare professionals from the American Heart Association/American Stroke Association. Stroke. 2016;47:e98–e169.
2. Teasell R, Foley N, Salter K, et al. Evidence-based review of stroke rehabilitation: executive summary, 12th edition. Top Stroke Rehabil. 2009;16:463–88.
3. Bernhardt J, English C, Johnson L, et al. Early mobilization after stroke: early adoption but limited evidence. Stroke. 2015;46:1141–6.
4. Coletta EM, Murphy JB. The complications of immobility in the elderly stroke patient. J Am Board Fam Pract. 1992;5:389–97.
5. Krakauer JW, Carmichael ST, Corbett D, et al. Getting neurorehabilitation right: what can be learned from animal models? Neurorehabil Neural Repair. 2012;26:923–31.
6. Biernaskie J, Chernenko G, Corbett D. Efficacy of rehabilitative experience declines with time after focal ischemic brain injury. J Neurosci. 2004;24: 1245–54.
7. Schmidt A, Wellmann J, Schilling M, et al. Meta-analysis of the efficacy of different training strategies in animal models of ischemic stroke. Stroke. 2014;45:239–47.
8. Herisson F, Godard S, Volteau C, et al. Early Sitting in Ischemic Stroke Patients (SEVEL): a randomized controlled trial. PLoS One. 2016;11:e0149466.
9. Lynch E, Hillier S, Cadilhac D. When should physical rehabilitation commence after stroke: a systematic review. Int J Stroke. 2014;9:468–78.
10. AVERT Trial Collaboration group, Bernhardt J, Langhorne P, et al. Efficacy and safety of very early mobilisation within 24 h of stroke onset (AVERT): a randomised controlled trial. Lancet. 2015;386: 46–55.
11. Bernhardt J, Churilov L, Ellery F, et al. Prespecified dose-response analysis for A Very Early Rehabilitation Trial (AVERT). Neurology. 2016;86:2138–45.
12. Teasell R. Evidence-based benefit of rehabilitation after stroke. In: Selzer ME, Clarke S, Cohen LG, Kwakkel G, Miller RH, editors. Textbook of neural repair and rehabilitation. 2nd ed. Cambridge: Cambridge University Press; 2014.
13. Martino R, Foley N, Bhogal S, et al. Dysphagia after stroke: incidence, diagnosis, and pulmonary complications. Stroke. 2005;36:2756–63.
14. Poorjavad M, Jalaie S. Systemic review on highly qualified screening tests for swallowing disorders following stroke: validity and reliability issues. J Res Med Sci. 2014;19:776–85.
15. Trapl M, Enderle P, Nowotny M, et al. Dysphagia bedside screening for acute-stroke patients: the Gugging Swallowing Screen. Stroke. 2007;38: 2948–52.

Part III

Certain but Relatively Frequent Causes of Ischemic Stroke

Cerebral Venous Sinus Thrombosis 16

Beom Joon Kim

Abstract

Cerebral venous thrombosis (CVT) is caused by thrombosis and resultant occlusion of cerebral venous system, and its incidence rate is lower than ischemic stroke or intracerebral hemorrhage. CVT has a variety of presenting symptoms/signs and commonly poses diagnostic challenges. Its most frequent presentations are headache, symptoms with increased intracranial pressures, seizures, and any of cortical symptoms/signs. The confirmation of the diagnosis of CVT relies on the demonstration of thrombi in the cerebral veins/sinuses by relevant neuroimaging studies. Computed tomography may reveal venous thrombi, but magnetic resonance techniques with venography are more sensitive. Risk factors for CVT consisted of various thrombophilic conditions, either genetic or acquired, oral contraceptives, puerperium and pregnancy, infection, and malignancy. During the acute period, anticoagulation with heparin may be beneficial to CVT patients in spite of hemorrhages. Deteriorating cases despite full anticoagulation may benefit through local thrombolysis or thrombectomy. After the acute phase, patients remain on oral vitamin K antagonists for a variable period of time, depending on their inherent thrombotic risk. The prognosis of CVT is in general favorable.

Cerebral venous thrombosis (CVT) is an uncommon form of vascular disease which occurred in the brain. After the completion of multicenter collaboration registration study [1], stroke physicians became familiar to the disease. However, due to its low prevalence and variety in associated risk factors and presenting symptoms/signs, much of diagnostic strategy and treatment decision for CVT patients are still obscure. Also, CVT tends to occur in relatively younger age groups and associated with various medical and surgical conditions including pregnancy and autoimmune diseases, so that CVT patients may first be detected by non-neurologists [2]. In this

B.J. Kim, M.D., Ph.D.
Department of Neurology and Regional Cerebrovascular Center, Seoul National University Bundang Hospital, Room #8710, Bldg #2, Gumi-ro 173 beon-gil, Bundang-gu, Seonnam-si, Gyeonggi-do 13620, South Korea
e-mail: Kim.BJ.Stroke@gmail.com

S.-H. Lee (ed.), *Stroke Revisited: Diagnosis and Treatment of Ischemic Stroke*, Stroke Revisited, DOI 10.1007/978-981-10-1424-6_16

chapter, various clinical aspects of CVT will be discussed, including its pathogenesis, risk factors, diagnosis, and treatments.

16.1 What Is Cerebral Venous Thrombosis and Why It Occurs?

16.1.1 Anatomy of Cerebral Venous System

Approximately 70–80% of cerebral blood volume is known to reside in the venous system. The internal jugular vein usually drains two-thirds of the ipsilateral hemispheric venous blood from the superficial cerebral venous system and deep cerebral venous system (Fig. 16.1). The superficial cerebral venous system is consisted of superior sagittal sinuses and cortical veins, and the deep cerebral venous system is consisted of lateral sinuses, straight sinuses, sigmoid sinuses, and deep-seated veins.

The superficial cerebral venous system may be categorized into three venous groups: (1) mediodorsal group into superior sagittal sinus and straight sinus, (2) lateroventral group into lateral sinus, and (3) anterior group to cavernous sinus. The superficial cerebral venous system is well known for its anatomic variety, and it is important to distinguish anatomic variance from the occlusion of existing venous structures in CVT cases. Notable venous structures in the deep cerebral venous system are the internal cerebral vein, vein of Galen, and vein of Rosenthal; this system usually drains venous blood from the deep white matters and basal ganglia. Anatomic variance of deep cerebral venous system is not so much frequent as superficial system.

16.1.2 Structure of Cerebral Venous System and Cerebral Venous Thrombosis

Structural peculiarity of the anatomy of cerebral veins and venous sinuses is their lack of vascular valves and tunica muscularis. Bidirectional venous flow is permitted due to the lack of one-way valves, which usually pose a structural advantage for collateral drainage when any major veins are compressed or occluded. Also, there are multiple confluences in the entire cerebral venous system which give greater flexibility for collateral venous drainage. Lack of muscle layer in the venous sinuses and cerebral veins enables increased compliance for the volume of venous flow. Lastly, venous sinuses are located within the thick and tough dura mater, so that they are

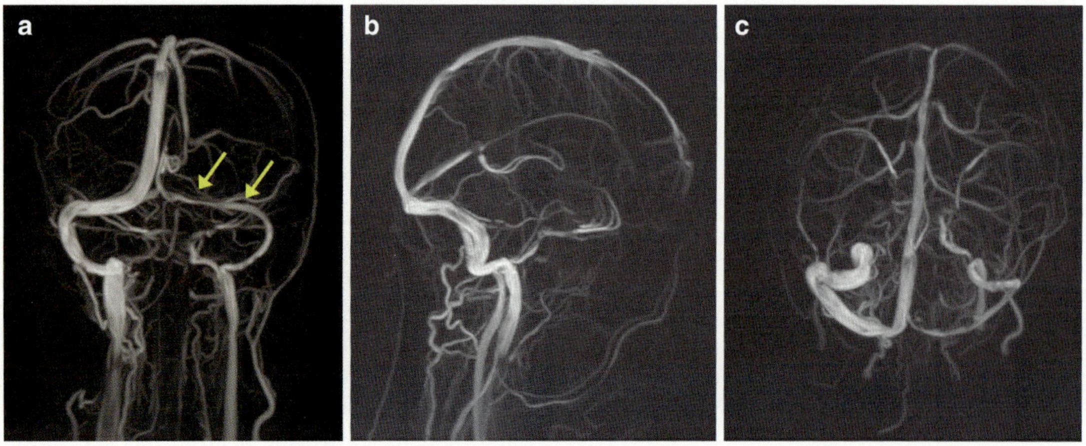

Fig. 16.1 Normal MR venography. Normal MR venography in anteroposterior view (**a**), lateral view (**b**), and cone-down view (**c**). Hypoplasia of transverse and downstream jugular vein (*yellow arrow*) is considered normal

protected when the intracranial pressure is elevated. Various prognoses in CVT patients may be explained by the above anatomic characteristics.

Superficial veins in the hemisphere usually drain venous blood to superior sagittal sinuses, which have large intravenous lumen with slow flow. The confluence of superficial cerebral veins and superior sagittal sinus may cause turbulence in the sinus. Also, fibrous septa in the inferior angle may also interfere with lamina venous flow. Both of the above may be underlying conditions for higher proportion of CVT in superior sagittal sinus or adjacent venous structures. Additionally, the intracranial venous system also receives venous drainage from the diploic vein, meningeal vein, and emissary veins, which drains blood from extracranial anatomic structures. Due to the drainage from extracranial structures, infective organisms from the face and scalp or chronic otitis media may spread into the intracranial venous system and cause CVT.

16.2 Risk Factors for Cerebral Venous Thrombosis

Risk factors associated with CVT are multiple (Table 16.1) [3]. Most of the associated factors are linked to the classic Virchow triad, including stasis of blood, changes in the vessel wall, and changes in the composition of the blood. The structural characteristics of the cerebral venous system discussed in the previous section may attribute to the stasis of blood inside of the venous system. Risk factors for CVT are usually prothrombotic conditions, including genetic or acquired, oral contraceptives, puerperium and pregnancy, infection, and malignancy. Subjects with predisposing genetic prothrombotic conditions may become more susceptible to CVT when exposed to any of the acquired causes, including oral contraceptives or puerperium. The most frequent genetic thrombophilias are G20210A prothrombin and factor V Leiden mutations, followed by protein C, S, and antithrombin III deficiencies. But the prevalence of genetic prothrombotic conditions may differ according to the ethnic groups of patients, so stroke physicians should use their caution before ordering a genetic test. Hyperhomocysteinemia is a risk factor for venous thrombosis, but the role of MTHFR/C677T mutation is under controversy. Anticardiolipin antibodies are found in 6% of CVT cases. According to the largest study of CVT patients, ISCVT, 34% of CVT patients had an inherited or acquired prothrombotic condition.

The most frequent risk factors in young women are oral contraceptive use and pregnancy/puerperium. During pregnancy and for 6–8 weeks after birth, women are at increased risk of venous thromboembolic events, such as deep venous thrombosis. Hypercoagulability worsens after delivery as a result of volume depletion and trauma. Additional risk factors are infection and instrumental delivery or cesarean section during the puerperium. CVT has also been reported in association with hormone replacement therapy, the day-after pill, and in vitro fertilization. The additional risk for CVT from oral contraceptive

Table 16.1 Potential risk factors associated with cerebral venous thrombosis

Prothrombotic conditions
Antithrombin III deficiency
Protein C deficiency
Antiphospholipid and anticardiolipin antibodies
Resistance to activated protein C and factor V Leiden
Mutation G20210A of factor II
Hyperhomocysteinemia
Pregnancy and puerperium
Oral contraceptives
Medications—androgen, danazol, lithium, vitamin A, IV immunoglobulin, ecstasy
Cancer related—local compression, hypercoagulable, antineoplastic drug
Parameningeal infections (ear, sinus, mouth, face, and neck)
Mechanical precipitants (complication of epidural blood patch, spontaneous intracranial hypotension, lumbar puncture)
Hematologic disorders (paroxysmal nocturnal hemoglobinuria, iron deficiency anemia, nephrotic syndrome, polycythemia, thrombocythemia)
Systemic disease (systemic lupus erythematosus, Behcet's disease, inflammatory bowel disease, thyroid disease, sarcoidosis)
Miscellaneous

use and pregnancy/puerperium may be augmented for young women with inherited thrombophilic conditions.

Other conditions associated with CVT are local or systemic infections including mastoiditis, sinusitis, or meningitis and medical conditions including cancer, iron deficiency anemia, thrombotic thrombocytopenic purpura, nephrotic syndrome, and systemic lupus erythematosus.

16.3 How to Diagnose Cerebral Venous Sinus Thrombosis

16.3.1 Why Venous Thrombosis Matters

Cerebral venous system is well known for its flexibility and compliance. However, thrombosis and occlusion of major venous sinuses would cause both localized venous stasis and generalized increment of intracranial pressure, both of which provoke symptoms/signs of CVT [4].

Thrombosis and occlusion of cerebral vein/venous sinus may cause localized infarction and edema in the brain parenchyma. The infarction is irrelevant to the alleged arterial vascular territories, which would be an important clue to suspect venous thrombosis. Pathologic specimen of CVT cases reveals localized edema, ischemic injuries, and petechial hemorrhages. Occasionally, frank hematoma may be documented.

Two types of cerebral edema may occur in CVT cases. First, ischemic injuries and associated cellular death may result in cytotoxic edema, which originated from the depletion of cellular energy source and failure of ATP-dependent membrane pumps. Second, vasogenic edema would cause diffuse but reversible stasis of interstitial and extracellular fluid, due to increased permeability of the blood-brain barrier and failure of venous drainage. Brain MR typically reveals mixed pattern of edematous brain in CVT patients.

Increased intracranial pressure is a frequent phenomenon of CVT. Thrombosis and occlusion of superior sagittal sinus will interfere with the absorption of cerebrospinal fluid through arachnoid villi to the sinuses. Occasionally, CVT patients may present only with symptoms/signs of increased intracranial pressure without any signs of parenchymal infarctions or edema.

16.4 Symptoms and Signs of CVT

The clinical presentation of CVT is highly variable and its mode of onset may be acute or subacute. Headache is the most frequent symptom of CVT, usually the initial one and may be the sole manifestation of CVT, found in more than 90% of afflicted cases. The most frequent type of headache is the intracranial hypertension type, a severe, generalized headache of progressive onset, worsening with Valsalva maneuvers and when lying down. However, focal and nonspecific headache found in the neck or posterior cranium may be associated with CVT. Also, isolated headache without focal neurological findings or papilledema occurs in up to 25% of patients with CVT. ISCVT study reported higher frequency of headache in women with oral contraceptive use or pregnancy/puerperium [5].

When focal brain injury occurs because of venous ischemia or hemorrhage, neurological symptoms/signs referable to the affected region are often present. Clinical manifestation of CVT may also depend on the location of thrombosis. Typically, cortical vein thrombosis produces motor and/or sensory deficits and seizures. Hemiparesis and aphasia are most common neurological deficits associated with CVT, but other cortical signs including sensory and visual symptoms may occur. Transient loss of vision may occur in association with episodes of intense headache. Psychosis, in conjunction with focal neurological signs, has also been reported, associated with thrombosis in the deep cerebral venous system. Patients with isolated thrombosis of the lateral sinus often present as isolated intracranial hypertension.

16.5 Diagnosis of Cerebral Venous Thrombosis

The confirmation of the diagnosis of CVT relies on the demonstration of thrombi in the cerebral veins or sinuses and establishment of association between the thrombi and presenting symptoms/

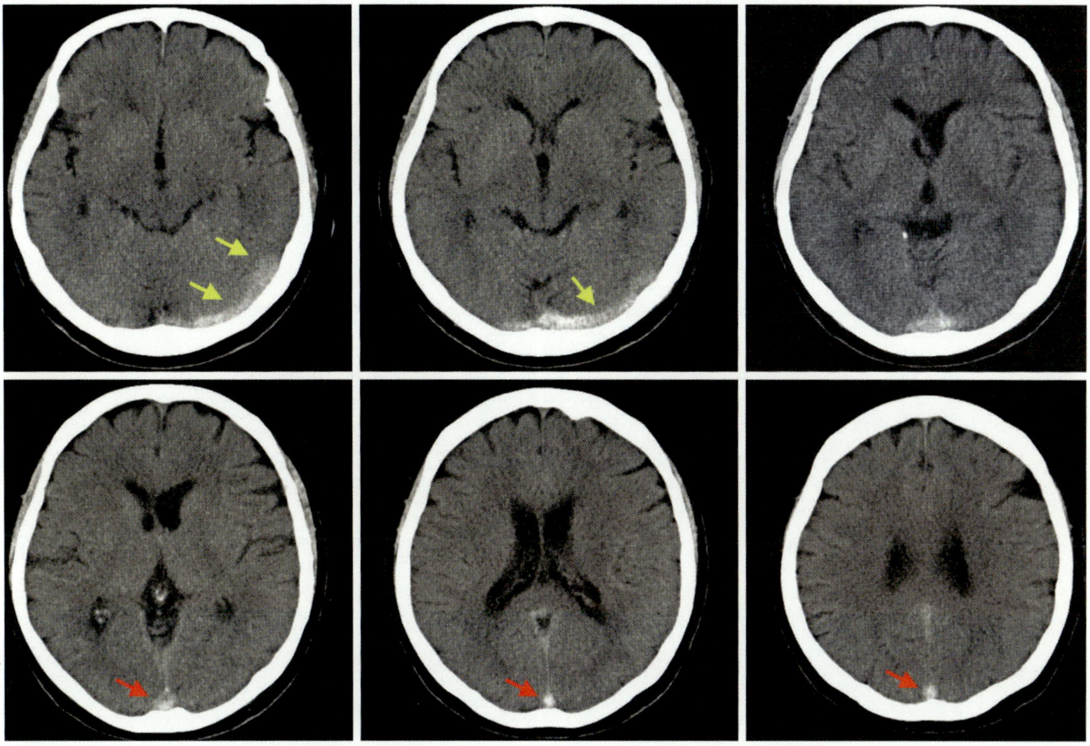

Fig. 16.2 Cerebral venous thrombosis depicted on computed tomography (CT). A 48-year-old male arrived to emergency room with acute fever and headache. To diagnose meningitis, his cerebrospinal fluid was taken and showed mildly elevated leukocyte and protein with normal glucose. He was discharged with symptomatic medication. He returned to emergency room with severe headache, visual blurring, and imbalance on gait, all of which are aggravated over 4–5 days. His body temperature was normal. To rule out secondary cause of headache, brain CT was taken. This non-contrast brain CT showed high-attenuation left transverse sinus (*yellow arrow*) and superior sagittal sinus (*red arrow*), which implies cerebral venous thrombosis

signs [6]. CVT should be included in the list of differential diagnosis when acute or subacute headache patients are presented with a sign of increased intracranial pressure, focal neurological deficits, or first seizure during the lifetime. The neuroimaging findings of CVT are rather characteristic, but when unsuspected, its feature may go unnoticed.

In the evaluation of patients suspected of CVT, computed tomography (CT) with contrast is useful (Fig. 16.2). CT with contrast is useful to visualize venous thrombi. CT would reveal parenchymal infarction or associated edema as a diffuse low-attenuation lesion. Parenchymal low-attenuation lesions may present with distinct topographies: bilateral parasagittal hemispheric lesions for superior sagittal sinus thrombosis, temporo-occipital lesions for lateral sinus thrombosis, and bilateral thalamic and caudate head lesions for internal cerebral vein thrombosis. All of the above are frequently irrespective of arterial vascular territories. Parenchymal lesions may be vanished through serial follow-ups of CT due to resorption of venous thrombosis. Direct signs of CVT may be found in about one-third of cases and include the cord sign (thrombosed cortical or deep vein), the dense triangle sign (visualization of the clot inside the sinus, usually in the posterior portion of superior sagittal sinus), and the empty delta sign with contrast dye.

Magnetic resonance imaging (MRI) combined with magnetic resonance venography (MRV) is currently the best method to confirm CVT and delineate resultant parenchymal infarcts and edema (Fig. 16.3). Visualization of venous thrombosis through MRI may be possible, as venous thrombi are isointense on T1-weighted images and hypointense on

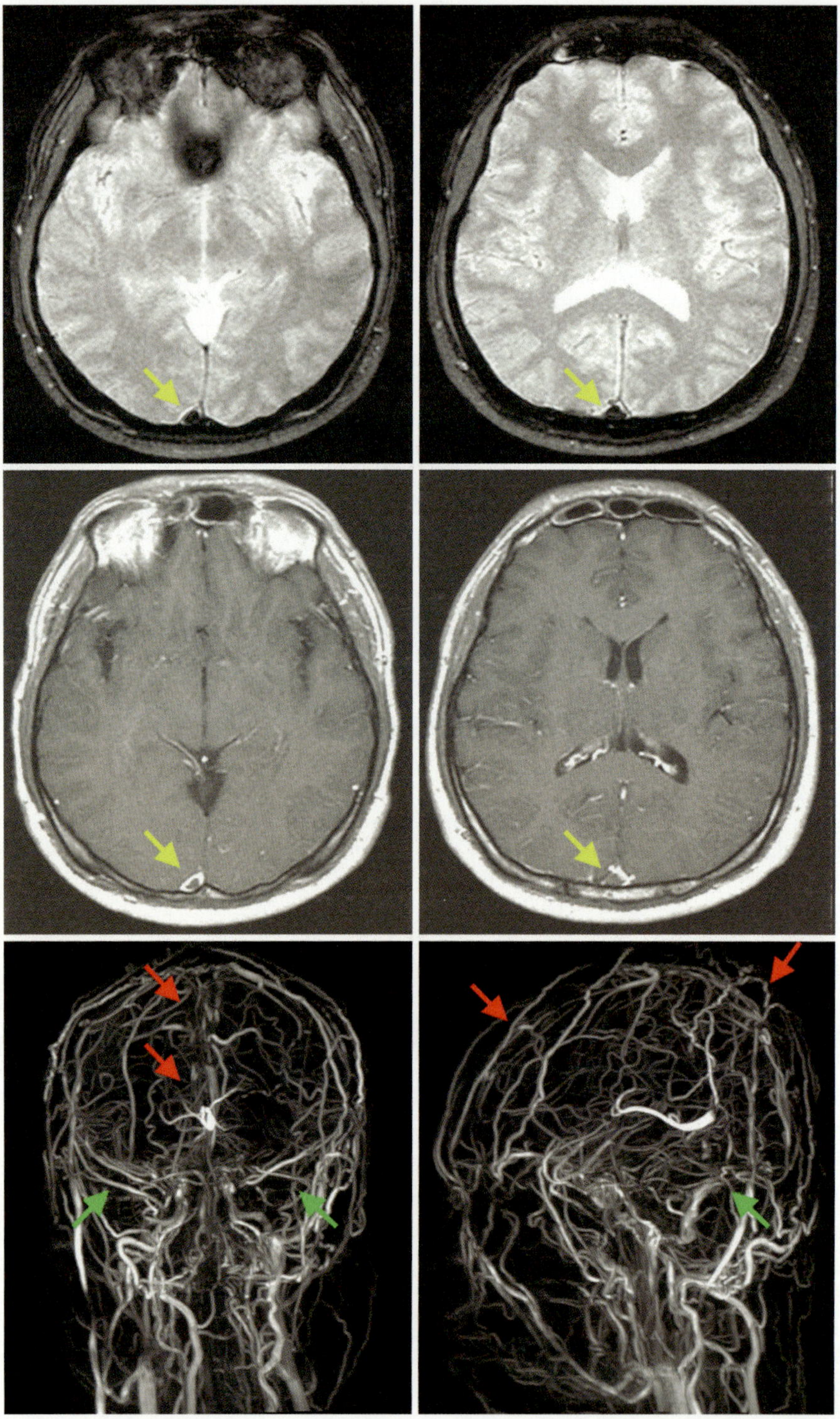

Fig. 16.3 Cerebral venous thrombosis on magnetic resonance imaging (MRI). Identical case of Fig. 16.2. Gradient-echo image (*upper panel*) and T1-weighted contrast image (*middle panel*) show venous thrombosis at superior sagittal sinus (*yellow arrow*). MR venography (*lower panel*) revealed extensive cerebral venous thrombosis at superior sagittal sinus (*red arrow*) and bilateral transverse sinuses (*green arrow*), both of which are obliterated and do not clearly show on the MR venography

T2-weighted images during the acute stage. After the acute stages, the signal intensity of thrombus may increase both on T1- and T2-weighted images. Echo-planar T2* susceptibility-weighted images (gradient-echo images) improve the visualization of thrombus with blooming signs. Diffusion-weighted images (DWI) and apparent diffusion coefficient (ADC) maps are useful to delineate the extent of infarcts, but DWI and ADC do not commonly match in a case of CVT, as there are mixed pathologies of cellular death and interstitial edema.

Detection of diagnosis of venous thrombi solely on MRI image may pose a diagnostic challenge, and confirmation of venous obstruction through MRV is required. MRV with time-of-flight (TOF) sequence demonstrates the absence of flow in the thrombosed venous structures. However, stroke physicians should keep in mind the anatomic variance in cerebral venous structures and should compare MRV with thrombus signals on MRI and patients' symptoms/signs [7].

Traditionally, venous angiography by transfemoral cerebral angiography is considered as a gold standard of CVT diagnosis, but currently it is not a mandatory tool due to its invasiveness and the advance of MRV techniques. Cerebral angiography is required when vascular anomaly is suspected or CVT is combined with subarachnoid hemorrhage to decide whether neuroendovascular intervention is warranted.

The utility of laboratory diagnosis of CVT is not established. D-dimer may be useful when suspicious of CVT but its specificity is quite low.

16.6 How to Treat Cerebral Venous Sinus Thrombosis

The aim of treating CVT is to remove venous thrombi and reanalyze the cerebral venous system, with additional symptomatic management for underlying thrombotic conditions and general supportive care. Antithrombotic treatment for CVT is consisted of anticoagulation and intravenous thrombolysis or thrombectomy [8].

There has been a fear of hemorrhagic complications by anticoagulation for CVT cases, as almost all the CVT patients have petechial hemorrhages over the venous infarction. However, anticoagulation treatment has its rationales for CVT such as preventing thrombus growth, facilitating recanalization, and preventing systemic thromboembolic complications including deep venous thrombosis or pulmonary embolization. Although there is a paucity of well-designed and sufficiently large clinical trials for this issue, currently available best evidence may be summarized that initial anticoagulation for CVT patients may be beneficial, in spite of slight increase in hemorrhagic complications. Anticoagulants are also safe to use in patients with intracranial hemorrhages, either intracerebral or subarachnoid, in patients with CVT. Unfractionated heparin or low molecular weight heparin may be used, and a few studies have supported the use of low molecular weight heparin, except in patients who are expected to undergo an invasive procedure. Direct thrombolysis or thrombectomy through endovascular venous access has been used and reported as an alternative for systemic thrombolysis or anticoagulation, although its efficacy and safety has not been thoroughly evaluated (Fig. 16.4) [9, 10].

Acute complications including seizure and increased intracranial pressures commonly occurred in CVT patients. Although preventive antiepileptic drugs are usually not recommended, seizure should be anticipated in CVT patients with immediate medication. Increased intracranial pressure may be managed through conventional treatment strategies such as mannitol or sedation. Craniectomy for extreme cases or herniated cases may be beneficial.

Following oral vitamin K antagonists, regardless of the presence of cerebral hemorrhage, is reasonable for prolonged use of anticoagulation. Antiplatelet agents may be utilized for those who have unacceptable condition for oral vitamin K antagonist, but there is no evidence for such alternative treatment. In patients with provoked CVT or with transient risk factors including well-controlled cancer pregnancy/puerperium, or oral contraceptive use, oral vitamin K antagonist would better be maintained for 3–6 months, with target international normalization ratio (INR) of 2.0–3.0.

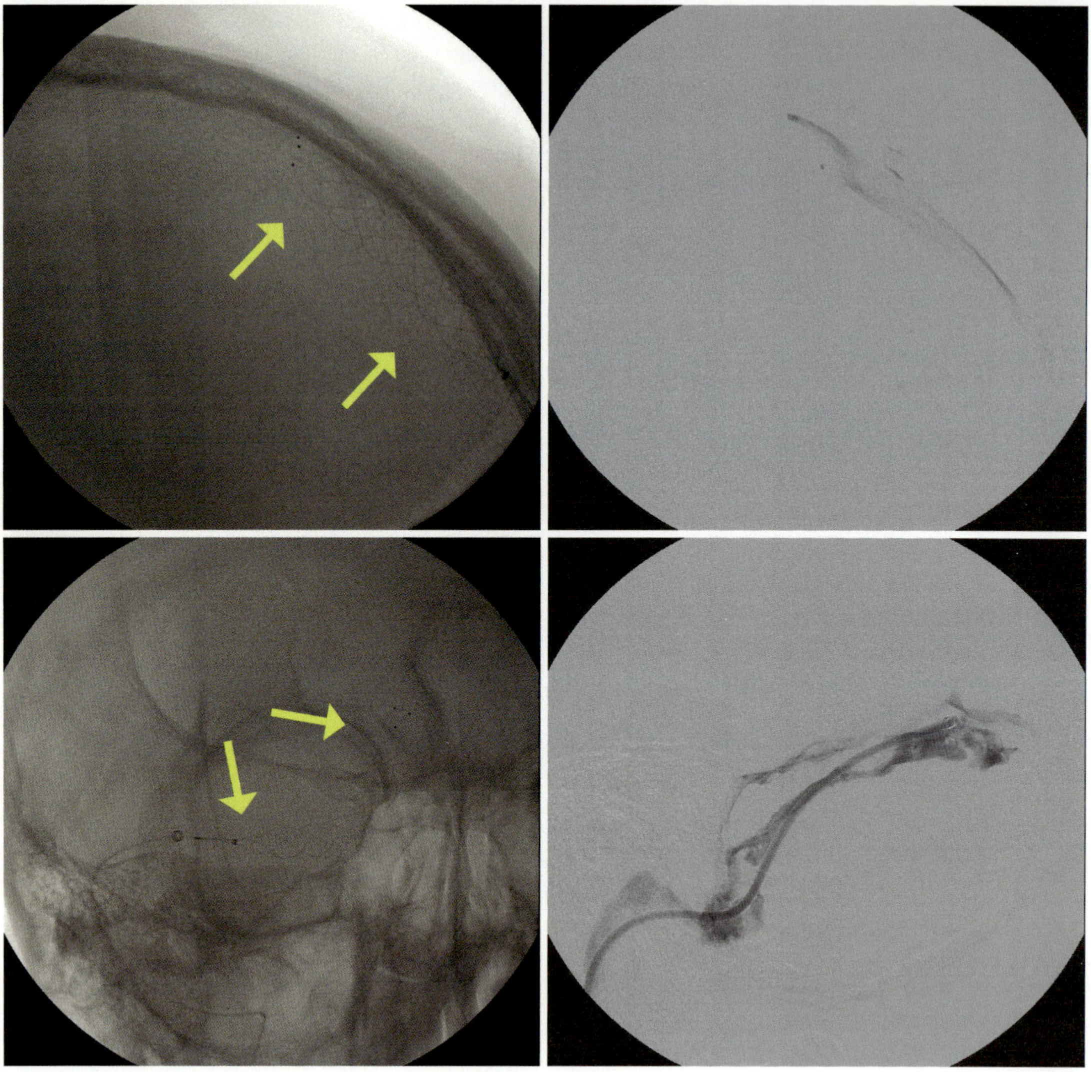

Fig. 16.4 Cerebral venous thrombosis treated by endovascular thrombolysis and stent-assisted thrombectomy. Identical case of Figs. 16.2 and 16.3. Due to the widespread venous thrombosis, the patient was treated with endovascular thrombolysis with urokinase of 400 K units and stent-assisted thrombectomy. Stent retriever (*yellow arrow*) is inserted in superior sagittal sinus (*upper panel*) and transverse sinus (*lower panel*). After the radiological intervention, his symptom started to relieve. Anticoagulation was initiated immediately with low-molecular-weight heparin followed by oral vitamin K antagonist. Follow-up MR venography taken 3 months after admission showed a normal venogram finding. Laboratory analyses revealed elevated anticardiolipin antibody titer

For patients with unprovoked CVT but without definite evidence of underlying thrombophilic conditions, oral vitamin K antagonist may be continued for 6–12 months. When a patient was documented to have severe thrombophilia or recurrent event of CVT or with past history of venous thrombosis in other vascular beds, indefinite oral vitamin K antagonist may be considered.

16.7 Prognosis After Cerebral Venous Thrombosis

Acute mortality after CVT is estimated to be around 6% for the first month, predominantly due to increased intracranial pressure and resultant herniation. However, long-term prognosis of CVT is more favorable than the conventional

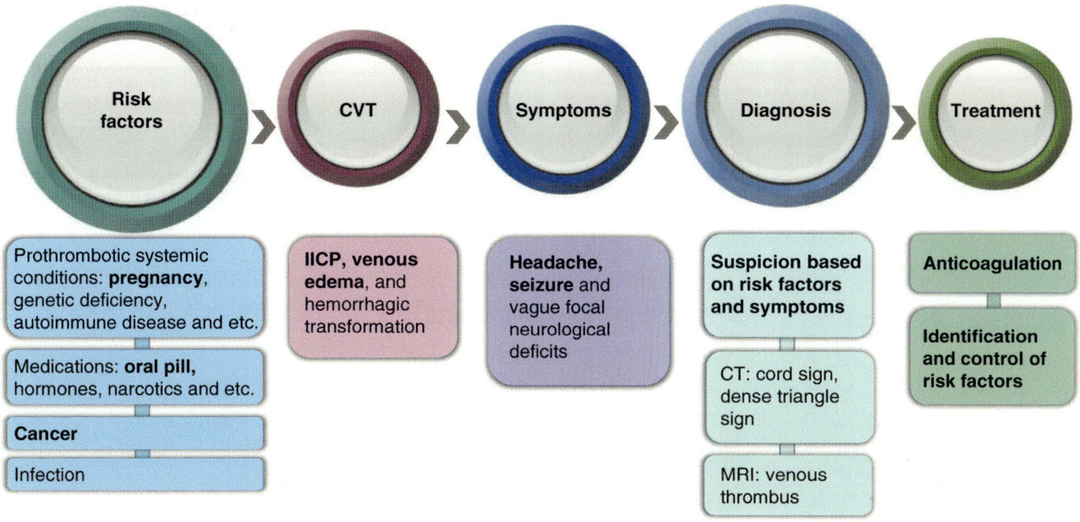

Fig. 16.5 A schematic diagram for understanding of cerebral venous thrombosis (*CVT* cerebral venous thrombosis, *IICP* increased intracranial pressure)

ischemic or hemorrhagic stroke, and good functional recovery may be expected in most of the afflicted cases. Poor prognosis factors after CVT are listed as increased age, decreased level of consciousness at presentation, seizure, deterioration of neurological symptoms/signs, and associated hemorrhagic strokes or cancer. In most cases, thrombosed veins/sinuses are reanalyzed. Collectively, a schematic diagram for understanding of CVT is shown (Fig. 16.5).

Suggestions from Current Clinical Practice Guidelines Patients with stroke caused by cerebral venous sinus thrombosis (CVT) are needed to receive anticoagulation, even in the presence of hemorrhagic transformation. The cause of thrombogenicity should be removed immediately, and anticoagulation for 3 months or more is appropriate. After then, antiplatelet therapy is reasonable, but the duration of treatment has not been established.

References

1. Ferro JM. Prognosis of cerebral vein and dural sinus thrombosis: results of the international study on cerebral vein and dural sinus thrombosis (ISCVT). Stroke. 2004;35:664–70.
2. Devasagayam S, Wyatt B, Leyden J, et al. Cerebral venous sinus thrombosis incidence is higher than previously thought: a retrospective population-based study. Stroke. 2016;47:2180–2.
3. Saadatnia M, Fatehi F, Basiri K, et al. Cerebral venous sinus thrombosis risk factors. Int J Stroke. 2009;4:111–23.
4. Gokhale S, Lahoti SA. Therapeutic advances in understanding pathophysiology and treatment of cerebral venous sinus thrombosis. Am J Ther. 2014;21:137–9.
5. Ferro JM, Canhão P. Cerebral venous sinus thrombosis: update on diagnosis and management. Curr Cardiol Rep. 2014;16:523.
6. Saposnik G, Barinagarrementeria F, Brown RD, et al. Diagnosis and management of cerebral venous thrombosis: a statement for healthcare professionals from the American Heart Association/American Stroke Association. Stroke. 2011;42:1158–92.
7. Patel D, Machnowska M, Symons S, et al. Diagnostic performance of routine brain MRI sequences for dural venous sinus thrombosis. AJNR Am J Neuroradiol. 2016:(Epub).
8. Einhäupl K, Stam J, Bousser MG, et al. EFNS guideline on the treatment of cerebral venous and sinus thrombosis in adult patients. Eur J Neurol. 2010;17:1229–35.
9. Viegas LD, Stolz E, Canhão P, et al. Systemic thrombolysis for cerebral venous and dural sinus thrombosis: a systematic review. Cerebrovasc Dis. 2014;37:43–50.
10. Siddiqui FM, Dandapat S, Banerjee C, et al. Mechanical thrombectomy in cerebral venous thrombosis: systematic review of 185 cases. Stroke. 2015;46:1263–8.

Stroke Caused by Cervical Artery Dissection

17

Stefan T. Engelter, Christopher Traenka, and Philippe A. Lyrer

Abstract

Cervical artery dissection (CAD) is the cause of stroke in 10–25% of young adults but occurs also in patients aged 60 years and older. Diagnosis of CAD requires the detection of characteristic CAD features in vascular imaging, most frequently by visualization of a mural hematoma. Magnetic resonance imaging has a higher sensitivity than neurosonography but can be falsely negative within the first days after CAD onset. The intramural bleeding is not a reason to withhold IV thrombolysis in patients with acute ischemic stroke attributable to CAD. Acute endovascular treatment has been shown feasible and might be considered an alternative to IV thrombolysis alone, worthwhile to be studied in more detail. Antiplatelets and anticoagulants are both used to prevent stroke in CAD patients. The findings of five large meta-analyses across observational data did not suggest any superiority of either treatment approach. Two randomized controlled trials do compare anticoagulation versus antiplatelets in CAD. One trial has been published, the other is

S.T. Engelter, M.D. (✉)
Department of Neurology and Stroke Center, University Hospital Basel and University of Basel, Petersgraben 4, CH-4031 Basel, Switzerland

Neurorehabilitation Unit, University of Basel, University Center for Medicine of Aging and Rehabilitation Basel, Felix Platter Hospital, Burgfelderstrasse 101, 4012 Basel, Switzerland
e-mail: stefan.engelter@usb.ch; stefan.engelter@fps-basel.ch

C. Traenka, M.D. • P.A. Lyrer, M.D.
Department of Neurology and Stroke Center, University Hospital Basel and University of Basel, Petersgraben 4, CH-4031 Basel, Switzerland

S.-H. Lee (ed.), *Stroke Revisited: Diagnosis and Treatment of Ischemic Stroke*, Stroke Revisited, DOI 10.1007/978-981-10-1424-6_17

ongoing, and participation is encouraged to increase the level of therapeutic evidence. Non-vitamin K oral anticoagulants have been used in few CAD patients. Currently, these direct oral anticoagulants should not be used in CAD patients except in the setting of properly designed studies. Angioplasty and stenting are usually reserved for CAD patients with recurrent ischemic events despite antithrombotic therapy, when hemodynamic infarction is impending in ruptured dissecting aneurysms or in iatrogenic CAD. If there are arguments against angioplasty and stenting in such patients, surgery might be considered.

Cervical artery dissection (CAD) is the cause of stroke in 10–25% of young adults. In average, CAD patients are aged approximately 45 years. In general, CAD is slightly more frequent among men (52–69%) than women. Men are on average roughly 5 years older than women, when they experience a CAD. In addition, CAD of the internal carotid artery shows a slight preference for male and older patients compared to the dissection of the vertebral artery [1]. CAD occurs also in patients aged 60 years and older. Mechanical triggers and pain occur less often in this age group than in younger patients. Convincing explanations for these observations are currently lacking. CADs are characterized by separation of the arterial wall layers by a blood accumulation, because of an intimal tear or less frequently due the rupture of vasa vasorum. Blood can separate the intima from the media, which may prompt a stenosis of the lumen, typically at the distal internal carotid artery or the V2/3—segment of the vertebral artery—locations that are different to those of atherosclerotic stenosis. Less frequently, blood dissects between the layers of media and the adventitia resulting in the formation of a dissecting aneurysm, usually without stenosis.

In about 40 of 100 patients, CAD occurs in the setting of a traumatic impact to the head or neck during the preceding 4 weeks. Most often, these traumatic events are mild or trivial and should more accurately be considered as mechanical trigger events [2]. In about 60% patients, CAD occurred spontaneously [2]. Ischemic stroke or transient ischemic attacks result mostly from thromboembolism or—less often—by hypoperfusion due to a hemodynamically relevant stenosis [3]. CAD is classified as extracranial or intracranial and, according to the site of the affected artery, as internal carotid artery dissection (ICAD) or vertebral artery dissection (VAD). In European populations, dissections seem to occur more likely in the extracranial segments of the internal carotid and vertebral arteries, while intracranial artery dissection appears to be more common than extracranial dissection in East Asian studies [4].

17.1 Clinical Presentation and Diagnosis

CADs may present with ischemic stroke or transient ischemic attacks, which is the case in approximately 2/3 of all CAD patients. Often, CAD patients present with a combination of ischemic events and local symptoms. The latter include Horner's syndrome, cranial nerve palsy, tinnitus, or cervical root impairment. In addition, these symptoms are often associated with headache or neck pain [1]. Neurovascular imaging is essential to confirm the diagnosis of CAD. The presence of at least one of the following neurovascular criteria is required: visualization of a mural hematoma, aneurismal dilatation, long tapering stenosis, intimal flap,

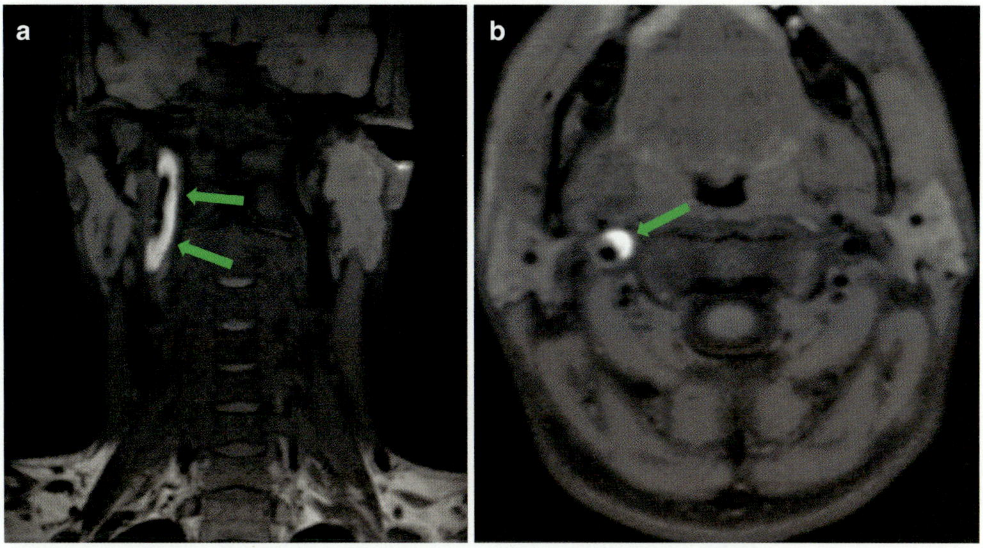

Fig. 17.1 T1-weighted, fat-suppressed magnetic resonance imaging of a 37-year-old female patient with multiple cervical artery dissections (right internal carotid artery and left vertebral artery (Fig. 17.2)). The *arrows* are indicating the T1 hyperintense signal of the mural hematoma of the right ICA in coronal plane sequences (**a**) and in axial plane sequences (**b**)

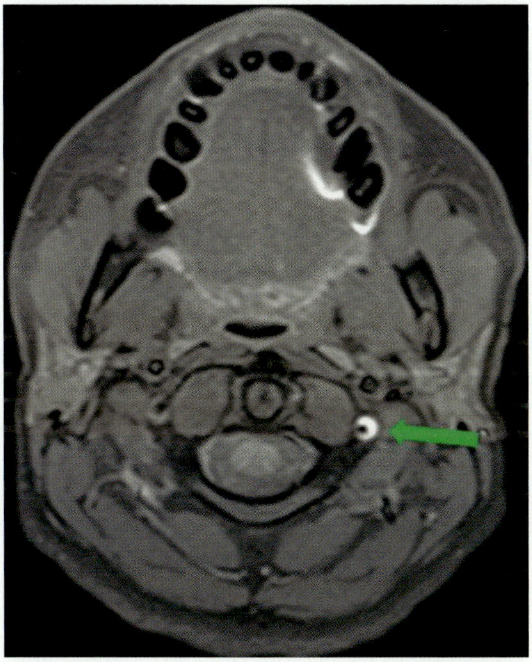

Fig. 17.2 T1-weighted, fat-suppressed magnetic resonance imaging of the same 37-year-old female patient as depicted in Fig. 17.1. The *arrows* are indicating the T1 hyperintense signal of the mural hematoma of the left vertebral artery (VA, axial plane sequences)

double lumen, or occlusion >2 cm above the carotid bifurcation revealing an aneurismal dilatation or a long tapering stenosis after recanalization in the internal carotid or vertebral artery [5, 6]. These imaging features are most accurately visualized by magnetic resonance imaging (MRI), with identification of mural hematoma by fat-suppressed T1 sequences (Figs. 17.1 and 17.2) [7]. CAD can be suspected by computed tomography findings, too. However, detection of the characteristic mural hematoma is usually not feasible [8]. Neurosonography can be used, too, in particular to detect mural hematoma (Figs. 17.3 and 17.4). Compared to MR imaging, neurosonography has a lower sensitivity in the diagnosis of CAD. However, MR can also be false negative, as it takes a few days until the blood is metabolized to methemoglobin. In these situations, neurosonography can be useful as it enables the visualization of the mural hematoma early. Neurosonography is also an ideal tool for follow-up studies and for reviewing the hemodynamic course of CAD.

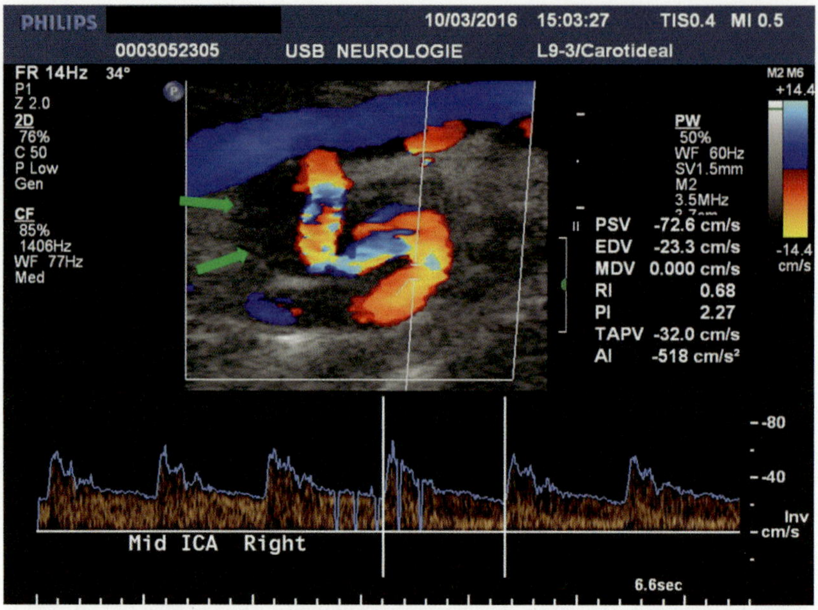

Fig. 17.3 Color duplex neurosonography of an internal carotid artery dissection (right ICA) of a 38-year-old male patient. The *arrows* are indicating the mural hematoma visualized as hypoechogenic structure in the kinked middle to distal ICA

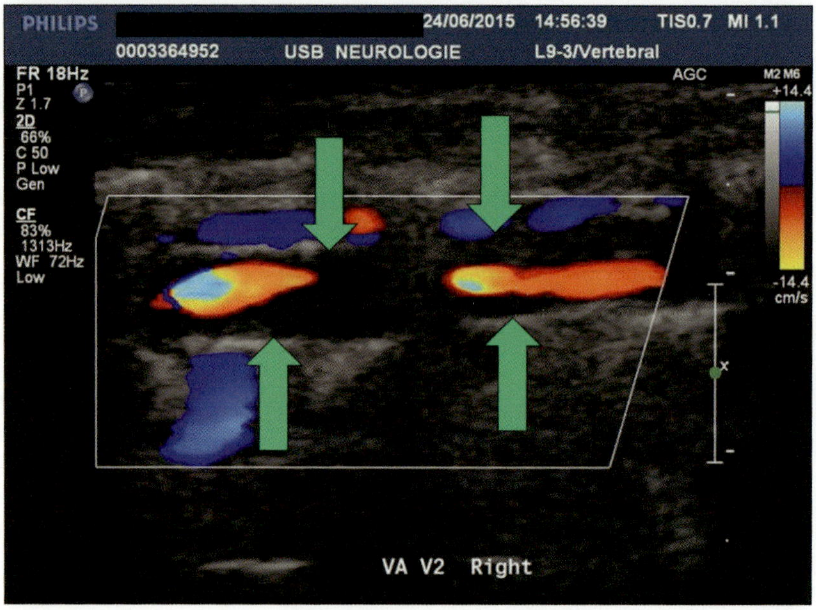

Fig. 17.4 Color duplex neurosonography of a vertebral artery dissection (*right*). The *arrows* are indicating the mural hematoma visualized as hypoechogenic structure in the wall of the V2 segment of the right vertebral artery

17.2 Treatment

17.2.1 Intravenous Thrombolysis in Cervical Artery Dissection

Intravenous thrombolysis (IVT) or endovascular recanalization therapy (EVT) has to be considered in patients with ischemic stroke attributable to CAD. At least in theory, due to the pathophysiology of CAD which is characterized by an intramural blood accumulation, there might be the risk of an enlargement of the mural hematoma of the dissected artery if treated with intravenous thrombolysis. This enlargement might cause hemodynamic worsening and might result in infarct growth. However, regarding the existing evidence on IVT in CAD, this seems to be a theoretical concern, and there is currently no convincing reason to withhold IVT or EVT in CAD patients. Though established as safe and efficacious in patients with acute ischemic stroke from different etiologies [9, 10], the evidence for the use of IVT in CAD patients is scarce and based on observational, nonrandomized data only. Current guidelines of acute stroke treatment do not recommend against IVT in CAD patients [11]. IVT or EVT increases the odds to induce recanalization of an occluded (dissected) artery or of a distal (intracranial) thrombosis in CAD patients, too.

IVT in patients with ischemic stroke due to CAD was compared to patients with stroke attributable to a cause other than CAD (i.e., non-CAD-stroke) in observational, registry-based studies [6, 12]. In one of these studies, CAD patients showed a slightly lower recovery rate—which reached statistical significance after adjustment for age, gender, and stroke severity—than patients with stroke due to another cause. Thirty-six percent of the CAD patients but 44% of the non-CAD patients had an excellent 3-month outcome (modified Rankin scale (mRS) score of 0 or 1) ($OR_{adjusted}$ 0.50 [95% CI, 0.27–0.95], $p = 0.03$) [6]. A possible explanation for the lower recovery rate might be a high rate (67.7%) of arterial occlusions caused by the dissection. More importantly, there was no signal of harm involved in IVT in CAD patients (i.e., hemorrhagic complications or recurrent infarction caused by IVT). Another study compared pooled data from observational IVT-treated CAD patients with those of a comparison group derived from the Safe Implementation of Thrombolysis in Stroke-International Stroke Thrombolysis Register (SITS-ISTR). The comparison group comprised of patients with manifold causes of stroke but were matched for age and stroke severity with the CAD patients [12]. Both groups did not differ with regard to 3-month mortality, the rate of symptomatic ICH, and the number of patients with excellent 3-month functional outcome.

In addition to the aforementioned reports of IVT-treated CAD patients compared to those with stroke due to causes other than CAD, there are also observational data on CAD patients treated with versus those treated without IVT. Analyses of the data set from the Cervical Artery Dissection and Ischemic Stroke Patients (CADISP) consortium showed identical rates of favorable recovery after CAD-related ischemic stroke in both IVT-treated and non-IVT-treated patients ($OR_{adjusted}$ 0.95 [95% CI, 0.45–2.00]). A meta-analysis across observational studies ($n = 10$) identified 174 CAD patients receiving IVT (or some other form of thrombolytic treatment, $n = 26$) who were compared to 672 CAD patients who did not receive thrombolysis. Most importantly, the odds for achieving a favorable 3-month outcome were similar in thrombolyzed and non-thrombolyzed CAD patients (OR 0.782 [95% CI, 0.49–1.33], $p = 0.441$). Interestingly, despite a higher rate of intracranial hemorrhage of all types (i.e., symptomatic or asymptomatic) among thrombolyzed CAD patients (OR 2.65 [95% CI, 0.49–1.33], $p = 0.042$), symptomatic hemorrhages were absent among the thrombolyzed CAD patients. Interestingly, the only case of a symptomatic intracranial hemorrhage occurred in one of the non-thrombolyzed CAD patients [13].

In conclusion, regarding the existing evidence on IVT in CAD—though purely observational—there is currently no convincing reason to withhold IVT in CAD patients. Further research is encouraged.

17.2.2 Endovascular Therapy in Cervical Artery Dissection

Endovascular thrombectomy with or without IVT is of benefit for patients with acute ischemic stroke caused by occlusion of the proximal anterior circulation, as shown in several randomized controlled trials, recently meta-analyzed [14]. Whether this includes patients with stroke attributable to CAD is unproven, as there is no evidence from randomized controlled trials. The current evidence on EVT in CAD is based on case series and small nonrandomized studies and should therefore be interpreted very cautiously. Such observational studies showed that the endovascular approach is feasible in CAD. In a series of 24 CAD patients treated with EVT (combined with or without IVT), favorable 3-month outcome (i.e., mRS 0–2) was as frequent in EVT-treated as compared to non-EVT-treated patients (OR 0.62 (0.12–3.14), $p = 0.56$). If compared to CAD patients receiving IVT only ($n = 11$), the odds of a favorable 3-month outcome in EVT-treated CAD patients were similar (OR 1.32 (0.16–10.72), $p = 0.79$). Likewise, there was no difference in the odds of a favorable 3-month outcome if EVT-treated CAD patients ($n = 24$) were compared to EVT-treated non-CAD patients ($n = 421$) (OR 0.58 (0.19–1.78), $p = 0.34$) [15]. A meta-analysis across five nonrandomized observational case series comparing IVT-treated to EVT-treated CAD patients found a similar likelihood of a favorable outcome (modified Rankin scale 0–2) in both groups (OR 1.41 [95% CI, 0.45–3.45], $p = 0.46$). Endovascular treatment might be particularly important in patients presenting with tandem occlusion (i.e., occlusion of the dissected artery and a distally located intracranial artery). In a retrospective study of EVT-treated patients with stroke due to different causes, 20 CAD patients with tandem occlusion which includes the internal carotid artery were compared to non-CAD patients with occlusion solely of a large intracranial artery. Recanalization rates did not differ between both groups. CAD patients recovered in 70%, while non-CAD patients did recover in 50%, a difference which however was not statistically significantly different ($p = 0.093$) [16]. As a limitation, comparisons were not adjusted for possible confounding variables (e.g., stroke severity) or imbalanced baseline characteristics. In a recent case series of 21 CAD patients treated with EVT reported, 15 (71%) recovered well at 90 days (i.e., mRS 0, 1 or 2) compared to 69 out of 133 (51%) CAD patients with IVT treatment reported in the literature. This difference (OR 1.38 [1.00—1.89]) was borderline significant ($p = 0.05$) [17] and might be considered as a signal that modern EVT might be as beneficial in stroke due to CAD as it has been shown in strokes with occlusion of a major intracranial artery in general.

In conclusion, as EVT is likely to increase the odds of recanalization of an occluded artery also in CAD patients, it is probably recommendable to use this approach also in CAD given the patient is otherwise eligible for this kind of therapy. Further research is encouraged.

17.3 Recurrent Ischemic Events and Prophylactic Antithrombotic Treatment in CAD

Under treatment with antithrombotic agents, first or recurrent cerebral ischemic events as well as bleeding complications do occur. The frequency of such events differed between studies (for details, see Table 17.1). There is still equipoise on whether anticoagulation or the antiplatelets should be used.

17.3.1 Observational Data

Five meta-analyses used observational data for comparisons between antiplatelets and anticoagulants in CAD patients [18–22]. These meta-analyses used different statistical approaches and showed conflicting results. No difference in occurrence of stroke or death was reported by Menon et al. in 2008 and by Chowdhury and coworkers [22]. A nonsignificant trend in favor of anticoagulants was reported in a Cochrane Review regarding the end point of death or disability at the end of follow-up (OR 1.77 [95% CI, 0.98–3.22], $p = 0.06$) [19]. Interestingly, major bleeding complication—such as symptomatic intracranial hemorrhage (5/627; 0.8%) or major extracranial hemorrhage (7/425; 1.6%)—occurred exclusively among CAD patients treated with anticoagulants. In turn, a beneficial effect of antiplatelets was reported by Sarikaya et al. for a composite outcome of ischemic stroke, intracranial hemorrhage, or death (RR 0.32 [95% CI, 0.12–0.64]) [21]. Table 17.1 shows details of the five meta-analyses. The differences of the key findings are explained by mainly methodological differences and a high risk of bias involved in

Table 17.1 Synopsis of meta-analyses across observational data comparing antiplatelets with anticoagulants in CAD

	Year	Site of dissection	Methodology	Number of patients	Key findings
Menon et al.	2008	ICA, VA	Meta-analysis	762	No significant difference in risk of: • death: antiplatelet 5/268 (1.8%), anticoag. 9/494 (1.8%), $p = 0.88$ • stroke: antiplatelet 5/268 (1.9%), anticoag. 10/494 (2.0%), $p = 0.66$
Lyrer and Engelter	2010	ICA	Cochrane system review	1285	Nonsignificant trend in favor of anticoagulants for: • death or disability (OR 1.77 [0.98 to 3.22][a] $p = 0.06$), (463 patients) no significant differences in odds • death (OR 2.02, 95% CI 0.62–6.60) • ischemic stroke (OR 0.63, 95% CI 0.21–1.86) (1262 patients) Sympt. intracranial hemorrhages (5/627; 0.8%) only with anticoag. Major extracranial hemorrhages (7/425; 1.6%) only with anticoag.
Kennedy et al.	2012	ICA, VA	Meta-analysis	1636	No significant differences in risk of: • re-stroke: antiplatelet 13/499 [2.6%], anticoag. 20/1137 [1.8%] • death: antiplatelet 5/499 [1.0%], anticoag. 9/1137 [0.80%]
Sarikaya et al.	2013	ICA, VA	Bayesian meta-analysis	1991	Antiplatelets lead significant reduction of composite outcome—ischemic stroke, intracranial hemorrhage, or death (3 months) • relative risk 0.32 [0.12–0.63][b]
Chowdhury et al.	2015	ICA, VA	Meta-analysis	1398	No significant differences for the odds of death, death and disability, ischemic stroke, symptomatic intracranial hemorrhage, major extracranial hemorrhage during follow-up

[a]Antiplatelets, aspirin, dipyridamole, clopidogrel; anticoagulants, unfractionated heparin, dalteparin, enoxaparin, tinzaparin, warfarin
[b]CIHD—the composite outcome CIHD includes the following efficacy and safety outcome measures during the 3-month treatment period: (1) occurrence of any stroke and new acute lesions on diffusion-weighted MRI; (2) any major extracranial hemorrhage, any symptomatic intracranial hemorrhage, and any asymptomatic micro-or macro-bleeds; and (3) death

observational explorative studies. Thus, meta-analyses across observational data will not answer the question, whether anticoagulants are superior or inferior to antiplatelets or whether they are equally beneficial treatment options in CAD. The answer of these clinically important questions requires evidence from randomized controlled trials.

17.3.2 Randomized Controlled Trials

There are two randomized controlled trials comparing anticoagulation versus antiplatelets in CAD. In 2015, the results of the Cervical Artery Dissection in Stroke Study (CADISS) have been published. CADISS was designed as a prospective feasibility study randomly assigning CAD patients to either antiplatelet therapy (aspirin, dipyridamole, or clopidogrel alone or in combination) or to anticoagulation therapy (heparin followed by warfarin with a target INR of 2–3) [23]. CADISS included 250 CAD patients, mainly presenting with stroke or transient ischemic attack ($n = 224$). Overall, the combined end point of ischemic stroke, death, or major bleeding was met in 2% (4 of 196) in the per-protocol population [23]. With regard to the primary outcome (ipsilateral stroke or death), there was no statistically significant difference between both groups (intention-to-treat population: OR 0.335 [95% CI, 0.006–4.233], $p = 0.63$). However, the single major bleeding complication in CADISS occurred in the anticoagulation group. Central reading of the patient baseline imaging confirmed CAD diagnosis in solely 197 of the 250 study participants. However, the main results of the study did not differ in the per-protocol population, either. Based on the very low event rates of the purely clinical primary outcome in this study, the authors calculated that 4876 patients per group would be needed to show significant differences between groups. The usage of imaging surrogate outcomes might help to overcome the feasibility issue in treatment trials comparing different antithrombotic agents in CAD patients. Such an approach is utilized in an ongoing prospective, randomized, open-labeled, multicenter trial investigating aspirin vs. anticoagulation in acute CAD. The "Biomarkers and Antithrombotic Treatment in Cervical Artery Dissection" (TREAT-CAD, NCT0204640, www.clinicaltrials.gov) trial uses a composite primary outcome including both clinical and imaging surrogate outcome measures for ischemic stroke as well as intracerebral hemorrhage. Including such surrogate imaging outcomes in the composite primary outcome is assumed to substantially reduce the target sample size of the study, which is useful to accomplish feasibility of the study. This assumption is based on the observation that new ischemic lesions visible on diffusion-weighted imaging (DWI) sequences were observed in 25% of CAD patients who had repeated brain MRI in an explorative study [24]. This frequency is much higher than the rate of clinical apparent strokes reported in CADISS or in the aforementioned meta-analysis across observational studies. Thus, the target sample size of TREAT-CAD is estimated to be $n = 169$ patients. The TREAT-CAD study had started recruitment in 2013. The 100th patient was recruited in September 2016. Participation is encouraged to increase the level of therapeutic evidence. Study completion is expected at the end of 2018. Table 17.2 displays details of CADISS and TREAT-CAD. Non-vitamin K oral anticoagulants have been used in a few patients. Currently, these direct oral anticoagulants should not be used in CAD patients except in the setting of properly designed studies.

17.3.3 Treatment Duration

There are no reliable data on the optimum duration of antithrombotic treatment in CAD. Yet, as the ideal duration of such a treatment has not been studied in clinical trials and is therefore unclear, the duration of treatment has to be based on clinical reasoning taking into account the knowledge about the time course of (1) recurrent ischemic events, (2) recanalization, and (3) recurrent dissections. Most ischemic events occur within the first 2–4 weeks [1, 19, 24]. Recanalization of initial occlusion or high-grade stenosis in a dissected artery can be expected in about 2/3 of such CAD patients within 6 months. Beyond 12 months, recanalization of an initially occluded artery is exceptional in CAD patients. There is a heterogeneity about the frequency of recurrent dissection in the literature. At least, it is agreed that usually a "recurrent" dissection affects the same type of artery but on the contralateral instead of the ipsilateral side. Furthermore, the risk of recurrent dissection seems to decrease substantially beyond the first weeks after CAD. While in up to 1/4 of all CAD patients, a recurrent dissection might be detected within the first 4 weeks—often clinically oligo-symptomatic or even asymptomatic—much lower rates (i.e., 0–8.3%) are reported thereafter [5]. Based on these observations—if anticoagulation is chosen as antithrombotic agent—it is mostly maintained for at least 3–6 months in a pragmatic approach. In the absence of ischemic events, hemorrhagic complications, and substantial stenosis at a follow-up visit 3 months or 6 months later, aspirin is often used instead of anticoagulants for another 6–9 months. Provided that (1) no ischemic event occurred under this treatment regimen, (2) there is full restitution of the dissected artery (MRI or neurosonography), and (3) there is no evidence of clinically silent ischemic lesions on MRI, it may be considered to stop

Table 17.2 Synopsis of randomized controlled trials comparing antiplatelets versus anticoagulants in cervical artery dissection

Study	Duration	Type	Treatment	Primary outcome	Main result (per protocol)/ current status	Sample size (*n*)	ClinicalTrial. gov identifier
CADISS	2005–2014	Randomized controlled prospective multicenter study	Antiplatetelets[a] vs. anticoagulants (see legend)	Ipsilateral stroke or death within 3 months from randomization	*Antiplatelets*: ipsilateral Stroke/death: 3/101 Major bleeds: 0/101 *Anticoagulants*: ipsilateral Stroke/death: 1/91 Major bleeds: −1/91	192 per protocol 250 intention to treat	NCT 00238667
TREAT-CAD	2013–2018	Randomized controlled open-label multicenter, non-inferiority trial with blinded assessment of outcome events	Aspirin 300 mg OD vs. vitamin K antagonists	Cerebrovascular ischemia, major hemorrhagic events, or death[b]	Recruiting	104[c] (target:169)	NCT 02046460

[a]Antiplatelets, aspirin, dipyridamole, clopidogrel; anticoagulants, unfractionated heparin, dalteparin, enoxaparin, tinzaparin, warfarin
[b]CIHD—the composite outcome CIHD includes the following efficacy and safety outcome measures during the 3-month treatment period: (1) occurrence of any stroke and new acute lesions on diffusion-weighted MRI; (2) any major extracranial hemorrhage, any symptomatic intracranial hemorrhage, and any asymptomatic micro-or macro-bleeds; and (3) death
[c]December 2, 2016

antithrombotic treatment. The same criteria can be applied if antiplatelets rather than anticoagulants were used as first antithrombotic treatment. In case of the development of an (asymptomatic) dissecting aneurysm at the site of the initially dissected artery, ongoing antiplatelet treatment is mostly preferred. This approach can be modified taking into account the vascular risk profile, comorbidities, and—most importantly—the patient's perspective. Given the absence of sound data on this issue, this approach is of unknown effectiveness and includes recommendations by others, as well as our own experiences [1].

Suggestions from Current Clinical Guidelines
Either antiplatelet or anticoagulant therapy is appropriate to patients with stroke caused by extracranial carotid or vertebral arterial dissection. The treatment duration has not been established, but maintenance for at least 3–6 months is appropriate. Priority between antiplatelet or anticoagulant therapy has not been understood and should be determined on an individual basis. For patients with medical treatment failure, angiographic intervention (i.e., angioplasty or stenting) or surgery might be considered.

References

1. Engelter ST, Traenka C, Von Hessling A, et al. Diagnosis and treatment of cervical artery dissection. Neurol Clin. 2015;33:421–41.
2. Engelter ST, Grond-Ginsbach C, Metso TM, et al. Cervical artery dissection: trauma and other potential mechanical trigger events. Neurology. 2013;80:1950–7.

3. Morel A, Naggara O, Touze E, et al. Mechanism of ischemic infarct in spontaneous cervical artery dissection. Stroke. 2012;43:1354–61.
4. Debette S, Compter A, Labeyrie MA, et al. Epidemiology, pathophysiology, diagnosis, and management of intracranial artery dissection. Lancet Neurol. 2015;14:640–54.
5. Debette S, Leys D. Cervical-artery dissections: predisposing factors, diagnosis, and outcome. Lancet Neurol. 2009;8:668–78.
6. Engelter ST, Rutgers MP, Hatz F, et al. Intravenous thrombolysis in stroke attributable to cervical artery dissection. Stroke. 2009;40:3772–6.
7. Rodallec MH, Marteau V, Gerber S, et al. Craniocervical arterial dissection: spectrum of imaging findings and differential diagnosis. Radiographics. 2008;28:1711–28.
8. Ben Hassen W, Machet A, Edjlali-Goujon M, et al. Imaging of cervical artery dissection. Diagn Interv Imaging. 2014;95:1151–61.
9. Wardlaw JM, Murray V, Berge E, et al. Thrombolysis for acute ischaemic stroke. Cochrane Database Syst Rev. 2014;29:CD000213.
10. Emberson J, Lees KR, Lyden P, et al. Effect of treatment delay, age, and stroke severity on the effects of intravenous thrombolysis with alteplase for acute ischaemic stroke: a meta-analysis of individual patient data from randomised trials. Lancet. 2014;384:1929–35.
11. Jauch EC, Saver JL, Adams HP Jr, et al. Guidelines for the early management of patients with acute ischemic stroke: a guideline for healthcare professionals from the American Heart Association/American Stroke Association. Stroke. 2013;44:870–947.
12. Zinkstok SM, Vergouwen MD, Engelter ST, et al. Safety and functional outcome of thrombolysis in dissection-related ischemic stroke: a meta-analysis of individual patient data. Stroke. 2011;42:2515–20.
13. Lin J, Sun Y, Zhao S, et al. Safety and efficacy of thrombolysis in cervical artery dissection-related ischemic stroke: a meta-analysis of observational studies. Cerebrovasc Dis. 2016;42:272–9.
14. Goyal M, Menon BK, van Zwam WH, et al. Endovascular thrombectomy after large-vessel ischaemic stroke: a meta-analysis of individual patient data from five randomised trials. Lancet. 2016;387:1723–31.
15. Jensen J, Salottolo K, Frei D, et al. Comprehensive analysis of intra-arterial treatment for acute ischemic stroke due to cervical artery dissection. J Neurointerv Surg. 2016 Jun 10 [Epub ahead of print].
16. Marnat G, Mourand I, Eker O, et al. Endovascular management of tandem occlusion stroke related to internal carotid artery dissection using a distal to proximal approach: insight from the RECOST study. AJNR Am J Neuroradiol. 2016;37:1281–8.
17. Haussen DC, Jadhav A, Jovin T, et al. Endovascular management vs intravenous thrombolysis for acute stroke secondary to carotid artery dissection: local experience and systematic review. Neurosurgery. 2016;78:709–16.
18. Menon R, Kerry S, Norris JW, et al. Treatment of cervical artery dissection: a systematic review and meta-analysis. J Neurol Neurosurg Psychiatry. 2008;79:1122–7.
19. Lyrer P, Engelter S. Antithrombotic drugs for carotid artery dissection. Cochrane Database Syst Rev. 2010;6:CD000255.
20. Kennedy F, Lanfranconi S, Hicks C, et al. Antiplatelets vs anticoagulation for dissection: CADISS nonrandomized arm and meta-analysis. Neurology. 2012;79:686–9.
21. Sarikaya H, da Costa BR, Baumgartner RW, et al. Antiplatelets versus anticoagulants for the treatment of cervical artery dissection: Bayesian meta-analysis. PLoS One. 2013;8:e72697.
22. Chowdhury MM, Sabbagh CN, Jackson D, et al. Antithrombotic treatment for acute extracranial carotid artery dissections: a meta-analysis. Eur J Vasc Endovasc Surg. 2015;50:148–56.
23. Investigators Ct, Markus HS, Hayter E, et al. Antiplatelet treatment compared with anticoagulation treatment for cervical artery dissection (CADISS): a randomised trial. Lancet Neurol. 2015;14:361–7.
24. Gensicke H, Ahlhelm F, Jung S, et al. New ischaemic brain lesions in cervical artery dissection stratified to antiplatelets or anticoagulants. Eur J Neurol. 2015;22:859–65.

Antiphospholipid Antibody Syndrome

18

Ana Rodríguez Sanz, Melissa Báez Martínez,
Ángel Robles Marhuenda,
and Patricia Martínez-Sánchez

Abstract

Antiphospholipid antibody syndrome (APS) is a systemic autoimmune disease defined by recurrent thromboembolic events and/or pregnancy morbidity in the presence of medium- or high-titer antiphospholipid (aPL) antibodies, including anticardiolipin antibodies (aCLs), anti-β2-glycoprotein 1 (aβ2GP1) antibodies, and lupus anticoagulant (LA). The pathogenic mechanisms that lead to neurological and systemic clinical manifestations associated with aPL are only partially understood, although it is thought that aPLs have thrombogenic properties, increasing thrombus formation in the venous and arterial circulation. Stroke has a strong impact on morbidity and mortality in APS, especially in young patients. An overall aPL prevalence of 6.8% has been reported in patients with stroke, and a prevalence of 20% has been observed in patients with stroke younger than 45 years. In addition, cerebral manifestations, including infarcts, are observed in more than 50% of patients with catastrophic APS. The primary stroke mechanisms are thrombotic or embolic arterial occlusion affecting mainly small- and medium-sized vessels. Regarding treatment, clinical guidelines recommend antiplatelet therapy for patients with ischemic stroke or transient ischemic attacks who meet the criteria for APS

A.R. Sanz, M.D. • M.B. Martínez, M.D.
Á.R. Marhuenda, M.D.
P. Martínez-Sánchez, M.D., Ph.D. (✉)
Department of Neurology and Stroke Centre, La Paz University Hospital, Autonoma of Madrid University, IdiPAZ Health Research Institute (ARS, MBM, PMS), Paseo de la Castellana 261, PC: 28046 Madrid, Spain

Department of Internal Medicine, La Paz University Hospital, Autonoma of Madrid University, IdiPAZ Health Research Institute (ARM), Madrid, Spain
e-mail: patrindalo@hotmail.com

S.-H. Lee (ed.), *Stroke Revisited: Diagnosis and Treatment of Ischemic Stroke*, Stroke Revisited, DOI 10.1007/978-981-10-1424-6_18

with a level of evidence A. Anticoagulant therapy might be considered, depending on the perception of risk of recurrent thrombotic events and bleeding. Cerebral ischemic vascular events are the most frequent recurrent thrombotic events in patients with APS. The role of serum levels of aCL as markers of stroke severity and outcome is unknown.

Antiphospholipid antibody syndrome (APS) is a systemic autoimmune disease that clinically manifests as recurrent thromboembolic events and/or pregnancy morbidity with the elevated levels of antiphospholipid (aPL) antibodies, including anticardiolipin antibodies (aCLs), anti-β2-glycoprotein 1 (aβ2GP1s) antibodies, and lupus anticoagulant (LA) [1]. First recognized in patients with systemic lupus erythematosus (SLE) and later in other autoimmune disorders as "secondary" APS, however, it is now well known that the development of this syndrome might be independent of other underlying diseases, thus being termed "primary APS." Another subset has been described, characterized by an accelerated form of APS with multiple vascular occlusive events, usually affecting small vessels and resulting in multiorgan failure, termed "catastrophic" APS; it represents less than 1% of all patients with APS.

The Euro-Phospholipid Project is a multicenter, consecutive, prospective design of a cohort of 1000 patients with APS, derived from 13 European countries and followed up for 10 years. It showed that deep venous thrombosis (38.9%), stroke (19.8%), pulmonary embolism (14.1%), superficial thrombophlebitis (11.7%), transient ischemic attacks (TIAs) (11.1%), and obstetric morbidity (including both fetal and maternal complications) were the most common manifestations of the syndrome [2].

The importance of neurological manifestations was predicted in the original description of the syndrome in 1983. They reported the aPL positivity was related to a spectrum of neuropsychiatric manifestations, including cerebral ischemia, dementia, migraine, convulsions, chorea, transverse myelitis, and Guillain-Barre´ syndrome [3].

Interestingly, in the Euro-Phospholipid Project, strokes and transient ischemic attacks were the most frequent recurrent thrombotic events—given they appeared in 2.4 and 2.3% of the total cohort, respectively [2]. The aPL antibodies are found in 6.8% of patients with stroke, and especially a prevalence of 20% has been observed in the young patients (age <45 years) [4]. Neurological manifestations such as stroke, encephalopathy, and seizure were observed in 62% patients in the European Catastrophic Antiphospholipid Antibody Syndrome (CAPS) registry, with 13% mortality of stroke in this registry [5]. These data reveal the strong impact of stroke on morbidity and mortality within the syndrome, especially in young patients.

18.1 Pathogenesis of APS

The pathogenic mechanisms associated with clinical manifestations of aPL are understood partly. Several in vitro and in vivo animal studies reported that the aPL antibodies are pathogenic drivers in APS. The thrombogenic properties of aPL antibodies induce venous and arterial thrombosis. However, the exact mechanisms that produce autoantibodies and mediate disease related to thrombosis remain unclear. In spite of the heterogeneous families of aPL, similar HLA class allele associations have been identified. It has been known that the association with HLA-DR4, HLA-DR7, and HLA-DRw is the most relevant in the APS patients. The β2GP1, also known as a plasma apolipoprotein, is the primary autoantigen for aPL antibodies, which mediates the interaction with aPL on target cells such as platelets, monocytes, endothelial cells, and trophoblasts [6]. Additionally, the β2GP1-dependent aCL IgG-positive finding can lead to a twofold increase in the risk of a stroke occurrence within 15 years of follow-up compared with β2GP1-dependent aCL IgG-negative finding. The effects of aPL antibodies on hemostatic reactions include inhibition of the fibrinolytic system and activation of the coagulation cascade by various mechanisms that will be explained subsequently within the specific mechanisms of stroke.

18.2 Mechanisms of Stroke

Arterial occlusion can be thrombotic or embolic affecting small-, medium-, or large-size vessels (Table 18.1) [7].

18.2.1 Thrombotic Mechanism

Arterial thrombosis in patients with APS more frequently affects small- and medium-sized vessels. The exact mechanism is still unknown, although there are data suggesting that aPL induces thrombosis through any one or more of several mechanisms [7]:

- Interaction of aPL with proteins affected in clotting pathway, such as prothrombin, factor X, protein C, and plasmin, might hinder inactivation of procoagulant factors and impede fibrinolysis [7, 8].
- Binding and activation of platelets [7] that increase expression of glycoprotein 2b–3a and synthesis of thromboxane A2 [8].
- Interaction of aPL with endothelial cells and inducing expression of procoagulant, proinflammatory, and intercellular cell adhesion molecules (ICAM-1, VCAM-1, E-selectin) [7, 8].
- Upregulation of tissue factor transcription in endothelial cells and monocytes, thus activating the extrinsic pathway of the coagulation, increases resistance to activated protein C and binds to annexin A5. The binding of annexin A5 to anionic phospholipid on the surface of the cell makes them unavailable to other coagulation factors, thus exerting an anticoagulant activity. It is an important thrombogenic mechanism that the aPL antibodies disrupt the annexin A5 anticoagulant shield [9].
- Activation of the complement cascade [7].

In summary, interaction of antiphospholipid antibodies with endothelial cells, monocytes, and platelets induces a procoagulant state that is primarily mediated by the increased synthesis of tissue factor and thromboxane A2. Induction of procoagulant state and activation of the complement cascade can provoke thrombotic events (Fig. 18.1) [8].

Moreover, the prevalence of vascular risk factors such as tobacco or estrogens is more than 50% in patients with APS, and the coexistence of these factors is related to thrombotic event. This could be relevant in patients with clinical manifestations highly suggestive of APS but with persistently negative conventional aPLs, classified as "seronegative APS." Several studies reported noncriteria antibodies that have been proposed to be relevant to APS and that could be potentially involved in the classification criteria of APS [10].

Table 18.1 Mechanisms of stroke in antiphospholipid antibody syndrome

Mechanism	Affected vessel size	Pathogenesis
Thrombotic	Small Medium Large	1. Expression of molecular protein adhesion in endothelial cells, monocytes, and platelets 2. Increased tissue factor production 3. Interactions of aPL with proteins implicated in clotting regulation 4. Complement activation
Embolic	Medium Large	1. Left-sided cardiac valvular anomalies: (a) Deposition of immune complexes (b) Vegetations (Libman-Sacks endocarditis) (c) Valve dysfunction 2. Intracardiac thrombus

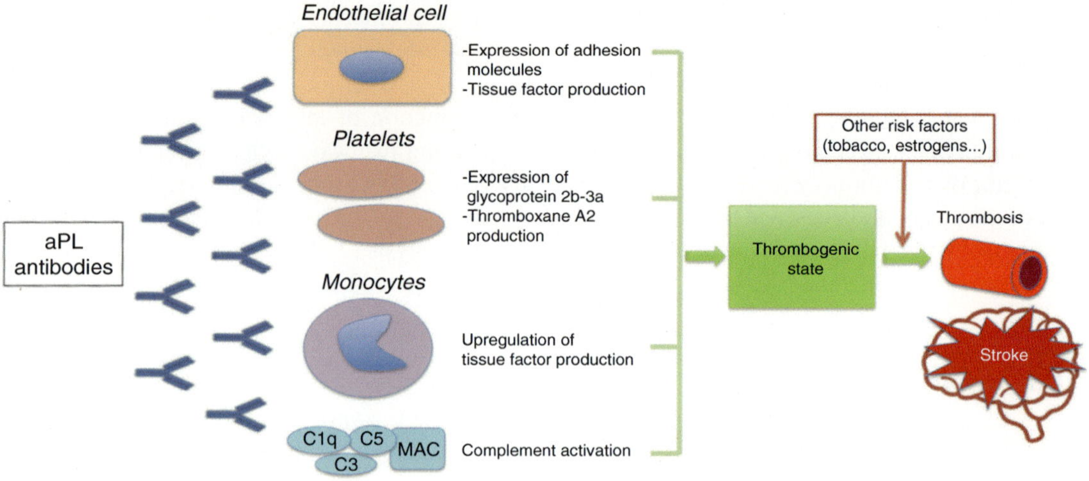

Fig. 18.1 Thrombotic mechanisms in antiphospholipid antibody syndrome (*aPL* antiphospholipid antibodies, *MAC* membrane attack complex)

Sneddon's syndrome (SS) is a rare, progressive noninflammatory thrombotic arteriopathy affecting small- and medium-sized vessels. This disease is characterized by the combination of livedo reticularis and various neurological problems including cerebrovascular diseases. Approximately 40–50% of patients with SS are aPL positive, which suggests that SS is part of the clinical spectrum of primary aPL syndrome and the pathogenic mechanism would probably be thrombotic. However, SS patients with aPL negative might have a distinct entity or perhaps a group of various disorders. However, the developed thrombotic mechanisms in aPL-negative SS patients are still unclear. Several possible mechanisms associated with thrombosis are reported including activated protein C resistance, platelet aggregation, increased thromboglobulin levels, the change of tissue plasminogen activator to inhibitor ratio, antithrombin III deficiency, and protein S deficiency. In large studies, these abnormalities have not been identified; therefore, it is unclear at present [11].

On other hand, some patients with APS have had multiple white matter lesions that commonly involved both lobes of the brain asymmetrically. These lesions could be asymptomatic (silent brain infarcts), but they are frequently associated with attentional and cognitive impairment. This mechanism might be related to microvascular thrombosis.

18.2.2 Embolic Mechanisms

The cardiac involvement such as left-sided cardiac valvular anomalies and, rarely, intracardiac thrombus is associated with thromboembolic events in APS patients. The cardiac involvement in APS has prevalence of more than 80% using highly sensitive techniques such as transesophageal echocardiogram (TEE). The irregular thickening of the valve leaflets due to the deposition of immune complexes, vegetation (Libman-Sacks endocarditis), and valve dysfunction is known as the main valvular pathologies. Although the valvular impairment mechanisms caused by aPLs remains unclear, the antibodies are thought to be an important factor for the formation of thrombi on the valvular endothelium. In addition, a higher aCL titer and a history of arterial thrombosis are associated with valvular heart diseases. The mostly involved valve is the mitral valve, followed by the aortic and tricuspid valves. The TEE is recommended in patients with high clinical suspicion of embolic source for identifying the intracardiac embolic source. The recurrent thrombotic events and a high IgG aCL titer could be a reflection of the aggravation or the development of cardiac abnormalities despite optimal antithrombotic treatment. The prevalence of intracardiac thrombus in APS patients is rare (~4% patients), which is more likely to develop on the right side, regardless of the type of heart chambers [7].

18.3 Diagnosis

The diagnosis of APS is based on clinical criteria of pregnancy morbidity or thromboembolism and laboratory findings of medium- or high-titer aPLs that are present on two or more abnormal blood test results with at least 12 weeks apart between tests (Table 18.2) [1].

Table 18.2 Revised classification criteria for antiphospholipid antibody syndrome [1]

Clinical criteria (one or more) 1. Vascular thrombosis: One or more objectively confirmed episodes of arterial, venous, or small-vessel thrombosis occurring in any tissue or organ 2. Pregnancy morbidity: (a) One or more unexplained deaths of a morphologically normal fetus at or beyond the 10th week of gestation (b) One or more premature births of a morphologically normal neonate before the 34th week of gestation due to eclampsia, preeclampsia, or placental insufficiency (c) Three or more unexplained consecutive spontaneous abortions before the 10th week of gestation
Laboratory criteria (one or more, present in two or more occasions at least 12 weeks apart using recommended procedures) 1. Lupus anticoagulant, detected according to the guidelines of the International Society on Thrombosis and Hemostasis 2. Anticardiolipin antibody of IgG and/or IgM isotype, present in a medium or high titer (greater than 40 GPL or MPL or greater than the 99th percentile), measured by a standardized ELISA 3. Anti-β2-glycoprotein-1 antibody of IgG and/or IgM isotype, present in a titer greater than the 99th percentile, measured by a standardized ELISA

Reproduced by permission of Journal of Thrombosis and Haemostasis [1]

Because the aPL level could be transiently increased by ischemic events or other medical conditions such as viral infections, lymphoproliferative disorders, Crohn's disease, or various drugs (phenytoin, quinine, amoxicillin), it is necessary to confirm the high aPL titer at least 12 weeks after the stroke to rule out other causes of increased aPL level.

Antibodies against β2-glycoprotein I (anti-β2-GPI) and cardiolipin (aCL), together with the LA functional assay, are the three laboratory tests considered in the revised criteria for the diagnosis of the syndrome [1]. Although thrombocytopenia, livedo reticularis, valvular heart lesions, and nephropathy are common clinical features in APS, these are not formally involved in the consensus of diagnostic criteria. Moreover, APS patients are more likely to have aPL antibodies than LA, aCL, and anti-β2-GPI, relevant antibodies against prothrombin, other proteins, or phospholipids that are not also included in the current consensus criteria.

There is a limit to the measurement method of aPL. Generally, at least two phospholipid-dependent coagulation tests are widely used as screening tests of LA. Patients on oral anticoagulants or unfractionated heparin therapy may have false-positive results for LA because prolonged clotting times on screening and confirmatory testing can be similarly prolonged. Despite the techniques that can overcome these limitations, testing for LA should ideally be done after discontinuing antithrombotic agents or anticoagulation. The enzyme-linked immunosorbent assay (ELISA) methods are common methods for detection of both aCL and anti-β2-GPI antibodies. However, there are still significant batch-to-batch variability problems because of not standardized assay methods.

The American Stroke Association recommends testing for aPL in patients with TIA or ischemic stroke who have other features of APS, such as livedo reticularis, obstetric complications, unexplained thrombocytopenia, or prolongation of coagulation test, with no alternative explanation for their ischemic event [12].

18.4 Treatment

Antithrombotic therapies are needed in the APS patients with high risk of recurrent thromboembolism. Pharmacological agents include antiplatelets such as low-dose aspirin and anticoagulant drugs such as vitamin K antagonists (VKA), heparin, or its derivatives.

Adequately controlled studies evaluating treatment of elevated aCL to prevent a first stroke are not available. The Antiphospholipid Antibody Acetylsalicylic Acid (APLASA) study did not find a reduction in the rate of first thrombotic events with low-dose aspirin (81 mg/d) over placebo in persistently aPL-positive asymptomatic individuals. In addition, antiplatelets are not indicated for primary stroke prevention in people who have persistently increased aPL titer [13].

On the other hand, only a few studies have investigated the relationship between the aPL antibodies and the risk of recurrent thromboembolic events after TIA or stroke. These studies showed wide variability in the prevalence of aPL, from 6 to 46%, and inconsistent findings for an association with increased risk for recurrent stroke. There remains a lack of consensus regarding optimal antithrombotic management of patients with ischemic stroke and aPL [12]. Further complicating the picture is the balance between thrombosis and hemorrhage in an individual patient with APS, who might have concomitant thrombocytopenia and other comorbidities contributing to increased bleeding risks. It is important to estimate the individual risk of bleeding for preventing complications and good outcome. Common major bleeding predictors include prolonged international normalized ratio (INR) values above 4.0, concomitant aspirin treatment with polypharmacy, old age (>75 years), history of gastrointestinal tract bleeding, malignancy, and uncontrolled high blood pressure.

In the randomized controlled Antiphospholipid Antibodies and Stroke Study (APASS), aspirin at a dose of 325 mg daily was shown to be as effective as low-intensity anticoagulation (target INR 1.4–2.8) in the secondary prevention of stroke among aPL-positive patients [12]. In 2009, Okuma first shed light on the combination of low-dose aspirin with moderate intensity anticoagulation as a therapeutic option in patients with stroke with a definite diagnosis of APS. This randomized controlled trial showed a lower incidence of recurrent stroke among patients treated with low-dose aspirin plus warfarin compared with those receiving low-dose aspirin alone, with a cumulative stroke-free survival of 74% compared with 25%. Given this conflicting picture, the task force at the 13th International Congress on Antiphospholipid Antibodies could not reach a consensus about the optimal management of arterial thrombosis. Eight of the 13 members of the task force recommended that patients with definite APS and arterial thrombosis should be treated with warfarin with INR over 3.0 or a combination of moderate anticoagulation (INR 2.0–3.0) and aspirin. Low-dose aspirin would be reserved for patients with stroke who have a low-risk profile and reversible thrombotic risk factors [13].

The American Heart Association/American Stroke Association guidelines [12] recommend antiplatelet therapy for patients with ischemic stroke or TIA who meet the criteria for APS with a level of evidence A. Anticoagulant therapy might be considered depending on the perception of risk of recurrent thrombotic events and bleeding.

New-generation oral anticoagulants (NOACs) are emerging new class of anticoagulant drugs because, unlike warfarin, they do not need for regular international normalized ratio (INR) monitoring. Moreover, NOACs have fewer drugs, dietary, and alcohol interactions compared to warfarin. However, further supportive strategies are needed for the NOAC management in APS patients. There are few ongoing randomized controlled clinical trials evaluating the treatment effect of rivaroxaban compared with low-intensity anticoagulation in the management of APS. The Rivaroxaban in Antiphospholipid Syndrome trial has been promoted by a UK group and is a phase II/III study that has recruited APS patients with a history of venous thromboembolism. In Spain, a phase III trial has begun on 218 patients with venous or arterial events; and recently, an Italian trial considering triple-positive patients with APS only will start recruiting [14].

On the other hand, there are limited therapeutic options for patients who have recurrent stroke despite high-intensity warfarin. In these patients, addition of an antiplatelet agent or low molecular weight heparin could be possible therapeutic options. The possibility that the INR might not reflect the true anticoagulant intensity in patients with APS should be considered, and the measurement of amidolytic factor X levels might be useful to assess the true intensity of warfarin anticoagulation in this circumstance [15]. For cases in which anticoagulation has failed, other available therapeutic options include combining anticoagulation with immunosuppression and/or immunomodulation with modalities including rituximab hydroxychloroquine and statins, although there is not enough evidence of their efficacy.

18.5 Prognosis

Antiphospholipid antibody-related vascular events have a strong clinical impact in terms of morbidity and mortality. This chronic and disabling condition usually presents in early adulthood. In a large European cohort, the median age at disease onset was 31 years, and stroke accounted for 13% of deaths at a mean age of 42 years. The highest morbidity is attributed to neurologic damage.

Recurrent stroke is one of the complications we can see in outcomes of patients with APS after a first ischemic stroke. The process by which APS causes recurrent stroke or TIA is thought to be either thrombotic or embolic. In the thrombotic process, in situ thrombus formation is due to the hypercoagulable state associated with APS, in which aPL activated platelet function or prostaglandin activity and the resulting metabolites stimulate the chemoreceptors of the vascular endothelium. On the other hand, Fulham et al. [16] reported seven patients with aPL whose multiple cerebral infarctions were proven to be cardiogenic. They speculate that cardiac valvular lesions—in particular, nonbacterial thrombotic endocarditis—play an important role in the pathogenesis of recurrent ischemic stroke in patients with APS. A recent publication reported a 77-year-old woman with atrial fibrillation treated with warfarin who had recurrent ischemic stroke in various brain areas. A complete blood analysis was performed and primary APS was later confirmed. Although APS is not frequent in stroke patients older than 70 years, a broader study should be undertaken to exclude an APS of late onset in all patients with a recurrent stroke regardless of age.

On the other hand, an observational study investigated treatment effect with aspirin 100 mg and low molecular weight heparin (LMWH) on outcome in APS women with previous ischemic stroke during pregnancy. Despite combination therapy daily during the pregnancy, there was a significant risk of obstetrical complications including mainly preeclampsia and preterm delivery and an increased risk of recurrent cerebral ischemia in women complicated by preeclampsia. Therefore, several authors believe that anticoagulation should be given rigorously during pregnancy, especially in the context of preeclampsia, to prevent recurrence of ischemic stroke [17].

Finally, understanding of the relationship between aPL level and stroke severity and outcome is limited. In 1998, Verro et al. reported 27 patients with cerebrovascular ischemic symptoms who were found to have high positive aCL levels of the IgG isotype on one or more occasions. However, higher IgG aCL titer is not associated with poor prognosis, severe neurological symptoms, and recurrent ischemic events. However, a recent observational study, which included young stroke patients with APS, suggests that serum levels of IgM aCL within 48 h of hospital admission may be positively associated with stroke severity, and levels of IgG anti-b2GPI are also related to the outcome [18].

Suggestions from Current Clinical Practice Guidelines Incidence of stroke or transient ischemic attack (TIA) caused by antiphospholipid antibody syndrome (APS) is increasing, but the routine tests for confirmation of APS in stroke or TIA with undetermined cause are not mandatory. Treatment of APS-related stroke has not been established, and the recommendation is dependent upon results from several small-sized hospital-based studies. In general, antiplatelet therapy is enough to prevent recurrence of stroke in the patients with APS who fulfill the APS criteria. In some severe cases, long-term anticoagulation may be needed.

References

1. Miyakis S, Lockshin MD, Atsumi T, et al. International consensus statement on an update of the classification criteria for definite antiphospholipid syndrome (APS). J Thromb Haemost. 2006;4:295–306.
2. Cervera R, Boffa M-C, Khamashta MA, et al. The Euro-Phospholipid Project: epidemiology of the antiphospholipid syndrome in Europe. Lupus. 2009;18:889–93.
3. Hughes GR. Thrombosis, abortion, cerebral disease and the lupus anticoagulant. Br Med J (Clin Res Ed). 1983;287:1088–9.
4. Rodrigues CE, Carvalho JF, Shoenfeld Y. Neurological manifestations of antiphospholipid syndrome. Eur J Clin Invest. 2010;40:350–9.
5. Bucciarelli S, Espinosa G, Cervera R. The CAPS Registry: morbidity and mortality of the catastrophic antiphospholipid syndrome. Lupus. 2009;18:905–12.
6. Comarmond C, Cacoub P. Antiphospholipid syndrome: from pathogenesis to novel immunomodulatory therapies. Autoimmun Rev. 2013;12:752–7.
7. Panichpisal K, Rozner E, Levine SR. The management of stroke in antiphospholipid syndrome. Curr Rheumatol Rep. 2012;14:99–106.
8. Ruiz-Irastorza G, Crowther N, Branche W, et al. Antiphospolipid syndrome. Lancet. 2010;376: 1498–509.
9. Carecchio M, Cantello R, Comi C. Revisiting the molecular mechanism of neurological manifestations in antiphospholipid syndrome: beyond vascular damage. J Immunol Res. 2014;2014:239398.
10. Nayfe R, Uthman I, Aoun J, et al. Seronegative antiphospholipid syndrome. Rheumatology. 2013;52:1358–67.
11. Wu S, Xu Z, Liang H. Sneddon's syndrome: a comprehensive review of the literature. Orphanet J Rare Dis. 2014;9:215.
12. Kernan WN, Ovbiagele B, Black HR, et al. Guidelines for the prevention of stroke in patients with stroke and transient ischemic attack: a guideline for healthcare professionals from the American Heart Association/American Stroke Association. Stroke. 2014;45:2160–236.
13. Meschia JF, Bushnell C, Boden-Albala B, et al. Guidelines for the primary prevention of stroke: a statement for healthcare professionals from the American Heart Association/American Stroke Association. Stroke. 2014;45:3754–832.
14. Chighizola CB, Moia M, Meroni PL. New oral anticoagulants in thrombotic antiphospholipid syndrome. Lupus. 2014;23:1279–82.
15. Keeling D, Mackie I, Moore GW, et al. Guidelines on the investigation and management of antiphospholipid syndrome. Br J Haematol. 2012;157:47–58.
16. Fulham MF, Gatenby P, Tuck RR. Focal cerebral ischemia and antiphospholipid antibodies: a case for cardiac embolism. Acta Neurol Scand. 1994;90:417–23.
17. Fischer-Betz R, Specker C, Brinks R, et al. Pregnancy outcome in patients with antiphospholipid syndrome after cerebral ischaemic events: an observational study. Lupus. 2012;21:1183–9.
18. Rodríguez-Sanz A, Martínez-Sánchez P, Prefasi D, et al. Antiphospholipid antibodies correlate with stroke severity and outcome in patients with antiphospholipid syndrome. Autoimmunity. 2015;48:275–81.

Cancer-Related Stroke

19

Hyung-Min Kwon

Abstract

Cancers are often associated with hypercoagulability, and patients with malignancy are at risk for the development of cancer-related stroke. Patients with concomitant cancer and acute ischemic stroke show more frequent multiple arterial lesions in diffusion-weighted imaging, and the levels of the D-dimer have a tendency to increase. Malignant cells activate the coagulation cascade by multiple mechanisms, i.e., tissue factor expression, inflammatory cytokines, and procoagulant expression. The causes of this spoiled coagulation are related to patient characteristics and specific cancer-related characteristics or treatment-related factors. Trousseau's syndrome is the second leading cause of death in cancer patients, after death from cancer itself. Appropriate prophylaxis and treatment of cancer-related thromboembolism reduce morbidity and mortality, increase survival rate, and improve patients' quality of life. Low-molecular-weight heparin is the drug of choice for the management of venous thromboembolism in patients with cancer and is an effective and safe drug of prevention and treatment according to the international scientific guidelines. Studies evaluating the efficacy and safety of novel oral anticoagulants for the prevention of cancer-related thrombosis in high-risk patients and in the long-term management of ischemic stroke are expected.

Cancer-related thrombosis was first described in 1865 by French physician Armand Trousseau [1]. Since its discovery, the combination of cancer and hypercoagulable states is often termed Trousseau's syndrome (TS) because Trousseau's report is considered the first report that described an association between cancer and hypercoagulation. Cancers are often associated with hypercoagulability, and patients with malignancy are at risk for the development of cancer-associated thrombosis.

H.-M. Kwon, M.D., Ph.D.
Department of Neurology, SMG-SNU Boramae Medical Center, Seoul National University College of Medicine, Seoul, South Korea
e-mail: hmkwon@snu.ac.kr

S.-H. Lee (ed.), *Stroke Revisited: Diagnosis and Treatment of Ischemic Stroke*, Stroke Revisited, DOI 10.1007/978-981-10-1424-6_19

After Trousseau, Sack reported that TS was chronic disseminated intravascular coagulation (DIC) associated with nonbacterial thrombotic endocarditis (NBTE) and arterial thrombosis in patients with malignancy in 1977 [2]. Currently, the term "TS" is often used to describe a hypercoagulable state in patients with cancer and cancer-related thrombosis.

Our comprehension of thrombosis in patients with malignancy has altered from an incidental event to a major cause of morbidity and mortality directly associated with cancer. Embolic strokes are the commonest etiology of stroke in patients with malignancy, due partially to hypercoagulable condition, while large artery atherosclerosis amounts to only 22% of strokes in this population [3]. Besides acute cerebral infarction, TS can present as an NBTE or migratory thrombophlebitis. In advanced or metastatic cancer, a hypercoagulable or prothrombotic condition is a frequent complication and may be encountered as a various clinical thromboembolism and cerebral infarction [4].

19.1 Clinical Presentation of Cancer-Related Stroke

The cardinal clinical manifestations of cancer-associated thrombosis include arterial thrombosis, pulmonary embolism, deep vein thrombosis, and chronic DIC associated with NBTE.

Cerebral arteries and upper and lower extremities are the common sites of arterial thrombosis in patients with malignancy. It has been reported that the incidence of arterial thrombosis is estimated to be 2–5%, accounting for 10–30% of all thrombotic complications [5, 6]. The cerebrum and cerebellum are frequently injured by arterial thrombosis due to the rich distribution of the procoagulants, thromboplastin, combined with low levels of the anticoagulation factors in the brain epithelium.

Ischemic stroke occurs very infrequently as the first manifestation of a cancer. However, cerebrovascular disease occurs frequently in cancer patients, with 15% of cancer patients experiencing a thromboembolic event after their initial cancer diagnosis [4]. The number of people living with cancer is increasing with an increase in life expectancy, and improvements in treatment modality have contributed to improved survival. As a result, the proportion of patients who have malignancy is expected to increase among all stroke patients.

19.2 Various Stroke Mechanism in Cancer Patients

In several studies, patients with cancer and acute ischemic stroke simultaneously showed more frequent multiple arterial lesions in diffusion-weighted imaging [7, 8]. In the absence of an established embolic source, ischemic stroke related to the cancer-associated hypercoagulation accounts for most of cases. When there is no explainable cause of stroke, cancer-associated hypercoagulable infarction should be considered particularly. In addition, levels of the D-dimer were higher in the cryptogenic group than in the conventional stroke mechanism group. Therefore, laboratory findings and diffusion-weighted image lesion patterns can be helpful in the early identification of embolic source in cancer patients.

Microembolic signals on transcranial Doppler ultrasound in cancer patients with ischemic stroke, especially in those without conventional stroke mechanisms, may be observed with a high prevalence [9]. A microembolic signal was found in around 50 % of acute ischemic stroke patients with cancer but more frequently in patients without conventional stroke mechanism (58%) than in those with conventional stroke mechanism (33%). Furthermore, elevated D-dimer levels were independently associated with embolic signals and decreased dramatically with the use of anticoagulants [9]. Thus, the detection of a microembolic signal by transcranial Doppler ultrasound may provide hints about the cancer-specific stroke mechanism related to the hypercoagulable state.

Table 19.1 Risk factors for cancer-associated thrombosis

Patient characteristics	Treatment-related factors	Cancer-related factors
Older age Prolonged immobility Prior history of thrombosis Elevated leukocyte and platelet counts Acute infection Comorbidity Obesity	Chemotherapy Hormonal agents Growth factors Antiangiogenic agents Major surgery Central venous catheters	Primary site of cancer Stage of cancer Compression of directly invasion of large vessels Mucin from adenocarcinoma Tissue factor expression

19.2.1 Nonbacterial Thrombotic Endocarditis (NBTE)

NBTE is a disease characterized by the presence of vegetations on cardiac valves, which consist of fibrin and platelet aggregates and are devoid of inflammation or microorganism. NBTE, also known as marantic endocarditis, can affect various internal organs or peripheral arteries. Among TS patients, a diagnosis of NBTE is usually not made while they are alive but is made at postmortem due to the limitation of diagnostic tools. Patients with adenocarcinoma have a fivefold higher risk for NBTE than patients with other cell types of malignant tumors according to the previous report [10]. The frequency of NBTE in one case series report was low (1/10), because only transthoracic echocardiography was available for the detection of NBTE [8]. In that study, a half of patients had adenocarcinoma (5/10), which is consistent with the previous report.

NBTE should be suspected in all stroke patients who have an underlying cancer and are best diagnosed with transthoracic or transesophageal echocardiography. Histologically, the cusps of the heart valve are covered with small wartlike materials. Small- to medium-sized vegetations are formed with a uniform eosinophilic appearance devoid of visible inflammatory cells or bacteria.

19.3 Pathophysiology and Risk Factors

The complete pathophysiology of cancer-associated thrombosis remains unknown. The pathogenesis and risk factors of cancer-associated thrombosis are divided into the following three categories: patient characteristics, treatment-related factors, and cancer-specific factors (Table 19.1) [11].

In regard to cancer-related factors, malignant brain tumors, hematological malignancies, and adenocarcinomas of the pancreas, stomach, ovary, uterus, lungs, and kidneys were related to highest risk for development of venous thromboembolism (VTE) through large epidemiological studies [12]. Moreover, advanced stage or metastatic cancer has been shown to be associated with an increased risk of VTE compared with early-stage or localized cancers. Besides, direct compression or invasion of large blood vessels due to the tumor itself is one of the important causes of cancer-associated thrombosis.

Malignant cells themselves activate the coagulation cascade through multiple mechanisms, i.e., inflammatory cytokines, tissue factor (TF) expression, and procoagulant expression by cancer cells. When monocytes or macrophages interact with cancer cells, they release tumor necrosis factor, interleukin-1, and interleukin-6, causing endothelial damage and disruption (Fig. 19.1). Moreover, cancer cells activate monocytes or macrophages to release TF. TF directly induces the conversion of factor VII to factor VIIa, leading to the subsequent activation of the extrinsic pathway of the coagulation cascade, which brings out thrombin generation and thrombosis. Procoagulants are expressed by cancer cells and normal cells. It directly accelerates the conversion of factor X to factor Xa. In one side, advanced stage cancer cells often express large amount of sialic acid-rich glycoproteins. The sialic acid in mucin from adenocarcinomas can cause a direct nonenzymatic activation of factor X [13]. To prevent cancer cell-related thrombosis

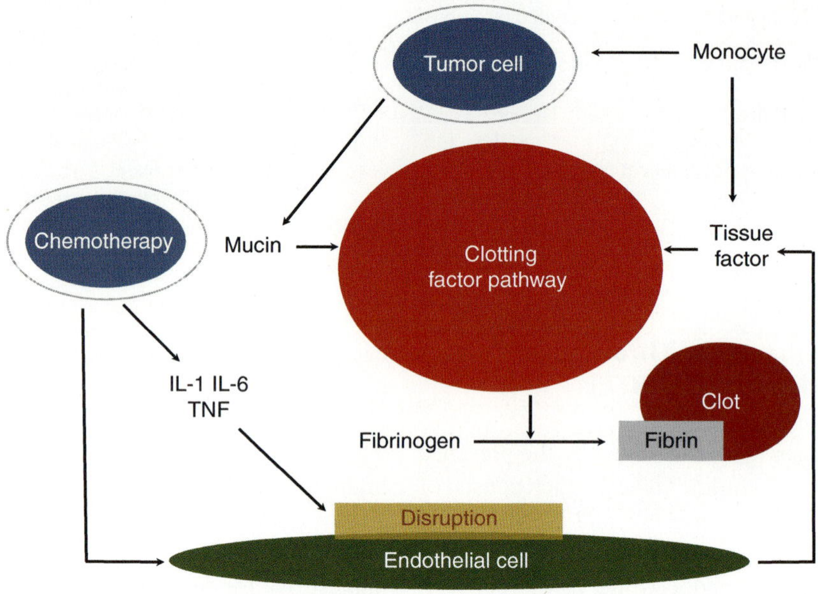

Fig. 19.1 Multiple mechanisms in Trousseau's syndrome. When cells of the monocyte or macrophage interact with malignant cells, they release tumor necrosis factor, interleukin-1, and interleukin-6, causing endothelial damage and disruption. Monocytes or macrophages are also induced by cancer cells to release tissue factor. Tissue factor directly induces activation of clotting factor pathway resulting in thrombosis. The interaction between tumor cells and macrophages also activates platelets and clotting factor pathway, which leads to the generation of thrombin and thrombosis. The mucin and procoagulants produced from adenocarcinomas cause activation of clotting factor pathway. In addition, aggressive chemotherapy itself increases the risk of thrombosis

through various mechanisms, unfractionated heparin is considered much more effective than warfarin.

19.4 Management of Cancer-Related Stroke

Regardless of underlying mechanisms, the primary approach to treating TS is to eliminate the causative tumor as soon as possible. Treatment and prevention of cancer-associated thrombosis should focus on reducing mortality and morbidity and improving the quality of life in patients with malignancy. Furthermore, benefits of anticoagulation therapy should always surpass the risk of bleeding because the bleeding is the most harmful or devastating effect of anticoagulant use.

For a long time, warfarin has been the standard therapy for chronic anticoagulation but in the cancer population is highly associated with bleeding complication, recurrent venous thromboembolism, and drug–nutrient and drug–drug interactions. Low-molecular-weight heparin (LMWH) is generally preferred to unfractionated heparin because LMWH does not need frequent monitoring with blood tests. Several randomized controlled trials compared the efficacy and safety of LMWH with warfarin for the treatment of VTE. The Comparison of Low-Molecular-Weight Heparin versus Oral Anticoagulant Therapy (CLOT) study published in 2003 was the largest randomized controlled multicenter trial [14]. This study enrolled 672 patients (336 patients in the dalteparin group and 336 patients in the oral-anticoagulant group) with cancer and acute VTE, and it compared 6 months of treatment with warfarin and the LMWH dalteparin at a dose of 200 IU/kg body weight, administered once daily subcutaneously. The probability of recurrent thromboembolism at 6 months was 17% in the warfarin group and 9% in the dalteparin group. The hazard ratio for recurrent thromboembolism in the dalteparin group as compared with the oral-anticoagulant group was 0.48 over the 6-month study period, which was statistically significant [14]. No significant differences between the dalteparin and warfarin groups were detected in the rate of bleeding (14 and 19%, respectively) and the mortality rate at 6 months (39 and 41%, respectively). Based on this result, LMWH is recommended for both the initial and maintenance therapies of cancer-associated thrombosis by major international guidelines (Table 19.2) [15, 16].

It is well known that recurrent thrombosis is frequently encountered in cancer patients because of the increased life expectancy and availability of advanced treatment modality. Therefore, long-term management of cancer-associated thrombosis is of importance. LMWH is the preferred anticoagulant agent even for long-term treatment as well as initial management in patients with cancer and thromboembolism since some data indicate that it reduces the recurrence rate of thromboembolism. For the reasons stated above, LMWH is generally recommended as the first-line anticoagulant therapy for the first 3 months following the diagnosis of thromboembolism according to current international guidelines [15].

There is no definite consensus on the management of cancer-related stroke. It is necessary to consider patients' condition, age, and the availability of anticoagulant agents. Recently, novel oral anticoagulants such as factor Xa inhibitors (e.g., rivaroxaban, apixaban, and edoxaban) and direct thrombin inhibitors (e.g., dabigatran) are emerging as candidate agents for the management of VTE and arterial thrombosis in patients with cancer. They have more advantages because they have fewer food–drug and drug–drug interactions than warfarin and do not require regular monitoring of the blood test to achieve a proper therapeutic anticoagulant effect. However, until now there is little data proving the efficacy and safety of these agents for the management of cancer-associated stroke and VTE. Clinical trials evaluating the efficacy and safety of novel oral

Table 19.2 Guidelines on treatment of venous thromboembolism in patients with cancer

	NCCN 2014	ASCO 2014
Acute management		
LMWH	Dalteparin 200 U/kg OD Enoxaparin 1 mg/kg BID	Recommended for the initial 5–10 days of treatment for DVT and PE inpatients with CrCl > 30 mL/min
Fondaparinux	5 mg (<50 kg), 7.5 mg (50–100 kg), 10 mg (>100 kg) OD	
UFH	APTT-adjusted infusion (target APTT 2–2.5× control)	
Chronic management		
LMWH	Recommended for first 6 months as monotherapy without warfarin in patients with proximal DVT or PE and metastatic or advanced cancer	Recommended for long-term therapy for DVT and PE
Warfarin	2.5–5 mg every day initially with dynamic dosing strategy (INR value targeted at 2–3)	Acceptable for long-term therapy if LMWH is not available.(target INR, 2–3)
NOACs		Not recommended
Duration of therapy	Minimum 3 months	At least 6 months Extended anticoagulation with LMWH or VKA beyond 6 months for patients with: • metastatic disease • receiving chemotherapy • recurrent thrombosis

NCCN National Comprehensive Cancer Network, *ASCO* American Society of Clinical Oncology, *OD* once-daily dosing, *BID* twice-daily dosing, *DVT* deep vein thrombosis, *PE* pulmonary embolism, *LMWH* low-molecular-weight heparin, *NOACs* novel oral anticoagulants, *VKA* vitamin K antagonist anticoagulants for cancer-related stroke and thromboembolism are needed.

Suggestions from Current Clinical Practice Guidelines Clinical suspicion on hidden malignancy is critical in diagnosis of cancer-related stroke or transient ischemic attack (TIA). When stroke or TIA has no apparent cause, hidden malignancy might be associated, especially in patients with elevated D-dimer levels. Low-molecular-weight heparin is generally recommended for prevention of further stroke. Other anticoagulants such as warfarin or new oral anticoagulants have not been studied yet.

References

1. Trousseau A. Plegmasia alba dolens. Clinique Medicale de l'Hotel Dieu de Paris. 1865;5:281–332.
2. Sack GH Jr, Levin J, Bell WR. Trousseau's syndrome and other manifestations of chronic disseminated coagulopathy in patients with neoplasms: clinical, pathophysiologic, and therapeutic features. Medicine (Baltimore). 1977;56:1–37.
3. Cestari DM, Weine DM, Panageas KS, et al. Stroke in patients with cancer: incidence and etiology. Neurology. 2004;62:2025–30.
4. Rogers LR. Cerebrovascular complications in cancer patients. Neurol Clin. 2003;21:167–92.
5. Sanon S, Lenihan DJ, Mouhayar E. Peripheral arterial ischemic events in cancer patients. Vasc Med. 2011;16:119–30.
6. Di Nisio M, Ferrante N, Feragalli B, et al. Arterial thrombosis in ambulatory cancer patients treated with chemotherapy. Thromb Res. 2011;127:382–3.
7. Kim SG, Hong JM, Kim HY, et al. Ischemic stroke in cancer patients with and without conventional mechanisms a multicenter study in korea. Stroke. 2010;41:798–801.
8. Kwon HM, Kang BS, Yoon BW. Stroke as the first manifestation of concealed cancer. J Neurol Sci. 2007;258:80–3.
9. Seok JM, Kim SG, Kim JW. Coagulopathy and embolic signal in cancer patients with ischemic stroke. Ann Neurol. 2010;68:213–9.
10. Chomette G, Auriol M, Baubion D. Non-bacterial thrombotic endocarditis—autopsy study, clinicopathological correlations. Ann Med Interne. 1980;131:443–7.
11. Elyamany G, Alzahrani AM, Bukhary E. Cancer-associated thrombosis: an overview. Clin Med Insights Oncol. 2014;8:129–37.
12. Wun T, White RH. Epidemiology of cancer-related venous thromboembolism. Best Pract Res Clin Haematol. 2009;22:9–23.
13. Bick RL. Cancer-associated thrombosis. N Engl J Med. 2003;349:109–11.
14. Lee AY, Levine MN, Baker RI. Low-molecular-weight heparin versus a coumarin for the prevention of recurrent venous thromboembolism in patients with cancer. N Engl J Med. 2003;349:146–53.
15. Streiff MB, Bockenstedt PL, Cataland SR. Venous thromboembolic disease. J Natl Compr Canc Netw. 2013;11:1402–29.
16. Lyman GH, Bohlke K, Khorana AA, et al. Venous thromboembolism prophylaxis and treatment in patients with cancer: American society of clinical oncology clinical practice guideline update 2014. J Clin Oncol. 2015;33:654–6.

Moyamoya Disease

20

Tackeun Kim and Chang Wan Oh

Abstract

Moyamoya disease (MMD) is a rare disease, with typical characteristics including progressive stenosis or occlusion of the bilateral internal carotid artery and accompanying basal collateral formation. Although MMD only accounts for a small portion of stroke in the elderly, it is the most common cause of pediatric stroke in East Asia. East Asian regional predilection and female predominance are well-known epidemiologic features, and the age of onset follows a bimodal distribution. The affected blood vessel shows intimal hyperplasia with shrinkage of the outer diameter. Owing to stenosis or occlusion, cerebral perfusion decreases, resulting in ischemic symptoms that include transient ischemic attack or cerebral infarction. In these cases, cerebral revascularization surgery is effective to prevent stroke reoccurrence and neurological deterioration. The fragility of fine collateral vascular networks is another problem. These are prone to rupture leading to intraventricular or intracerebral hemorrhage. Cerebral revascularization surgery can reduce the extent of fragile collaterals by augmenting cerebral blood flow. One study reported that extensive bilateral direct bypass surgery could prevent further hemorrhage by decreasing blood flow through fragile collaterals. Another reported option to prevent further hemorrhage is endovascular obliteration of the aneurysm (or pseudoaneurysm) at the site of hemorrhage.

Moyamoya disease (MMD) is characterized by progressive stenosis or occlusion at the internal carotid artery (ICA) bifurcation. Typically, MMD affects the bilateral ICAs, including the adjacent anterior cerebral arteries (ACAs) and middle cerebral arteries (MCAs), which is accompanied by the formation of abnormal vascular networks at the base of the brain. Due to the shape of

T. Kim • C.W. Oh, M.D., Ph.D. (✉)
Department of Neurosurgery, Seoul National University Bundang Hospital,
82, Gumi-ro 173 Beon-gil, Bundang-gu, Seongnam-si, Gyeonggi-do 13620, South Korea
e-mail: wanoh@snu.ac.kr

S.-H. Lee (ed.), *Stroke Revisited: Diagnosis and Treatment of Ischemic Stroke*, Stroke Revisited, DOI 10.1007/978-981-10-1424-6_20

collateral vessels, the disease was named "moyamoya" (puff of smoke) in Japanese. Although MMD is a rare cause of stroke in the elderly, it is the most common cause of pediatric stroke, especially in East Asia. Geographical predilection and female predominance are well-known epidemiologic features and onset peaks at two distinct ages. Many studies have contributed to the understanding of MMD pathophysiology. Although some potential causative genetic alterations have been discovered, the etiology of MMD is largely unknown. Thus, there is currently no specific treatment to halt or prevent progression of the disease. However, for patients with ischemic symptoms related to impaired hemodynamics, surgical cerebral blood flow augmentation can prevent stroke reoccurrence.

20.1 Epidemiology

The geographic and ethnic differences in MMD incidence or prevalence rates have been well described by previous epidemiologic studies. Most notable is the higher incidence and prevalence in East Asian countries, especially Korea and Japan. The highest reported incidence of MMD was 4.3 per 100,000 people per year in Korea in 2013 [1]. The prevalence was 18.1 per 100,000 people in 2013. Both the incidence and prevalence have gradually increased from 2.7 to 6.5, respectively, since 2005. In Japan, the incidence was measured as 0.54 and 0.94 by nationwide survey and local investigation, respectively [2, 3]. The incidence in China (0.43) and Taiwan (0.20) was also higher than that in other countries. Although not fully understood, different genetic backgrounds may play a role in these regional differences. Incidence and prevalence rates have increased in more recent data using chronological comparisons.

Female predominance is a consistent finding among MMD epidemiological reports. Although there was a subtle difference in the reported sex ratio, the male-to-female incidence ratio was about 1:2. Familial moyamoya disease accounts for approximately 5–15% of cases. The age of onset typically shows a bimodal distribution. A first peak is consistently reported at 5–15 years old, and a second peak occurs from 35–60 years old.

20.2 Genetics of MMD

There have been many studies to elucidate the causative genetic factors of MMD owing to regional differences in incidence rates and its similarities to hereditary disorders such as neurofibromatosis, sickle cell anemia, etc. Several genetic studies of MMD have been performed using various techniques. Chromosomes 3p24-26, 6, and 8q21-22 were suggested as potential loci related to MMD [4]. Recently, ring finger protein 213 (RNF213) located at 17q25 was suggested to be the susceptibility gene for MMD [5]. Among the Japanese population, the RNF213 mutation was identified in most patients with familial MMD and over 70% of sporadic MMD cases. Similarly, the impact of this mutation was described in a Korean study [6]. Many RNF213 studies reported two types of mutations, p. R4810K and p.4859K; however, these two mutations represented the same alteration in protein level (rs112735431).

In contrast, several variants of the RNF213 gene in different locations have been found to be potential genetic mutation in Caucasian and South Asian individuals with MMD [7]. Also, the relationship between clinical presentation (i.e., ischemic or hemorrhagic stroke) and genetic alteration has been documented. Throughout these findings, the RNF213 mutation seems to be strongly linked to MMD. However, the precise mechanism of pathogenesis is not yet fully understood, and further studies are warranted.

20.3 Pathophysiology

MMD usually affects the distal ICA to the proximal ACA and MCA. The intima of this segment shows fibrocellular thickening and accompanying waving of internal elastic laminae. These vascular changes are believed to be mainly related to intimal hyperplasia (proliferation of the smooth

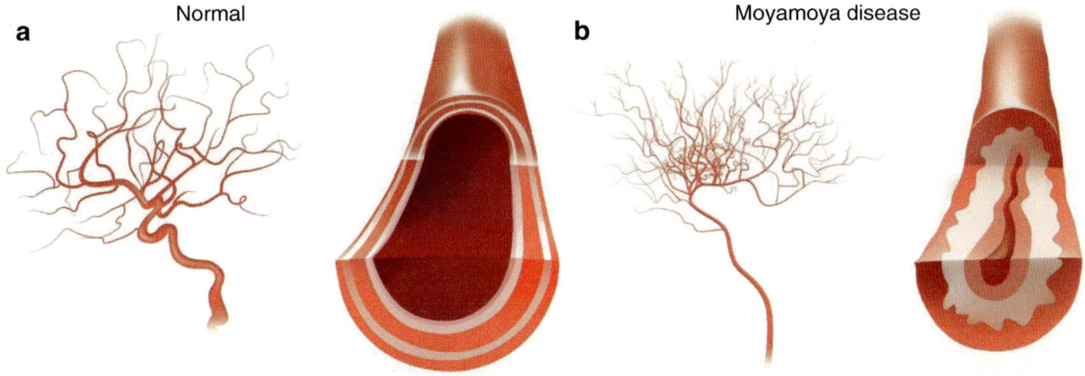

Fig. 20.1 A schematic illustration showing gross and microscopic morphology of moyamoya vessels (**b**) as compared with normal vascular anatomy (**a**)

muscle or endothelium), and the endothelial lining of vessel lumen remains intact (Fig. 20.1). Thus, ischemic stroke related to MMD is usually hemodynamic rather than embolic infarction. It is considerably different than atherosclerotic intracranial stenosis, which is accompanied by destruction of the endothelium causing primarily thromboembolic stroke. On the other hand, the outer diameter of the affected segment narrows, which can be interpreted as a sequence of constrictive remodeling. Although the main cause of these changes and anatomical predilection is not fully known, the contribution of hemodynamics, which causes constrictive remodeling, has emerged as a hypothesis from laboratory-based studies.

Prominent vascular proliferation, especially at the base of the brain (so-called moyamoya vessels), is another main pathological finding of MMD. These collateral vessels experience several histological changes as they compensate for hypoperfusion from stenosis/occlusion of the ICA bifurcation. Fibrin deposition, fragmented elastic laminae, and thinned media contribute to the fragility of these vascular networks, which sometimes leads to the formation of an aneurysm. While progressive stenosis or occlusion can cause hemodynamic impairment and subsequent ischemic stroke, fragile vascular network formation is related to hemorrhagic stroke. The basal collateral vascular networks mainly arise from lenticulostriate and choroidal arteries, including anterior and lateral posterior ones. Rupture of these collateral arteries usually causes intraventricular hemorrhaging, since these arteries run along ventricular walls.

20.4 Diagnosis

The guidelines for diagnosis were made by the Japanese Ministry of Health and Welfare [8]. The key elements of diagnosis are as follows: (1) bilateral stenosis/occlusion at the terminal ICA, (2) bilateral abnormal vascular network at the base of the brain, and (3) unknown etiology. While pediatric MMD patients rarely have other medical problems influencing intracranial stenosis, adult patients should be carefully diagnosed and considered for other steno-occlusive conditions.

The diagnosis of MMD is solely made from imaging studies. Although spatial resolution of magnetic resonance imaging (MRI) had been greatly improved and accepted as the primary diagnostic modality for selective cases, digital subtraction angiography (DSA) still remains the most reliable diagnostic tool, because steno-occlusive changes are often overestimated and basal collateral vessels are underestimated by MRI. Suzuki et al. proposed an angiographic staging system, which consisted of six stages. However, it is not clear whether this system reflects MMD progression and classifies clinical significance.

20.5 Clinical Features and Treatments

Ischemic symptoms, including transient ischemic attack (TIA) and cerebral infarction, are the most important presentations of MMD. This is due to cerebral hypoperfusion caused by stenosis or occlusion of the ICA, ACA, and MCA. Thus, infarction in the anterior circulation is more common than the posterior circulation. However, stenotic change of the posterior cerebral artery (PCA) and related hypoperfusion have also been reported to a considerable extent, up to 30%. TIA symptoms can be induced by lowering the partial pressure of carbon dioxide in the arterial blood, such as during hyperventilation and crying. Dehydration can also aggravate hemodynamic impairments. Several modalities, such as perfusion computed tomography (CT), single-photon emission computed tomography (SPECT), and positron emission tomography (PET), can be used to evaluate hemodynamic status. The acetazolamide challenge test provides additional information regarding vascular reactivity known as "vascular reserve capacity."

Cerebral revascularization surgery is usually recommended for symptomatic patients with impaired hemodynamics. Surgical revascularization involves augmentation of intracranial blood flow using the external carotid artery (ECA) system and is classified into indirect and direct revascularization. In the former surgery, the surface of the brain is covered with various connective tissues (e.g., dura matter, periosteum, muscular fascial, etc.) connected with the ECA system. The lateral side of the brain (usually near the central sulcus) can be covered using the parietal branch of the superficial temporal artery (STA) and adjacent connective tissue (encephaloduroarteriosynangiosis (EDAS)). By the same principle, the flap that includes the occipital artery (OA) can cover PCA territories. For augmenting ACA territories, periosteum on the frontal bone is used for covering. Neovascularization from covered connective tissue connected to the brain surface needs time to form gradual synangiosis from the ECA system to the ICA system.

For direct revascularization, usually the STA is used as a donor artery and is anastomosed with the cortical branch of the MCA (M3 or M4) (Fig. 20.2). In the case of PCA insufficiency, the OA to M4 or PCA branches can also be considered. In a recent report, combined bypass surgery at the MCA territory also resulted in hemodynamic improvements in the ACA territory, especially in patients with preoperative-related symptoms [9]. Various indirect methods can be combined during most of the direct revascularization procedures. Compared with indirect revascularization, blood flow is augmented immediately after anastomosis. Owing to altered autoregulation and vascular reactivity, an abrupt increase in blood flow can cause hyperperfusion syndrome, which elicits various symptoms during the early postoperative period. Increased vascular permeability derived from chronic ischemia is another possible mechanism to explain hyperperfusion syndrome. Although lowering systemic blood pressure may seem plausible, it can cause ischemic stroke, because hyperperfusion is a local phenomenon associated with global hypoperfusion. Rather, adequate use of fluids and maintaining systemic blood pressure according to preoperative levels may be appropriate to prevent further damage from both ischemic and hemorrhagic stroke. Direct or combined bypass for adult MMD patients with ischemic presentation is effective for preventing stroke reoccurrence. The calculated number needed to treat for preventing further stroke was 11 [10]. According to a recent meta-analysis study, indirect revascularization showed similar efficacy [11]. For pediatric patients, respective annual stroke rates after direct and indirect revascularization were 0.2 and 1.6%, which were considerably lower incidence rates compared to adults [12].

Involuntary movement, mainly chorea, is another presentation of patients with MMD. The interruption of basal ganglia-thalamocortical circuits by diffuse hemispheric hypoperfusion may play a role in developing chorea, although the mechanism is not yet fully elucidated. Direct revascularization is useful for prompt relief of this symptom, and indirect revascularizatio is also effective but takes several months.

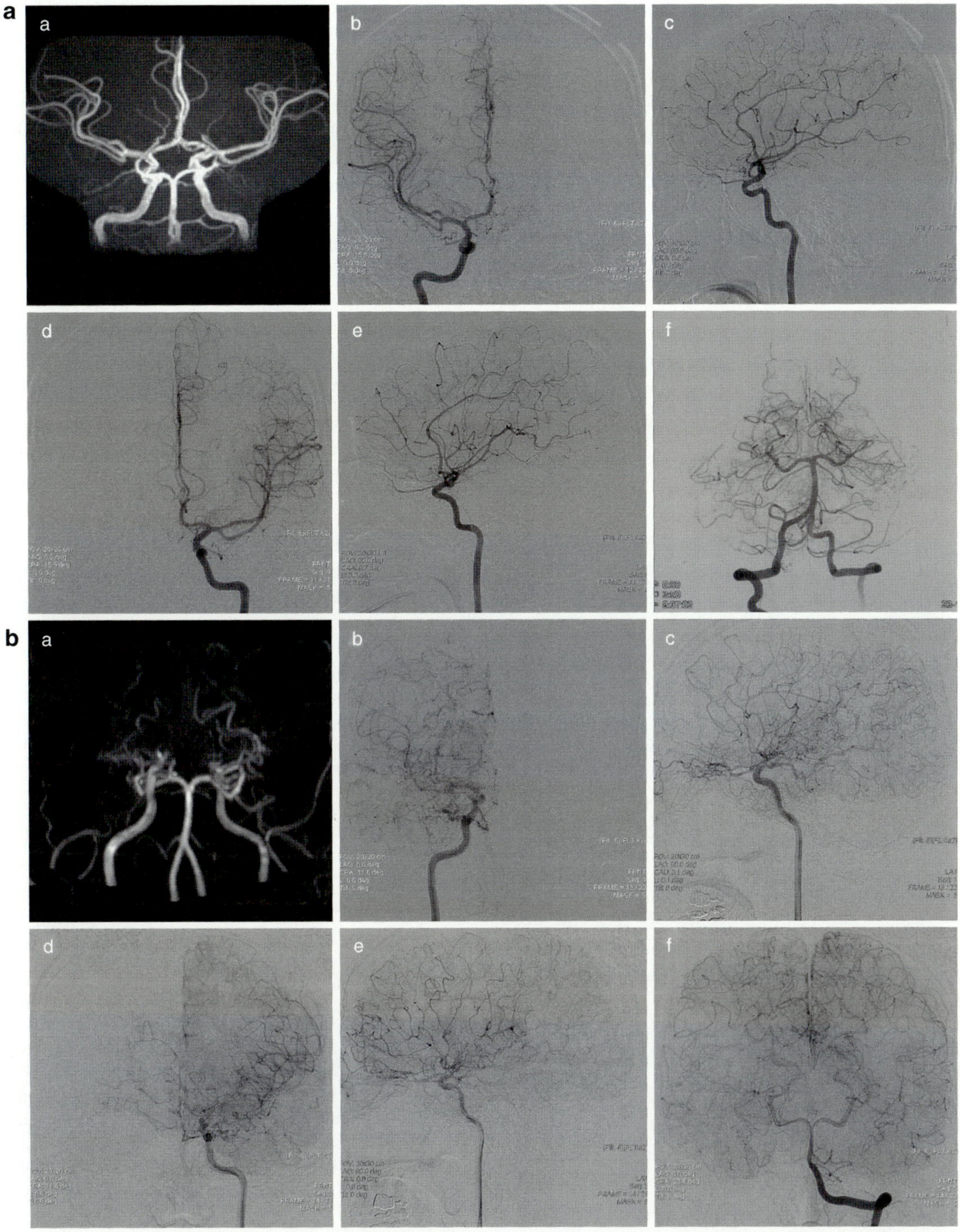

Fig. 20.2 Angiography comparison of a normal adult and a moyamoya patient. (**a**) A normal adult: findings of magnetic resonance angiography (*a*) and findings of digital subtraction angiography (*b–f*). (**b**) (*a*) A moyamoya patient with typical findings: findings of magnetic resonance angiography (*a*) and findings of digital subtraction angiography (*b–f*). Angiography shows stenosis of the bilateral terminal ICA and fine collateral networks. Leptomeningeal collaterals from posterior circulation are prominent in moyamoya patient (*f*) compared to normal adult

Additionally, some patients suffer from headaches, and hypoperfusion is thought to be a potential cause. The progressive recruitment and redistribution of blood flow is also referenced as a cause. Revascularization surgery may improve headache symptoms by flow augmentation.

Intracranial hemorrhage, including intraventricular (IVH) and intracerebral hemorrhage (ICH), is an initial manifestation in about one third of MMD patients. This type of hemorrhage is thought to be due to the fragile collateral vessels and subsequent aneurysm formation described earlier. Although controversial, previous investigations have reported the efficacy of preventing further hemorrhaging by direct or indirect revascularization surgery [13]. Additionally, a randomized controlled study showed that bilateral combined revascularization surgery could prevent further hemorrhaging [14]. Since blood flow augmentation can lower the burden of basal collateral channels, revascularization surgery may reduce the extent of fragile vascular networks. In some cases, an initial diagnostic workup with DSA shows the hemorrhage focus—a pseudoaneurysm arising from basal collateral vessels. Although collateral arteries are very small in diameter and tortuous, successful endovascular embolization for pseudoaneurysm has been reported [15]. However, sufficient evidence is still lacking for it to be considered as standard treatment.

Subarachnoid hemorrhage (SAH) can occur in MMD patients by rupture of saccular aneurysms in the circle of Willis. The most common concurrent intracranial aneurysm is a basilar artery (BA) bifurcation or superior cerebellar artery (SCA) aneurysm. The vertebrobasilar system is an important source of compensating hypoperfusion caused by bilateral stenosis or occlusion of the ICAs. According to quantitative blood flow measurements, the vertebrobasilar system contributes up to 50% of total intracranial blood flow. This excessive hemodynamic stress is a well-known risk factor for aneurysm formation. Thus, initial DSA workup has another important role for detecting aneurysms of the posterior circulation.

Suggestions from Current Clinical Practice Guidelines There has been no specific medical treatment for moyamoya disease. For patients with recurrent ischemic events, antiplatelet therapy might be considered, but their efficacy has not been tested in controlled trials. Anticoagulation is generally not accepted because of the risk of intracerebral hemorrhage. It is understood that revascularization surgery is the only therapeutic option for moyamoya disease. There has been no controlled trials on direct versus indirect revascularization technique, and the selection or combination of the techniques is basically decided on the individual basis. Indirect techniques are preferable in younger children cases. Transcranial Doppler is reasonable to monitor the cerebral hemodynamic status in asymptomatic patients with moyamoya disease.

References

1. Kim T, Lee H, Bang JS, et al. Epidemiology of moyamoya disease in Korea: based on national health insurance service data. J Korean Neurosurg Soc. 2015;57:390–5.
2. Kuriyama S, Kusaka Y, Fujimura M, et al. Prevalence and clinicoepidemiological features of moyamoya disease in Japan: findings from a nationwide epidemiological survey. Stroke. 2008;39:42–7.
3. Baba T, Houkin K, Kuroda S. Novel epidemiological features of moyamoya disease. J Neurol Neurosurg Psychiatry. 2008;79:900–4.
4. Ikeda H, Sasaki T, Yoshimoto T, et al. Mapping of a familial moyamoya disease gene to chromosome 3p24.2-p26. Am J Hum Genet. 1999;64:533–7.
5. Liu W, Morito D, Takashima S, et al. Identification of RNF213 as a susceptibility gene for moyamoya disease and its possible role in vascular development. PLoS One. 2011;6:e22542.
6. Kim EH, Yum MS, Ra YS, et al. Importance of RNF213 polymorphism on clinical features and long-term outcome in moyamoya disease. J Neurosurg. 2016;124:1221–7.
7. Cecchi AC, Guo D, Ren Z, et al. RNF213 rare variants in an ethnically diverse population with Moyamoya disease. Stroke. 2014;45:3200–7.
8. Fukui M. Guidelines for the diagnosis and treatment of spontaneous occlusion of the circle of Willis ('moyamoya' disease). Research Committee on Spontaneous Occlusion of the Circle of Willis (Moyamoya Disease) of the Ministry of Health and Welfare, Japan. Clin Neurol Neurosurg. 1997;99(Suppl 2):S238–40.

9. Cho WS, Kim JE, Paeng JC, et al. Can combined bypass surgery at middle cerebral artery territory save anterior cerebral artery territory in adult moyamoya disease? Neurosurgery. 2017;80:431–8.
10. Kim T, Oh CW, Kwon OK, et al. Stroke prevention by direct revascularization for patients with adult-onset moyamoya disease presenting with ischemia. J Neurosurg. 2016;124:1788–93.
11. Kim H, Jang DK, Han YM et al. Direct bypass versus indirect bypass in adult moyamoya angiopathy with symptoms or hemodynamic instability: A meta-analysis of comparative studies. World Neurosurg. 2016;94:273–84.
12. Kim T, Oh CW, Bang JS, et al. Moyamoya disease: treatment and outcomes. J Stroke. 2016;18:21–30.
13. Ahn JH, Wang KC, Phi JH, et al. Hemorrhagic moyamoya disease in children: clinical features and surgical outcome. Childs Nerv Syst. 2012;28:237–45.
14. Miyamoto S, Yoshimoto T, Hashimoto N, et al. Effects of extracranial-intracranial bypass for patients with hemorrhagic moyamoya disease: results of the Japan Adult Moyamoya Trial. Stroke. 2014;45:1415–21.
15. Kim SH, Kwon OK, Jung CK, et al. Endovascular treatment of ruptured aneurysms or pseudoaneurysms on the collateral vessels in patients with moyamoya disease. Neurosurgery. 2009;65:1000–4.

Central Nervous System Vasculitis

21

Adam J. Brown and Rula A. Hajj-Ali

Abstract

Central nervous system (CNS) vasculitis is an uncommon disease that results in vasculitis of the CNS or spinal cord and a rare cause of stroke. CNS vasculitis is categorized into primary angiitis of the CNS (PACNS) or secondary CNS vasculitis and represents a wide spectrum of neurological signs such as headache, seizure, mental changes, and focal neurological deficit. Although no diagnostic criteria has been validated prospectively, the diagnosis of CNA vasculitis is based on a combination of laboratory findings such as elevations in cerebrospinal fluid protein and white blood cells, imaging such as magnetic resonance imaging and cerebral angiography, and histology from a brain biopsy. A variety of mimics of CNS vasculitis need to be ruled out prior to the diagnosis being made, including reversible cerebral vasoconstriction syndrome, infectious causes and malignancy. Prompt diagnosis of CNS vasculitis and urgent treatment with glucoroticoids or immunosuppressive agents such as cyclophosphamide are critical to prevent poor outcome.

Central nervous system (CNS) vasculitis is a form of vasculitis that occurs in the CNS or spinal cord and can be broadly divided into primary angiitis of the CNS (PACNS) or secondary CNS vasculitis. PACNS is a vasculitis confined to the CNS without systemic involvement, while secondary CNS vasculitis reflects a vasculitic process that is secondary to either a systemic vasculitis or a systemic inflammatory/infectious disease.

CNS vasculitis is a rare and potentially life-threatening form of vasculitis. Patients can present with a variety of symptoms from headaches, altered mental status, to an acute and recurrent strokes. Multiple challenges face the diagnosis and recognition of this disease; these include the protean nonspecific symptoms at presentation, the rarity of the disease, and the lack of specific imaging and laboratory diagnostic findings; further, many diseases can mimic CNS

A.J. Brown, M.D.
Department of Rheumatic and Immunologic Diseases
Cleveland Clinic, 9500 Euclid Avenue, Desk A50,
Cleveland, OH 44195, USA
e-mail: BROWNA22@ccf.org

R.A. Hajj-Ali, M.D. (✉)
Department of Rheumatologic and Immunologic
Disease, Cleveland Clinic Main Campus,
9500 Euclid Avenue, Cleveland, OH 44195, USA
e-mail: hajjalr@ccf.org

S.-H. Lee (ed.), *Stroke Revisited: Diagnosis and Treatment of Ischemic Stroke*,
Stroke Revisited, DOI 10.1007/978-981-10-1424-6_21

vasculitis, and most patients suspected of the disease will be found to have a different disorder [1].

21.1 Clinical Presentation

The clinical presentation of CNS vasculitis is variable, but headache (58–63%) and altered mental status (30–71%) appear to be the most common [2]. It is not uncommon for the initial clinical presentation of CNS vasculitis to be stroke (40%) or TIA (30–50%) [2, 3]. Headaches are usually chronic and insidious in contrast to the thunderclap variety associated with aneurysmal subarachnoid hemorrhage or reversible cerebral vasoconstriction syndrome (RCVS). Other symptoms include visual field deficits, focal neurologic changes, seizures, as well as constitutional symptoms in a minority of patients. The age range of patients who present with CNS vasculitis is broad, ranging from the pediatric population to the elderly with a median of approximately 50 years [1].

The prevalence of CNS vasculitis is not well studied, but the annual incidence of PACNS is estimated to be 2.4 cases per million [2]. Vasculitis is an uncommon cause of stroke although CNS vasculitis presents as a stroke in 40% of the cases [3]. Kempster et al. retrospectively explored the prevalence of primary and secondary cerebral angiitis among patients, all ages, presenting with stroke to a single center over a 10-year period [4]. Among the 7475 strokes, 13 initially were worked up for vasculitis because of suspicions found on MRI, including multiple infarcts, or arterial narrowing on vascular imaging. Two of these patients were eventually diagnosed with RCVS, four with non-vasculitis stroke, one with acute disseminated encephalomyelitis; six patients had the final diagnosis of vasculitic ischemic stroke, four had systemic symptoms, only one had PACNS. The incidence of vasculitic stroke was 0.13% of all stroke presentations (these included patients with systemic vasculitis) and 0.02% was PACNS. Importantly, this study included all patients evaluated for stroke regardless of age; if the age range is narrowed to a younger patient population, the percentage of CNS vasculitis causes of stroke would increase.

21.2 Primary Angiitis of the CNS

The initial description of primary angiitis of the CNS described a homogeneous clinicopathologic finding of granulomatous angiitis on brain tissue; thus the term granulomatous angiitis of the CNS (GACNS) emerged to describe the original reports. Thereafter, distinct disease subsets have been identified. Currently, no prospective study has been performed to stratify any disease subsets in regard to different outcomes or optimal treatments regimens. In this section we review different subset of PACNS.

21.2.1 GACNS

GACNS accounted for 59% of cases in a larger series of PACNS [3]. MRI findings are consistently abnormal in these patients and show multiple ischemic foci in both hemispheres with an inflammatory pattern seen on cerebrospinal fluid (CSF). The histologic findings are characteristic of granulomatous inflammation affecting small vessels of brain tissue. Cerebral angiography is often normal in GACNS likely because of the small vessel sizes that are involved [5].

21.2.2 Lymphocytic PACNS

Lymphocytic PACNS has similar radiographic and clinical findings of GACNS, but histology distinguishes the two subtypes by findings of lymphocytic infiltrate on brain tissue [5]. It is very important to emphasize that findings of lymphocytic vasculitis on pathology should prompt the treating physician for a thorough evaluation of the brain tissue to rule out any of the CNS vasculitis mimics especially angiocentric lymphoproliferative diseases.

21.2.3 Angiographically Defined PACNS

This subtype is characterized by medium to large intracranial vessel involvement which results in angiographic abnormalities. Issuing a diagnosis of CNS vasculitis based on cerebral vascular imaging can be very problematic and should only be certain after a vigilant workup has been completed to rule out radiologic mimics [5]. In such instances, the diagnostic confidence is enhanced by finding a CSF inflammatory pattern; nonetheless, revisiting the diagnosis of PACNS is essential if an unfavorable outcome ensues after initiation of treatment. Brain biopsies are usually normal in this entity likely secondary to the sampling challenge of the affected medium/large cerebral vessels.

21.2.4 Mass Lesion Presentation of PACNS

PACNS is estimated to present as a mass lesion in approximately 5%–15% of cases, making it a very rare presentation [3, 6]. The symptoms are similar to what is described in other subsets of PACNS with headache being the most common feature, but patients with a mass lesion tend to present earlier (within 1 month) compared to 6 months or more as in other forms of PACNS. In a study of 38 patients with PACNS presenting as a mass lesion, CSF was abnormal in 14 out of the 21 (66%) patients who had CSF sampled. Cerebral angiography was abnormal in 8 out of 14 patients (57%) with finding of mass effect in the majority. The diagnosis of mass lesion presentation of CNS vasculitis should only be made by histologic finding after ruling out malignancy and infectious causes; granulomatous angiitis on pathology occurs in 53% while lymphocytic vasculitis in 47%, with positive staining for amyloid present in 34% [6].

21.2.5 Amyloid-β-Related Cerebral Angiitis

Cerebral amyloid angiopathy (CAA) is characterized by deposition of amyloid-β in the leptomeningeal vessels, usually within the media and adventitia. Cerebral amyloid deposition in the brain is a broad category of diseases most commonly associated with dementia in the elderly. A spectrum of neurologic diseases associated with CAA ranges from noninflammatory to inflammatory brain diseases with or without vasculitis. Aβ-related angiitis (ABRA) is a subset of CAA with an associated vascular inflammatory infiltrate in response to the amyloid deposition. The vasculitis is usually transmural and is occasionally granulomatous [7]. In a systematic review of inflammatory CAA, neuropathologic findings indicated an ABRA pattern in 35.2% (vasculitic inflammation with or without granuloma) of the cases with an overlap pattern of inflammation and vasculitis in 50% [8].

The amyloid in ABRA is composed of the same amino acid peptides seen in neuritic plaques in Alzheimer's disease. These amyloid depositions can lead to vessel wall fragility leading to intracerebral hemorrhage. Many of these patients are diagnosed after presenting with intracerebral hemorrhage [7]. Patients with ABRA had a lower median age at diagnosis, fewer incidences of stroke and altered cognition, and a lower rate of intercerebral hemorrhage compared to patients with just CAA. Abnormal CSF was noted in the vast majority of patients with ABRA with protein being most likely to be elevated in 96% of patients. Of note, leptomeningeal enhancement on MRI was more common in patients with ABRA, and response to immunosuppressants is more favorable in ABRA compared to CAA [7].

Table 21.1 Secondary CNS vasculitis

Systemic vasculitis	Henoch-Schönlein purpura, Kawasaki disease, granulomatosis with polyangiitis, microscopic polyangiitis, eosinophilic granulomatosis with polyangiitis, polyarteritis nodosa, Behçet's disease
Systemic rheumatologic disease	Systemic lupus erythematosus (usually a vasculopathy), dermatomyositis, scleroderma, rheumatoid arthritis, Cogan's, inflammatory bowel disease, sarcoidosis

21.3 Secondary Forms of CNS Vasculitis

More common than PACNS is a systemic disease that can result with secondary CNS involvement which is referred to as CNS vasculitis. Table 21.1 lists systemic rheumatologic diseases that have known to be associated with CNS vasculitis. Neurologic involvement in systemic disease is usually a late manifestation of the disease and rarely present at onset.

21.4 Evaluation of Patients Suspected with CNS Vasculitis

The clinical presentation of CNS vasculitis is protean which often causes a delay in diagnosis. In our practice CNS vasculitis is primarily suspected after an unexplained neurologic deficit, stroke, or multi-strokes in younger-aged patients with no cardiovascular risk factors and when an abnormal cerebrovascular study emerges while working up a patient with neurologic abnormalities. In most instances, an alternative diagnosis is made giving the rarity of the CNS vasculitis.

Diagnostic criteria for PACNS were proposed in 1988 by Calabrese and Mallek (Table 21.2) [9]. Although not validated prospectively, these criteria remain the mainstay of the workup of patients with PACNS. These criteria emphasize the importance or ruling many mimics of the disease before making the diagnosis of PACNS.

Table 21.2 Diagnostic criteria for primary angiitis of the central nervous system

The presence of an acquired and otherwise unexplained neurologic deficit
• With presence of either classic angiographic or histopathologic features of angiitis within the CNS
• And no evidence of systemic vasculitis or any condition that could elicit the angiographic or pathologic features

21.4.1 Laboratory Testing

Laboratory testing in PACNS are normal giving the isolated nature of the disease. Inflammatory markers such as sedimentation rate and C-reactive protein are normal in PACNS. Abnormalities in inflammatory markers should prompt an evaluation for a systemic involvement whether inflammatory or infectious. Autoimmune serologies, such as antinuclear antibodies (ANA), rheumatoid factor (RF), and antineutrophilic cytoplasmic antibodies (ANCA), are also negative in PACNS. These serologic tests are often requested during the evaluation of CNS vasculitis, but should be indicated in the right clinical setting to assist in ruling in or refuting a systemic inflammatory disease diagnosis. Evaluation for an infectious process by blood cultures and/or serology and PCR, for suspected bacterial endocarditis or other infectious diseases. In patients who have unexplained multiple strokes, coagulation studies and antiphospholipid testing are essential for evaluation. Other laboratory testing should be tailored according to the individual exposures and risk factors of the patient.

21.4.2 Cerebrospinal Fluid Studies

Cerebrospinal fluid findings are abnormal in 81–90% of cases of CNS vasculitis; in a cohort of 101 patients, 88% of the CSF tests showed at least one abnormality, with the majority of cases being a mildly increased protein, white blood cells (WBC), or both [2, 3, 10]. In the combined series published by Calabrese et al., the average CSF white blood cell count was 60 cells/high-power field (hpf), with the highest reported value of 330 cells/hpf. The average protein level was 118 mg/dL, with a maximum value seen of 825 mg/dL [9]. Other series have reported lower values with medium CSF white blood cell count of 5 cells/μL (range of 0–535 cells/μL) and a median total protein of 0.7 g/dL (range of 0.15–1.03 g/dL) [2]. This discrepancy of CSF findings among the cohorts could be related to the contamination of some cohorts with cases of RCVS, thus making the amount of pleocytosis seen in CNS vasculitis CSF samples artificially lower. CSF is a vital component of the workup for CNS vasculitis, but it is important to note that abnormalities seen in the CSF are not specific for CNS vasculitis, and it's critical that other causes of CSF pleocytosis such as infection be ruled out.

21.4.3 Magnetic Resonance Imaging

Magnetic resonance imaging (MRI) is a very sensitive modality in the diagnosis of CNS vasculitis. In the Mayo cohort of patients, 97% of patients with CNS vasculitis had MRI abnormalities with ischemic infarcts being the most common (53%). The majority of MRI abnormalities follow a supratentorial distribution. Infratentorial lesions in the absence of supratentorial lesions are extremely rare. Radiographic lesions are distributed evenly in subcortical white matter, cortical gray matter, deep white matter, and cerebellum (Fig. 21.1a). One third of the cases can have gadolinium enhancement (Fig. 21.1b). CNS vasculitis can also present with a mass lesions found on MRI mimicking a neoplasm in upwards of 5–15% [2, 3]. MRI has the highest sensitivity compared to any other imaging modality and should be the neuroimaging of choice in the first step in evaluating a patient with CNS vasculitis. Importantly these lesions are not specific for the diagnosis of CNS vasculitis and can be seen in other neurologic disease such as demyelinating or ischemic disorders.

21.4.4 Cerebral Vascular Studies

Cerebral angiography is part of the diagnostic criteria proposed by Calabrese and Mallek (Table 21.2). The classic finding of CNS vasculitis is either vascular narrowing or focal dilations, which can alternate causing the appearance of a "string of beads" that are typically bilateral. The middle cerebral artery is affected the most, with an average of 2.3 lesions per patient compared to the anterior cerebral artery of 0.2 lesions per patient and the posterior cerebral artery of 0.7 lesions per patient [10] (Fig. 21.1c). It is important to understand that angiography provides information on the contour and the lumen of the vessels without providing the underlying cause of the abnormality thus limiting its specificity to as low as 30% for the diagnosis of CNS vasculitis [11]. Multiple noninflammatory etiologies can cause the classic findings of CNS vasculitis such as infection, vasospasm, atherosclerosis, fibro muscular dysplasia, malignancies, or neurofibromatosis.

Cerebral angiography is the most invasive of imaging studies, but up to this point provides the most sensitive spatial and temporal resolution of the vessel anatomy. Angiography can be falsely negative, as the imaging modality resolution is limited to vessels larger than 0.2 mm; thus small-vessel vasculitis can be missed. In various cohorts of CNS vasculitis, the sensitivity of angiography ranges between 50 and 90% [2, 3]. Other vascular modalities such as magnetic resonance angiography (MRA) and computed angiography (CTA) have much lower spatial resolution compared to cerebral angiography and are more useful in large- and medium-sized vessels (Fig. 21.1d). Other vascular modalities such as high-resolution MRI (HR-MRI) have emerged in the field of CNS vasculitis. HR-MRI focuses on the vessel wall and provides more information than lumenography and can be helpful in differentiating patients with CNS vasculitis and RCVS.

21.4.5 Brain Biopsy

Although biopsy is not mandated for the diagnosis of CNS vasculitis, it is extremely important to consider this diagnostic modality in each case as it is the only definitive way of making the diagnosis. Brain biopsy not only ensures the diagnosis of CNS vasculitis but it can reveal an

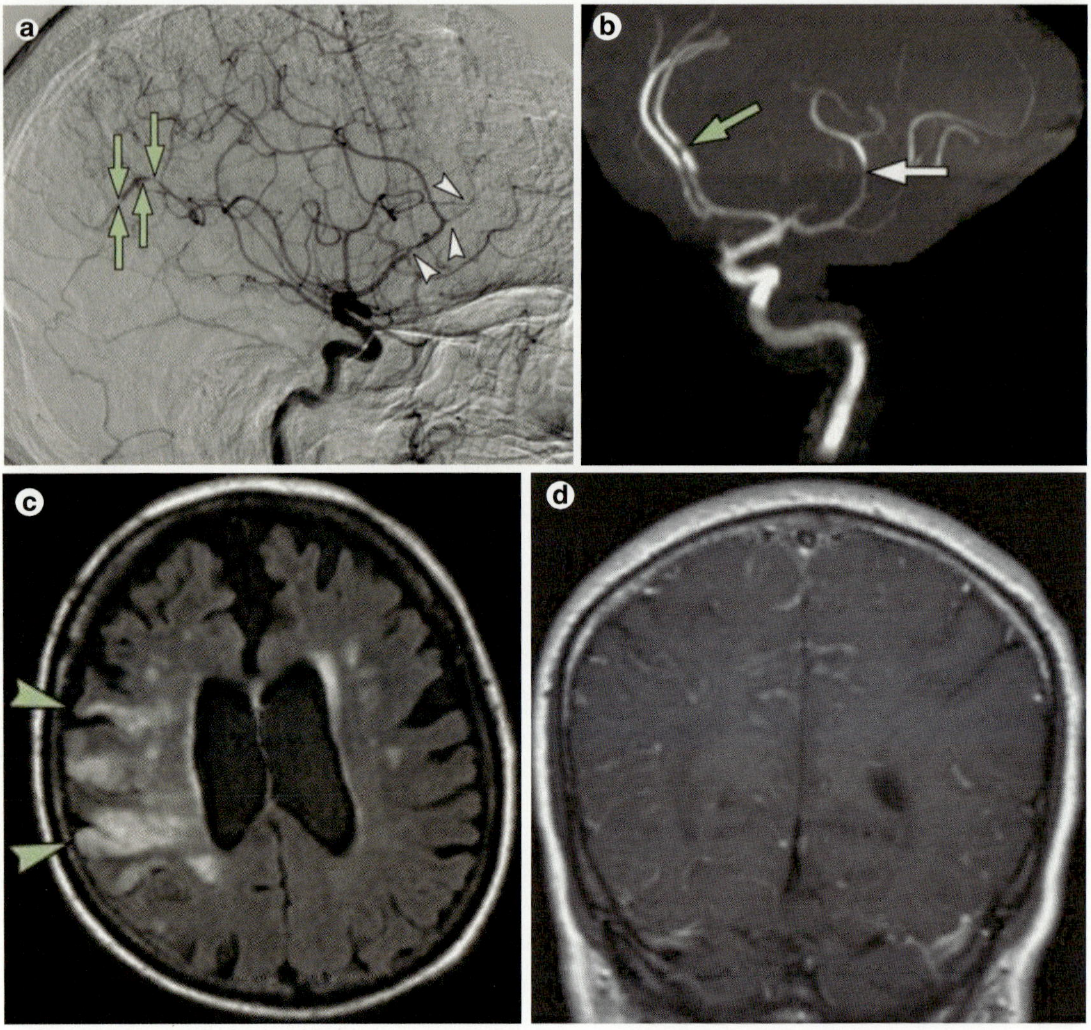

Fig. 21.1 Imaging of patients with primary CNS vasculitis. (**a**) Cerebral angiogram shows alternating stenosis and dilatation of the distal middle cerebral artery (*arrows*) and the anterior cerebral artery (*arrowheads*). (**b**) Magnetic resonance angiography of the brain shows a short segment stenosis of the anterior cerebral artery (*green arrow*) and stenosis of the distal middle cerebral artery (*white arrow*). (**c**) Fluid-attenuated inversion recovery (FLAIR)-weighted MRI shows a large abnormality within the right cerebral hemisphere consistent with ischemia (*arrowheads*). (**d**) MRI shows diff use, asymmetric, nodular, and linear leptomeningeal enhancement, with dura only slightly affected. Reproduced by permission of Lancet (Salvarani et al. Lancet 2012;380:767–777)

alternative diagnosis. A meta-analysis reported in 2015 revealed a diagnostic yield of brain biopsy of 74.7% for suspected PACNS [12]. In this report a brain biopsy for suspected PACNS had the highest yield compared to other indications. Furthermore, alternative diagnosis can be found in 30% to 39% of the biopsies [13]; these include cerebral amyloid angiopathy, viral meningoencephalitis, CNS lymphoma, demyelination, and other miscellaneous diagnoses such as posterior reversible encephalopathy syndrome, progressive multifocal leukoencephalopathy, and Alzheimer's disease. These studies highlight the importance of histologic confirmation of the diagnosis which can reveal an alternative diagnosis in many cases. False negatives are possible and have been reported as high as 47% likely secondary to the skipped lesion nature of the vasculitic process and inaccessible locations for biopsy [11]. It is not clear if there is a difference in diagnostic yield between the different surgical techniques obtaining the biopsy. In the retrospective study of 29 biopsy samples, there was no difference in biopsy yield between open and closed technique [13].

Three histologic patterns are generally recognized in CNS vasculitis: granulomatous, lymphocytic, and necrotizing. Granulomatous angiitis is characterized by destructive mononuclear inflammation with well-formed granulomas and multinucleated giant cells. Granulomatous angiitis usually affects the small and medium leptomeningeal and cortical arteries [14]. The inflamed vessels cause ischemia and stroke once they become narrowed, occluded, and thrombosed preventing flow to their vascular territory [14] (Fig. 21.2a). Lymphocytic inflammation has similar findings to granulomatous, except a lymphocytic predominant infiltrate instead of a mononuclear infiltrate, and without associated granulomas (Fig. 21.2b). Lymphocytic infiltrate can also be seen in malignancy and infections. In these circumstances a more diligent workup should be performed on the pathologic tissue to rule out an infectious or malignant process. Necrotizing vasculitis is characterized by necrotizing vasculitis with transmural fibrinoid necrosis. Necrotizing vasculitis usually involves small muscular arteries with disruption of the internal elastic lamina (Fig. 21.2c).

21.4.6 Other Evaluations

Echocardiogram is a useful test and commonly performed in patients with suspected CNS vasculitis to rule out a structural abnormality, atrial myxoma, or endocarditis as an etiology of stroke. Prolonged EKG monitoring with a holter monitor may be needed to rule out an arrhythmic source of emboli.

21.5 Mimics of Central Nervous System Vasculitis

21.5.1 RCVS

The most common mimicker of CNS vasculitis is RCVS. RCVS is a reversible vasospastic process that occurs in the cerebral vessels causing acute debilitating headaches and occasional strokes or hemorrhages. RCVS is often considered in patients being evaluated for CNS vasculitis because of the similarities seen on MRI and cerebral angiography between the two disorders. Importantly RCVS is not an inflammatory condition and will not respond to immunosuppressant medications.

The classic presentation RCVS is a sudden "thunderclap headache" which is seen at presentation in 78–100% of the cases and can be accompanied by focal deficits [15]. There is an association of RVCS with conditions such as pregnancy, migraines, as well as drugs and medications such as sumatriptan, pseudoephedrine, selective serotonin reuptake inhibitors, and marijuana, among others [15]. In the cohort of 139 patients, recent exposure to vasoconstrictive drug was seen in 42% of patients and recent pregnancy in 9% [16].

The hallmark of RCVS is demonstration of vasoconstriction and subsequent resolution of constriction by means of imaging the cerebral blood vessels. The characteristic appearance of cerebral angiographic studies in RCVS is the diffuse "string of beads" indicating segmental narrowing and dilatation, which is also the classic appearance for CNS vasculitis. The vascular distribution is usually bilateral and diffuse and includes anterior and posterior circulation [15] (Fig. 21.3a). The vascular abnormalities seen on angiography are not specific for RCVS but reversibility of the findings are. In a study of 139 patients with RCVS, vascular abnormalities completely reversed in 74% of patients and partially reversed in 24% of patients within 4–12 weeks upon follow-up imaging [16] (Fig. 21.3b).

Stroke is a major complication of RCVS. In the cohort of 139 patients with RCVS, isolated ischemic infarcts were the most common lesion observed in 27% of cases, isolated convexity subarachnoid hemorrhage in 16%, and isolated intracerebral hemorrhage in 6% [16]. In another cohort of 162 patients with RCVS, approximately 33–50% of patients developed intracerebral hemorrhage, subarachnoid hemorrhage, ischemic stroke, and posterior reversible leukoencephalopathy [17] (Fig. 21.3c–e).

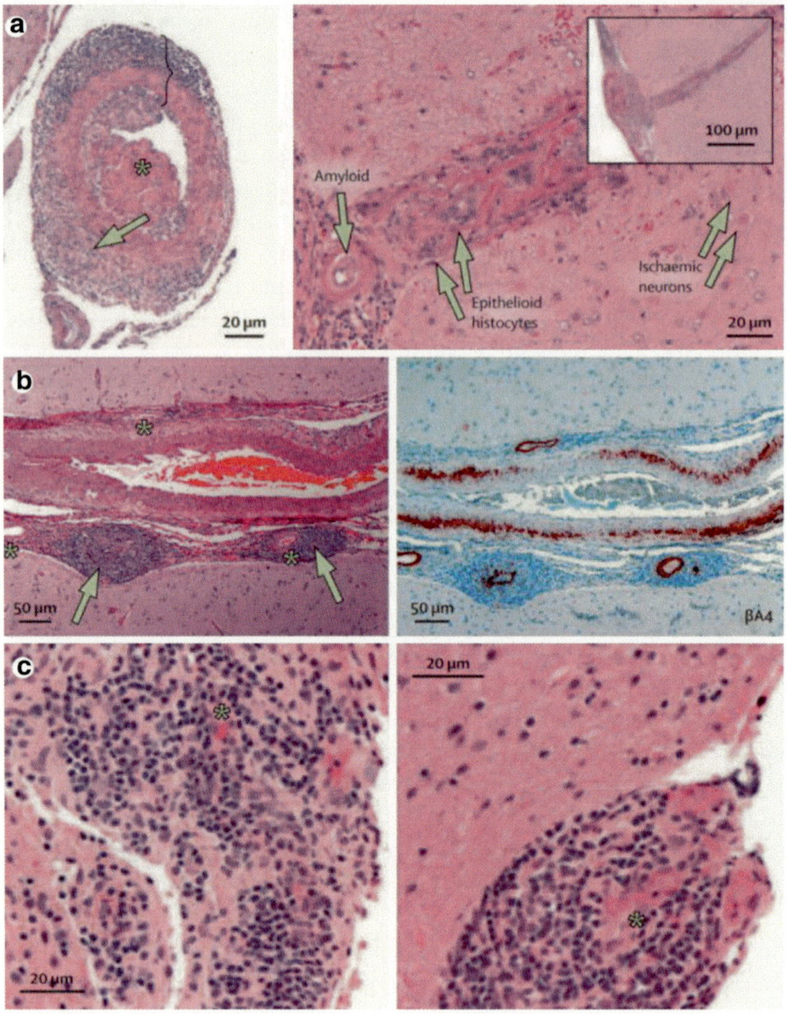

Fig. 21.2 Histopathological features of primary CNS vasculitis. (**a**) Granulomatous pattern of primary CNS vasculitis. Left-hand image shows transmural inflammation of a leptomeningeal artery with prominent mononuclear (*bracket*) and granulomatous (*arrow*) adventitial inflammation and focal fibrin thrombus formation (*asterisk*; hematoxylin and eosin [H&E] stain). Inset picture on right shows noticeable thickening and luminal obliteration of several leptomeningeal vessels (H&E stain). The right-hand image shows focal collections of epithelioid histiocytes arranged in granuloma-like aggregates. Where the lumen is preserved, the vessel wall is thickened by an amorphous eosinophilic material (amyloid). Ischemic neurons can be seen in the adjacent parenchyma (H&E stain). (**b**) Granulomatous pattern with amyloid angiopathy in primary CNS vasculitis. Left-hand image shows destructive vasculitis with well-formed granulomas in leptomeningeal vessels (*arrows*) and wall thickening with eosinophilic material (*asterisk*; H&E stain). The right-hand image shows amyloid-β deposits in all vessels (immunoperoxidase stain for βA4 amyloid). (C) Lymphocytic pattern of primary CNS vasculitis. Left-hand and right-hand images show substantial thickening and luminal obliteration (asterisks mark lumen remnant) of several leptomeningeal vessels. The infiltrate is predominated by lymphocytes, but has few histiocytes and granulocytes. Granuloma-like features are not seen (H&E stain). (**d**) Necrotizing pattern of primary CNS vasculitis. Left-hand image shows a small leptomeningeal artery with transmural acute inflammation (H&E stain). Right-hand image shows segmental transmural fibrinoid necrosis (*asterisk*), which displays as red-staining material in the vessel wall (Masson's trichrome). Hemorrhage and acute infarction are evident in the underlying cortical parenchyma (right-hand image, *bottom*). Reproduced by permission of Lancet (Salvarani et al. Lancet 2012;380: 767–777)

Fig. 21.2 (continued)

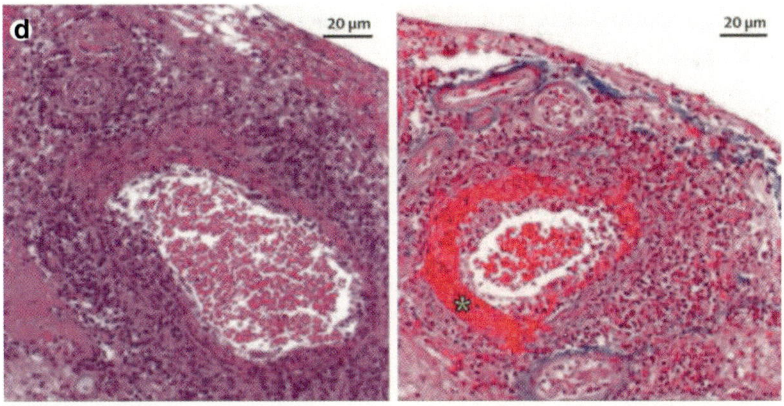

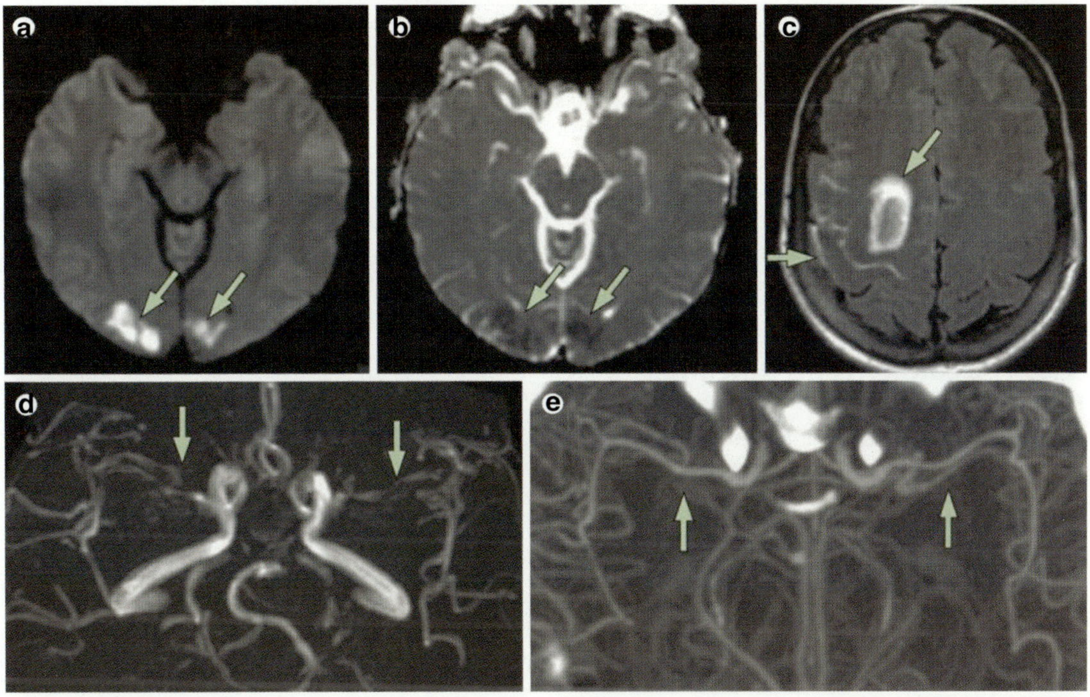

Fig. 21.3 Reversible cerebral vasoconstriction syndrome. A 47-year-old woman developed an abrupt onset, "worst-ever" headache during a bowel movement. The headache resolved over hours but recurred the next day and was associated with right-sided visual blurring. Her medical history included common migraine headaches and depression, for which she took fluoxetine. Examination findings were notable for normal blood pressure and right superior quadrantanopia. Blood tests showed a normal erythrocyte sedimentation rate, negative toxicological screen, negative rheumatological panel tests, normal antiphospholipid antibody concentrations, and no evidence of infections such as herpes-zoster virus or HIV. A brain MRI was done 3 days after symptom onset. Diffusion-weighted imaging (**a**) and corresponding apparent diffusion-coefficient maps (**b**) showed bilateral infarctions in the middle and posterior cerebral artery watershed territories. Fluid-attenuated inversion recovery images (**c**) showed a right parietal lobar hemorrhage and convexity subarachnoid hemorrhage overlying the right cerebral hemisphere. Magnetic resonance angiography (**d**) showed severe constriction of the bilateral middle and posterior cerebral arteries and their branches. Diagnostic considerations at this stage included primary angiitis of the CNS (PACNS) and reversible cerebral vasoconstriction syndrome (RCVS). The abrupt onset of severe headaches, and the presence of bilateral watershed infarcts and lobar and cortical subarachnoid hemorrhage, suggested RCVS as the likely diagnosis. Hence, brain biopsy and empirical immunosuppressive treatment were withheld. A follow-up head CT angiogram (**e**) done 9 days after symptom onset showed significant improvement in the caliber of the intracerebral arteries, indicating the dynamic nature of the vasoconstriction and confirming the diagnosis of RCVS. The patient remained asymptomatic over a 6-month follow-up period. Reproduced by permission of Lancet Neurology [5]

A distinctive feature of RVCS compared to CNS vasculitis is a benign CSF (unless associated with subarachnoid bleed) as well as the dramatic presentation of intense headache seen in RCVS compared to the inflammatory pattern of the CSF and the indolent headache in CNS vasculitis. This is an important distinction as RCVS will not require a biopsy to diagnose and does not respond to immunosuppressive medications.

21.5.2 Other Mimics

Multiple diseases can mimic the appearance of CNS vasculitis on imaging as well as laboratory markers like CSF pleocytosis. The majority of these entities are considered "noninflammatory," but multiple infections can cause an inflammatory vasculitis that is not autoimmune in etiology and must be ruled out in the workup of suspected CNS vasculitis. See Table 21.3.

Table 21.3 Mimics of primary angiitis of the CNS

Neoplasms	Intravascular lymphoma
	Gliomatosis cerebri
Infectious	Varicella-zoster virus, HIV, Epstein-Barr virus, cytomegalovirus, hepatitis C virus, parvovirus B19, enterovirus
	Syphilis
	Progressive multifocal leukoencephalopathy (JC virus)
	Tuberculosis
	Neuroborreliosis
	Aspergillosis, nocardiosis, cryptococcus, histoplasmosis
Noninflammatory vascular disease	Fibromuscular dysplasia
	Moyamoya disease
	Radiation vasculopathy
	Premature intracranial atherosclerosis
	RCVS
	Intracranial dissection
Genetic conditions	Retinal vasculopathy with cerebral leukoencephalopathy
	Kohlmeier-Degos disease
Endotheliopathy	Susac syndrome
Demyelinating diseases	Multiple sclerosis
	Acute disseminated encephalomyelitis
Multifocal cerebral Thromboembolism	Cholesterol atheroembolism
	Subacute bacterial endocarditis
	Left atrial myxoma
	Antiphospholipid antibody syndrome (Sneddon's syndrome)
Autoantibody-mediated inflammatory brain disease	Anti-NMDA receptor encephalitis
	Neuromyelitis optica
Hereditary stroke disorders	CADASIL

21.6 Treatment and Outcomes

Considering the rarity of CNS vasculitis, no prospective randomized controlled trials exist to evaluate different treatment modalities. The available treatment data has been gathered from retrospective patient cohorts and case reports. In one of the largest retrospective patient cohorts, including 163 patients with PACNS, 43% of the patients received only glucocorticoids with good outcome in 85% of these patients. The remainder of the patients received a combination of glucocorticoids and cyclophosphamide with good outcome in 81% of these patients as measured by the Rankin scale [3, 18]. In the French cohort of 52 patients with CNS vasculitis, 85% received a combination of cyclophosphamide and glucocorticoids, with a mortality rate of 6% [19].

In terms of glucocorticoid dosing, the dosing regimens have been adapted from treatment of small-vessel systemic vasculitis and usually comprise an induction and remission phase followed by a maintenance of remission phase. The induction phase often includes pulse dose methylprednisone 1 g for 1–3 days followed by prednisone 1 mg/kg/day with a taper of 10% every 2 weeks. In addition other immunosuppressive agents are used in the induction phase such as cyclophosphamide or mycophenolate mofetil. The choice among both agents depends on the severity of the disease and the certainty of the diagnosis. Cyclophosphamide can be administered either oral/continuous of 2 mg/kg/day or as intermittent intravenous pulses of 15 mg/kg/day every 4 weeks with dose adjustments for renal function. Induction agents are used from 3 to 6 months depending on the patient's response, with more severe disease often being treated for 6 months, although there is no clear consensus of what constitutes severe disease. Once the patient achieves remission, a less toxic second-line medication is used such as azathioprine or mycophenolate mofetil. The duration of maintenance therapy is unknown, and long-term immunosuppression is favored by the authors.

Other treatment considerations that have been attempted with CNS vasculitis include anti-TNF therapy and rituximab, but the data on these treatment modalities are extremely limited to case reports and should not be generalized at this point.

Prior to effective treatment regimens, PACNS was considered a disease with a high mortality rate. However, with more effective therapy, we have witnessed better outcome in these patients. In a study assessing the long-term outcome of patients with PACNS with a median follow-up of 5.5 years, 27 patients were surveyed by patient-centered questionnaires. Using the Barthel Index, 19 of 27 patients (70.4%) scored 85 or more, indicating mild disability. Meanwhile, five (18.5%) patients scored 25 or less, indicating severe disability. Using the European quality of life questionnaire (EuroQOL), 14 of 27 patients (51.9%) had no problems with mobility, 18 (66.7%) had no problems with self-care, and15 (55.6%) had no problems with usual activities. Approximately 70% of patients had minimal or no depression using both the physician health questionnaire for depression and EuroQOL. This study indicated that most patients had mild long-term disability and minimal to no depression, which may be reflective of the advances of treatment.

Conclusion

A diagnosis of PACNS and secondary CNS vasculitis is still challenging in many different aspects due to its protean clinical presentation, lack of definitive surrogate markers, and non-specific imaging findings. A diagnosis of PACNS requires a very thorough evaluation to exclude infection, malignancy, systemic autoimmune disease, systemic vasculitis, non-inflammatory vasculopathy, and other CNS inflammatory diseases. This evaluation cannot be accomplished without CSF studies. Vascular imaging studies are important tools to prove vasculopathy but are not specific for vasculitis. A brain biopsy remains a golden standard for the diagnosis and is sometimes useful to establish an alternative diagnosis.

Suggestions from Current Clinical Practice Guidelines There are no recommended guidelines on these issues.

References

1. Birnbaum J, Hellmann DB. Primary angiitis of the central nervous system. Arch Neurol. 2009;66:704–9.
2. Salvarani C, Brown RD Jr, Calamia KT, et al. Primary central nervous system vasculitis: analysis of 101 patients. Ann Neurol. 2007;62:442–51.
3. Salvarani C, Brown RD Jr, Christianson T, et al. An update of the Mayo Clinic cohort of patients with adult primary central nervous system vasculitis: description of 163 patients. Medicine. 2015;94:e738.
4. Kempster PA, McLean CA, Phan TG. Ten year clinical experience with stroke and cerebral vasculitis. J Clin Neurosci. 2016;27:119–25.
5. Hajj-Ali RA, Singhal AB, Benseler S, et al. Primary angiitis of the CNS. Lancet Neurol. 2011;10:561–72.
6. Molloy ES, Singhal AB, Calabrese LH. Tumour-like mass lesion: an under-recognised presentation of primary angiitis of the central nervous system. Ann Rheum Dis. 2008;67:1732–5.
7. Salvarani C, Hunder GG, Morris JM, et al. Abeta-related angiitis: comparison with CAA without inflammation and primary CNS vasculitis. Neurology. 2013;81:1596–603.
8. Castro Caldas A, Silva C, Albuquerque L, et al. Cerebral amyloid angiopathy associated with inflammation: report of 3 cases and systematic review. J Stroke Cerebrovasc Dis. 2015;24:2039–48.
9. Calabrese LH, Mallek JA. Primary angiitis of the central nervous system. Report of 8 new cases, review of the literature, and proposal for diagnostic criteria. Medicine. 1988;67:20–39.
10. Pomper MG, Miller TJ, Stone JH, et al. CNS vasculitis in autoimmune disease: MR imaging findings and correlation with angiography. AJNR Am J Neuroradiol. 1999;20:75–85.
11. Duna GF, Calabrese LH. Limitations of invasive modalities in the diagnosis of primary angiitis of the central nervous system. J Rheumatol. 1995;22:662–7.
12. Bai HX, Zou Y, Lee AM, et al. Diagnostic value and safety of brain biopsy in patients with cryptogenic

neurological disease: a systematic review and meta-analysis of 831 cases. Neurosurgery. 2015;77:283–95.
13. Torres J, Loomis C, Cucchiara B, et al. Diagnostic yield and safety of brain biopsy for suspected primary central nervous system angiitis. Stroke. 2016;47:2127–9.
14. Hajj-Ali RA, Calabrese LH, et al. Central nervous system vasculitis. Curr Opin Rheumatol. 2009;21:10–8.
15. Mehdi A, Hajj-Ali RA. Reversible cerebral vasoconstriction syndrome: a comprehensive update. Curr Pain Headache Rep. 2014;18:443.
16. Singhal AB, Hajj-Ali RA, Topcuoglu MA, et al. Reversible cerebral vasoconstriction syndromes: analysis of 139 cases. Arch Neurol. 2011;68:1005–12.
17. Topcuoglu MA, Singhal AB. Hemorrhagic reversible cerebral vasoconstriction syndrome: features and mechanisms. Stroke. 2016;47:1742–7.
18. Pagnoux C, Hajj-Ali RA. Pharmacological approaches to CNS vasculitis: where are we at now? Expert Rev Clin Pharmacol. 2016;9:109–16.
19. de Boysson H, Zuber M, Naggara O, et al. Primary angiitis of the central nervous system: description of the first fifty-two adults enrolled in the French cohort of patients with primary vasculitis of the central nervous system. Arthritis Rheumatol. 2014;66:1315–26.

Genetic Causes of Ischemic Stroke

22

Jay Chol Choi

Abstract

Monogenic disorders in which ischemic stroke is the main clinical feature are rare, but the number of reported cases is increasing as the clinical features become widely known and diagnostic examinations are more readily available. The exact diagnosis of such monogenic disorders causing ischemic stroke is important for patients and clinicians because clinical courses are different from those of sporadic ischemic stroke, timely treatment can be useful in certain disorder, and genetic counselling is crucial in reproductive planning and education. In this chapter, clinical features, neuroradiological findings, and stroke mechanisms of monogenic disorders causing ischemic stroke are reviewed. The disorders reviewed here are cerebral autosomal dominant arteriopathy with subcortical infarcts and leukoencephalopathy (CADASIL), cerebral autosomal recessive arteriopathy with subcortical infarcts and leukoencephalopathy (CARASIL), autosomal dominant retinal vasculopathy with cerebral leukodystrophy (RVCL), Fabry disease, sick cell disease, homocystinuria, and other inherited connective tissue disorders causing ischemic stroke. This chapter will help clinicians readily identify monogenic disorders causing ischemic stroke by their characteristic clinical features and stroke mechanisms.

Monogenic disorders account for up to 7% of all ischemic stroke according to a recent report. The exact diagnosis of monogenic disorders causing ischemic stroke is important because clinical courses are different from those of sporadic ischemic stroke, timely treatment can be useful in certain disorder, and genetic counselling is crucial in reproductive planning and education [1, 2, 3]. In young stroke patients, certain clinical features, neuroradiological findings,

J.C. Choi, M.D., Ph.D.
Department of Neurology, Jeju National University, Jeju-si, Jeju-do, South Korea

Jeju Regional Cardio Cerebrovascular Center, Jeju National University Hospital, 15 Aran 13 gil, Jeju-si, Jeju-do 63241, South Korea
e-mail: jaychoi@jejunu.ac.kr

S.-H. Lee (ed.), *Stroke Revisited: Diagnosis and Treatment of Ischemic Stroke*, Stroke Revisited, DOI 10.1007/978-981-10-1424-6_22

and subtype of ischemic stroke can be very helpful in clinical suspicion of monogenic disorder causing ischemic stroke as well as relevant family history. This chapter summarized clinical, genetic, and neuroradiological findings of cerebral autosomal dominant arteriopathy with subcortical infarcts and leukoencephalopathy (CADASIL), cerebral autosomal recessive arteriopathy with subcortical infarcts and leukoencephalopathy (CARASIL), autosomal dominant retinal vasculopathy with cerebral leukodystrophy (RVCL), Fabry disease, sickle cell disease, homocystinuria, and other inherited connective tissue disorders causing ischemic stroke. This chapter will help clinicians readily identify monogenic disorders causing ischemic stroke by their characteristic clinical features and stroke mechanisms (Table 22.1).

Table 22.1 Characteristics of monogenic disorders causing ischemic stroke

	Prevalence	Inheritance	Gene	Stroke incidence	Mechanism of ischemic stroke	Other neurovascular complications	Other clinical features
CADASIL	2/100,000	AD	*NOTCH3*	60–84%	SVD	ICH	Migraine, psychiatric symptom, dementia
CARASIL	Rare	AR	*HTRA1*	50%	SVD	–	Alopecia, low back pain
RVCL	Rare	AD	*TREX1*	Unknown	SVD	–	Progressive visual loss, psychiatric symptoms
COL4A1-related SVD	Rare	AD	*COL4A1*	20%	SVD	ICH, cerebral aneurysm	Porencephaly, infantile hemiparesis cataracts, retinal vascular tortuosity, retinal hemorrhage
FD	1/17,000–11,700	X-linked	*GLA*	4–13%	SVD/LVD/CE	Dolichoectasia	Acroparesthesia, hypohidrosis angiokeratomas, corneal opacity, cardiac involvement
Sickel cell disease	1/500 African Americans	AR	*HBB*	24%	LVD	ICH	Hemolytic anemia, acute chest syndrome, intermittent claudication
Homocystinura	1/344,000	AR	*CBS*	15%	LVD	–	Ectopia lentis, mental retardation, seizure, tall and slender marfanoid features, thromboembolic events
HHT	1–2/100,000	AD	*ENG* *ACVRL1*	10%	Paradoxical embolism	Cerebral AVM	Telangiectasia, recurrent epistaxis, pulmonary AVM
vEDS	Rare	AD	*COL3A1*	10%	Dissection	ICH due to arterial rupture, carotid-cavernous fistula	Distinctive facial features, frequent bruises

Table 22.1 (continued)

	Prevalence	Inheritance	Gene	Stroke incidence	Mechanism of ischemic stroke	Other neurovascular complications	Other clinical features
PXE	1/100,000	AD/AR	*ABCC6*	7–15%	LVD/SVD	Cerebral aneurysm	Yellow-orange papules, intermittent claudication, angioid retinal streak, abdominal angina, and gastrointestinal hemorrhage
Marfan syndrome	1/5000	AD	*FBN1*	10–20%	Dissection/ CE	–	Skeletal manifestations, ectopia lentis, aortic dissection
NF 1	1/3000–4000	AD	*NF1*	Rare	LVD	–	Café-au-lait spots, multiple cutaneous neurofibromas, scoliosis, and iris Lisch nodules

AD autosomal dominant, *AR* autosomal recessive, *SVD* small-vessel disease, *LVD* large-vessel disease, *CE* cardioembolism, *ICH* intracerebral hemorrhage

22.1 CADASIL

CADASIL is one of the most frequent monogenic disorders of the cerebral small blood vessels caused by mutations in the *NOTCH3* gene on chromosome 19q12.40 [4]. CADASIL has been reported worldwide in all ethnic groups with a prevalence approximately 2 per 100,000. In patients with ischemic stroke, CADASIL mutation was found in 0.5–4% of the patients. The main clinical features are recurrent stroke, migraine, psychiatric disturbance, and progressive cognitive deficit [5].

Ischemic stroke is the most frequent manifestation and affects 60% to 84% patients with CADASIL. The mean age at stroke onset is fifth decade and most of the patients show typical lacunar syndrome such as pure motor or pure sensory strokes, dysarthria or clumsy hand syndrome, and ataxic hemiparesis. Occlusive diseases of large cerebral arteries were present 20–30% of the patients, but symptomatic stenosis was rare. In general, hemorrhagic stroke has been described only sporadically in patients with CADASIL. However, recent studies from East Asia found that 25% of symptomatic patients with CADASIL had intracerebral hemorrhages (ICHs), and the presence of ICH was closely related to the number of cerebral microbleeds (CMBs). The patients with ICH had worse clinical outcome compared with those patients without ICH.

Recurrent stroke was reported in almost 70% of the patients who experienced an initial stroke. Eventually recurrent subcortical strokes result in vascular parkinsonism and pseudobulbar palsy in some patients. Although vascular risk factors have been found infrequently in patients with CADASIL in large clinical series, hypertension and smoking were associated with increased risk of stroke in CADASIL. Cognitive deficit is reported in approximately 60% patients, and majority of them develop dementia by age 65 years. Migraine is the most frequent early symptom that occurs in 22% to 77% patients. Migraine usually begins around age 20 years and will develop in 90% patients by age 40 years. Basilar migraine, hemiplegic migraine, or migraine with prolonged aura have been reported in patients with CADASIL. Psychiatric symptoms occur in 20% to 41% patients with CADASIL and mood disorders are most common. Other uncommon manifestations are epileptic seizures, acute reversible

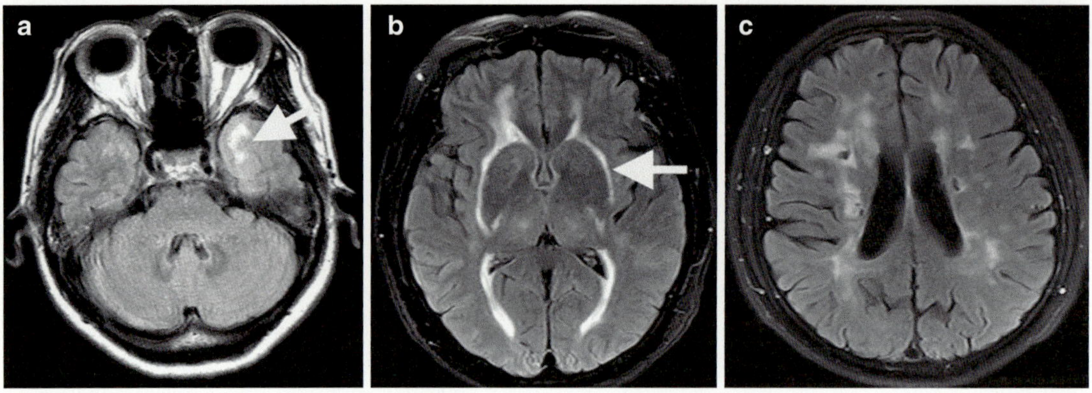

Fig. 22.1 Typical brain MRI findings in CADASIL. FLAIR images demonstrated high-signal intensity lesions in the anterior temporal lobe (**a**) and bilateral external capsules (**b**). Multiple lacunar infarctions (**c**) are noted on bilateral periventricular or deep white matter. Reproduced by permission of Journal of Clinical Neurology [5]

encephalopathy, and high risk of neurological complications following catheter angiography. As a pathognomonic finding, granular osmiophilic material can be observed in the walls of affected arterioles of the brain, and it can be also observed in skin and muscle, which is very useful for pathologic diagnosis. Brain magnetic resonance imaging (MRI) of patients with CADASIL frequently shows progressive white matter hyperintensity (WMH), multiple lacunar infarcts, and CMBs. The involvement of the anterior temporal lobe and external capsule is reported to be unique in comparison to that in the sporadic form of WMH (Fig. 22.1).

22.2 CARASIL

CARASIL is a single-gene disorder of cerebral small blood vessels with autosomal recessive inheritance. This disorder is caused by mutations in the *HTRA1* gene encoding HtrA serine peptidase/protease 1 (HTRA1) [6]. Since the first report from a Japanese family in 1976, the disorder has been mainly reported in Japan. However, a small number of cases in patients from other ethnicities have also been reported recently. Compared with CADASIL, CARASIL seems to be much rarer because approximately only 50 patients have been reported so far.

The frequent clinical features are early-onset lacunar stroke, progressive cognitive deficit, gait disturbance, alopecia, and low back pain. Lacunar stroke, reported in approximately 50% patients, is the most frequent finding of CARASIL and is usually observed in the basal ganglia or brainstem. Cognitive decline is the second-most common symptom, and almost all patients will suffer from dementia when they reach 30 to 40 years of age. Alopecia can be found in almost 90% patients and it is the most frequent early manifestation of the disorder. Hair loss usually begins at adolescence and involves the entire scalp. Low back pain is present in approximately 80% patients and usually begins at 20 to 40 years of age. Migraine-like headache has not been reported with CARASIL. Brain MRI findings are similar to that in CADASIL patients. In cerebral small arteries, extensive degeneration of vascular smooth muscle cells and reduction in the mural extracellular matrix are found, but granular osmiophilic materials or amyloid deposition has not been observed.

22.3 RVCL

Hereditary vascular retinopathy, cerebroretinal vasculopathy, and hereditary endotheliopathy with retinopathy, nephropathy, and stroke (HERNS) were initially known as separate autosomal dominant disorders. The disorders present with various combinations of Raynaud phenomenon, migraine, cranial pseudotumor, and mild kidney or liver dysfunction in addition to vascular retinopathy as a common feature. Recently three disorders were localized to a same locus in chromosome 3p21, and these are now collectively called as autosomal dominant RVCL [7]. The disorder is caused by C-terminal heterozygous, frameshift mutations in *TREX1* gene encoding a DNA-specific 3′ to 5′ exonuclease DNase III. Progressive visual loss usually starts at 20 to 30 years of age. Neurologic deficits present as stroke-like episodes following visual loss and consisted of multifocal cortical and subcortical dysfunction. Brain MRI can disclose multifocal WMH lesions even before neurological symptoms. The lesions can turn into contrast-enhancing lesions with edema, later at the time of focal neurologic deficit.

22.4 COL4A1-Related Cerebral Small-Vessel Disease (SVD)

Mutations in a gene encoding type IV collagen α1 (COL4A1) were initially known to cause porencephaly and infantile hemiparesis; however, these mutations have been later found to cause cerebral SVD even in adulthood. In addition to infantile hemiparesis, lacunar stroke or ICH affects approximately 20% of patients with the mean age of onset of stroke at 36 years [8]. Typically, ICH was often recurrent and provoked by minor trauma, activity, or anticoagulant use. Asymptomatic intracranial aneurysm was also found frequently, while migraine was reported in 30% cases with a mean age of onset at 30 years.

22.5 Fabry Disease

Fabry disease (FD) is an X-linked disorder of glycosphingolipid metabolism, and the disorder is caused by defective lysosomal α-galactosidase A activity [9]. Due to deficiency of the enzyme, globotriaosylceramide accumulates within the lysosomes of various organs, such as the blood vessels, kidneys, heart, and dorsal root ganglia. Lysosomal α-galactosidase A is encoded by the *GLA* gene on chromosome Xq22, and more than 500 pathogenic mutations have been reported in the *GLA* gene so far. Incidence of the disorder has been estimated to be 1 per 17,000 to 117,000 in the general population, but the average prevalence was 4.5% in men and 3.4% in women among patients with cryptogenic stroke.

In the classic form of FD with no detectable α-galactosidase A, patients initially present with angiokeratomas, acroparesthesia, hypohidrosis, and corneal opacity in childhood or adolescence, and subsequently patients can suffer from progressive vascular disease of the heart, kidneys, and brain. About 60% to 80% patients complain of burning pain in the extremities (acroparesthesia), and autonomic dysfunctions such as hypohidrosis, cardiac arrhythmia, or intestinal motility disorder occur if patients have concurrent autonomic neuropathy. Cerebrovascular complications usually develop between the age of 20 and 50 years and overall affects 4.3–13.2% of patients with FD. Ischemic stroke in patients with FD can be classified as either large artery or small-vessel disease. Patients with FD also have a cardiogenic embolism due to cardiac arrhythmia, ischemic heart disease or valvular heart disease. Recurrent strokes are frequent, occurring in 76% to 86% patients. Dolichoectasia of vertebral or basilar arteries is the most frequent angiographic findings. Almost all patients will have WMH on brain MRI at more than 55 years of age, and the pattern of WMH involvement is similar to that of sporadic cerebral SVD. Other evidences of cerebral SVD, including lacunar infarcts, and CMBs have also been reported in patients with FD. So-called pulvinar sign refers to the hyperintensity in the pulvinar on T1-weighted images, and it was reported to be present in 23% patients with FD (Fig. 22.2) [10].

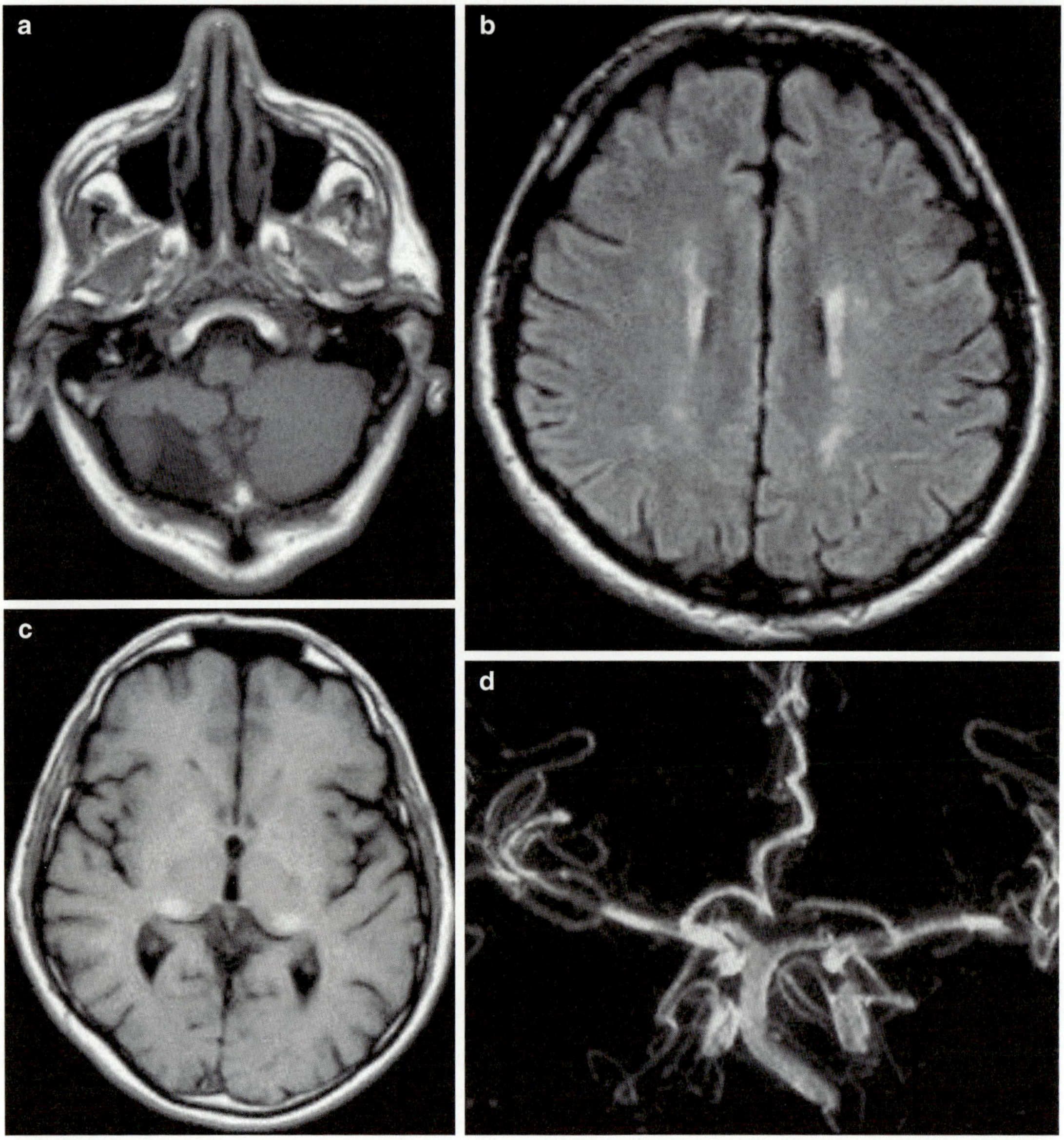

Fig. 22.2 MRI abnormalities in Fabry disease. (**a**) T1-weighted axial MRI section showing a cerebellar infarct. (**b**) Fluid-attenuated inversion recovery (FLAIR)-weighted axial MRI section showing multiple white matter lesions in the cerebral hemispheres. (**c**) T1-weighted axial MRI section showing symmetrical high signal in the pulvinar region. (**d**) Time of flight magnetic resonance angiography showing ectatic vessels. Reproduced by permission of Lancet Neurology (Fellgiebel A et al. Lancet Neurol 2006;5:781–795)

22.6 Sickle Cell Disease

Sickle cell disease is caused by a point mutation at chromosome 11p15.5 that results in substitution of valine for glutamic acid in β-chain of hemoglobin. The point mutation resulted in abnormal hemoglobin (HbS) which led to abnormal aggregation of hemoglobin on deoxygenation. Morphologically, red blood cells are distorted into an elongated "sickle" shape due to the abnormal aggregation of hemoglobin. The disease is inherited as autosomal recessive pattern. Sickle cell disease affects millions of people throughout the world and is particularly common among those whose ancestors came from sub-Saharan Africa, Spanish-speaking regions in the Western Hemisphere (South America, the Caribbean, and Central America), Saudi Arabia, India, and Mediterranean countries such as Turkey, Greece, and Italy.

Most patients with sickle cell disease have hemolytic anemia with hematocrit from 15 to 30% with and reticulocytosis. Vessel occlusion due to sickle cells causes unique clinical manifestations. Intermittent vessel occlusions in various organs produce painful ischemia characterized by acute pain, tenderness, fever, tachycardia, and anxiety. Patients may present with acute chest pain, tachypnea, fever, cough, and arterial oxygen desaturation. This acute chest syndrome is probably caused by vaso-occlusion within pulmonary vasculature.

Risk of stroke was estimated to be at 11% at 20 years age, 15% at 30 years, and 24% in 45 years of age [11]. The incidence of overt stroke in children with sickle cell disease is approximately 1% per year. Both ischemic and hemorrhagic stroke can occur in patients with sickle cell disease. Incidence of ischemic stroke was highest in patients younger than 20 years of age and adults more than 30 years of age. In contrast, the risk of hemorrhagic stroke was highest in patients 20 to 29 years of age and was low in children and older patients. Recurrence of ischemic stroke has been reported in two-thirds of patients, and most of them occurred within 2–3 years of the initial event. Risk factors for ischemic stroke were prior transient ischemic attacks, low hemoglobin concentrations, recent acute chest syndromes, and high blood pressure.

Ischemic strokes are caused by various pathomechanisms. As many as 86% of stroke patients with sickle cell disease showed intracranial large artery occlusive disease on angiography. Some patients showed moyamoya-like basal collateral vessels. As a result, most patients had infarct patterns consistent with major intracranial arterial occlusion or border-zone infarction. Histologic examination of those intracranial arteries exhibited nonatherosclerotic arteriopathy characterized by intimal hyperplasia, smooth muscle cell proliferation, fragmentation of the internal elastic lamina, and superimposed thrombus. Silent infarcts can also be seen in 17–35% of children with sickle cell disease and are usually distributed in the white matter of the frontal and parietal lobes. Hemorrhagic strokes are probably caused by rupture of fragile collateral vessels like those hemorrhages from moyamoya disease.

Hemoglobin electrophoresis is inexpensive, and it can be used as an initial screening test for hemoglobinopathy. The mutant hemoglobin can be more specifically characterized by an isoelectric focusing and/or high-pressure liquid chromatography. The genetic tests are available at several investigational laboratories. Flow velocities measured with transcranial Doppler correlated well with angiography and were inversely related with hematocrit. In children with sickle cell disease, the risk of stroke increased with mean velocity of middle cerebral artery greater than 170 cm/s, and guidelines strongly recommended transfusion in all patients with elevated mean velocity of middle cerebral artery greater than 200 cm/s. Transfusion therapy exhibited a 9% absolute and 92% relative risk reduction for prevention of a first stroke over a 2-year follow up. The transfusion also decreased the risk of new silent infarction. There are several complications associated with long-term transfusion such as transmission of infections and hemosiderosis. Recently oral chelating therapy using deferasirox showed similar efficacy to parenteral deferoxamine. In a recent non-inferiority trial, hydroxyurea with phlebotomy was compared with standard transfusion and oral iron chelation with deferasirox. No stroke occurred among 66 patients on transfusion/chelation, whereas 7 (10%) out of 67 patients on hydroxyurea/phlebotomy developed stroke [12]. Although the risk of stroke was still within non-inferiority margins, transfusion and chelation remained as a standard treatment for preventing stroke in patients with sickle cell disease.

22.7 Homocystinuria

Homocystinuria is an autosomal recessive disorder of cystathionine β-synthase deficiency with estimated frequency in 1 in 344,000. Clinical manifestations include myopia, lens dislocation (ectopia lentis), osteoporosis, mental retardation, seizure, tall and slender marfanoid features, and thromboembolic events (ischemic stroke, myocardial infarction, pulmonary embolism). Thromboembolism can occur in about 25% of patients with homocystinuria before age 16 years and 50% of by 30 years. Stroke was the most common thromboembolic events which accounts for 30% of all thromboembolic events. The possible mechanisms underlying thromboembolism were premature atherosclerosis associated with endothelial dysfunction and hypercoagulable state. According to the case reports, the main causes of ischemic strokes were carotid artery thrombosis, dissection, and arteriopathy mimicking fibromuscular dysplasia. Homocysteine can be measured reliably both in urine and in blood for diagnostic purpose, and activity of cystathionine β-synthase can be measured in cultured fibroblast. For treatment, pyridoxine phosphate (vitamin B6) should be administered 100–600 mg per day. Antiplatelet agents are also used frequently to prevent recurrent stroke prevention.

22.8 Hereditary Hemorrhagic Telangiectasia

Hereditary hemorrhagic telangiectasia (HHT), or Osler-Weber-Rendu disease, is an autosomal dominant disorder characterized by vascular malformations in mucocutaneous tissue, viscera, and the central nervous system (CNS). Prevalence of the disorder is estimated about 1–2 per 100,000. HHT has been linked to two genes; *ENG* gene is located in chromosome 9q33-q34.1 (HHT1), and *ACVRL1* gene is localized on chromosome 12q11-q14 (HHT2). Clinical presentation of HHT is quite heterogeneous, and there seems to be no clear phenotypic difference according to the involved genetic locus. Telangiectasia is frequently observed in the oral or nasal mucosa, tongue, lip, finger tips, and gastrointestinal mucosa. Recurrent epistaxis is the most common and early presentation followed by gastrointestinal hemorrhage. Multiple telangiectasias develop later on at the hands, face, and oral cavity (Fig. 22.3) [13]. Arteriovenous malformations (AVMs) are mainly found in the lungs, CNS, liver, and gastrointestinal tract. Pulmonary AVM is present approximately in one-third of patients with HHT, and 30–40% of them develop ischemic stroke or brain abscess. In patients presented with ischemic stroke due to pulmonary AVM, HHT should be suspected because as many as 70% of patients with pulmonary AMVs will have HHT. AVM can be found along the CNS in approximately 10% of patients with HHT.

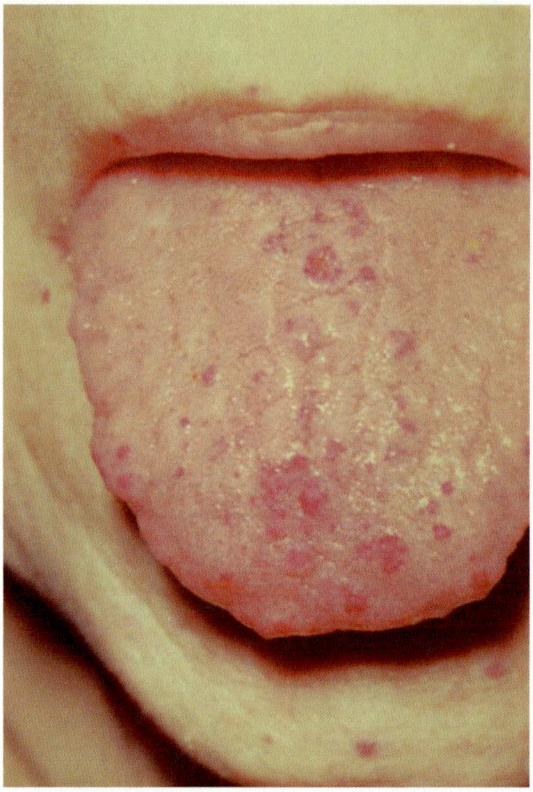

Fig. 22.3 Telangiectases on the tongue. Multiple telangiectatic lesions are seen on the tongue in a patient with HHT. Reproduced by permission of Journal of Neurology [13]

22.9 Vascular Ehlers-Danlos Syndrome

Vascular Ehlers-Danlos syndrome (vEDS), formerly known as type IV EDS, is characterized by distinctive facial features, thin translucent skin, excessive bruising, and rupture of vessels or viscera. Distinctive facial features include sunken cheeks, bulging eyes with periorbital pigmentation, thin nose and upper lip, and lobeless ears (Fig. 22.4) [14]. Unlike classical EDS, skin and

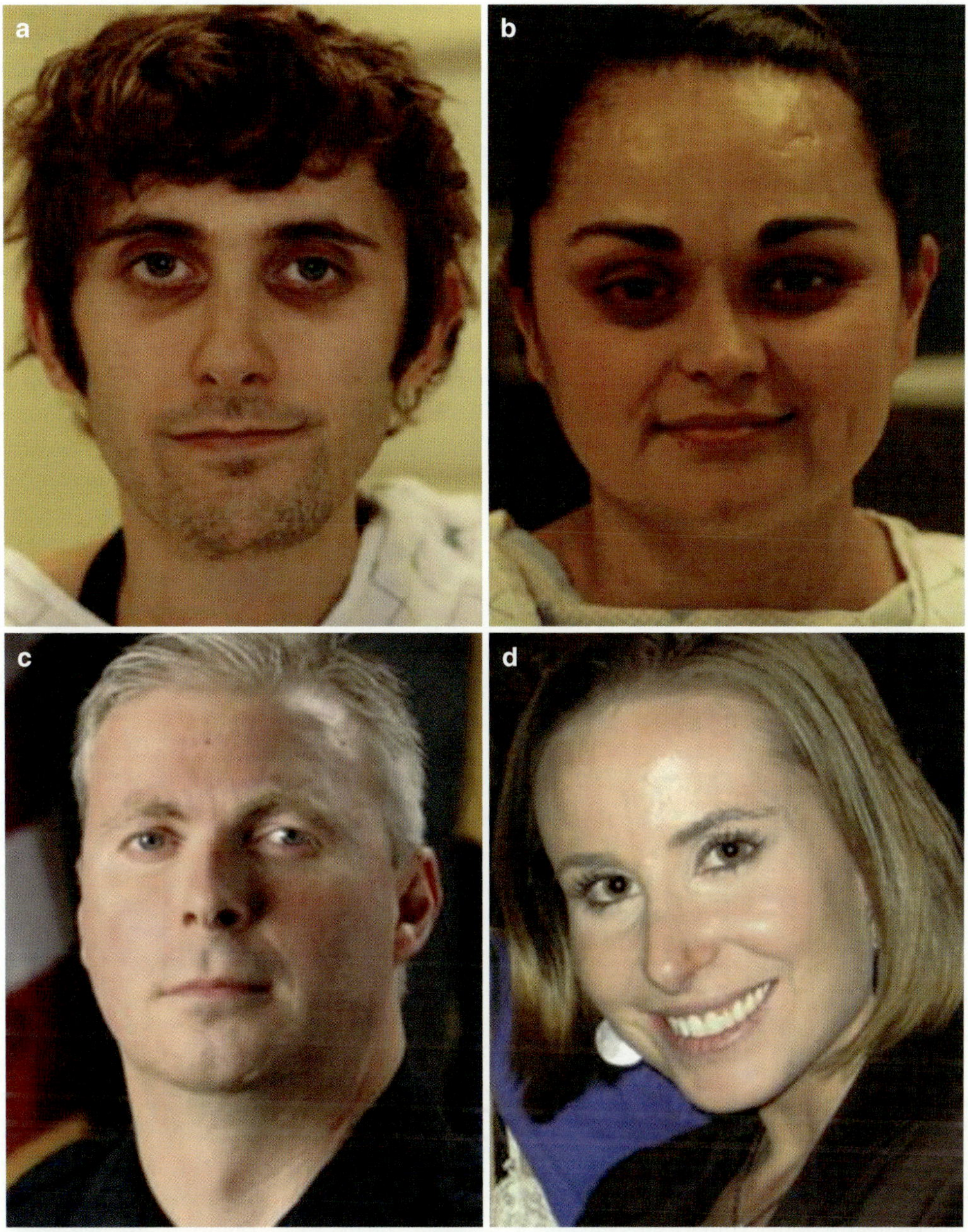

Fig. 22.4 Spectrum of facial features in individuals with vascular Ehlers-Danlos syndrome (vEDS) shows variability among patients and does not necessarily correlate with the severity of the underlying arterial pathology. These four individuals died of vascular complications. (**a**) Caucasian man (MIN mutation, c.2553 + 1delG) presenting with characteristic vEDS facies, including proptotic eyes, long and thin nose, minimal subcutaneous facial fat, and a triangular-shaped face. (**b**) Hispanic woman (MIN mutation, c.3545G>A p.G1182E) with mildly proptotic eyes, a long thin nose, and a hypotrophic forehead scar, but otherwise normal facial features. (**c**) Caucasian man (MIN mutation, c.2870G>T, p.G957D) with downslanting palpebral fissures, long thin nose, thin lips, and attached pinna. (**d**) Caucasian woman (c.665G>T, p. G222V) presenting with a long thin nose but otherwise normal facial features. Written consent was obtained at the time of enrollment for clinical photography and use in medical education. MIN, mutations that lead to minimal (10%–15%) normal type III collagen production. Reproduced by permission of Journal of Vascular Surgery (Shalhub S et al. J Vasc Surg. 2014;60:160–169)

joint symptoms can be mild in vEDS. Bruises are frequent and often can result in massive hematoma. Vascular complications such as spontaneous arterial rupture, dissection, and arteriovenous fistula can occur anywhere with a predilection for midsized arteries. Because of intestinal wall involvement, patients with vEDS can develop gastrointestinal perforation.

The disorder is inherited as an autosomal dominant pattern and resulted from mutations in the *COL3A1* gene on chromosome 2q32.2. The mutations led to defects in procollagen type III which is one of the essential components of walls of arteries and hollow visceral organ.

Cerebrovascular complications were present approximately in 10% of patients with vEDS, and the mean age at presentation was around 28 years. The most common presentations were carotid-cavernous fistula, intracranial aneurysm, carotid or vertebral artery dissection, and arterial rupture. Conventional catheter angiography is associated with high risk of arterial hematoma and dissection (up to 70%), and therefore noninvasive test should be used to investigate cerebral vasculature. Carotid-cavernous fistula is usually caused by rupture of aneurysm or transmural dissection of the cavernous segment of internal carotid artery, and most of them develop spontaneously without history of trauma. Because of high rate of complication with catheter angiography, endovascular embolization should be done with great caution. In addition to the formation of carotid-cavernous fistula, intracranial aneurysms may present with subarachnoid hemorrhages. Dissection can occur in any intracranial or extracranial arteries, and its occurrence can be iatrogenic after angiography. Surgical mortality was also very high reaching almost 40% in patients with vEDS undergoing neurovascular surgery. In a randomized clinical trial, celiprolol, a β(1)-adrenoceptor antagonist with a β(2)-adrenoceptor agonist action, was effective in preventing vascular event in patients with vEDS.

22.10 Pseudoxanthoma Elasticum

Pseudoxanthoma elasticum (PXE) is an inherited disorder of the connective tissue mainly involving the elastic fibers of the skin, eyes, gastrointestinal tract, and cardiovascular system. The prevalence of PXE was estimated to be approximately 1 in 100,000. The defective gene has been localized in the chromosome 16p13.1 and the gene codes for an ATP-binding cassette protein multidrug resistance-associated protein 6 (ABCC6). The disorder can be transmitted as either autosomal dominant or autosomal recessive pattern. The characteristic skin lesions are round, oval, or linear yellow-orange papules resembling xanthoma and are usually found in flexor aspect of the neck, axillar, and groin. Another characteristic ocular finding is an angioid streak that occurs in approximately 85% of patients with PXE (Fig. 22.5) [15]. Due to involvement of medium-sized peripheral arteries, patients may suffer from intermittent claudication, hypertension, abdominal angina, and gastrointestinal hemorrhage. The most frequent cardiac manifestation was mitral valve prolapse.

In patients with PXE, ischemic stroke usually begins at fifth or sixth decade when many of them had other vascular risk factors like hypertension. Ischemic stroke is caused by either occlusion of large intracranial or extracranial arteries or small-vessel disease associated with hypertension. In some patients, moyamoya-like collateral blood vessels from external carotid artery can be seen with occlusion of internal carotid artery. Intracranial aneurysm with or without aneurysmal SAH have been also reported in patients with PXE. Although dissection of cervical arteries has been observed in several patients with PXE, the association between PXE and arterial dissection is unclear.

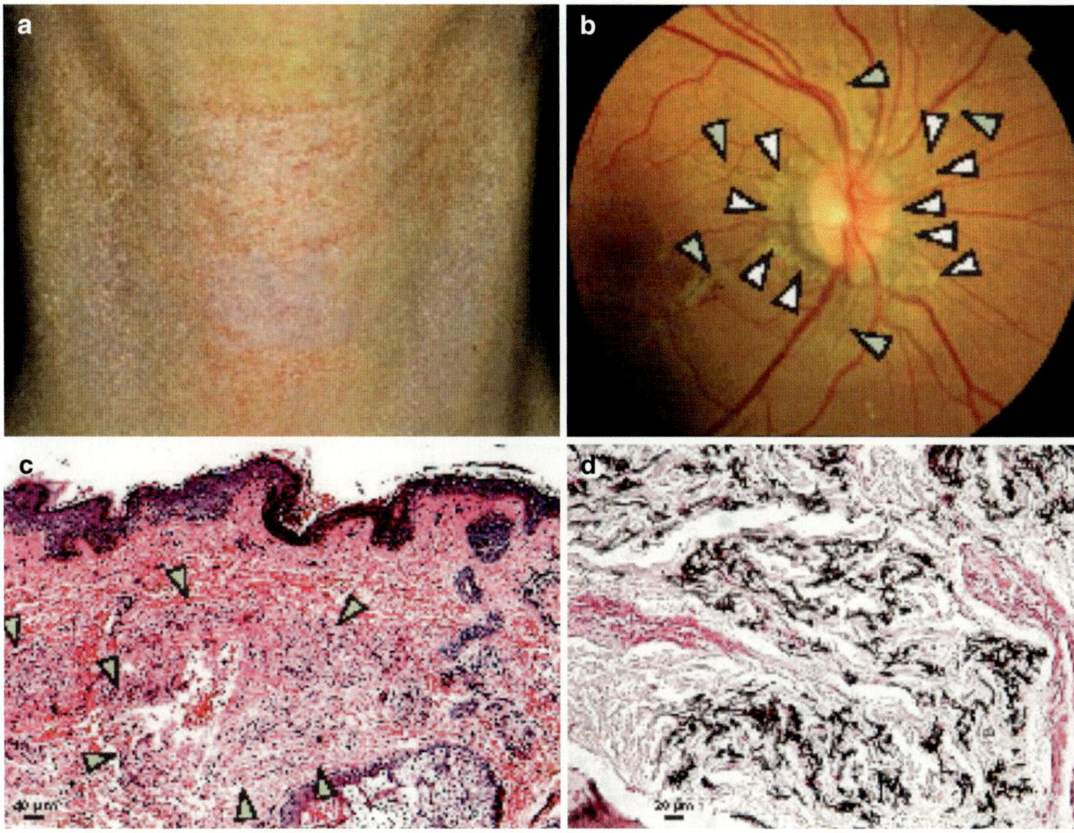

Fig. 22.5 Pseudoxanthoma elasticum. (**a**) Photograph of the neck of our patient showing several yellowish waxy papules. (**b**) Direct ophthalmoscopy of the right eye showing characteristic angioid streaks (green arrowheads) with nasal drusen (white arrowheads). (**c**) Histological examination of the skin biopsy showed fragmentation of elastic fibers (green arrowheads) in the reticular dermis. (**d**) Calcium deposits in the elastic fibers confirmed by von Kossa stains. Reproduced by permission of Lancet (Ko JH et al. Lancet. 2013;381:565)

22.11 Marfan Syndrome

Marfan syndrome is a connective tissue disorder with an autosomal dominant inheritance. The disorder is caused by mutations in the *FBN1* gene localized to chromosome 15q21.1 which led to defective fibrillin-1 and extracellular matrix glycoprotein found in vessel wall and ciliary zonule. The disorder is known to affect about 1 in 10,000 individuals. Marfan syndrome is characterized by skeletal manifestations including tall stature with disproportionately long bones in the limb compared with trunk, prognathism, high-arched palate, kyphoscoliosis, pectus excavatum, and joint hypermobility. Major ocular finding is lens dislocation which affects about 50% of patients. Cardiovascular involvement is a major cause of morbidity and mortality and includes aortic root dilatation, aortic dissection, and mitral valve prolapse. Ischemic strokes are usually caused by extension of aortic dissection to brachiocephalic trunk or common carotid arteries. Although intracranial aneurysms have been reported in patients with Marfan syndrome, the prevalence of aneurysm was not different from that of general population in large cohort or autopsy studies.

22.12 Neurofibromatosis Type 1

Neurofibromatosis type 1 (NF1) is an autosomal dominant disorder caused by mutations of *NF1* gene located on chromosome 17q11.2. Neurofibromatosis 1 (NF1) is characterized by multiple café-au-lait spots, multiple cutaneous neurofibromas, scoliosis, and iris Lisch nodules. Neurologic manifestations include optic nerve glioma, other primary brain tumors, and malignant peripheral nerve sheath tumors and vasculopathy. Stroke rarely affected in adults with NF1. In children or adolescence, occlusive diseases of intracranial or extracranial arteries due to intimal proliferation have been reported. Many of them also exhibited moyamoya pattern of collateral flow.

Suggestions from Current Clinical Practice Guidelines There are no recommended guidelines on these issues.

References

1. Majersik JJ, Skalabrin EJ. Single-gene stroke disorders. Semin Neurol. 2006;26:33–48.
2. Schievink WI, Michels VV, Piepgras DG. Neurovascular manifestations of heritable connective tissue disorders. A review. Stroke. 1994;25: 889–903.
3. Choi JC. Genetics of cerebral small vessel disease. J Stroke. 2015;17:7–16.
4. Joutel A, Corpechot C, Ducros A, et al. Notch3 mutations in CADASIL, a hereditary adult-onset condition causing stroke and dementia. Nature. 1996;383:707–10.
5. Choi JC. Cerebral autosomal dominant arteriopathy with subcortical infarcts and leukoencephalopathy: a genetic cause of cerebral small vessel disease. J Clin Neurol. 2010;6:1–9.
6. Hara K, Shiga A, Fukutake T, et al. Association of HTRA1 mutations and familial ischemic cerebral small-vessel disease. N Engl J Med. 2009;360:1729–39.
7. Ophoff RA, De Young J, Service SK, et al. Hereditary vascular retinopathy, cerebroretinal vasculopathy, and hereditary endotheliopathy with retinopathy, nephropathy, and stroke map to a single locus on chromosome 3p21.1-p21.3. Am J Hum Genet. 2001;69:447–53.
8. Lanfranconi S, Markus HS. COL4A1 mutations as a monogenic cause of cerebral small vessel disease: a systematic review. Stroke. 2010;41:e513–8.
9. Kolodny E, Fellgiebel A, Hilz MJ, et al. Cerebrovascular involvement in Fabry disease: current status of knowledge. Stroke. 2015;46:302–13.
10. Moore DF, Ye F, Schiffmann R, et al. Increased signal intensity in the pulvinar on T1-weighted images: a pathognomonic MR imaging sign of Fabry disease. AJNR Am J Neuroradiol. 2003;24:1096–101.
11. Ohene-Frempong K, Weiner SJ, et al. Cerebrovascular accidents in sickle cell disease: rates and risk factors. Blood. 1998;91:288–94.
12. Ware RE, Helms RW, SWiTCH Investigators. Stroke with transfusions changing to hydroxyurea (SWiTCH). Blood. 2012;119:3925–32.
13. Razvi SS, Bone I. Single gene disorders causing ischaemic stroke. J Neurol. 2006;253:685–700.
14. Schievink WI, Limburg M, Oorthuys JW, et al. Cerebrovascular disease in Ehlers-Danlos syndrome type IV. Stroke. 1990;21:626–32.
15. Plomp AS, Florijn RJ, Ten Brink J, et al. ABCC6 mutations in pseudoxanthoma elasticum: an update including eight novel ones. Mol Vis. 2008;14:118–24.

Part IV

Secondary Prevention of Stroke

23 Identification of Vascular Risk Factors

Keun-Sik Hong

Abstract

Patients with stroke or transient ischemic attack are at high risk of recurrent stroke and other vascular events, and the risk is particularly increased during the early period after acute stroke or transient ischemic attack. The identification of vascular risk factors would be the first step to initiate the risk management. Since physiological parameters are altered by acute stroke and covert risk factors might be unrecognized even with standard diagnostic investigations during the limited time period of acute stroke admission, special considerations are required for the identification and diagnosis of vascular risk factors in patients with acute stroke or transient ischemic attack. During the past decades, the implementation of vascular prevention therapies with proven efficacy from clinical trials into clinical practice have reduced the risk of recurrent stroke and other vascular events in patients with stroke or transient ischemic attack. In addition, the benefit of risk reduction increases with greater achievement of optimal risk factor controls.

Patients who experienced a stroke or a transient ischemic attack (TIA) are at high risk of subsequent vascular events including recurrent stroke, myocardial infarction, and vascular death. In stroke patients, the long-term annual risk is about 3% to 4% for recurrent stroke, about 2% for myocardial infarction, and about 2% for nonstroke vascular death [1, 2]. The risk for recurrent stroke is particularly high within the first year after an index stroke: about 3% at 30 days and about 11% at 1 year [3].

Many risk factors independently and interactively contribute to developing strokes, largely by their link to atherothrombosis or embolism. The American Stroke Association and American Heart Association classify the stroke risk factors according to their potential for modification and evidence level based on data from observational studies and clinical trials: generally nonmodifiable

K.-S. Hong, M.D., Ph.D.
Department of Neurology and Stroke Center, Inje University Ilsan Paik Hospital, 2240 Daewha-dong, Ilsanseo-gu, Goyang City, Gyeonggi-do 411-706, South Korea
e-mail: nrhks@paik.ac.kr

S.-H. Lee (ed.), *Stroke Revisited: Diagnosis and Treatment of Ischemic Stroke*, Stroke Revisited, DOI 10.1007/978-981-10-1424-6_23

Table 23.1 Vascular risk factors

Category	Risk factors
Non-modifiable risk factors	Age, sex, race/ethnicity, low birth weight, family history of stroke/transient ischemic attack
Well-documented and modifiable risk factors	Hypertension, smoking, diabetes, dyslipidemia, atrial fibrillation, carotid stenosis, prior stroke, other cardiovascular disease, physical inactivity, obesity, postmenopausal hormonal therapy, oral contraceptive use, dietary-nutrition, excessive alcohol consumption, sickle cell disease
Less well-documented and potentially modifiable risk factors	Migraine with aura, metabolic syndrome, infection and inflammation, sleep-disordered breathing, hypercoagulability, drug abuse, hyperhomocysteinemia

risk factors, well-documented and modifiable risk factors, and less well-documented or potentially modifiable risk factors (Table 23.1) [4]. Generally nonmodifiable risk factors are well known to increase the risk of stroke, but effective interventions to modify the risk are not available in general. Well-documented and modifiable risk factors include those for which multiple epidemiological observational studies have indicated strong associations with the increased risk of stroke and large randomized trials have demonstrated the reduction of stroke with modification. Less well-documented or potentially modifiable risk factors are those with less clear evidence for their association with stroke risk from observational studies or for the benefit of their modification from clinical trials.

Identifying risk factors for stroke is the first step to initiate optimal preventive therapies and also help determine the risk of vascular events in individual patients. There has been a great advance in the stroke prevention therapies including antihypertensive therapy, antiplatelet or anticoagulation therapies, carotid intervention, and statins. During the last decades, the risk of recurrent stroke and major vascular events in patients with stroke or TIA has declined [5]. As achieving optimal risk factor levels increases, the benefit of vascular event risk reduction increases. Definitions of individual vascular risk factors are generally identical for both the stroke and general populations. However, acute stroke influences on physiological parameters and the limited time period of acute stroke admission might be insufficient to identify covert risk factors, and thereby special considerations are required for the identification and diagnosis of vascular risk factors in patients with acute stroke or TIA.

23.1 Hypertension

Hypertension is the most common and important risk factor for stroke, and 60–70% of stroke patients have hypertension. However, elevated blood pressure is common in acute stroke patients even in those without underlying hypertension. During the first 1–2 days, an elevated blood pressure > 140/90 mmHg is observed in about 75% of patients with acute ischemic stroke and in more than 80% of patients with acute primary intracerebral hemorrhage. More than 50% of patients with acute stroke have systolic blood pressure > 160 mmHg. The elevated blood pressure is attributed to several factors, including neuroendocrine system-related stress response to acute stroke, stroke-related injury in autonomic center, increased intracranial pressure, or inadequately treated or untreated hypertension before the index stroke. The elevated blood pressure usually decreases spontaneously over the first week but sometimes over a few weeks in patients with severe stroke [6]. Therefore, the diagnosis of hypertension in patients with acute stroke can be made if patients have a history of use of antihypertensive agents or physician diagnosis before their strokes. For patients without a history of hypertension, the diagnosis can be made when the mean blood pressure in repeated measurements after the acute stage of stroke is ≥140/90 mm Hg.

23.2 Diabetes

Diagnosis of diabetes can be made if patients have a history of diabetes treatment of diagnosis before their strokes. For patients who do not have a clear history of prior diabetes, diabetes can be made by (1) an HbA1c value ≥6.5% on repeated tests, (2) a fasting plasma glucose level ≥ 126 mg/dL (7.0 mmol/L) on repeated tests, (3) a 2-h plasma glucose ≥200 mg/dL during a 75-g oral glucose tolerance test on repeated tests, or (4) typical hyperglycemic symptoms associated with a random plasma glucose ≥200 mg/dL.

About one-third of patients with acute stroke have prior or newly diagnosed diabetes. However, 44–68% of patients with acute stroke have hyperglycemia, and patients with severe stroke are more likely to have hyperglycemia. Underlying diabetes, the release of cortisol and norepinephrine in response to stroke-related stress, and relative insulin deficiency due to increased lipolysis in acute stroke contribute to hyperglycemia in acute stroke. Elevated glucose levels usually decline during the first week. Therefore, the diagnosis of new diabetes based on glucose level should be determined at least after 1 week from stroke onset. In contrast, HbA1c level reflects the 3-month average plasma glucose concentration and is less affected by acute stroke. Therefore, HbA1c level rather than glucose level would be better to newly diagnose diabetes and to assess pre-stroke glycemic status.

23.3 Dyslipidemia

The previous National Cholesterol Education Program Adult Treatment Panel III set an LDL cholesterol target goal based on the patient's risk category determined by the presence of atherosclerotic disease and major risk factors and then recommended how to achieve the target goal. In contrast, the updated 2013 American College of Cardiology and the American Heart Association guidelines do not specify a target LDL cholesterol goal. Instead, the guidelines recommend high-intensity statin (lowering LDL cholesterol by approximately ≥50%) or moderate-intensity statin (lowering LDL cholesterol by approximately 30–50%) in four major statin benefit groups who are at high risk of atherosclerotic cardiovascular disease events [7]. According to these guidelines, patients with ischemic stroke or TIA presumed to be of atherosclerotic origin are indicated for high-intensity statin therapy irrespective of their LDL cholesterol levels. For patients with ischemic stroke of non-atherosclerotic origin (cardioembolism, other determined etiology), statin therapy should be individualized based on their LDL cholesterol level, presence of diabetes, and 10-year estimated risk of atherosclerotic cardiovascular disease events. For patients with hemorrhagic stroke, there is debate on the risk and benefit of statin. Furthermore, in patients who were taking statins before their hemorrhagic strokes, the decision is more complex regarding whether to resume statins or not. After taking into consideration both the risks of future atherosclerotic cardiovascular disease events and recurrent hemorrhagic stroke, the decision should be individualized.

It is generally recommended to assess lipid profile during the acute stroke admission, and in-hospital LDL cholesterol levels can be used to guide decisions regarding long-term statin therapy. Since statin trials generally excluded patients with acute stroke, the benefit of statins in acute stage of ischemic stroke or TIA has not been confirmed. Observational studies and meta-analyses have suggested that statin therapy initiated during the acute ischemic stroke or TIA was associated with better functional outcome with a minimal risk. Furthermore, acute stroke hospitalization is a good opportunity to initiate statins and to increase the patients' adherence.

23.4 Atrial Fibrillation

Twenty to twenty-five percentage of patients with ischemic stroke or TIA have atrial fibrillation (AF), and long-term oral anticoagulation is strongly recommended otherwise contraindicated. AF is newly detected in about 10% of patients with acute ischemic stroke or TIA. Therefore, 12-lead electrocardiography (ECG) should be tested in all patients. However, covert paroxysmal AF is not easily detected by standard ECG. Patients who have stroke or TIA of presumed embolic origin should be additionally evaluated with 24-h ambulatory ECG monitoring, continuous ECG monitoring during stroke unit admission, or transesophageal echocardiography to detect occult AF.

However, despite cardiac evaluations and neuroimaging studies, 20–25% of patients have no clear embolic source, categorized as embolic stroke of undetermined source (ESUS). For these patients, outpatient prolonged ECG monitoring (generally up to 30 days) can be considered. The 30-Day Cardiac Event Monitor Belt for Recording Atrial Fibrillation After a Cerebral Ischemic Event (EMBRACE) trial demonstrated that, in patients with ESUS despite of standard tests including 24-h ECG monitoring, the noninvasive ambulatory ECG monitoring with a 30-day event trigger recorder compared to the standard 24-h ECG monitoring significantly improved the detection of AF. Within 90 days after randomization, AF was newly detected in 16.1% of the long-term monitoring group versus 3.2% in the 24-h ECG monitoring group [8]. In the Cryptogenic Stroke and Underlying AF (CRYSTAL AF) trial, the long-term ECG monitoring with an insertable cardiac monitor detected new AF in 8.9% of patients with ESUS, whereas the routine practice detected new AF in 1.4% of patients with ESUS within 6 months [9].

23.5 Cardiac Evaluation

Stroke and coronary heart disease share common risk factors and pathophysiologic mechanisms. In addition, some cardiac conditions as well as AF are potential sources of cerebral embolism. More than one-third patients with ischemic stroke have overt or covert significant coronary artery stenosis. Therefore, during the acute stroke admission, transthoracic echocardiography can be considered as a routine examination to evaluate potential cardiac embolic sources and left ventricle wall motion. Patients with stroke or TIA are at high risk of coronary event as well as recurrent stroke, and the average 10-year risk of myocardial infarction is about 20% [2]. For patients who have a 10-year coronary heart disease risk >20%, or have significant stenosis in the major cerebral arteries, noninvasive testing for coronary artery disease may be considered [10].

23.6 Proximal Carotid Stenosis

Proximal carotid stenosis accounts for about 15% of ischemic stroke or TIA. Earlier large randomized trials and their meta-analysis confirmed that carotid endarterectomy (CEA) in addition to best medical therapy compared to best medical therapy alone in patients with >50% symptomatic stenosis significantly reduced the risk of recurrent stroke. Carotid angioplasty and stenting (CAS) has emerged as a therapeutic alternative to CEA [11].

For patients with TIA or acute ischemic stroke in the territory of internal carotid artery, noninvasive vascular imaging should be conducted to assess the carotid stenosis using duplex carotid ultrasonography, magnetic resonance angiography (MRA), or computed tomography angiography (CTA). The most common cause of carotid stenosis is atherosclerosis. Because atherosclerosis is a systemic disease, the presence of carotid stenosis indicates a high atherosclerotic burden. Patients with carotid stenosis are likely to have atherosclerosis in the non-cerebral vascular beds, including coronary artery, aorta, and peripheral artery, and are at increased risk of other atherosclerotic cardiovascular disease events including myocardial infarction and vascular death as well as stroke. In addition to carotid stenosis, carotid plaque and intima-media thickness (IMT) are markers of systemic atherosclerosis and associated with future atherosclerotic cardiovascular disease events, particularly coronary events. Therefore, irrespective of carotid stenosis, carotid evaluation in patients with acute stroke or TIA might be reasonable to assess the long-term risk of atherosclerotic cardiovascular disease events.

Duplex carotid ultrasonography is noninvasive and widely available. Rather than luminal area or diameter, the peak systolic velocity in the internal carotid artery and the ratio of the peak systolic velocity in the internal carotid artery to that in the ipsilateral common carotid artery are usually recommended to assess the degree of stenosis. In the presence of carotid plaque narrowing lumen, a peak systolic velocity of 125 to 230 cm/s indicates 50–69% stenosis, and >230 cm/s suggests >70% stenosis [12]. However, duplex carotid ultrasonography has several disadvantages. The diagnostic accuracy is operator dependent. Subtotal and total occlusion cannot be differentiated, and arterial calcification potentially limits the accurate assessment. The velocity is usually increased if the contralateral carotid artery is occluded. Furthermore, duplex carotid ultrasonography does not provide information regarding the steno-occlusion in the intracranial cerebral arteries.

MRA is useful to assess carotid stenosis. MRA has several advantages over duplex carotid ultrasonography. MRA combined with MRI allows to confirm acute stroke, to assess stroke severity, and to evaluate intracranial vessels. Compared to duplex carotid ultrasonography and CTA, MRA is less affected by arterial calcification. However, MRA usually overestimates the degree of stenosis and cannot be obtained in some patients who are not cooperative, have claustrophobia, or have incompatible implanted pacemakers or defibrillators.

CTA compared to duplex carotid ultrasonography and MRA usually more accurately measures the degree of stenosis by directly imaging the arterial lumen. CTA also can provide intracranial vessel images. However, major disadvantages are radiation and need for injection of contrast dye. Like with duplex carotid ultrasonography, dense calcification interferes the accurate assessment of stenosis with CTA.

Conventional angiography is the gold standard method but is largely replaced by noninvasive tests as a screening modality. For the measurement of carotid stenosis, there was a discrepancy between the North American Symptomatic Carotid Endarterectomy Trial and the European Carotid Surgery Trial. Currently, the method adopted by the North American Symptomatic Carotid Endarterectomy Trial is recommended as a standard measurement for carotid stenosis.

23.7 Hypercoagulability

Hypercoagulability related to inherited or acquired disorders potentially leads to thromboembolism in arterial or venous system in the brain. Hypercoagulability is generally associated with venous thrombosis and rarely associated with arterial thromboembolism in adults. However, in younger patients who have recurrent cerebral arterial thromboembolism without traditional vascular risk factors, hypercoagulability can be a potential mechanism. Because laboratory results tested in the acute stage of stroke are at risk of false positive, repeated testing after the acute phase should be considered to confirm diagnosis. Detailed description is provided in other chapters.

23.8 Impact of Risk Factor Control

Stroke is a highly preventable disorder. The INTERSTROKE study which was an international, multicenter, case-control study showed that 88% of all strokes were attributable to ten risk factors including hypertension, regular physical activity, waist-to-hip ratio, ratio of ApoB to ApoA1, smoking status, diet risk score, cardiac causes, diabetes mellitus, psychosocial factors, and alcohol intake (in order of the magnitude of population-attributable risk) [13]. Large population-based studies conducted in developed countries have shown that the incidence of first-ever stroke declined, largely attributed to the improvement of risk factor controls during the past decades.

With the introduction of secondary vascular prevention therapies with proven efficacy into clinical practice, the recurrent stroke and major vascular events in stroke survivors have declined over the five decades: per decade, the annual risk declined by ≈1.0% for recurrent stroke and by ≈1.3% for major vascular events [5]. Overall risk factor control is of great importance. In the analysis of data from the SPARCL (Stroke Prevention by Aggressive Reduction in Cholesterol Levels) trial which was a secondary stroke prevention trial testing high-dose atorvastatin, patients who achieved optimal levels of lipid profiles and blood pressure had a relative risk reduction of 65% for recurrent stroke and 75% for major vascular events compared to patients who achieved none [14]. Similarly, in another study analyzing data of the VISP (Vitamin Intervention for Stroke Prevention) trial which was a secondary stroke prevention trial testing multivitamin to lower homocysteine level, patients who took all of antihypertensive agents, lipid modifiers, and antithrombotic agents had a relative risk reduction of 61% for recurrent stroke and 61% for major vascular events compared to patients who did not take any agent [15].

Conclusion

Control of vascular risk factors are highly effective for the prevention of primary and secondary stroke and other vascular events. Identifying the vascular risk factors is the first step of the risk management. Hurdles and solutions in identification of risk factors are illustrated in Fig. 23.1. The acute stroke admission is a good opportunity to initiate the whole process to reduce future vascular events including recurrent stroke.

Suggestions from Current Clinical Practice Guidelines Diagnostic criteria of vascular risk factors in health adult persons is widely accepted, but there is no standard guideline for diagnosis of vascular risk factors during acute stroke period. Regarding blood pressure, diagnostic definition of hypertension is not documented in stroke patients without previous hypertension history, but it is reasonable that blood pressure control is initiated "after the first several days" to stroke patients with sustained increased blood pressure (>140/90 mm Hg). In addition, diagnosis of dyslipidemia is more confusing in stroke patients. Thus, definition of dyslipidemia has not been suggested in stroke, and indication of statin therapy has been recommended: (1) ischemic stroke or transient ischemic attack caused by large artery atherosclerosis and (2) low-density lipoprotein cholesterol level ≥ 100 mg/dL. Finally, in terms of diabetes, its diagnosis is relatively simple as compared with hypertension and

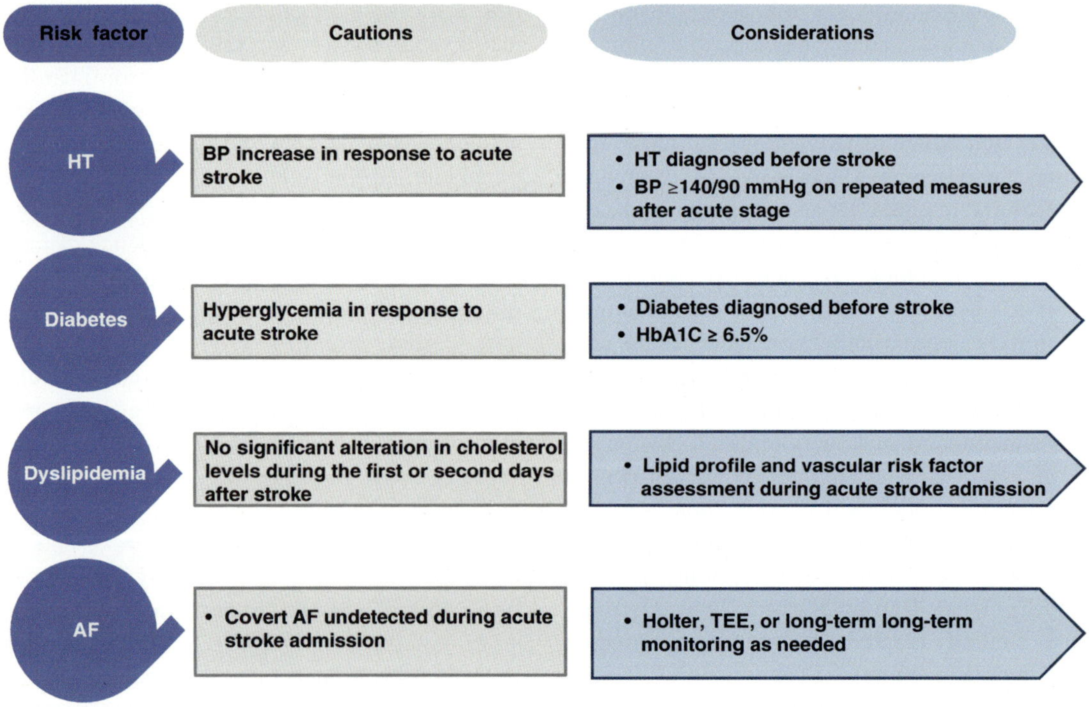

Fig. 23.1 A schematic diagram showing risk factor identification in acute ischemic stroke

dyslipidemia. In general, HbA1c test (≥6.5%) is recommended because it may be more accurate than other screening tests in the immediate post-stroke period.

References

1. Kernan WN, Ovbiagele B, Black HR, et al. Guidelines for the prevention of stroke in patients with stroke and transient ischemic attack: a guideline for healthcare professionals from the American Heart Association/American Stroke Association. Stroke. 2014;45:2160–236.
2. Touzé E, Varenne O, Chatellier G, et al. Risk of myocardial infarction and vascular death after transient ischemic attack and ischemic stroke: a systematic review and meta-analysis. Stroke. 2005;36:2748–55.
3. Mohan KM, Wolfe CD, Rudd AG, et al. Risk and cumulative risk of stroke recurrence: a systematic review and meta-analysis. Stroke. 2011;42:1489–94.
4. Meschia JF, Bushnell C, Boden-Albala B, et al. Guidelines for the primary prevention of stroke: a statement for healthcare professionals from the American Heart Association/American Stroke Association. Stroke. 2014;45:3754–832.
5. Hong KS, Yegiaian S, Lee M, et al. Declining stroke and vascular event recurrence rates in secondary prevention trials over the past 50 years and consequences for current trial design. Circulation. 2011;123:2111–9.
6. Qureshi AI. Acute hypertensive response in patients with stroke: pathophysiology and management. Circulation. 2008;118:176–87.
7. Stone NJ, Robinson JG, Lichtenstein AH, et al. 2013 ACC/AHA guideline on the treatment of blood cholesterol to reduce atherosclerotic cardiovascular risk in adults: a report of the American College of Cardiology/American Heart Association Task Force on Practice Guidelines. Circulation. 2014;129(25 Suppl 2):S1–S45.
8. Gladstone DJ, Spring M, Dorian P, et al. Atrial fibrillation in patients with cryptogenic stroke. N Engl J Med. 2014;370:2467–77.
9. Sanna T, Diener H-C, Passman RS, et al. Cryptogenic stroke and underlying atrial fibrillation. N Engl J Med. 2014;370:2478–86.
10. Adams RJ, Chimowitz MI, Alpert JS, et al. Coronary risk evaluation in patients with transient ischemic attack and ischemic stroke: a scientific statement for healthcare professionals from the Stroke Council and the Council on Clinical Cardiology of the American Heart Association/American Stroke Association. Stroke. 2003;34:2310–22.
11. Brott TG, Halperin JL, Abbara S, Bacharach JM, et al. Guideline on the management of patients with extracranial carotid and vertebral artery disease. Stroke. 2011;42:e464–540.
12. Grant EG, Benson CB, Moneta GL, et al. Carotid artery stenosis: gray-scale and Doppler US diagnosis—Society of Radiologists in Ultrasound Consensus Conference. Radiology. 2003;229:340–6.
13. O'Donnell MJ, Xavier D, Liu L, et al. Risk factors for ischaemic and intracerebral haemorrhagic stroke in 22 countries (the INTERSTROKE study): a case-control study. Lancet. 2010;376:112–23.
14. Amarenco P, Goldstein LB, Messig M, et al. Relative and cumulative effects of lipid and blood pressure control in the Stroke Prevention by Aggressive Reduction in Cholesterol Levels trial. Stroke. 2009;40:2486–92.
15. Park JH, Ovbiagele B. Optimal combination secondary prevention drug treatment and stroke outcomes. Neurology. 2015;84:50–6.

Hypertension Management in Acute Ischemic Stroke

24

Mi Sun Oh

Abstract

Hypertension is the leading risk factor for ischemic stroke. Baseline blood pressure (BP) in the setting of acute ischemic stroke is closely related clinical outcomes. High BP is also associated with an increased risk of recurrent stroke. The management of hypertension in ischemic stroke is determined by timing, the use of thrombolysis, medical comorbidities, and the subtypes of ischemic stroke. In this chapter, we review the current evidences and guidelines for acute stroke. Additionally, based on current evidences, we discuss the optimal strategy of hypertension management in the acute and subacute/chronic stages of ischemic stroke.

Hypertension is a major modifiable risk factor for ischemic stroke. Blood pressure (BP) management is an important intervention for prevention of first and recurrent ischemic stroke. The management of hypertension should be determined based on the timing, the stroke subtype, the use of thrombolysis, and the concurrent comorbidity. However, how best to treat acute hypertensive response during the early phase of acute ischemic stroke is less well established. In this chapter, we review controversy and guidelines for management of BP in acute ischemic stroke. Our discussion is subdivided to address important questions and management guideline about the early BP management in acute ischemic stroke and chronic BP management for secondary prevention of ischemic stroke.

24.1 Acute Hypertensive Response in Patients with Ischemic Stoke

24.1.1 Characteristics of Acute Hypertensive Response

Acute hypertensive response commonly occurs in patients with ischemic stroke within the first 24 h of stroke onset. This hypertensive response is characterized by high prevalence, self-limiting nature, and prognostic significance.

M.S. Oh, M.D.
Department of Neurology, Hallym University Sacred Heart Hospital, Hallym University College of Medicine, Anyang, South Korea
e-mail: iyyar@hallym.ac.kr

S.-H. Lee (ed.), *Stroke Revisited: Diagnosis and Treatment of Ischemic Stroke*, Stroke Revisited, DOI 10.1007/978-981-10-1424-6_24

- High prevalence: Acute hypertensive response has been reported in around 75% ~ 80% of patients with ischemic stroke on admission to the hospital [1, 2]. In the International Stroke Trial (IST), mean systolic blood pressure (SBP) within 48 h of stroke onset was 160 mm Hg, and 82% of patients had acute hypertensive response based on the WHO definition of hypertension (SBP > 140 mm Hg).
- Self-limiting nature: The acute hypertensive response tends to spontaneously decline without antihypertensive therapy in the first few hours after stroke onset and continues to decrease by an average BP 20/10 mm Hg over the following hours or days [3]. The mechanisms of the spontaneous BP reduction have not been elucidated, but are likely to relate, to least in part, to the initial rise in BP. The rapid BP lowering presumably has been allowed in parallel with the decrease of the stimulus that results in the temporary increase in BP.
- Prognostic significances: Both high and low BP are associated with an increased risk of death and disability in patients with acute ischemic stroke. A post hoc analysis of patients with acute ischemic stroke enrolled in the IST demonstrated a U-shaped relationship of initial BP with outcomes, indicating that a higher rate of death or dependency was seen in patients with either high or low initial SBP [1]. For every 10 mm Hg increase in SBP above 150 mm Hg, death at 14 days increased by 3.8%, and for every 10 mm Hg decrease below 150 mm Hg, death at 14 days and dependency at 6 months after stroke onset increased by 17.9% and 3.6%, respectively. An initial SBP of 140 to 179 mm Hg, with the nadir at 150 mm Hg, resulted in the lowest frequency of worse outcomes. This relationship has been confirmed by several subsequent studies. Another study found the similar findings of a U-shaped association between initial BP and early neurological deterioration, but found that the risk was lowest in those with an initial BP of around 180/100 mm Hg [4].

24.1.2 Mechanisms of Acute Hypertensive Response

The acute hypertensive response is multifactorial and still not well understood. Several mechanisms and factors have been proposed, including fallowing:

- Related factors: Pre-existing chronic hypertension, headache, urine retention, psychological stress of hospitalization, pain, infection, infarct topography, stroke subtype, stroke severity, or raised intracranial pressure.
- Brain injury: The transient or permanent damage or compression of specific regions in the brain that play a role in regulating the neuroendocrine leads to disrupt normal autonomic control and hence exaggerate sympathetic response. The increased sympathetic outflow, coupled with the impairment of parasympathetic activity, leads to elevated endogenous catecholamines, vasoconstriction, and increased systemic vascular resistance.
- Selfish brain: Acute hypertensive response may reflect a compensatory or protective physiologic response to maintain cerebral perfusion and to increase blood flow to salvageable tissue in the ischemic penumbra.

24.1.3 Impact of Acute Hypertensive Response

Although the association between the early BP and outcomes has been confirmed in multiple studies, it remains unclear whether acute hypertensive response is protective or detrimental to further injury of ischemic brain. Thus, there is debate whether the early BP lowering is protective or harm to patients with acute ischemic stroke.

24.1.3.1 Cons of Treating Acute Hypertensive Response

- Acute hypertensive response is self-limiting nature in the first several days, and moreover it is protective response in order to improve cerebral blood flow (CBF) to the ischemic penumbra defending the brain from the further ischemia.

- Cerebral autoregulation becomes dysfunctional in the ischemic tissue because cerebral resistance vessels are dilated to near or total capacity to increase CBF in response to tissue ischemia and acidosis. As a result, because of impaired regional autoregulation, the CBF in the ischemic tissue tends to passively be dependent on perfusion pressure and more sensitive to changes in systemic BP. In the penumbra, even small reductions in systemic BP may cause reduction of CBF to critical levels, resulting in exacerbation of permanent ischemic brain damage. Hence, pharmacological reduction of BP during the acute phase of stroke may have to be done cautiously in order to maintain the CBF and reduce the possibility of infarction extension and worsened outcome.

24.1.3.2 Pros of Treating Acute Hypertensive Response

- During the early phase of ischemic stroke, untreated elevated BP may cause further neurological damage by hemorrhagic transformation, increasing intracranial pressure, or worsening cerebral edema.

24.2 Management of Acute Hypertensive Response During the Early Phase of Ischemic Stroke

Regardless of several large randomized clinical trials evaluating the safety and efficacy of the early BP lowering with various antihypertensive agents in the setting of acute ischemic stroke, results from these trials are controversial. These controversies could arise, at least in part, from different study designs including subtype of acute stroke (ischemic stroke, hemorrhagic stroke, or both), administrated type of antihypertensive agents (oral or intravenous), degree and speed of BP reduction, and the regarding time of BP lowering. We briefly summarized designs and results of trials in Table 24.1. I present a brief summary of these trials that disclaim, support, or show neutral results about the BP lowering during the acute phase of ischemic stroke.

24.2.1 Con Studies Against Early BP Lowering

The Low-Dose Beta Blockade in Acute Stroke (BEST, 1988) [5]: The BEST trial revealed a higher rate of mortality among patients who were treated by beta-blocker therapy within 48 h of symptom onset.

The Intravenous Nimodipine West European Stroke Trial (INWEST, 2000) [6]: The INWEST trial found a significant correlation between prominent DBP lowering with intravenous nimodipine and worsening of clinical outcomes at 21 days after stroke onset. Higher rates of death and disability were statistically significant associated with a decrease in DBP > 20% or DBP < 60 mm Hg. A subsequent meta-analysis of the studies of oral nimodipine started within 48 h after stroke onset also showed that the BP lowering with oral nimodipine did not improve functional outcome at 3 months but was significantly associated with higher rates of mortality.

The Scandinavian Candesartan Acute Stroke Trial (SCAST, 2011) [3]: In the SCAST trial, BP was significantly lower in the treatment group, 147/82 mm Hg for the candesartan group vs. 152/84 mm Hg for the placebo group. However, there was no significant difference in the composite outcome of vascular death, myocardial infarction, or stroke during the first 6 months, but a nonsignificant trend toward worse functional outcome at 6 months. The study concluded BP lowering with candesartan showed no benefit in patients with acute stroke. If anything, the evidence suggested a harmful effect. In addition, subgroup analysis of the SCAST demonstrated that large SBP change was associated with the increased risk of early adverse event and early neurological deterioration.

The Valsartan Efficacy on Modest Blood Pressure Reduction in Acute Ischemic Stroke (VENTURE, 2015) [7]: Valsartan started within 48 h after stroke onset did not reduce rates of death or dependency and vascular events at 3 months, but significantly increased the risk of early neurological deterioration at 7 days.

Table 24.1 Summary of clinical trials on the role of early BP lowering in acute ischemic stroke

	Study design	Patients included	No. of patients with ischemic stroke	Intervention vs. control	Mean time from stroke onset to randomization, h	Outcome assessments	Results
Con studies against BP lowering							
BEST, 1988	Randomized trial	Any stroke within 48 h after stroke	NA 302 (any stroke)	Propranolol, or atenolol vs. placebo 21 days or until discharge	NA	Neurologic recovery, discharge state, functional outcome, death at 30 days and 6 months	Higher death rate in the treatment arm at 6 months and no difference of neurologic recovery and functional outcome at 6 months
INWEST, 2000	Randomized, double-blinded, placebo-controlled trial	Ischemic stroke within 24 h in the carotid artery territory	295	Intravenous nimodipine vs. placebo 21 days	11	Death or dependency (BI < 60) at day 21 days	Higher rate of death and worse neurologic recovery by reduction of diastolic BP (>20%) after high-dose nimodipine
SCAST, 2011	Randomized, double-blinded, placebo-controlled trial	Any stroke within 30 h after stroke, SBP ≥140 mm Hg	1733	Candesartan vs. placebo for 7 days	NA	mRS > 2 at 6 months, vascular events at 6 months	No beneficial effect but a trend toward increased risk of vascular events and worsening functional outcome at 6 months in the treatment arm
VENTURE, 2015	Randomized, open, blinded end point, controlled trial	Ischemic stroke within 48 h after stroke, SBP 150 to 185 mm Hg	372	Valsartan vs. no antihypertensive agents for 7 days	NA	Death or functional dependency (mRS > 2) at 90 days; END at 7 days, vascular events and BI at 90 days	No beneficial effect in death or dependency at 90 days but trend to increased risk of END in the treatment arm
Pro studies supporting BP lowering							
ACCESS, 2003	Randomized, double-blinded, placebo-controlled trial	Ischemic stroke within 36 h, SBP ≥ 200 mm Hg and DBP ≥ 110 mm Hg	339	Candesartan vs. placebo for 7 days	30	Vascular events and death at 12 months; BI at 3 months	No difference in functional dependency at 3 months but reduction of vascular events and death at 1 y in the treatment arm

CHHIPS, 2009	Randomized, double-blinded, placebo-controlled trial	Any stroke within 36 h after stroke, SBP > 160 mm Hg	99	Labetalol, or lisinopril vs. placebo for 14 days	NA	mRS > at 14 days	No difference in death or neurologic recovery at 2 weeks but reduction in death at 3 months with treatment group
Studies with neutral results							
COSSACS, 2010	Randomized, open, blinded end point trial	Any stroke within 48 h after stroke, pre-existing, hypertension agents	444	Continuous or stop pre-existing antihypertensive agents for 14 days	NA	Death or functional dependency (mRS > 3) at 14 days	No difference in death or dependency at 2 weeks No difference in death or recurrent stroke at 6 months
PRoFESS substudy, 2009	Randomized, double-blinded, placebo-controlled trial	Ischemic stroke within 72 h after stroke, SBP 121 to 180 mm Hg	1360	Telmisartan vs. placebo for 90 days	58	mRS at 30 days, death at 90 days; stroke recurrence, combined vascular at 90 days	No difference in dependency, death, or recurrent stroke at 3 months
CATIS, 2014	Randomized, open, blinded end point, controlled trial	Ischemic stroke within 48 h after stroke, SBP 140 to 220 mm Hg	4071	Antihypertensive agents vs. discontinue all antihypertensive agents during hospitalization	15	mRS at 14 days (or discharge) and 90 days; vascular events, recurrent stroke, and death at 90 days	No difference in death and dependency at 14 days or at discharge No difference in death or dependency at 3 months
ENOS, 2015	Randomized, open, blinded end point, controlled trial	Any stroke within 48 h after stroke, SBP 140 to 220 mm Hg	3342	Transdermal GTN vs. no transdermal GTN for 7 days/ continuing vs. stop antihypertensive agents	NA	mRS > 2 at 90 days after enrolment	Neutral effect on functional outcome at 90 days, but some benefit in a subgroup of administration within 6 h

BEST Low-Dose Beta Blockade in Acute Stroke, *INWEST* Intravenous Nimodipine West European Stroke Trial, *SCAST* the Scandinavian Candesartan Acute Stroke Trial, *VENTURE* Valsartan Efficacy on Modest Blood Pressure Reduction in Acute Ischemic Stroke, *ACCESS* Acute Candesartan Cilexetil Therapy in Stroke Survivors, *CHHIPS* Controlling Hypertension and Hypotension Immediately Post Stroke, *COSSACS* Continue or Stop Post-Stroke Antihypertensives Collaborative Study, *PRoFESS* the Prevention Regimen for Effectively Avoiding Second Stroke, *CATIS* China Antihypertensive Trial in Acute Ischemic Stroke, *ENOS* Efficacy of Nitric Oxide in Stroke, *SBP* systolic blood pressure, *DBP* diastolic blood pressure, *GTN* glyceryl trinitrate, *NA* not available, *BI* Barthel index, *mRS* modified Rankin scale, *END* early neurological deterioration

24.2.2 Pro Studies Supporting Early BP Lowering

The Acute Candesartan Cilexetil Therapy in Stroke Survivors (ACCESS, 2003) [8]: The ACCESS trial showed that, in the absence of BP lowering, candesartan for 7 days initiated within 24 h of stroke onset significantly reduced the morality and vascular events at 12 months. The trial concluded that candesartan is safe to use in the acute setting of ischemic stroke and may have therapeutic benefits, irrespective of lowering BP effect.

The Controlling Hypertension and Hypotension Immediately Post-Stroke (CHHIPS, 2009) [9]: In the CHHIPS trial, there was no difference in 14-day mortality and disability. However, the rate of 90-day mortality was reduced in receiving antihypertensive therapy, but clinical significance was borderline. In addition, there was no increase in adverse event (early neurological deterioration) in the treatment group receiving oral and sublingual lisinopril and oral and intravenous labetalol.

24.2.3 Studies with Neutral Results

- The Continue or Stop Post-Stroke Antihypertensives Collaborative Study (COSSACS, 2010) [10]: The COSSACS trial was aimed at establishing the safety and efficacy of stopping vs. continuing prior prescribed antihypertensive agents in acute ischemic stroke. Continuation of antihypertensive agents did not reduce death or dependency at 2 weeks, cardiovascular event rate, or mortality at 6 months. Furthermore, lower BP in those who continued antihypertensive agents were not associated with an increased risk in adverse events. These neutral results might be because the study was underpowered owing to early termination of the trial.
- In a substudy of the Prevention Regimen for Effectively Avoiding Second Strokes trial (PRoFESS substudy, 2009) [11]: In a substudy of the PRoFESS trial, treatment with telmisartan in 1360 patients enrolled within 72 h appeared to be safe without increasing adverse events, but was not associated with a significant effect on functional dependency, death, or stroke recurrence. The results of a substudy of the PROFESS trial suggest that it is safe to initiate antihypertensive therapy in the first 72 h after acute ischemic stroke.
- The second trial is the China Antihypertensive Trial in Acute Ischemic Stroke (CATIS, 2014) [12]: The CATIS trial concluded that the early BP lowering with antihypertensive agents had no effect on the incidence of death and major disability at 14 days or at hospital discharge when compared with the absence of treatment. There was also no difference in the rate of death or major disability at 3 months between the two groups.
- The Efficacy of Nitric Oxide in Stroke trial (ENOS, 2015) [13]: The ENOS trial demonstrated that there was a neutral effect on modified Rankin Score at 90 days with either glyceryl trinitrate (GTN) compared with no GTN or continuing prestroke antihypertensive drugs compared with stopping them temporarily. However, some benefit was reported in the subgroups given GTN within 6 h of stroke onset.
- Data from recent meta-analysis of 13 randomized controlled BP lowering trials in acute ischemic stroke showed a neutral effect of early BP lowering in the setting of acute ischemic stroke on the prevention of death, functional dependency, and recurrent vascular events including stroke [14].

24.2.4 Management of BP

Optimizing hypertensive managements in acute ischemic stroke are discussed based on the currently available evidence including results of these summarized clinical trials. The key clinical questions of early BP lowering in the setting of acute ischemic stroke include following.

When to start BP lowering? The meta-analysis of oral nimodipine trials showed a benefit from nimodipine when given within 12 h after stroke onset, no benefit between 12 and 24 h, and worse outcome when initiated after 24 h. In the SCAST, the benefit of candesartan was seen in a small subgroup started within 6 h, but when the later treatment was initiated, the more did candesartan seem to result in harm regarding the composite vascular events. Recent results of a subgroup analysis of ENOS study also found that the transdermal GTN was safe to administer and significantly associated with improved functional outcome and few deaths when treated within 6 h of stroke onset [15]. However, CHHIPS, COSSACS, CATIS, and VENTURE trials that started treatment later were all neutral or negative effect, even with a small benefit in secondary outcomes. These results, taken together, suggest that there is a small benefit in the earlier BP treatment and trend toward less benefit with increasing time to treatment. The effectiveness of the earlier BP lowering may be proven by forthcoming trials on the earlier management of hypertension in the acute phase of stroke including the earlier Rapid Intervention with Glyceryl Trinitrate in Hypertensive Stroke Trial (RIGHT) and Field Administration of Stroke Therapy-Magnesium (FAST-MAG) trial.

How fast and how much to lower BP? In the INWEST trial, the high-dose intravenous nimodipine was associated with death and dependency when DBP was lowered by more than 20% within the first 48 h after stroke onset. In post hoc analysis of the SCAST trial, large SBP decrease of more than 28 mm Hg was also significantly associated with poor functional outcome at 6 months. However, the CHHIPS trial showed that the gradually moderate BP lowering seems safe and even protective. A difference of SBP with 10 mm Hg over 24 h reduced 90-day mortality, and this did not increase early neurological deterioration at 72 h. So the rapid and large reduction of BP seems to be dangerous for patients with acute ischemic stroke. These results support a cautious BP lowering with gradual titration and modest reduction to more aggressive BP treatment targets. Current consensus guidelines recommend that a cautious BP reduction by below 15% of initial BP for the first 24 h of stroke onset should be as gradual and as modest reduction.

Is it safe to lower BP in patients with large artery stenosis? BP reduction is associated with an increased risk of early neurological deterioration and worse outcomes in some studies. The data from VENTURE trial showed the association between the early BP reduction with valsartan and the early neurological deterioration within 7 days, particularly in patients with subtype of large artery atherosclerotic stroke or significant large artery stenosis, although a causal relationship had not been demonstrated conclusively. Conversely, several data showed that BP reduction is safe in terms of early neurological deterioration and functional outcome, even in the presence of carotid artery stenosis [13]. To date, there is no specific prospective randomized trial to evaluate the impact of protocol of BP lowering in the specific subtypes of ischemic stroke. However, it is cautious to aggressive BP lowering in patients with significant large artery disease combined to poor collateral flow on vascular imaging.

Which drugs to select? Another aspect further considered is which class of antihypertensive medication is appropriate for management of acute hypertensive response, but there is no clear answer to this question as yet. Direct acting cerebral vasodilators adversely affect CBF and may be potential to increase ICP. The calcium channel blocker nimodipine had a positive effect when given orally within 12 h, but a negative effect when given intravenously in the INWEST trial. The angiotensin-converting enzyme inhibitor (ACEI) had a positive effect in the CHHIPS trial, but a neutral effect in the CATIS trial. Other trials of the angiotensin-receptor antagonist during the acute phase of stroke have shown that the drug possibly was associated with a worse outcome in the SCAST and VENTURE trials. The mixed alpha-/beta-receptor blocker (labetalol) showed a low rate of 3-month mortality in the CHHIPS trial; conversely the oral beta-blocker agents (propranolol, atenolol) were associated with a higher rate of mortality in the BEST. A recent Cochrane review addressed BP lowering in acute stroke concluded that none of BP lowering agents affected in either mortality or functional outcome [15]. In general, antihypertensive agents that have rapid onset of action and are short acting and easy to titrate are most relevant in the setting of acute ischemic stroke. The AHA/ASA guidelines recommend antihypertensive agents for acute hypertensive response that are either intravenous or transdermal agents with easy titration to consider ability to swallow (Table 24.2).

Whether previous antihypertensive agents to continue or to stop? Last issue is whether previous antihypertensive drugs should be continued or stopped temporarily during the acute phase after stroke in patients who have chronic hypertension. The COSSACS trial reported that the continuing antihypertensive agents after stroke did not change death or dependency at either 2 weeks or 6 months after stroke. The results from the ENOS trial also demonstrated that there was no difference in the rates of death or dependency and functional outcomes for continue and stop groups, but rather some secondary outcomes were worse in patients who continued their BP lowering agents. To date based on the data from these trials, it seems reasonable to stop previous BP lowering agents until patients with acute stroke are medically and neurologically stable.

Current guidelines recommend a cautious approach of BP lowering for ischemic stroke patients who are not lytic candidates, avoiding BP lowering unless BP exceeds 220/120 mm Hg at which point antihypertensive agent may be initiated (Table 24.3) [16, 17]. An exception is when other end-organ damages such as aortic dissection, acute heart failure, or hypertensive encephalopathy

Table 24.2 Pharmacological agents for early BP lowering in ischemic stroke

	Class	CBF change	Dose	Onset of action	Duration of action
Labetalol	Adrenergic antagonist beta-blocker	…	5–20 mg bolus every 15 min, up to 300 mg	5–10 min	3–6 h
Nicardipine	Calcium channel blocker	+	5–15 mg/h, increase by 2.5 mg/h every 5–10 min	5–10 min	0.5–4 h
Nitroglycerine	Nitrate	+	10–400 mg/min	1–2 min	3–5 min
Sodium nitroprusside	Nitrate	++	0.2–10 mg/kg/min	<1 min	2–5 min
Esmolol	Beta adrenergic blocker	…	250 μg/kg bolus followed by 25 to 300 g/kg/min	5 min	9 min
Enalapril	ACE inhibitor	…	1.25–5 mg every 6 h	15 min	1–4 h

CBF cerebral blood flow, *ACE* angiotensin-converting enzyme, + increase or favorable effects, ++ substantial increase or favorable effects, – decrease or negative effects, … no documented direct effect

Table 24.3 Management of hypertension in ischemic stroke

	AHA/ASA guideline (2014)	ESO guideline (2008)
Early BP lowering in the acute setting		
Patients eligible for IV tPA	• For BP > 185/110 mm Hg before initiating fibrinolytic therapy: administer IV labetalol or nicardipine	• If BP of 185/110 mm Hg or higher, lowering before thrombolysis
During and after IV tPA	• BP goal ≤180/105 mm Hg for at least the first 24 h after IV tPA	• NA
Patients treated with IAT	• Until other data become available, previously described BPs in patients undergoing other acute interventions to recanalize occluded vessels, including IAT	• NA
Patients not eligible for acute reperfusion therapy	• For SBP > 220 mm Hg or DBP > 120 mm Hg, administer labetalol IV or nicardipine as IV infusion, aiming for a 10%–15% reduction of BP	• No recommendation of routine BP lowering following acute stroke • Cautious BP lowering in patients with extremely high BPs (>220/120 mm Hg) on repeated measurements, or with severe cardiac failure, aortic dissection, or hypertensive encephalopathy

Table 24.3 (continued)

	AHA/ASA guideline (2014)	ESO guideline (2008)
Initiation or restarting BP therapy	• Initiation of antihypertensive therapy within 24 h of stroke onset • Reasonable restarting antihypertensive medications after the first 24 h for patients who have pre-existing hypertension and neurologically stable unless a specific contraindication to restarting treatment is known	• NA
Optimal antihypertensive medications	• No data available to guide selection of medications • Reasonable choices on general consensus, rapid- and short-acting antihypertensive medications (Table 5.3.4)	• NA
Management of hypertension for secondary stroke prevention		
Previously untreated patients with SBP ≥ 140 mm Hg or DBP ≥ 90 mm Hg	• BP reduction is recommended for prevention of recurrent stroke • Initiation of BP lowering after the first several days	• BP be checked regularly • BP lowering is recommended after the acute phase, including in patients with normal BP
Previously treated patients with known hypertension	• Resumption of BP therapy beyond the first several days	
Patients with SBP < 140 mm Hg and DBP < 90 mm Hg	• Initiation of BP therapy is of uncertain benefit	
Goals for target BP level	• Goals for target BP level or reduction from pretreatment baseline are uncertain and should be individualized • Reasonable to achieve a SBP < 140 mm Hg and a DBP < 90 mm Hg	
Lifestyle modification	• Salt restriction; weight loss; the consumption of a diet rich in fruits, vegetables, and low-fat dairy products; regular aerobic physical activity; and limited alcohol consumption	
Optimal drug regimen	• In recommended level, the uncertainty of optimal drug regimen • In available data, useful diuretics or the combination of diuretics and an angiotensin-converting enzyme inhibitor • The choice of specific drugs and targets should be individualized on the basis of characteristic drug and patients (extracranial cerebrovascular occlusive disease, renal impairment, cardiac disease, and DM)	
Specific indications		
Recent lacunar stroke	• Reasonable to target SBP of <130 mm Hg	• NA
Intracranial artery atherosclerotic stroke (50% to 99% stenosis of a major intracranial artery)	• Reasonable to maintenance of SBP <140 mm Hg	

tPA tissue plasminogen activator, *BP* blood pressure, *NA* not available, *SBP* systolic blood pressure, *DBP* diastolic blood pressure, *IAT* intra-arterial thrombolysis, *DM* diabetes mellitus warrant urgent BP lowering. The recommended medications for acute hypertensive response are either intravenous or transdermal agents with rapid onset and short duration of action to allow precise titration (Table 24.2). A reasonable goal for target BP is to initially lower BP by 15% of initial BP during the first 24 h of stroke onset with close monitoring for neurological deterioration related to BP lowering. The optimal time after stroke onset to start or restart long-term antihypertensive therapy has not been established, but both characteristics of patient and stroke including collateral blood flow, subtype of ischemic stroke, large artery stenosis or occlusion, comorbid illnesses, and ability to swallow must be taken into account. Despite that, it is reasonable to initiate BP lowering after the first 24 h of stroke onset because most of cases including further ischemic injury in penumbra and hemorrhagic transformation are common within the first 24 h.

24.3 Management of Acute Hypertensive Response in Patients Treated with Recanalization Therapy

The acute hypertensive response in patients who received intravenous tissue plasminogen activator (IV tPA) for ischemic stroke is frequently transient and resolves after successful recanalization [18]. Elevated BPs before and after administration of IV tPA are associated with an increased risk of hemorrhagic transformation (HT). The Safe Implementation of Thrombolysis in Stroke-International Stroke Thrombolysis Register (SITS-ISTR) showed higher symptomatic HT rate and worse outcomes in patients with elevated SBP. Interestingly, a U-shaped relationship was noted between SBP and death and dependency, with the best outcome observed in the nadir 141 and 150 mm Hg up to 24 h after IV tPA [19]. Another retrospective observational study demonstrated that acute hypertensive response occurred predominantly within the first 6 h of administration of IV tPA, but, if treated adequately, is not associated with an increased risk of HT [20]. Early BP lowering with rapidly acting antihypertensive agents appears for safety and beneficial thrombolysis among patients with acute ischemic stroke.

A pilot study of evaluating the factors associated with HT after the administration of IV tPA revealed that the elevated DBP increased the risk of HT [21]. Therefore, the investigators of the National Institute of Neurological Disorders (NINDS) study did not enroll patients with uncontrolled elevated BP. In a post hoc analysis of NINDS trial, there was no difference in rates of neurological worsening or deaths at 24 h and in rates of favorable outcomes at 3 months between hypertensive patients who received antihypertensive therapy (intravenous nitroprusside or labetalol) but no rtPA within 24 h of randomization and hypertensive patients who received neither antihypertensive therapy nor tPA. The post hoc analysis concluded that antihypertensive therapy before thrombolysis did not adversely affect the rate of favorable outcome at 3 months. Conversely, elevated BP and use of antihypertensive therapy after thrombolysis was significantly associated with a lower rate of favorable outcome at 3 months.

Current guidelines recommend the reduction of BP according to the eligibility on the NINDS tPA trial, in which a BP goal of <185/110 mm Hg should be achieved prior to initiating IV tPA and a BP of <180/105 mm Hg must be maintained in patients who received IV tPA (Table 24.3). The AHA/ASA guidelines also recommend the use of intravenous labetalol and nicardipine as the first-line antihypertensive agents. However, to date, there is not enough data from prospective randomized trial to establish the optimal BP protocol to decrease the risk of HT in patients who treated with IV tPA. The ongoing ENhanced Control of Hypertension ANd Thrombolysis strokE stuDy (ENCHANTED) may help to resolve this issue [22]. The ENCHANTED trial was designed to evaluate tissue plasminogen activator dose and/or BP lowering treatment initiated during the first 6 h after stroke. Patients were randomized to early aggressive BP lowering arm (130–140 mm Hg) or the guideline-recommended level of BP (180 mm Hg in SBP target) in patients receiving IV tPA.

Data to guide recommendations for the management of acute hypertensive response in patients undergoing intra-arterial (IA) recanalization are very limited. Recent recommendations are based on expert-derived opinion and general principles defined by observational studies [23, 24]. Prior to the procedure, the goal of BP level is not to exceed 185/110 mm Hg, especially if IA plus IV tPA is planned. During the procedure, the target BP level within 10%–20% of the baseline BP is reasonable if IA recanalization is used as monotherapy or less than 180/105 mm Hg if used with IV tPA. In the post-procedure period, the optimum BP should be titrated according to the degree of arterial recanalization. If successful reperfusion (≥thrombolysis in cerebral ischemia 2b) is achieved, then goal of BP level may be to a SBP of 120 to 140 mm Hg to reduce the risk of reperfusion hemorrhage. However, in cases of partial reperfusion, it is reasonable to maintain a SBP up to 185 mm Hg for 24 to 48 h to augment the collateral blood flow. Until more definitive data become available, the AHA/ASA's current guidelines recommend that the protocol of BP therapy for patients who received IV tPA should be followed in patients who underwent other acute interventions to recanalize occluded vessels, including IA (Table 24.3). Overall algorithm of hypertension in acute stage was illustrated in Fig. 24.1.

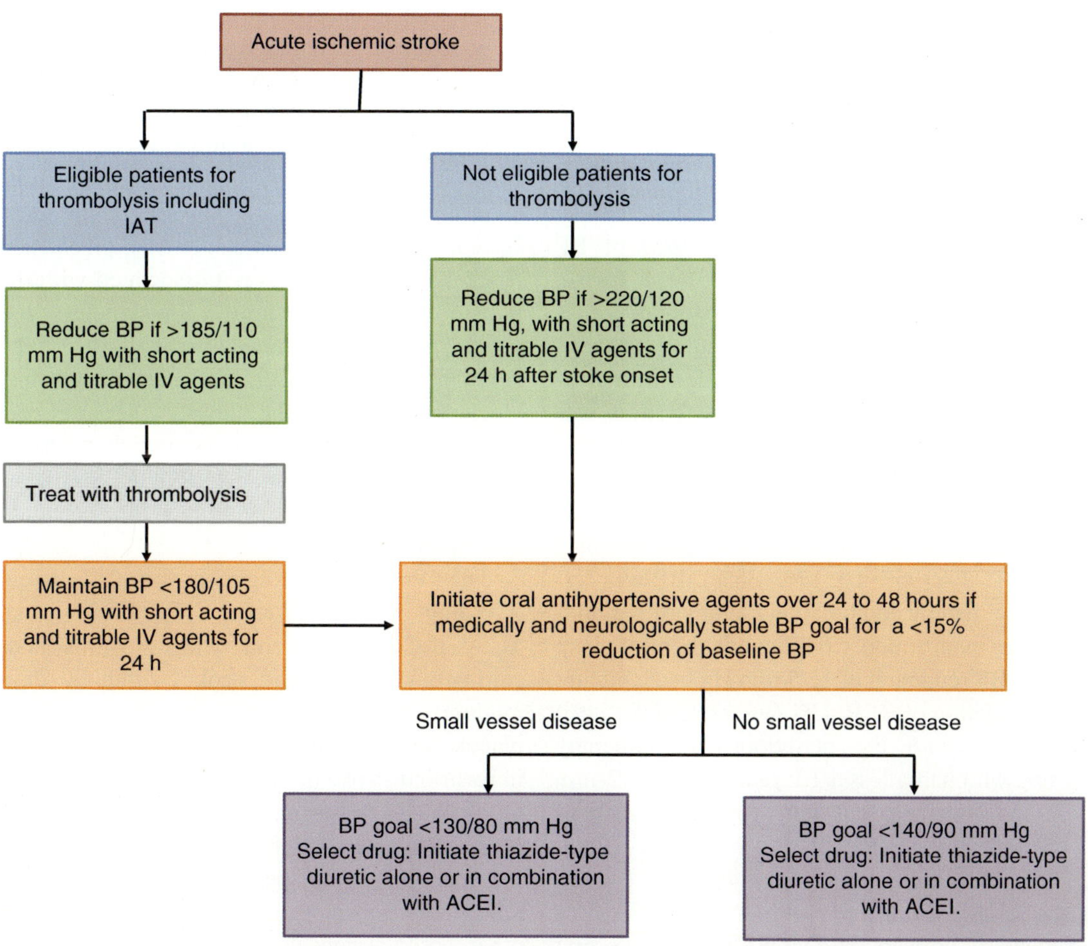

Fig. 24.1 An algorithm for hypertension management guideline

24.4 Hypertension Management to Prevent Recurrent Stroke

Hypertension is the most important modifiable risk factor to reduce recurrent stroke, accounting for 25% of attributable risk [25, 26]. However, to date, only a few randomized controlled trials have assessed BP lowering for secondary prevention of stroke in patients with stroke (Table 24.4).

The first major trial to demonstrate the effectiveness of hypertension management in secondary prevention of stroke in patients with prior stroke or TIA was the Post-Stroke Antihypertensive Treatment Study (PATS) trial [27]. This Chinese trial was a randomized, double-blinded, and placebo-controlled trial, which randomized 5665 patients with a history of any stroke or TIA to indapamide or placebo. A mean BP reduction of 12.4 mm Hg in the indapamide group significantly reduced the incidence of stroke compared with a BP reduction of 6.7 mm Hg in the placebo group (relative risk reduction [RRR], 30%; 95% confidence interval [CI], 14%–43%).

The Perindopril Protection Against Recurrent Stroke Study (PROGRESS) was large trial to clarify the association between degree of BP reduction and risk reduction of recurrent stroke. This trial randomized over 6000 patients with a history of TIA or any stroke to antihypertensive regimen of perindopril, in combination with indapamide, or placebo [28]. Randomization was stratified according to the treating physician's discretion of diuretic therapy. The BP reduction of 9/4 mm Hg in the treatment group compared with placebo reduced fatal or nonfatal stroke by a RRR of 28% (95% CI, 17%–38%). BP was further declined by combination therapy of perindopril plus indapamide. Combination therapy group with a BP reduction of 12/5 mm Hg had a greater risk reduction of RRR 43% (95% CI, 30%–54%) compared with the perindopril monotherapy group who had a lesser BP reduction of 5/3 mm Hg and nonsignificant benefit on prevention of recurrent stroke (RRR, 5%; 95% CI, 19%–23%).

The Morbidity and Mortality after Stroke, Eprosartan Compared with Nitrendipine for Secondary Prevention (MOSES) was the first trial to compare the relative benefit of particular class of antihypertensive agents for secondary prevention of stroke [29]. The trial randomized 1405 hypertensive patients with previous history of stroke or TIA to 600 mg daily of eprosartan or 10 mg daily of nitrendipine. BP reduction was similar in the two groups with a reduction of 13/3 mm Hg in the eprosartan group and 16/7 in the nitrendipine group. The composite events (death, cardiovascular events, or cerebrovascular events) were less frequent among the eprosartan group (incidence density ratio, 0.75; 95% CI, 0.66–0.96). There was a significant reduction of cerebrovascular disease including stroke or TIA (incidence density ratio, 0.75; 95% CI, 0.58–0.97); however, the most of the benefit of in cerebrovascular events in the eprosartan group was due to a reduction in the rate of TIA, with no significant difference in ischemic strokes.

The meta-analysis of ten randomized trials demonstrated that larger reductions in SBP tended to be associated with greater reduction in risk of recurrent stroke [27]. In particular, BP lowering with diuretics in alone or combination with ACEI significantly reduced the risk of stroke recurrence. However, BP lowering with renin system inhibitors, β-blockers, or calcium channel blockers used alone was not associated with the reduction of stroke recurrence; nonetheless, statistical power was limited, particularly for the assessment of β-blockers and calcium channel blockers. Therefore, the current guidelines recommend the combination of a diuretics and ACEI based on the results from the PROGRESS trial as first-line antihypertensive agents for secondary prevention of stroke.

The Prevention Regimen for Effectively Avoiding Second Strokes (PRoFESS) trial assessed 20,332 patients with previous noncardioembolic ischemic stroke within 90 days randomized to either telmisartan 80 mg daily or placebo [30]. There was no significant reduction in recurrent stroke (hazard ratio [HR], 0.95; 95% CI: 0.86 to 1.04) or major cardiovascular events (HR, 0.94; 95% CI: 0.87 to 1.01) during a mean 2.5-year follow-up period. Nonadherence to telmisartan and more aggressive treatment with other antihypertensive medications in the placebo group reduced the difference in BP between

Table 24.4 Summary of clinical trials on the management of hypertension for secondary stroke prevention

	Study design	Patients included	No. of patients	Intervention vs. control	Mean follow-up, year	Mean SBP reduction	Risk reduction of cerebrovascular events
PATS, 1995	Randomized, double-blinded, placebo-controlled trial	Recent TIA or any stroke within the prior 30 months with and without hypertension	5665	Indapamide 2.5 mg daily vs. placebo	2	SBP by 12.4/6.7 mm Hg	RRR 30% (95% CI, 14%–43%)
PROGRESS, 2001	Randomized, double-blinded, placebo-controlled trial	TIA or any stroke within the prior 5 years (mean 8 months) with and without hypertension	6105	Perindopril 4 mg daily alone vs. placebo	3.9	SBP by 9/4 mm Hg	RRR 28% (95% CI, 17%–38%)
				Perindopril 4 mg daily plus indapamide 2.5 mg daily vs. placebo		SBP by 12.3/5.0 mm Hg	RRR 43% (95% CI, 30%–54%)
MOSES, 2005	Randomized, open, blinded end point, controlled trial	TIA or any stroke within the prior 2 y with hypertensive patients	1405	Eprosartan 600 mg daily vs. nitrendipine 10 mg daily	2.5	SBP by 13.2/16 mm Hg	RRR 25%, Incidence density ratio, 0.75 (95% CI, 0.58–0.97)
PRoFESS, 2008	Randomized, double-blinded end point, controlled trial	IS within the prior 3 months (mean 15 days) with and without hypertension	20,332	Telmisartan 80 mg daily vs. placebo	2.5	SBP by 38/2.0 mm Hg	Hazard ratio 0.95 (95% CI, 0.86–1.04; $P = 0.23$)
SPS3, 2013	Randomized, open-label, controlled trial	MRI-defined symptomatic lacunar infarction within the prior 6 months	3020	SBP target of less than 130 vs. 130–149 mm Hg	3.7	After 1 year, mean SBP 127 mm Hg (95% CI, 126–128)/ mean SBP 138 mm Hg (95% CI, 137–139)	Hazard ratio 0.81 (95% CI, 0.64–1.03; $P = 0.08$)

PATS Post-Stroke Antihypertensive Treatment Study, *PROGRESS* Perindopril Protection Against Recurrent Stroke Study, *MOSES* Morbidity and Mortality After Stroke, Eprosartan Compared with Nitrendipine for Secondary Prevention, *PRoFESS* Prevention Regimen for Effectively Avoiding Second Strokes, *SPS3* Secondary Prevention of Small Subcortical Strokes, *TIA* transient ischemic attack, *SBP* systolic blood pressure, *RRR* relative risk reduction, *CI* confidence interval the treatment groups (SBP of 5.4 mm Hg at 1 month and 4.0 mm Hg at 1 year) and may have reduced the impact of treatment on stroke recurrence. In addition, the authors attributed the lack of benefit in the BP lowering to the lower mean BP reduction in the study group than PROFESS study and modest BP reduction in the telmisartan group. Although previous trials have proven the benefits of BP reduction for secondary prevention of stroke, whether there is superior benefit of BP lowering by a certain amount or to optimal BP goal remains uncertain.

Recently published Secondary Prevention of Small Subcortical Strokes (SPS3) trial demonstrated the role of aggressive BP lowering in patients with a recent symptomatic MRI-confirmed lacunar infarct [31]. All 3020 patients were randomized to either the lower-target group of SBP (<130 mm Hg) or the higher-target group of SBP (range 130–149 mm Hg). Primary outcome was all recurrent stroke. There were almost 20% nonsignificant reductions in all stroke (HR, 0.81; 95% CI, 0.64–1.03; $P = 0.08$), disabling or fatal stroke (HR, 0.81; 95% CI, 0.53–1.23; $P = 0.32$), and the composite outcome of myocardial infarction or vascular death (HR, 0.84; 95% CI, 0.68–1.04; $P = 0.32$) with the lower target. In addition, the rate of intracerebral hemorrhage was significantly reduced (HR, 0.37; 95% CI, 0.15–0.95; $P = 0.03$). Serious adverse events were not different between the lower-target BP lowering and the higher-target BP lowering group. The results from the SPS3 trial suggest that a target BP of <130 mm Hg was not only safe and well-tolerated, but also reduced the risk of recurrent stroke, especially hemorrhagic stroke over a period of 3–4 years. The SPS3 trial suggest lower BP goal in patients with recent lacunar infarct than those with other subtype of ischemic stroke.

The 2014 AHA/ASA's recent guideline recommends that an "absolute target BP level and reduction are uncertain and should be individualized." The guideline also recommends that the target level of BP lowering in patients with recent small vessel disease is 130/80 mm Hg based on results from the SPS3 trial. However, to date, there is no data from large randomized trials to establish guideline of hypertension management for secondary prevention of stroke in patients with other subtypes of ischemic stroke except those with small vessel disease. Recent study reported that patients who had ischemic stroke or TIA attributable to 70%–99% stenosis of a major intracranial artery, and in whom an aggressive medical management strategy including the achievement of a SBP < 140 mm Hg, had fewer recurrent cerebrovascular events compared with those who had a similar medical management strategy plus intracranial angioplasty and stenting [32]. Another subgroup analysis in nonsurgical controls from the Carotid Occlusion Surgery Study (COSS) study reported lower recurrent stroke in the individuals maintaining a follow-up BP of 130/85 mm Hg or lower in patients with symptomatic carotid artery occlusion and hemodynamic cerebral ischemia [33]. Further studies are necessary to establish the individualized hypertension management in consideration of specific subtype of ischemic stroke, major large artery occlusion, and comorbidities.

Conclusions

Regardless of active research, an optimal strategy for hypertension management in acute stroke remains unclear. Current guidelines for BP management in acute stroke are based largely on expert opinion and a paucity of high-quality evidence. Recent evidences suggest that active BP lowering in acute ischemic stroke is feasible and safe, but data showing an effect on death or functional outcome are controversial. Early BP reduction in ischemic stroke is cautious because inducing large or rapid BP changes in penumbral, at-risk tissue with altered cerebral autoregulation may be causative of secondary brain injury. Therefore, antihypertensive agents that have rapid onset and are short acting and easy to titrate are preferred in the setting of acute stroke. As the current evidence is insufficient to guide the choice of antihypertensive agents, selection of drugs should be decided on a case-by-case basis in consideration of pharmacological and patient's characteristics. Based on the current evidences, an optimal strategy of BP therapy might be to withheld antihypertensive agents in the first 12 to 24 h after stroke onset and then to initiate oral antihypertensive agents beyond 24 to 48 h to avert secondary injury. It is ensured that long-term hypertension treatment for secondary prevention of recurrent stroke will be transitioned when medical and neurological stability is achieved. Furthermore, different strategies are required to manage hypertension for secondary prevention of recurrent stroke in different subtypes of ischemic stroke. Overall, many questions remain about hypertension management of patients with ischemic stroke; thus additional studies are necessary to establish the optimal strategy of high BP management.

Suggestions from Current Clinical Practice Guidelines In general, it is recommended that blood pressure is not actively controlled until reaching >220/120 mm Hg, and it is reasonable that blood pressure control is initiated "after the first several days" to stroke patients with sustained increased blood pressure (>140/90 mm Hg). For patients who are eligible for intravenous fibrinolysis, blood pressure should be slowly lowered to <185/110 mm Hg.

References

1. Leonardi-Bee J, Bath PMW, Phillips SJ, et al. Blood pressure and clinical outcomes in the international stroke trial. Stroke. 2002;33:1315–20.
2. CAST (Chinese Acute Stroke Trial) Collaborative Group. CAST: randomised placebo-controlled trial of early aspirin use in 20,000 patients with acute ischaemic stroke. Lancet. 1997;349:1641–9.
3. Sandset EC, Bath PM, Boysen G, et al. The angiotensin-receptor blocker candesartan for treatment of acute stroke (SCAST): a randomised, placebo-controlled, double-blind trial. Lancet. 2011;377:741–50.
4. Castillo J, Leira R, García MM, et al. Blood pressure decrease during the acute phase of ischemic stroke is associated with brain injury and poor stroke outcome. Stroke. 2004;35:520–6.
5. Barer DH, Cruickshank JM, Ebrahim SB, et al. Low dose beta blockade in acute stroke ("BEST" trial): an evaluation. Br Med J (Clin Res Ed). 1988;296:737–41.
6. Ahmed N, Nasman P, Wahlgren NG. Effect of intravenous nimodipine on blood pressure and outcome after acute stroke. Stroke. 2000;31:1250–5.
7. Oh MS, Yu KH, Hong KS, et al. Modest blood pressure reduction with valsartan in acute ischemic stroke: a prospective, randomized, open-label, blinded-endpoint trial. Int J Stroke. 2015;10:745–51.
8. Schrader J, Luders S, Kulschewski A, et al. The ACCESS study: evaluation of acute candesartan cilexetil therapy in stroke survivors. Stroke. 2003;34:1699–703.
9. Potter JF, Robinson TG, Ford GA, et al. Controlling hypertension and hypotension immediately post-stroke (CHHIPS): a randomised, placebo-controlled, double-blind pilot trial. Lancet Neurol. 2009;8:48–56.
10. Robinson TG, Potter JF, Ford GA, et al. Effects of antihypertensive treatment after acute stroke in the Continue or Stop Post-Stroke Antihypertensives Collaborative Study (COSSACS): a prospective, randomised, open, blinded-endpoint trial. Lancet Neurol. 2010;9:767–75.
11. Bath PM, Martin RH, Palesch Y, et al. Effect of telmisartan on functional outcome, recurrence, and blood pressure in patients with acute mild ischemic stroke: a PRoFESS subgroup analysis. Stroke. 2009;40:3541–6.
12. He J, Zhang Y, Xu T, et al. Effects of immediate blood pressure reduction on death and major disability in patients with acute ischemic stroke: the CATIS randomized clinical trial. JAMA. 2014;311:479–89.
13. ENOS Trial Investigators, Bath PM, Woodhouse L, et al. Efficacy of nitric oxide, with or without continuing antihypertensive treatment, for management of high blood pressure in acute stroke (ENOS): a partial-factorial randomised controlled trial. Lancet. 2015;385:617–28.
14. Lee M, Ovbiagele B, Hong KS, et al. Effect of blood pressure lowering in early ischemic stroke: meta-analysis. Stroke. 2015;46:1883–9.
15. Bath PM, Krishnan K. Interventions for deliberately altering blood pressure in acute stroke. Cochrane Database Syst Rev. 2014;10:CD000039.
16. Jauch EC, Saver JL, Adams HP Jr, et al. Guidelines for the early management of patients with acute ischemic stroke: a guideline for healthcare professionals from the American Heart Association/American Stroke Association. Stroke. 2013;44:870–947.
17. European Stroke Organisation (ESO) Executive Committee. Guidelines for management of ischaemic stroke and transient ischaemic attack 2008. Cerebrovasc Dis. 2008;25:457–507.
18. Delgado-Mederos R, Ribó M, Rovira A. Prognostic significance of blood pressure variability after thrombolysis in acute stroke. Neurology. 2008;71:552–8.
19. Ahmed N, Wahlgren N, Brainin M, et al. Relationship of blood pressure, antihypertensive therapy, and outcome in ischemic stroke treated with intravenous thrombolysis: retrospective analysis from Safe Implementation of Thrombolysis in Stroke-International Stroke Thrombolysis Register (SITS-ISTR). Stroke. 2009;40:2442–9.
20. Aiyagari V, Gujjar A, Zazulia AR, et al. Hourly blood pressure monitoring after intravenous tissue plasminogen activator for ischemic stroke: does everyone need it? Stroke. 2004;35:2326–30.

21. Levy DE, Brott TG, Haley EC Jr, et al. Factors related to intracranial hematoma formation in patients receiving tissue-type plasminogen activator for acute ischemic stroke. Stroke. 1994;25:291–7.
22. Huang Y, Sharma VK, Robinson T, et al. Rationale, design, and progress of the ENhanced Control of Hypertension ANd Thrombolysis strokE stuDy (ENCHANTED) trial: An international multicenter 2×2 quasi-factorial randomized controlled trial of low- vs. standard-dose rt-PA and early intensive vs. guideline-recommended blood pressure lowering in patients with acute ischaemic stroke eligible for thrombolysis treatment. Int J Stroke. 2015;10: 778–88.
23. Leslie-Mazwi TM, Sims JR, Hirsch JA, et al. Periprocedural blood pressure management in neurointerventional surgery. J Neurointerv Surg. 2011;3:66–73.
24. Tarlov N, Nien YL, Zaidat OO, et al. Periprocedural management of acute ischemic stroke intervention. Neurology. 2012;79(13 Suppl 1):S182–91.
25. Hong KS, Yegiaian S, Lee M, et al. Declining stroke and vascular event recurrence rates in secondary prevention trials over the past 50 years and consequences for current trial design. Circulation. 2011;123: 2111–9.
26. Park TH, Ko Y, Lee SJ, et al. Identifying target risk factors using population attributable risks of ischemic stroke by age and sex. J Stroke. 2015;17:302–11.
27. Liu L, Wang Z, Gong L, et al. Blood pressure reduction for the secondary prevention of stroke: a Chinese trial and a systematic review of the literature. Hypertens Res. 2009;32:1032–40.
28. PROGRESS Collaborative Group. Randomised trial of a perindopril-based blood-pressure-lowering regimen among 6,105 individuals with previous stroke or transient ischaemic attack. Lancet. 2001;358:1033–41.
29. Schrader J, Lüders S, Kulschewski A, et al. Morbidity and mortality after stroke, eprosartan compared with nitrendipine for secondary prevention: principal results of a prospective randomized controlled study (MOSES). Stroke. 2005;36:1218–26.
30. Yusuf S, Diener HC, Sacco RL, et al. Telmisartan to prevent recurrent stroke and cardiovascular events. N Engl J Med. 2008;359:1225–37.
31. SPS3 Study Group, Benavente OR, Coffey CS et al. Blood-pressure targets in patients with recent lacunar stroke: the SPS3 randomised trial. Lancet. 2013;382:507–15.
32. Derdeyn CP, Chimowitz MI, Lynn MJ, et al. Aggressive medical treatment with or without stenting in high-risk patients with intracranial artery stenosis (SAMMPRIS): the final results of a randomised trial. Lancet. 2014;383:333–41.
33. Powers WJ, Clarke WR, Grubb RL, et al. Lower stroke risk with lower blood pressure in hemodynamic cerebral ischemia. Neurology. 2014;82:1027–32.

25 Diabetes Management After Stroke

Seung-Hoon Lee and Dong-Wan Kang

Abstract

Together with hypertension and dyslipidemia, diabetes is an important conventional risk factor for vascular events, including stroke. The prevalence of diabetes has increased dramatically worldwide, and its importance has increased. Diabetes is a prognosticator that influences both the incidence and recurrence of stroke and functional outcome and survival poststroke. Therefore, it is critical to diagnose diabetes as early as possible from the initial hospitalization and to maintain normoglycemia appropriately. During the chronic stage of stroke, the principles of diabetes management are not different from those for diabetes without stroke. Although numerous antidiabetic agents have been developed in recent years, it is difficult for stroke physicians to completely understand the therapeutic principles. In this chapter, we will guide you through the essence of diabetes management during the acute and chronic stages of stroke.

This chapter describes treatment during the acute stage and long-term management of diabetes in ischemic stroke patients. Diabetes is an important vascular risk factor with a rapidly increasing prevalence and critical impact on stroke. Since many excellent antidiabetic drugs have been developed, the therapeutic principles of diabetes have become increasingly complex. For physicians treating acute stroke, it is imperative to be familiar with the latest diabetes care principles. However, stroke physicians who do not have a deep knowledge of diabetes are more likely to be exposed to biased treatment because of the availability of numerous antidiabetic drugs and the influence of the pharmaceutical companies' marketing. However, stroke physicians should not only rely on consulting with diabetes physicians, without any prior knowledge. In this chapter, we will guide you in the practical ways of diabetes management after stroke for most readers except diabetes specialists.

S.-H. Lee, M.D., Ph.D., F.A.H.A., (✉)
D.-W. Kang, M.D.
Department of Neurology, Seoul National University Hospital, Seoul, South Korea
e-mail: sb0516@snu.ac.kr

S.-H. Lee (ed.), *Stroke Revisited: Diagnosis and Treatment of Ischemic Stroke*,
Stroke Revisited, DOI 10.1007/978-981-10-1424-6_25

25.1 The Effect of Diabetes on Stroke

Diabetes is a well-established and strong risk factor for stroke that has a negative impact on the natural course of stroke, i.e., its progression, recovery, recurrence, and prognosis. The paradox associated with alcohol, obesity, or smoking, which might produce some positive effects on vascular events in other aspects, is not at all relevant for diabetes. The risk of stroke in diabetic patients is about 2–3 times higher than in nondiabetic individuals. As diabetes is a common disease affecting more than 300 million people worldwide, considering the prevalence of diabetes, one in eight or nine cases of stroke can be attributed to diabetes [1]. While the effect of diabetes on stroke development is greater at an older age, it is also understood that impaired glucose tolerance (IGT)—the prediabetes stage—also has a slightly higher risk of stroke, albeit not as much as diabetes. Hence, the early diagnosis and management of diabetes are more important now than ever.

The negative effects of diabetes on stroke outcome have been mainly attributed to persistent and excess hyperglycemia. Hyperglycemia, which occurs after a stroke, either due to diabetes or not, causes additional damage to the brain tissue during the acute stroke period. However, in nondiabetic patients, hyperglycemia that is generally caused by a stress response is transient during the acute stage and not severe enough to have a significant effect on the outcome. In this context, we must understand the pathophysiology of the harmful effects of hyperglycemia [2]. First, hyperglycemia causes anaerobic glycolysis leading to direct tissue damage by promoting lactic acidosis. Second, hyperglycemia-induced mitochondrial dysfunction leads to apoptosis-like cell death in ischemic penumbra. Finally, hyperglycemia activates lipoxygenase and cyclooxygenase pathways and increases expression of several pro-inflammatory cytokines; this in turn may promote sterile inflammation. Some clinical studies indicate that hyperglycemia might increase the infarct volume measured on magnetic resonance imaging and induce hemorrhagic transformation and poor outcome. The abovementioned mechanisms induced by hyperglycemia are likely to work in clinical circumstances. Hyperglycemia during the acute stroke period may be an epiphenomenon due to an acute stress response especially in nondiabetic patients, but the consensus is that excessive hyperglycemia should be adjusted to an appropriate level.

Diabetes has a strong effect on the long-term outcome after stroke. Stroke patients with diabetes are more likely to have recurrent strokes, about two times more than nondiabetic patients. In addition, diabetes is associated with increased long-term functional deficit and mortality after stroke. Therefore, stroke physicians should not limit the treatment of diabetes only to the early stages of stroke. Continuous management of diabetes is an essential part of poststroke management due to its long-lasting harmful effects on the recovery phase after a stroke.

25.2 Differential Influence of Diabetes on Stroke Mechanism

Stroke occurs by a variety of mechanisms. Acute coronary syndrome is mostly caused by atherosclerosis, while stroke is a syndrome of various causes, including three major etiologies: large artery atherosclerosis (LAA), small vessel occlusion (SVO), and cardioembolism (CE). Hyperlipidemia affects most strongly in LAA, but hypertension is the most important factor in SVO. Atrial fibrillation is the most common cause of cardioembolism. It is interesting to understand how diabetes affects each stroke subtype in this respect. Unfortunately, few studies have been successful in this regard; a single-center-based study [3] and a meta-analysis [4] have provided some insight into the impact of diabetes on the stroke subtypes. These studies revealed that diabetes was a major risk factor for LAA but has little effect on SVO and CE. Is this differential effect expected?

The most common complications of diabetes—also termed as diabetic triopathy—are retinopathy, neuropathy, and nephropathy. These are all microvascular complications due to diabetes, while stroke and acute coronary syndromes typically present as macrovascular complications. In diabetes, microvascular complications are more common and important, and it is often the case that the effect of diabetes on stroke is the greatest in lacunar infarction or intracerebral hemorrhage because these conditions are typical manifestations of cerebral small vessel diseases. However, diabetes has little effect on cerebral small vessel diseases and has the greatest impact on LAA-related stroke. How do we interpret this? Since there have been no studies or opinions to explain this discrepancy, we hope you will read it now, considering that it is my opinion to correct the misunderstanding about diabetes.

As microvascular complication, the blood vessels involved by diabetes are anatomically capillaries. Diabetic microvascular complications occur because of a long-term progressive decrease in the function of the organs due to diminished capillary circulation in a certain area of the retina, neuron, or nephron. The characteristics of these diseases include vascular involvement at the capillary level and the progressive decrease in organ function. In stroke, lacunar infarction or intracerebral hemorrhage is caused by small vessel disease. The small vessels referred to here are not capillaries but penetrating arteries (small-sized arteries or large-sized arterioles) with diameters of 100–800 micrometers. In fact, stroke rarely occurs due to capillary level problems except during cerebral cavernous malformation-related hemorrhage. Penetrating arteries are the blood vessels most affected by long-standing hypertension, as the arterial blood pressure is transmitted to these vessels without any significant loss. On the other hand, at the capillary level, blood pressure sharply declines, so hypertension results in little damage to these vessels. Therefore, SVO in stroke is completely different from the microvascular complications caused by diabetes in terms of the level of the affected vessels. Nevertheless, due to the term "microvascular," many researchers and physicians have a confusion that the lacunar infarction of stroke is a part of the microvascular complications of diabetes or that it is strongly related, due to a lack of understanding of vascular anatomy and diabetes in the brain. Hypertension-induced physical damage and secondary degeneration (called arteriolosclerosis or lipohyalinosis) are the main cause of SVO, and the influence of diabetes is limited in this condition. The main mechanism of vascular compromise in diabetes is metabolic derangement caused by hyperglycemia. It is understood that the effects of diabetes on LAA may be associated with facilitation of atheroma progression induced by long-standing hyperglycemia.

Let me summarize my opinion as follows: first, diabetes induces microvascular complications due to metabolic dysfunction caused by hyperglycemia, which leads to disruption of capillary microcirculation. Second, at the large artery level, metabolic dysfunction due to hyperglycemia increases progression or vulnerability of atheromatous plaques. Finally, at the level of penetrating arteries, the physical damage caused by blood pressure is the most critical factor. Long-standing hypertension plays a major role in stroke development, but diabetes does not. Understanding of these differential impacts of diabetes on systemic vascular beds will be a great help in risk factor control to prevent different vascular events.

25.3 Diabetes Management During Acute Stroke Period

25.3.1 Patients with Diabetes

About 10–20% of stroke patients have diabetes, and many of them are diagnosed with previously unrecognized diabetes. The diagnosis of diabetes is based on the following: (1) fasting glucose level (≥126 mg/dL), (2) oral glucose tolerance test (≥200 mg/dL at 2 h), (3) HbA1c level (≥6.5%), and (4) a random plasma glucose (≥200 mg/dL in a patient with classic symptoms of hyperglycemia or hyperglycemic crisis) [5]. HbA1c is very useful in the diagnosis of unrecognized diabetes in patients with stroke. Diabetes is generally diagnosed by fasting glucose level, but this is likely to be increased due to stress hyperglycemia in acute stroke. HbA1c is little altered by acute stroke.

How do we control hyperglycemia in diabetic patients with acute stroke? The American Stroke Association guidelines recommend that glucose-lowering therapy be initiated when blood glucose is greater than 200 mg/dL (11 mmol/L) and should be maintained at 140–180 mg/dL [6, 7]. There are few comparative studies on the different classes of glucose-lowering therapy in acute stroke, so the protocol for this should be adjusted according to the circumstances and experience in each center. If glycemic control with non-insulin antidiabetic agent is tolerable, these drugs need not be changed to insulin therapy. Since non-insulin antidiabetic agents are difficult to titrate quickly, insulin therapy might be more effective if hyperglycemia persists in the early stages of stroke. Patients who have extreme or persistent hyperglycemia, are critically ill, or require endovascular therapy or enteral tube feeding may require an intravenous insulin injection on admission. In this situation, capillary glucose should be checked hourly until the insulin drip rate is stabilized. When the glycemic condition improves, it should be changed to basal-bolus subcutaneous insulin injection. Basal-bolus injection rather than insulin sliding is recommended, because insulin sliding is a reactive approach to blood glucose treatment, resulting in a roller-coaster effect, whereas basal-bolus insulin injection may proactively regulate glucose levels. Table 25.1 is an example of a basal-bolus subcutaneous insulin injection protocol [8].

How do we treat the stroke patients with unrecognized diabetes? There is no reason why the treatment of these patients should be different from those with already known diabetes. It should be remembered that more severe hyperglycemia may occur in patients with unrecognized diabetes. If the treatment of hyperglycemia is delayed, the long-term prognosis of the patient may be worse.

Table 25.1 Example of a subcutaneous insulin injection regimen

I. Check capillary blood glucose
1. "Before meals and at bedtime" or "before meals, bedtime, and 03:00"
2. "Every 6 h" for patients on continuous tube feeds or NPO
II. Scheduled subcutaneous insulin
1. Total daily dose of insulin
(a) 0.4–0.5 units/kg body weight
(b) Recommend use ½ daily dose as basal and other ½ as prandial
2. Basal insulin
(a) Glargine once daily
(b) Detemir once or twice daily
(c) NPH twice daily
3. Prandial insulin
(a) Lispro, aspart, or glulisine immediately before or after meals
(b) Regular insulin 30 min prior to meals
(c) Patients with inconsistent oral intake: give reduced prandial dose of insulin based on the percent of meal ingested (e.g., if 50% of calories are ingested, give 50% of the dose)
4. Supplemental/correction insulin (regular insulin, lispro, aspart, glulisine) added to dose of scheduled insulin
(a) Before meals, add supplemental insulin dose (# of units) from table below to scheduled insulin dose
(b) At bedtime, add ½ of supplemental insulin dose

Blood glucose (mg/dL)	Insulin sensitive	Usual	Insulin resistant
<141	0	0	0
141–180	1	2	4
181–220	2	4	6
221–260	4	6	8
261–300	6	8	10
301–350	8	10	12
351–400	10	12	14
>400	12	14	16

Usual column: patients expected to eat all or most of his/her meals
Insulin sensitive column: patients not able to eat, elderly patients
Insulin resistant column: patients receiving corticosteroids
Select appropriate column for supplemental insulin in case of persistent hyperglycemia or hypoglycemic episode
Reproduced by permission of Endocrinology and Metabolism Clinics of North America

25.3.2 Nondiabetic Patients

Hyperglycemia after stroke also occurs frequently in nondiabetic patients. One meta-analysis reported that hyperglycemia during the acute stroke period increased inhospital or 30-day mortality by about threefold [9]. In this analysis, it is difficult to conclude that hyperglycemia produced an independent negative effect because more severe stroke is associated with higher glucose levels. Therefore, there has been a long debate about whether hyperglycemia should be controlled in nondiabetic patients. There has been only one clinical trial to address this question, the GIST-UK trial [10]. In this study, patients with hyperglycemia after stroke (diabetic 17%, nondiabetic 83%) received a glucose-potassium-insulin infusion (n = 464) in the treatment group, while the control group received a saline infusion (n = 469). Outcomes of this study were 90-day death and severe disability. Unfortunately, the study was terminated early because of delayed recruitment and limitations of financial resources. In this underpowered study, blood glucose control with insulin infusion had no effect on the outcomes. There have been no other studies examining this issue, so the effect of blood glucose control in acute stroke cannot be concluded. However, insulin therapy did not show any tendency of improvement in nondiabetic stroke patients in this study, and we do not need to make any fuss about it. In our opinion, if blood glucose is episodically over 200 mg/dL in nondiabetic patients, it is better to observe it without treatment. Blood glucose control should be considered if the level is consistently above 200 mg/dL and should be maintained at 140–180 mg/dL according to the current guideline recommendation. The possibility of unrecognized diabetes should be investigated using HbA1c.

25.4 Long-Term Management of Diabetes After Stroke

Most clinical practice guidelines or textbooks on stroke rarely get into the specifics of diabetes management. They usually refer readers to the current guidelines from diabetes organizations such as the American Diabetes Association. In fact, there is no reason for long-term management of diabetes to be different in the presence or absence of stroke. Based on the principles of diabetes management, it may not be so difficult even to stroke physicians. However, the actual situation during the acute stage of stroke is not so comfortable for them, because of the complicated categories of diabetes medications and the new drugs that become available each year, and diabetes physicians often intervene in consultation. The situation may vary greatly from one country to another, but such consultations often exacerbate a simple problem. Unfamiliar with stroke situations, they may easily provide an insulin prescription during the acute stage, although the use of non-insulin antidiabetic agents is preferable, and the insulin therapy might persist for a long time without being noticed by the stroke physicians. Insulin therapy should be restricted to special situations or to patients with advanced diabetes, because of the risk of frequent hypoglycemia and low compliance due to its invasiveness. In this case, diabetes control may become worse, and the possibility of recurrence of the vascular event may increase. Even with a diabetes consultant, stroke physicians must understand the basics of diabetes care and the concept of antidiabetic drug use. This is because diabetes management is a long and distant voyage from the beginning to prevent the patient from driving the wrong way.

Before going into the details on diabetes care, just remember one principle. Stroke causes stress hyperglycemia. If needed, insulin therapy should be used temporarily to control this but should be discontinued when the patient is stable. In the same way, when the dosage of non-insulin antidiabetic agent is increased during the acute stage, it should be reduced during the chronic stage. Glucose monitoring should be performed frequently at least during the 3 months after stroke along with appropriate adjustment of antidiabetic medications. The following is a summary of the core content of long-term diabetes management. We have tried to describe the approach of antidiabetic medications from mild to severe diabetes to make it as easy as possible, even if you are unfamiliar with diabetes care.

25.4.1 Principles of Diabetes Management After Stroke

After the acute stroke period, glycemic control focuses on long-term diabetes care for secondary prevention of stroke. Pharmacological treatments are not different from general glucose-lowering therapy, and glycemic goals are also the same. However, we should carefully consider the patient's neurological disability (e.g., dysphagia, cognitive dysfunction, and motor weakness) and other medications to develop an effective treatment strategy and achieve good drug adherence.

25.4.2 Lifestyle Management

Lifestyle management is essential for all patients during the entire treatment period. It is even more important than taking any antidiabetic medications. Diabetes is a disease that requires more thorough lifelong self-management than any other conventional vascular risk factor such as hypertension or dyslipidemia. Thus, physicians should educate and support patients to manage diabetes by themselves through self-monitoring of blood glucose, diet and weight control, physical activity, and quitting smoking. Appropriate lifestyle management is effective not only in reducing weight, improving the quality of life, and reducing medical costs but also in reducing HbA1c, which is the ultimate goal of diabetes.

Specifically, every diabetic patient should receive individualized nutritional therapy or counseling. To adhere to a healthy eating pattern, nutritional diet should focus on personal and cultural preferences. Diabetic patients should also exercise at a moderate-to-vigorous intensity at least three times per week for more than 150 min, and this physical activity should not be discontinued for two consecutive days. All kinds of cigarettes including electronic cigarettes should be stopped. Emotional support is also essential, and screening for distress from diabetes can help physicians to intervene in the early stages of distress.

25.4.3 Non-insulin Antidiabetic Agents

It is best to follow the ADA/European Association for the Study of Diabetes guidelines for treatment with non-insulin antidiabetic agents (Fig. 25.1) [11]. As soon as stress hyperglycemia after stroke is stabilized, long-term management should begin. HbA1c is the standard for assessing long-term glycemic control. In general, HbA1c should be as low as 7%, but 8% is acceptable when patients have a history of severe hypoglycemia, a short life expectancy, or comorbidities such as vascular complications.

For initial monotherapy, metformin is first recommended unless there is a contraindication. This is because it is cheap and has high efficacy, low risk of weight gain and hypoglycemia, and evidence of cardiovascular risk reduction. In addition, moderate chronic kidney disease (eGFR $\geq$30 mL/min/1.73 m^2) patients can also use metformin. In case of gastrointestinal trouble as a side effect of metformin, consider changing medications to another class. Physicians should keep in mind that metformin can cause vitamin B12 deficiency. They should regularly check vitamin B12 levels and suspect vitamin B12 deficiency in cases of anemia or peripheral neuropathy in patients taking metformin.

If HbA1c does not reach the target by 3 months, consider dual therapy by adding a second medication to metformin. Dual therapy from the beginning is also possible for patients with HbA1c $\geq$9% since a submaximal dose of combination therapy is more effective than a maximal dose of monotherapy and has fewer side effects. There are many types of non-insulin antidiabetic agents both currently available and under development that are known to decrease HbA1c by about 1%, albeit demonstrating slight differences in their efficacies. Since there is no clearly superior medication, the choice should be made based on personal preference, cost, comorbidity, and especially side effects such as hypoglycemia and weight gain. Currently, non-insulin antidiabetic agents are classified as a thiazolidinedione, dipeptidyl peptidase 4 (DPP-4) inhibitor,

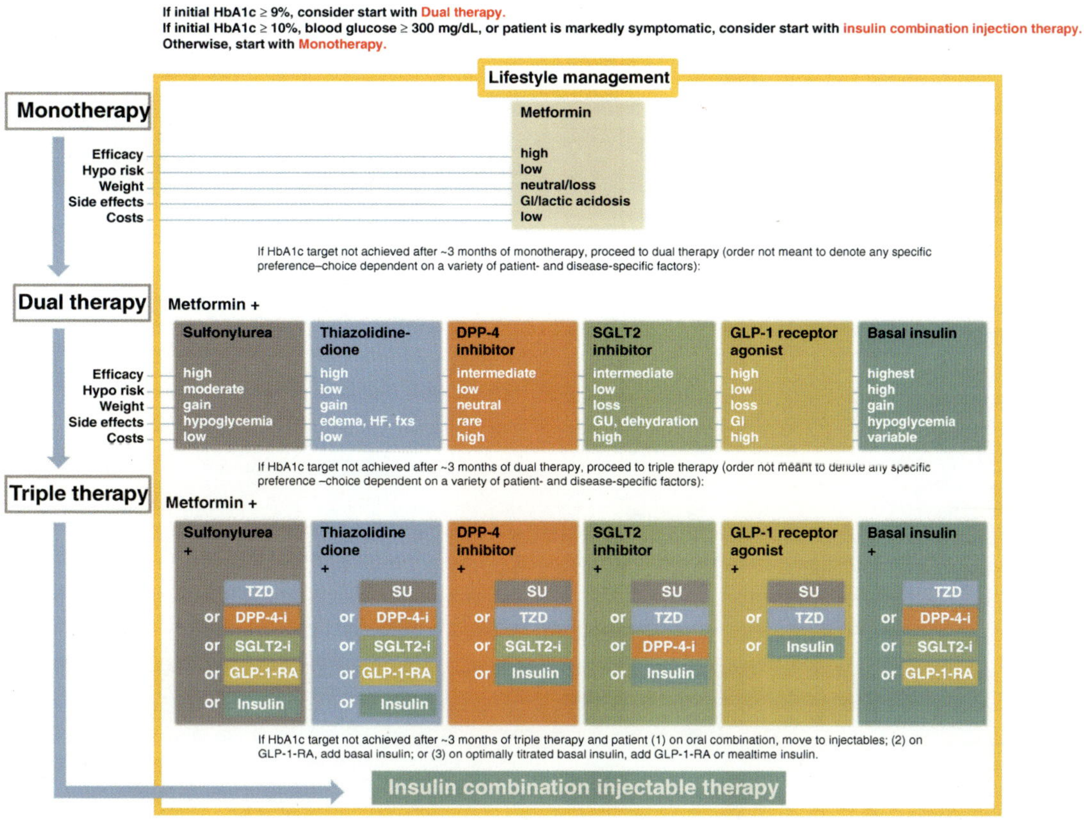

Fig. 25.1 The stepwise approach to antidiabetic agents for patients with type 2 diabetes. Lifestyle management should be encouraged in all steps. Start monotherapy first unless special conditions are written on top of the figure and advance to the bottom as needed. The order of the medications is not meant to denote any specific preference (See Fig. 25.2 for insulin combination injectable therapy.) Abbreviations: *HbA1c* glycated hemoglobin, *Hypo* hypoglycemia, *GI* gastrointestinal, *HF* heart failure, *fxs* fractures, *GU* genitourinary, *TZD* thiazolidinedione, *DPP-4-i* DPP-4 inhibitor, *SGLT2-i* SGLT2 inhibitor, *GLP-1-RA* GLP-1 receptor agonist, *SU* sulfonylurea (Reproduced by permission of Diabetes Care [11])

sodium-glucose cotransporter-2 (SGLT2) inhibitor, glucagon-like peptide-1 (GLP-1) receptor agonist, or sulfonylurea in addition to metformin. Basal insulin may be another option for dual therapy. Although most combinations are possible, the combination of DPP-4 inhibitor and GLP-1 receptor agonist is not recommended due to their similar mechanisms of action. The differential characteristics of each class of non-insulin antidiabetic agent are shown in Table 25.2.

If dual therapy is not effective at lowering HbA1c to a therapeutic target by 3 months, consider triple therapy. Again, as mentioned above, individualized consideration is needed to select the third medication, and other factors such as poor lifestyle management or drug compliance should be checked cautiously. For example, careless addition of medication to a patient with poor glycemic control due to irregular eating habits can increase the risk of hypoglycemia. Finally, insulin combination injectable therapy should be considered when triple therapy also fails to lower HbA1c to a target by 3 months or from the beginning of the pharmacologic treatment when (1) initial HbA1c ≥10%, (2) blood glucose ≥300 mg/dL, or (3) a patient is markedly symptomatic.

Table 25.2 Antidiabetic agents for use in diabetes

Class	Drug (brand name)	Effect on premeal glucose	Effect on postmeal glucose	Relative HbA1c lowering	Expected decrease in HbA1c	Hypoglycemia risk	Weight	Effect in CV outcome trial	Other therapeutic considerations
Metformin	Glucophage, Glumetza	++	+	↓↓	1.0–1.5%	Negligible	Neutral	–	– Improved cardiovascular outcomes in overweight subjects – Contraindicated if CrCl/eGFR <30 mL/min or hepatic failure – Vitamin B12 deficiency – GI side effects
Alpha-glucosidase inhibitor	Acarbose (Glucobay)	0	++	↓	0.6%	Negligible	Neutral	–	– GI side effects
DPP-4 inhibitor	Alogliptin (Nesina) Sitagliptin (Januvia) Saxagliptin (Onglyza) Linagliptin (Tradjenta)	+	++	↓↓	0.7%	Negligible	Neutral	Neutral	– Rare cases of pancreatitis
GLP-1 receptor agonist	Albiglutide (Eperzan) Dulaglutide (Trulicity) Exenatide (Byetta) Exenatide QW (Bydureon) Liraglutide (Victoza)	+	+++	↓↓ to ↓↓↓	1.0%	Negligible	↓↓	Superiority in T2DM patients with clinical CVD (liraglutide)	– Nausea, vomiting – Administration parenteral – Rare cases of pancreatitis – Parafollicular cell hyperplasia – Contraindicated with personal/family history of medullary thyroid cancer or multiple endocrine neoplasia syndrome type 2
Insulin secretagogue	**Sulfonylurea** Gliclazide (Diamicron, Diamicron MR) Glimepiride (Amaryl) Glyburide (Diabeta, Euglucon)	++	++	↓↓	0.8%	Minimal/moderate Moderate Significant	↑	–	– Relatively rapid BG-lowering response – Consider using other class(es) of antidiabetic agents first in patients at high risk of hypoglycemia (e.g., the elderly, renal/hepatic failure)
	Meglitinide Nateglinide (Starlix) Repaglinide (GlucoNorm)	+	++	↓ to ↓↓	0.7%	Minimal/moderate	↑	–	

Thiazolidinedione (TZD)	Pioglitazone (Actos) Rosiglitazone (Avandia)	++	+	↓↓	0.8%	Negligible	↑↑	Neutral	– Mild BP lowering – May induce edema and/or congestive heart failure – Contraindicated in patients with known clinical heart failure or evidence of left ventricular dysfunction – Higher rates of heart failure when combined with insulin – Higher occurrence of fractures – Possibility of increased risk of myocardial infarction with rosiglitazone – Rare risk bladder cancer with pioglitazone
SGLT2 inhibitor	Canagliflozin (Invokana) Dapagliflozin (Farxiga) Empagliflozin (Jardiance)	++	++	↓↓ to ↓↓↓	0.7–1.0%	Negligible	↓	Superiority in T2DM patients with clinical CVD (empagliflozin)	– Genital infections, UTI, hypotension, dose-related changes in LDL-C, caution with renal dysfunction and loop diuretics, dapagliflozin not to be used if bladder cancer, rare diabetic ketoacidosis

(continued)

Table 25.2 (continued)

Class	Drug (brand name)	Effect on premeal glucose	Effect on postmeal glucose	Relative HbA1c lowering	Expected decrease in HbA1c	Hypoglycemia risk	Weight	Effect in CV outcome trial	Other therapeutic considerations
Insulin	**Bolus (prandial) insulins** *Rapid-acting analogues* Aspart (NovoRapid) Glulisine (Apidra) Lispro (Humalog) *Short-acting* Regular (Humulin R) **Basal insulins** *Intermediate-acting* NPH (Humulin N) *Long-acting basal analogues* Detemir (Levemir) Glargine (Lantus) **Premixed insulins** Premixed regular NPH (Humulin 30/70) Biphasic insulin aspart (NovoMix 30) Insulin lispro/lispro protamine suspension (Humalog Mix25, Mix50)	+++	+++	↓↓↓	0.9–1.1%	Significant (highest with regular and NPH insulin)	↑↑↑	Neutral (glargine)	– Potentially greatest HbA1c reduction and no maximal dose – Numerous formulations and delivery systems – Allows for regimen flexibility

BG Blood glucose, *BP* blood pressure, *CrCl* creatinine clearance, *DPP-4* dipeptidyl peptidase 4, *eGFR* estimated glomerular filtration rate, *GI* gastrointestinal, *GLP-1* glucagon-like peptide-1

Reproduced by permission of Canadian Journal of Diabetes

25.4.4 Insulin Therapy

As previously mentioned, basal insulin alone is a convenient once-daily regimen and can be considered in combination therapy with metformin. Long-acting basal insulin such as glargine, detemir, and degludec has low risk of hypoglycemia. The starting dose of basal insulin is 10 units/day or 0.1–0.2 units/kg/day, and adjustment is needed according to fasting blood glucose.

Due to the progressive nature of type 2 diabetes, a large proportion of patients with type 2 diabetes eventually need a more intense insulin regimen with an additional prandial dose, i.e., insulin combination injectable therapy (Fig. 25.2). When the HbA1c target is not achieved after thorough

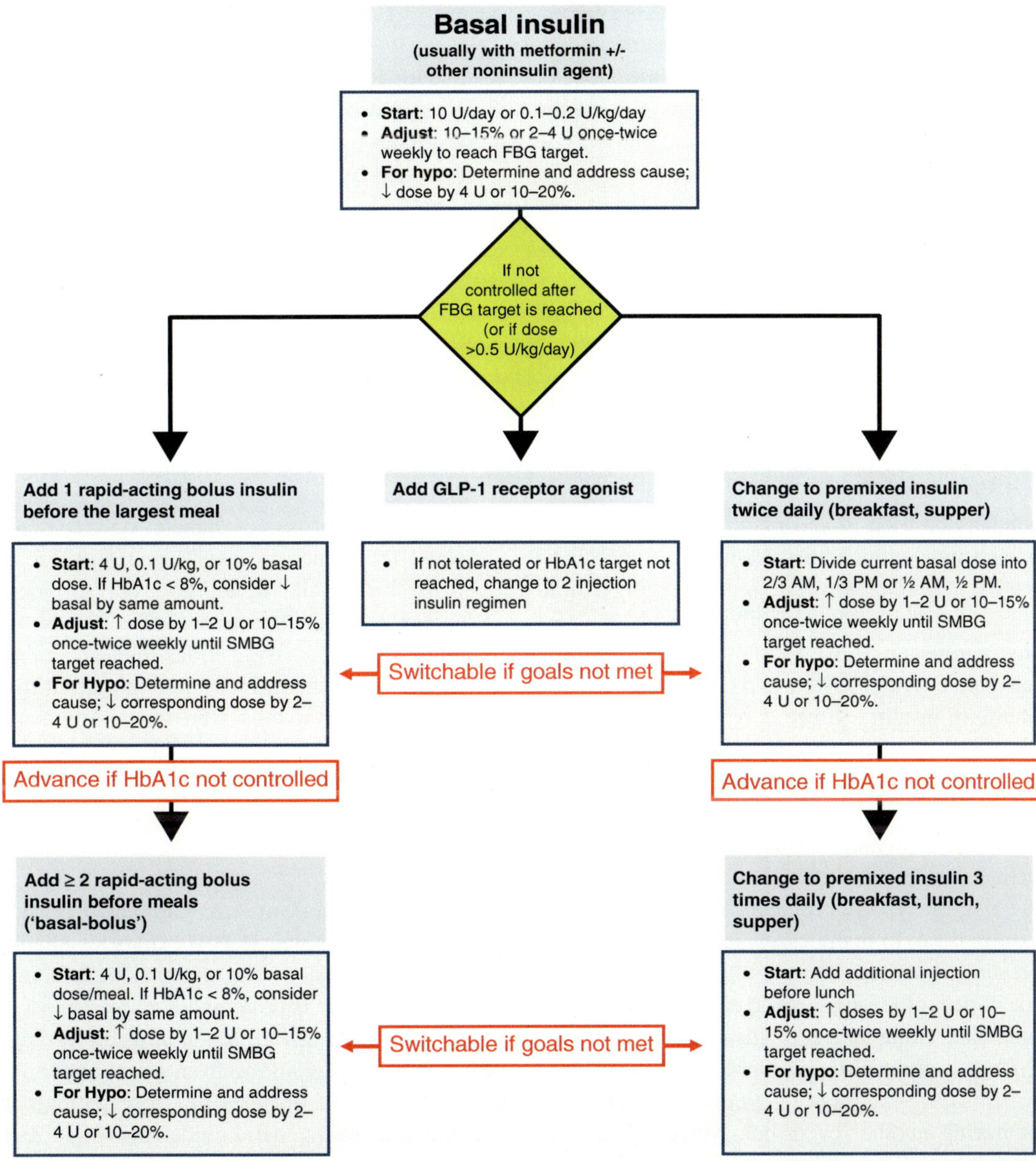

Fig. 25.2. The stepwise intensification of the insulin combination injectable therapy. Once an insulin combination injectable therapy is chosen, dose titration of both basal and bolus insulin is important based on self-monitoring of blood glucose. For insulin-treated patients, educating how to adjust insulin dose and avoid hypoglycemia is critically important as well as lifestyle management such as exercise and diet control. Abbreviations: *hypo* hypoglycemia, *U* unit(s), *HbA1c* glycated hemoglobin, *SMBG* self-monitoring of blood glucose (Reproduced by permission of Diabetes Care [11])

adjustment of basal insulin so that fasting blood glucose is in the range 80–130 mg/dL or after triple therapy, insulin combination injectable therapy should be considered as follows: (1) basal insulin + single rapid-acting insulin at the largest meal, (2) basal insulin + GLP-1 receptor agonist, or (3) two daily injections of premixed insulin. Metformin can be maintained, but other non-insulin antidiabetic agents, such as the sulfonylurea, DPP-4 inhibitor, and GLP-1 receptor agonists, are recommended to be discontinued to avoid an unnecessarily complex regimen. Since thiazolidinediones or SGLT2 inhibitors can help to lower the insulin dose, they may be adjunctively used carefully in case a large dose of insulin is required.

Rapid-acting bolus insulin, lispro, aspart, and glulisine, can be started with 4 units, 0.1 unit/kg, or 10% of basal dose before meals. If HbA1c <8% when the bolus insulin is started, the basal insulin dose can be reduced to avoid hypoglycemia. Then, increase the dose of rapid-acting bolus insulin for a target postprandial blood glucose <180 mg/dL, and decrease the dose when hypoglycemia occurs. Premixed insulin, such as NPH/regular 70/30, lispro 50/50, and aspart 70/30, is a formulation that contains both basal and prandial components. If one insulin combination injectable therapy is ineffective, consider selecting another regimen from the others. If it is still ineffective, consider the next step regimens: (1) basal-bolus regimen with ≥2 injections of bolus insulin and (2) three times daily premixed insulin regimen.

If you inevitably started insulin in the post-stroke diabetic patients, you should consider withdrawal or dose reduction of insulin by 10–20% at discharge. After acute illness, as both patient insulin sensitivity and activity levels rise, the risk of hypoglycemia increases at the same insulin dose. In many cases, insulin is carelessly prescribed after discharge, which is never good for a patient's long-term glycemic control and outcome. Compliance of insulin is worse than that of non-insulin antidiabetic agents. Once patients have experienced hypoglycemia, the fear of having another event can worsen their drug compliance. Thus, when patients are stabilized after a stroke, physicians must actively consider using non-insulin antidiabetic agents. If insulin therapy is still needed after discharge, patients must be educated about self-management of hypoglycemia. When hypoglycemic symptoms develop, patients should take half a cup of orange juice, 3–4 candies, or a tablespoon of sugar and be guided to reason out by themselves as to the cause of their hypoglycemia to prevent repeat events.

Conclusion

When a stroke patient is hospitalized, a stroke physician must establish an appropriate diagnosis and treatment plan for diabetes as early as possible. Unrecognized diabetes should be identified using HbA1c levels, and if positive, normoglycemia needs to be maintained during admission. For nondiabetic patients, transient hyperglycemia does not need to be controlled via glucose-lowering therapies. When insulin therapy is used temporarily in diabetic patients during the acute stage of stroke, stroke physicians should consider changing to non-insulin antidiabetic agents during the chronic phase. The negative effects of diabetes on the occurrence, recurrence, recovery, and survival of stroke are certain. In addition, due to recent increases in the prevalence of diabetes, its influence is increasing more than any other risk factor. In this context, it is important that the stroke physicians who deal with acute stroke fully understand diabetes treatment in the chronic stage of stroke as well as the acute stage.

Suggestion from Current Clinical Practice Guidelines Screening tests for diabetes should be conducted to all stroke or transient ischemic attack. HbA1c test is preferable (≥6.5%) in acute stroke period because of less confusion in diagnosis of diabetes resulting from stress hyperglycemia. Control of diabetes in stroke patients is not different from general guidelines (Figs. 25.1 and 25.2).

References

1. Luitse MJ, Biessels GJ, Rutten GE, et al. Diabetes, hyperglycaemia, and acute ischaemic stroke. Lancet Neurol. 2012;11:261–71.
2. Kruyt ND, Biessels GJ, Devries JH, et al. Hyperglycemia in acute ischemic stroke: pathophysiology and clinical management. Nat Rev Neurol. 2010;6:145–55.
3. Kim BJ, Lee SH, Kang BS, et al. Diabetes increases large artery diseases, but not small artery diseases in the brain. J Neurol. 2008;255:1176–81.
4. Schulz UG, Rothwell PM. Differences in vascular risk factors between etiological subtypes of ischemic stroke: importance of population-based studies. Stroke. 2003;34:2050–9.
5. American Diabetes Association. 2. Classification and diagnosis of diabetes. Diabetes Care. 2017;40:S11–24.
6. Jauch EC, Saver JL, Adams HP Jr, et al. Guidelines for the early management of patients with acute ischemic stroke: a guideline for healthcare professionals from the American Heart Association/American Stroke Association. Stroke. 2013;44:870–947.
7. Mccormick MT, Muir KW, Gray CS, et al. Management of hyperglycemia in acute stroke: how, when, and for whom? Stroke. 2008;39:2177–85.
8. Mcdonnell ME, Umpierrez GE. Insulin therapy for the management of hyperglycemia in hospitalized patients. Endocrinol Metab Clin North Am. 2012;41:175–201.
9. Capes SE, Hunt D, Malmberg K, et al. Stress hyperglycemia and prognosis of stroke in nondiabetic and diabetic patients: a systematic overview. Stroke. 2001;32:2426–32.
10. Gray CS, Hildreth AJ, Sandercock PA, et al. Glucose-potassium-insulin infusions in the management of post-stroke hyperglycaemia: the UK Glucose Insulin in Stroke Trial (GIST-UK). Lancet Neurol. 2007;6:397–406.
11. Inzucchi SE, Bergenstal RM, Buse JB, et al. Management of hyperglycemia in type 2 diabetes, 2015: a patient-centered approach: update to a position statement of the American Diabetes Association and the European Association for the Study of Diabetes. Diabetes Care. 2015;38:140–9.

26 Cholesterol Management After Stroke

Tae-Jin Song

Abstract

Dyslipidemia has generally been accepted as a cause of various cardio-cerebrovascular diseases (stroke, myocardial infarction, peripheral vascular disease) and is especially important factor for ischemic stroke. In stroke patients, underlying cause of dyslipidemia should be identified, and lifestyle modification together with medication is essential for the treatment. The first goal for treatment of dyslipidemia in ischemic stroke patients is to lower low-density lipoprotein cholesterol, and the secondary goal is to lower non-high-density lipoprotein cholesterol level. Based on the results of Stroke Prevention by Aggressive Reduction in Cholesterol Levels (SPARCL) study, which is the only randomized controlled study for secondary stroke prevention, moderate- to high-intensity statin is strongly recommended in patient with non-cardiogenic stroke. Preventive power of statin therapy is higher in large atherosclerosis stroke subtype than others. Moreover, statin treatment should be considered to prevent recurrent stroke, beyond treating dyslipidemia, as to its pleiotropic and protective mechanism. However, adverse effects of statin such as hepatotoxicity, myopathy, and increased blood glucose level are more frequent with intensive-dose statin. Therefore, careful consideration is mandatory for cholesterol management after stroke, particularly in statin.

Dyslipidemia is a major risk factor for ischemic stroke. There are many kinds of cholesterols in the blood such as total cholesterol, LDL, HDL, and TG. Among these, LDL cholesterol is well known as a risk factor for ischemic stroke and cardiovascular disease. In this chapter, cholesterol management in ischemic stroke patients mainly about LDL cholesterol and statin use will be discussed.

T.-J. Song, M.D., Ph.D.
Department of Neurology, Ewha Womans University School of Medicine, 1071 Anyangcheon-ro, Yangcheon-gu, Seoul 158-710, South Korea
e-mail: knstar@ewha.ac.kr

S.-H. Lee (ed.), *Stroke Revisited: Diagnosis and Treatment of Ischemic Stroke*, Stroke Revisited, DOI 10.1007/978-981-10-1424-6_26

26.1 Cholesterol Management After Stroke

Dyslipidemia can result from various kinds of disease conditions, and a secondary cause that elevates LDL cholesterol should be identified and treated. In recent guideline, making decision for treatment includes overall consideration of risk for cardiovascular disease and level of low-density lipoprotein (LDL). Coronary artery disease, peripheral vascular disease, ischemic stroke and atherosclerotic disease (aortic aneurysm, transient ischemic attack, severe carotid artery stenosis), or diabetes mellitus, risk factor for coronary artery disease (smoking, hypertension, low high-density lipoprotein [HDL] cholesterol, family history of early coronary artery disease, age), and LDL level are considered to decide treatment of dyslipidemia and can be a monitoring goal for the treatment. Statin is the first drug of choice to treat dyslipidemia, and goal level for the LDL cholesterol is determined considering the risk of cardiovascular disease. The primary goal for treatment is to lower LDL cholesterol to targeted level, and the secondary goal is to lower non-HDL cholesterol level [1].

Meanwhile, based on results of Stroke Prevention by Aggressive Reduction in Cholesterol Levels (SPARCL) study, which is the only randomized controlled study for secondary stroke prevention, moderate- to high-intensity statin is strongly recommended in patients with non-cardiogenic stroke [2]. SPARCL study included 4731 stroke or transient ischemic attack patients without coronary artery disease and compared atorvastatin 80 mg and placebo group, setting stroke recurrence as a primary end point. Subjects had history of stroke within 1–6 months before enrollment, mean age was 63 years old, and LDL-C level at the inclusion time was 133 mg/dL. Ischemic stroke patients were 67%, transient ischemic attack patients 30%, and hemorrhagic stroke patients 2%. In statin group, primary end point fatal and nonfatal stroke incidence showed 15% relative risk reduction in 5 years and 2.2% absolute risk reduction, and the number needed to treatment (NNT) was 230 in 1 year. This study was conducted to stroke patients due to large artery atherosclerosis, small artery occlusion, and other or undetermined etiology, excluding cardiogenic stroke. In the case of large artery atherosclerosis, carotid stenosis and non-stenosis group was separately compared using atorvastatin, and reduction of stroke incidence was higher in carotid stenosis group (RRR 33% vs. 10%). This result showed that effect of atorvastatin is different according to the subtype of stroke.

Based on the results of SPARCL, American Heart Association (AHA) and American Stroke Association (ASA) recommend statin use in the presence of cardiovascular disease or symptomatic atherosclerotic stroke, the goal for the treatment is LDL cholesterol lower than 100 mg/dL, and intensive treatment is recommended in high-risk patients with multiple risk factors. Also, atherosclerotic stroke patient without cardiovascular disease and with normal cholesterol level is recommended to use statins [1].

26.2 Controversy for Hemorrhagic Stroke

In epidemiologic studies, there is controversy whether dyslipidemia is a risk factor for stroke. But statin use, which is a typical treatment for dyslipidemia, is proven to lower the risk of stroke in many clinical studies. But association between low cholesterol level and intracranial hemorrhage in some studies gave a pause to aggressive use of high-dose statins. In particular, considering that the incidence of intracranial hemorrhage is higher in Korea compared to Western countries, it is a major concern. In Heart Protection Study using 40 mg of simvastatin, subgroup analysis on patients with history of stroke did not show reduction of total (both ischemic and hemorrhagic) stroke occurrence and raised the risk of intracranial hemorrhage. SPARCL provided evidence for statin treatment to prevent stroke recurrence, but risk of intracranial hemorrhage became an issue. In subgroup analysis for risk factor of intracerebral hemorrhage in SPARCL study, male and elderly patient had higher rate of intracerebral hemorrhage, and among the risk factors, history of old hemorrhage was highly associated. But the level of LDL cholesterol at the enrollment and follow-up did not appear to be associated with occurrence of intracranial hemorrhage [2]. In conclusion, careful approach is needed and further evidence is mandatory to clarify hemorrhagic risk from statin use.

26.3 Target Level of LDL Cholesterol for Stroke Prevention

Currently, there is no large data from randomized control study about LDL level and secondary prevention of stroke. Thus, target LDL level for the secondary prevention of stroke is uncertain. But post-analysis of SPARCL study showed low LDL cholesterol group below 70 mg/dL had 28% risk reduction (HR, 0.72; 95% CI, 0.59–0.89; $p = 0.0018$) of recurrent stroke without raising risk of intracranial hemorrhage (HR, 1.28; 95% CI, 0.78– 2.09; $p = 0.3358$). In the meta-analysis of 26 primary and secondary stroke prevention clinical trials about safety and effectiveness of aggressive LDL cholesterol-lowering therapy ($n = 170{,}000$), LDL cholesterol decreased by 1 mmol/l had an effect of 22% reduction of stroke incidence (RR, 0.78, 95% CI 0.76–0.80; $p < 0.0001$), and the risk of intracranial hemorrhage did not increase [3]. These studies recommend to control LDL cholesterol level in secondary prevention of stroke, but currently Treat Stroke to Target (TST) trial (ClinicalTrials.gov; unique identifier, NCT01252875) is progressing and yet to be concluded. For the effect of low-dose statin in Asian population, Japan Statin Treatment Against Recurrent Stroke (J-STARS, ClinicalTrials.gov; unique identifier, NCT00221104) using pravastatin 10 mg is currently progressing.

26.4 The New Guideline for Treatment of Dyslipidemia

AHA and ASA announced revised guideline for the prevention of stroke and transient ischemic attack recently [4]. It is based on 2013 ACC/AHA guideline, but some items have been changed and new recommendations are added. The new supplementary part is that statin should be given to patients with atherosclerotic stroke subtype or transient ischemic attack, even with clinically low risk of atherosclerotic cardio-cerebrovascular disease (ASCVD) and low LDL cholesterol level less than 100 mg/dL for its lipid-modifying effect. As 2013 ACC/AHA guideline did not suggest target level of LDL cholesterol, also the new guideline for secondary prevention of stroke did not include target level. For this guideline is based on randomized trials carried out only in the USA, there are some limitations to apply directly to Asian population, and additional data for rational difference is required for proper guideline.

The new ACC/AHA guideline has changed its target from measuring cholesterol level and selecting population for therapy and guiding drug dosage. Instead, guidelines defined statin benefit groups for drug treatment to reduce risk for atherosclerotic cerebrovascular disease: "Individuals with (1) clinical ASCVD, (2) primary elevations of LDL-C ≥190 mg/dL, (3) diabetes aged 40 to 75 years with LDL-C 70 to 189 mg/dL and without clinical ASCVD, or (4) without clinical ASCVD or diabetes and LDL-C 70 to 189 mg/dL and estimated 10-year ASCVD risk ≥7.5%." Clinical atherosclerotic cerebrovascular disease includes atherosclerotic ischemic stroke or TIA, a history of acute coronary syndromes, angina, or coronary or other peripheral revascularization. For individuals with clinical ASCVD and are ≤75 years of age, LDL-C ≥ 190 mg/dL, or have DM and a 10-year risk of ASCVD estimated at ≥7.5%, high-dose statin is recommended. Moderate-dose statin is recommended for the other groups (Fig. 26.1) (Table 26.1) [1].

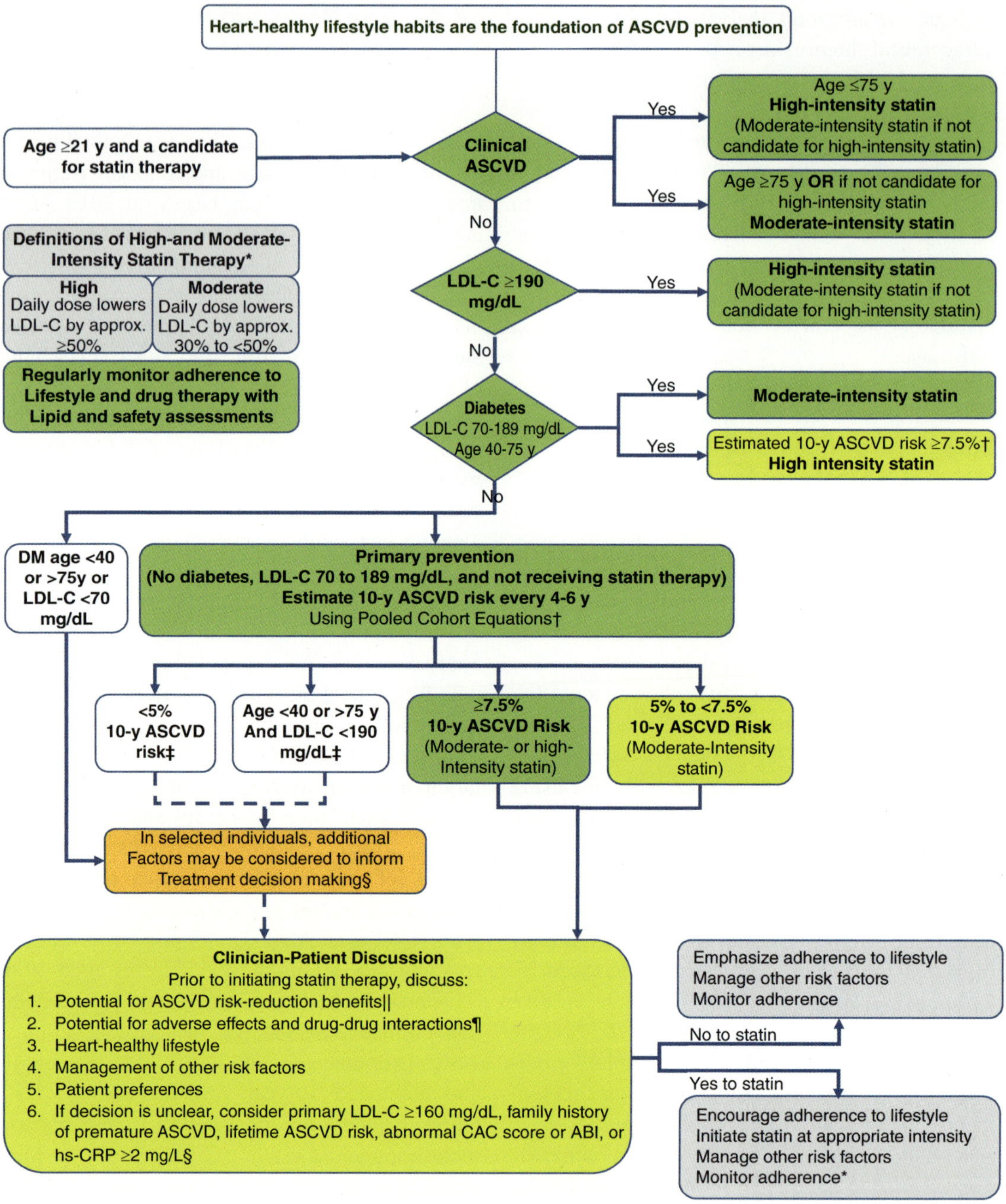

Fig. 26.1 Summary of statin initiation recommendations for the treatment of blood cholesterol to reduce atherosclerotic cardio-cerebrovascular disease (ASCVD) risk in adults [1]. Colors correspond to the classes of recommendation (green, Class I; yellow, Class IIa; orange, Class IIb). Assessment of the potential for benefit and risk from statin therapy for ASCVD prevention provides the framework for clinical decision making incorporating patient preferences. *Percent reduction in LDL-C can be used as an indication of response and adherence to therapy but is not in itself a treatment goal. †The pooled cohort equations can be used to estimate 10-year ASCVD risk in individuals with and without diabetes. The estimator within this application should be used to inform decision making in primary prevention patients not on a statin. ‡Consider moderate-intensity statin as more appropriate in low-risk individuals. §For those in whom a risk assessment is uncertain, consider factors such as primary LDL-C ≥ 160 mg/dL or other evidence of genetic hyperlipidemias, family history of premature ASCVD with onset <55 years of age

Table 26.1 High-, moderate-, and low-intensity statin therapy

High-intensity statin therapy	Moderate-intensity statin therapy	Low-intensity statin therapy
Daily dose lowers LDL-C, on average, by approximately ≥50%	Daily dose lowers LDL-C, on average, by approximately 30% to <50%	Daily dose lowers LDL-C, on average, by <30%
Atorvastatin (40)–80 mg Rosuvastatin 20 (40) mg	Atorvastatin 10 (20) mg Rosuvastatin (5) 10 mg Simvastatin 40 (80) mg Lovastatin 40 mg Fluvastatin XL 80 mg Fluvastatin 40 mg/bid Pitavastatin 2–4 mg	Simvastatin 10 mg Pravastatin 10–20 mg Lovastatin 20 mg Fluvastatin 20–40 mg Pitavastatin 1 mg

Reproduced by permission of Circulation [1]

26.5 Statin, HMG-CoA Reductase Inhibitor, Pharmacologic Characteristics of Statin

Statin has significant LDL-C-lowering effect, and it also has TG-lowering, HDL-C-uprising effect. Its side effects are relatively rare, and with good tolerability, statin is commonly used to treat dyslipidemia nowadays [5]. Currently used statin formulations are as follows (Table 26.2).

26.5.1 Action Mechanism

Statin inhibits HMG-CoA reductase (2-hydroxy-3-methylglurary1-coenzyme A reductase), which is a rate-limiting enzyme for synthesis of cholesterols. Consequentially, production of cholesterol in the liver decreases which leads to reduction of intracellular cholesterol level, and expression of LDL receptor in the liver cell surface makes cholesterols in the blood get into the liver cells and serum cholesterol level decreases. VLDL synthesis declines in the liver via LDL receptor which inducing VLDL elimination. TG level goes down, and apolipoprotein B-100 synthesis is inhibited. Statin actions in cholesterol synthesis pathway, reduction of farnesyl pyrophosphate, and isoprenylated protein synthesis by decreased geranylgeranyl pyrophosphate, which results in reduced activity of rhoA, ras, and rac1 inflammatory markers. Furthermore, statin ameliorates endothelial cell function by inhibiting cell proliferation related to atherosclerosis progression and reduction of high-sensitivity C-reactive protein (hs-CRP); thrombogenic factors and inflammatory factors make pleiotropic effects additive to anti-atherosclerotic effect. As cholesterol synthesis mainly occurs in the night, statin should be administrated before

in a first-degree male relative or <65 years of age in a first-degree female relative, hs-CRP ≥2 mg/L, CAC score ≥ 300 Agatston units, or ≥75th percentile for age, sex, and ethnicity (for additional information, see http://www.mesa-nhlbi.org/CACReference.aspx), ABI <0.9, or lifetime risk of ASCVD. Additional factors that may aid in individual risk assessment may be identified in the future. ||Potential ASCVD risk reduction benefits. The absolute reduction in ASCVD events from moderate- or high-intensity statin therapy can be approximated by multiplying the estimated 10-year ASCVD risk by the anticipated relative risk reduction from the intensity of statin initiated (~30% for moderate-intensity statin or ~45% for high-intensity statin therapy). The net ASCVD risk reduction benefit is estimated from the number of potential ASCVD events prevented with a statin, compared to the number of potential excess adverse effects. ¶Potential adverse effects. The excess risk of diabetes is the main consideration in ~0.1 excess cases per 100 individuals treated with a moderate-intensity statin for 1 year and ~0.3 excess cases per 100 individuals treated with a high-intensity statin for 1 year. In RCTs, both statin-treated and placebo-treated participants experienced the same rate of muscle symptoms. The actual rate of statin-related muscle symptoms in the clinical population is unclear. Muscle symptoms attributed to statin therapy should be evaluated. *ABI* indicates ankle-brachial index, *ASCVD* atherosclerotic cardiovascular disease, *CAC* coronary artery calcium, *hs-CRP* high-sensitivity C-reactive protein, *LDL-C* low-density lipoprotein cholesterol, *MI* myocardial infarction, and *RCT* randomized controlled trial. Reproduced by permission of Circulation [1]

Table 26.2 Effect and pharmacological characteristics of currently used statins

	Lovastatin	Pravastatin	Simvastatin	Fluvastatin	Atorvastatin	Rosuvastatin	Pitavastatin
Daily dose, mg	20–40	10–40	20–40	20–80	10–80	5–20	1–4
LDL-C TG HDL-C							
−24–−28% −8% 4%	20	20		40			1
−30–−36% −13–−10% 6%	40	40	20	80	10		2
−39–−45% −13–−23% 5–8%	80		40		20	5 ~ 10	4
−46–−52% −20–−28% 2–10%					40–80	20	
Metabolism	CYP3A4	sulfonylation	CYP3A4	CYP2C9	CYP3A4	CYP2C9	Glucuronidation, CYP2C9
Protein binding, %	>95	43–67	95–98	98	98	88	>99
Half-life, hour	2–4	2–3	1–3	0.5–3	13–30	19	−12
Hydrophilic	No	Yes	No	No	No	Yes	No
Excretion	Hepatobiliary	Hepatobiliary	Hepatobiliary	Hepatobiliary	Hepatobiliary	Hepatobiliary	Hepatobiliary
Renal excretion, %	10	20	13	<6	<2	28	15

sleep, but atorvastatin, rosuvastatin, pitavastatin have long half-life and thus morning administration is possible. Lovastatin drug absorption increases and reaches higher drug level when administrated with meal. LDL metabolism and statin action were briefly illustrated in Fig. 26.2.

26.5.2 Lipid-Modifying Effect

Statin is the most effective drug in lowering LDL-C (18–55%), also decreases TG (7–30%), and increases HDL-C (5–15%). Currently used statins have different dose-related lipid-lowering effects (Table 26.2). Statin has serum lipoprotein cholesterol-lowering effect by inhibiting cholesterol synthesis in the liver and decreasing serum low-density lipoprotein or TG-rich lipoproteins. Low-density lipoprotein cholesterol decreases in a log-linear dose-dependent pattern when treated with statin; double-dose statin has 6–7% more effects on lowering LDL-C than standard baseline dose (rule of six or seven).

26.5.3 Indication and Selection of Drugs

Other than IIa dyslipidemia with elevated LDL-C only, mixed dyslipidemia with elevated LDL-C and TG is also indicated to statin therapy. When choosing statin, pretreatment LDL-C level and target level according to the cardiovascular risk should be considered. In particular, high-risk groups with cardiovascular disease, high-dose statin with larger LDL-C-lowering effect, and drug with high-dose-related effects are considered.

26.5.4 Maintaining Statin

After 3 years after acute myocardial infarction, drug compliance was 50%. So, additional attentions are needed to continue the therapy. Discontinuation of statin leads to worsening of lipid profile including increased LDL-C to pretreatment level in 2–3 months. LDL-C level increases by 30–40% in 2–3 months after stopping taking statin. In addition, in case of acute coronary syndrome, discontinuation group had four times more frequent coronary events and deaths compared to statin treatment group and two times more frequent events than non-statin treatment group. This is probably due to anti-inflammatory, antithrombotic, anti-oxidative effect of statin rather than lipid-modifying effect. So, continued therapy is important, especially in acute phase of cardiovascular disease, as statin discontinuation increases coronary events and cardiovascular diseases and mortality [6].

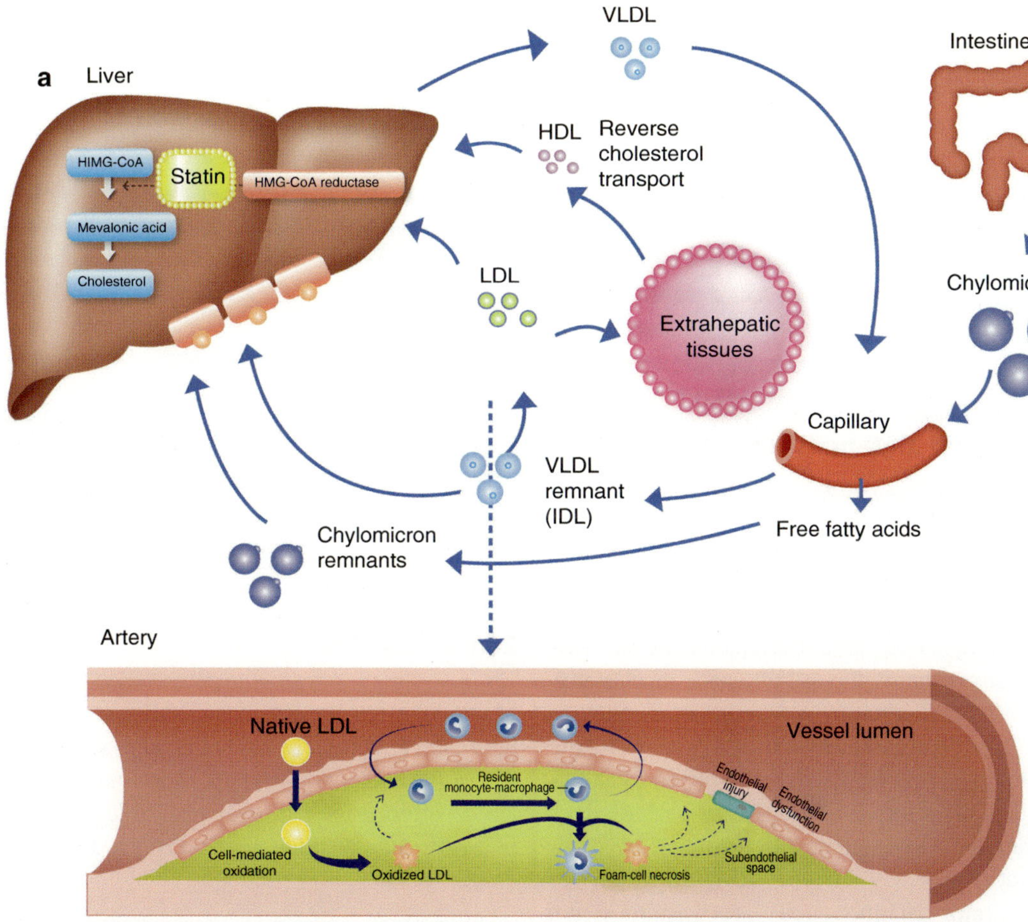

Fig. 26.2 LDL cholesterol and statin. (**a**) Normal cholesterol metabolism, contribution of LDL-C to generation of atherosclerosis, and mechanism of action of statin. (**b**) Statin: pleiotropic actions to protect vascular systems (*LDL-C* low-density lipoprotein cholesterol)

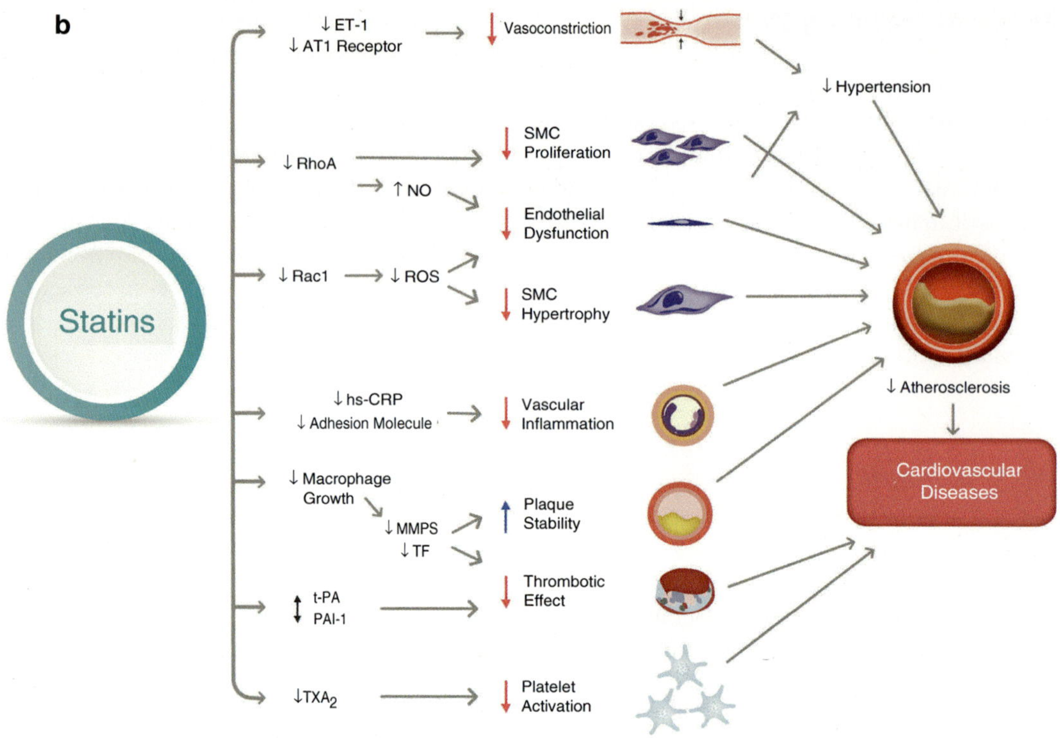

Fig. 26.2 (continued)

26.5.5 Characteristics and Metabolism of Statin

Statins can be divided into hydrophilic and lipophilic groups, and some insists that there are differences in lipid improvement effect in the liver, pleiotropic effect, and myopathy among groups. The examples of lipophilic statins are cerivastatin, simvastatin, fluvastatin, and atorvastatin, and hydrophilic statins are pravastatin, pitavastatin, and rosuvastatin. On the side of drug metabolism, pravastatin is metabolized by sulfation and therefore has the lowest risk of drug interaction. Fluvastatin is metabolized by cytochrome P450 2C9 subtype; lovastatin, simvastatin, atorvastatin, and cerivastatin are metabolized by cytochrome P450 3A4 subtype and may have some drug interactions. Rosuvastatin and pitavastatin have multiple metabolic pathways by various cytochrome P450 enzymes and also are metabolized by glucuronidation, which result in relatively low drug interaction side effects. Many trials have shown new-onset DM and worsening of glucose control with statins except for pravastatin, but its cause and mechanisms are still in investigation.

26.5.6 Side Effects

Most common side effects are indigestion, heartburn, and abdominal pain which can be found in 4% of patients, and the most serious side effects are hepatotoxicity and myopathy. Statin has relatively low rate of side effect, considered as a safe drug.

26.5.6.1 Hepatotoxicity

0.5–2% of the patients have elevated transaminase (AST, ALT), and it is proportional to the dose of drugs, which is reversible if discontinued. If statins are administrated with other medications with hepatotoxicity, the rate of side effects will increase. When transaminase is slightly elevated, there is no need to suspend taking medicine. If the level is higher than three times the normal range, temporary discontinuation is necessary. For resuming the drug, consider starting with lower dose of it and may switch to other medications when the enzyme level goes back to normal range. Liver function test should be done at 6 and 12 weeks after administration, and after that, repeat in 6 months.

26.5.6.2 Myopathy

Myalgia, lethargy, myoglobinuria, and creatine kinase level more than ten times the normal range can confirm the diagnosis. Occurrence rate is very low as 0.1–0.01%, but rhabdomyolysis has high mortality rate. Additional care is needed especially in old age, low body weight, renal failure, hypothyroidism, and alcohol addictive patients. Because statin is metabolized by cytochrome P450 3A4, combining it with cyclosporine, gemfibrozil, and erythromycin could raise the risk. If the creatine kinase level is lower than three times the normal range, drug can be maintained with regular checkup.

26.5.6.3 Diabetes Mellitus

In recent reports, statin increased new-onset diabetes mellitus. Most of new-onset diabetes mellitus occurred in patient with prediabetes status before taking statin, and high-dose group might have higher risk of new-onset diabetes mellitus. Therefore, checking fasting blood glucose level before taking statin might be helpful. In the meta-analysis of clinical trials, low/medium dose of statin group had 0.1% higher incidence of new-onset diabetes compared to the controls, and high-dose statin group had 0.3% higher incidence. The long-term effect of new-onset diabetes is uncertain, but protective effect of statin in high cardiovascular risk group is secure. So even if diabetes occurred during statin treatment, lifestyle modification including exercise, weight control, stopping smoking, and continuing statin treatment other than discontinuation is helpful for the prevention of cardiovascular disease.

26.5.7 Contraindications

Active or chronic liver diseases are absolute contraindication for statin. If a patient is pregnant, discontinuation of drug is recommended. Combined use of cyclosporine, macrolide, antifungal agent, and cytochrome P450 inhibitor is relative contraindication, and special care is needed.

26.5.8 Laboratory Studies Before and After Statin Treatment

26.5.8.1 Before Statin Treatment

Transaminase (AST, ALT) level should be checked before statin treatment. When ALT is higher than three times the normal range, do not start statin, and evaluation and treatment for liver diseases should be preceded and can be continued after normalization of liver enzyme level. Muscle enzyme (CK, creatine kinase) should be checked, and if baseline muscle enzyme is more than three times the normal range, look for the cause and decide whether to start statin.

26.5.8.2 Follow-Up After Statin Treatment

After 4–12 weeks, check cholesterol, triglyceride, and HDL for the lipid-modifying effect. If two consecutive LDL cholesterol levels are lower than 40 mg/dL, dose reduction may be considered. Twelve weeks and after, repeat follow-up in 3–12 months for monitoring effect of statin and liver toxicity. Regular checkup of muscle enzyme is not recommended.

26.5.8.3 Discontinuation of Statin

Two to three months after cessation, LDL cholesterol level increases to the level of pretreatment status. Also, pleiotropic effect of statin disappears in 1–2 days after discontinuation, so continued treatment is very important. Particularly, in the case of acute phase coronary syndrome or stroke, poor outcome was observed with statin withdrawal. Discontinuation should be done with special attention.

26.5.9 Ezetimibe

Ezetimibe is commonly used for combination therapy with statin. Ezetimibe can prohibit cholesterol absorption in the small intestine. During 7 years of follow-up after acute coronary syndrome, simvastatin 40 mg/ezetimibe 10 mg combination showed more significantly decreased LDL level and occurrence of major vascular disease outcome (about 6.4%) compared to those of simvastatin 40 mg in Improved Reduction of Outcomes: Vytorin Efficacy International Trial (IMPROVE-IT) study [7]. If physician fails to decrease LDL level to target goal, combination therapy with ezetimibe could be another option for preventing cardiovascular disease including stroke.

Suggestions from Current Clinical Practice Guidelines
Indication of statin therapy has been recommended in (1) ischemic stroke or transient ischemic attack caused by large artery atherosclerosis and (2) low-density lipoprotein cholesterol level ≥ 100 mg/dL in any ischemic stroke subtype.

References

1. Stone NJ, Robinson JG, Lichtenstein AH, et al. 2013 ACC/AHA guideline on the treatment of blood cholesterol to reduce atherosclerotic cardiovascular risk in adults: a report of the American College of Cardiology/American Heart Association ask force on practice guidelines. Circulation. 2014;129:S1–45.
2. Amarenco P, Bogousslavsky J, Callahan A, et al. High-dose atorvastatin after stroke or transient ischemic attack. N Engl J Med. 2006;355:549–59.
3. Baigent C, Blackwell L, Emberson J, et al. Efficacy and safety of more intensive lowering of LDL cholesterol: a meta-analysis of data from 170,000 participants in 26 randomised trials. Lancet. 2010;376:1670–81.
4. Kernan WN, Ovbiagele B, Black HR, et al. Guidelines for the prevention of stroke in patients with stroke and transient ischemic attack: a guideline for healthcare professionals from the American Heart Association/American Stroke Association. Stroke. 2014;45:2160–236.
5. Cholesterol Treatment Trialists' (CTT) Collaboration, Fulcher J, O'Connell R, et al. Efficacy and safety of LDL-lowering therapy among men and women: meta-analysis of individual data from 174,000 participants in 27 randomised trials. Lancet. 2015;385:1397–405.
6. Heeschen C, Hamm CW, Laufs U, et al. Withdrawal of statins increases event rates in patients with acute coronary syndromes. Circulation. 2002;105:1446–52.
7. Cannon CP, Blazing MA, Giugliano RP, et al. Ezetimibe added to statin therapy after acute coronary syndromes. N Engl J Med. 2015;372:2387–97.

Understanding Paradox of Risk Factors

27

Yerim Kim

Abstract

Although some indicators such as smoking, alcohol, and obesity increased stroke morbidity and mortality, recent researches have indicated that there is a paradoxical phenomenon between them. Smokers in ischemic stroke (IS) who received intravenous tissue plasminogen activator (tPA) had a significantly greater recanalization, reperfusion, and lower mortality. Smoking drops endogenous tPA release and makes circulating fibrinogen level to increase. As a result, the fibrin-rich clot in smokers may be more susceptible to fibrinolytic therapy. Regarding alcohol, heavy alcohol intake increases the risk of stroke or cardiovascular disease. However, some studies have found paradoxical effect of alcohol regarding J- or U-shaped relationship between alcohol consumption and mortality or morbidity. The mechanism remains unclear, but may be related to an increased blood concentration of high-density lipoprotein (HDL) cholesterol and adiponectin, insulin sensitivity, decreased levels of plasma fibrinogen, and a reduction of platelet aggregation. Finally, so-called obesity paradox supports that overweight or obese patients with cardio- or cerebrovascular diseases tend to have more favorable outcomes. Authors who support obesity paradox demonstrated that some protective cytokines and rennin-angiotensin-aldosterone system were attenuated in obese patients. However, there were some critical issues in these theories, and the exact patho-mechanisms were not elucidated yet. In conclusion, the paradoxes in stroke might be a mere epiphenomenon or a transitional process toward disastrous clinical outcomes. Therefore, physicians should consider intermediate confounders and should carefully apply these results to real clinical fields.

Y. Kim, M.D.
Department of Neurology, Gangdong Sacred Heart Hospital, Hallym University College of Medicine, 150, Seongan-ro, Gangdong-gu, Seoul 05355, South Korea
e-mail: brainyrk@hallym.or.kr

Stroke is the fourth-leading cause of death and a major health burden in the world. Despite advanced therapies for patients with acute ischemic stroke, control of risk factor remains the best method for preventing strokes. Smoking,

S.-H. Lee (ed.), *Stroke Revisited: Diagnosis and Treatment of Ischemic Stroke*, Stroke Revisited, DOI 10.1007/978-981-10-1424-6_27

alcohol, and obesity are well-known risk factors for cardio- and cerebrovascular disease. Because those factors increased morbidities and overall mortalities, physicians have recommended that patients should stop smoking and decrease alcohol consumptions and reduce their body weights. However, some studies have shown paradoxical findings that patients with those risk factors have lower mortality and morbidity. This phenomenon is referred to as a "paradox." Interestingly, the exact patho-mechanisms were not elucidated yet; researches exploring this paradox have been emerged in multiple disease categories.

27.1 Smoking Paradox

The so-called smoking paradox of an improved outcome after thrombolysis was first demonstrated in smokers in myocardial infarction (MI) in 1995 [1]. Although smoking is known to be a strong risk factor for atherosclerosis, MI, and sudden cardiac death, researchers have reported that smokers have better prognosis after thrombolysis compared with non-smokers in the reperfusion, unexpectedly [2]. The underlying mechanism of this phenomenon remains unclear. One proposing hypothesis was that smoking exposure alters clot formation dynamics and thrombus composition, consequently causing blood to become hypercoagulable. It has been suggested that higher risk of coronary artery disease in smokers is associated with increased intra-arterial fibrin concentrations. It is notable that smoking has been associated with (1) increased hematocrit, (2) platelet aggregation and activation, (3) elevated inflammatory markers, (4) vasoconstriction, (5) increased levels of fibrinogen, and (6) thrombin generation. These findings support that pathogenesis of vascular occlusion may be more thrombogenic than atherogenic in smokers and therefore more responsive to fibrinolytic therapy. In addition, epicardial coronary vasoconstriction may have occurred more frequently in smokers [3]. This hypothesis was also evaluated in the field of ischemic stroke (IS). Recent smokers in IS who received intravenous tissue plasminogen activator (tPA) had a significantly greater recanalization, reperfusion, and lower mortality [3, 4]. The tPA is a serine protease released from endothelial cells, which catalyzes the conversion of plasminogen to plasmin and responsible for clot formation. Smoking drops endogenous tPA release and makes circulating fibrinogen level to increase. As we mentioned above, although smoking may provoke coronary vessel occlusion, the fibrin-rich clot in smokers may be more susceptible to fibrinolytic therapy [3].

However, in a recent study (SYNTAX trial) reporting higher incidence of MI, sudden death in smokers had emphasized that interpretation of smoking paradox should be prudent. It is noteworthy that detailed smoking history reflecting changes of smoking status at serial time points was an independent predictor of poor clinical outcomes [5]. In previous studies, definition of smoking was ambiguous for the severity, duration, and changes in smoking patterns during follow-up. Because baseline smoking status may not provide appropriate information to predict the effect of smoking on clinical outcomes, there are some critical issues in smoking paradox. Furthermore, in many of the previous studies evaluating smoking paradox, smokers were younger, with a lower proportion of conventional vascular risk factors, and reduced number of medications [1]. We may assume that smokers might maintain their smoking habits because they were young and healthy. In SYNTAX cohort, smoking was more hazardous than age per increase in 10 years. Since SYNTAX trial analyzed patients with predominantly stable CAD, the results cannot be compared to the previous acute MI studies. However, despite that smoking paradox, smoking is associated with poor clinical outcomes after revascularization in patients with CAD or IS, and smoking cessation markedly attenuates mortality rates.

27.2 Alcohol Paradox

Alcohol accounts for approximately 5.1% of the global health burden and 3.3 million deaths worldwide either entirely or partially. There is a positive dose-response relationship between alcohol consumption and increased risk of cardio- or cerebrovascular disease [6]. Alcohol ingestion was known to be associated with (1) increased cardiac output, heart rate, systolic blood pressure, and pulse pressure, (2) reduced left ventricular contractile function and systemic vascular resistance, and (3) increased coronary blood flow in response to myocardial oxygen consumption. These findings contribute to cardio- or cerebrovascular disease in several ways: (1) provocation of cardiac arrhythmias and wall motion abnormalities which predispose to systemic/cerebral embolism, (2) induction of hypertension, and (3) platelet aggregation and clotting cascade activation [7]. Prior studies have reported that heavy alcohol intake increases the risk of stroke or cardiovascular disease. However, the effect of light-to-moderate alcohol drinking remains controversial. Therefore, some studies have found paradoxical effect of alcohol regarding J- or U-shaped relationship between alcohol consumption and mortality or morbidity. The mechanisms of this "alcohol paradox" remain unclear. However, some hypotheses include an increased blood concentration of high-density lipoprotein (HDL) cholesterol and adiponectin, insulin sensitivity, decreased levels of plasma fibrinogen, and a reduction of platelet aggregation [8].

There are a number of important limitations to this alcohol paradox. First, the definition of "light-to-moderate" amount of alcohol is ambiguous. In recent studies, three to four drinks (one drink = 10 g ethanol) per day were significantly related to a lower risk of ischemic stroke [9]. Second, various types of alcohol (wine, beer, soju, whiskey, gin, rum, vodka, etc.) might contain different materials and different dose of ethanol per glass. Third, the relationship between alcohol and outcome does not show linear correlation. Most of the studies do not consider baseline characteristics of subjects such as age, drinking habits (binge or heavy drinking), socioeconomic status, and the effect of accidents, violence, or suicide. The negative and positive effects of alcohol seem to depend not only on the amount of alcohol consumption but also on above variables. For example, young patients were more likely to have chances to exposure to external causes including accidents and violence [10]. Furthermore, regarding socioeconomic status, poor individuals appear to consume alcohol in fewer but heavier drinking habits and to consume other cheap liquors. Therefore, this J- or U-curve result might suggest that there might be other confounders between them.

Current guidelines recommend that heavy drinkers should reduce alcohol consumption. In case of drinking alcohol, light-to-moderate amounts of alcohol consumption (up to two drinks per day for men and up to one drink per day for nonpregnant women) may be reasonable.

27.3 Obesity Paradox

Obesity is known as a major health burden on the cardiovascular system, contributing to overall morbidity and mortality. Some considerable evidences suggest the adverse effects of obesity on cardiac structure/function and on central or peripheral hemodynamic status. Additionally, obesity seems to be related to increased C-reactive protein, insulin resistance, hyperleptinemia, and sympathetic nervous system activation. The adipocyte plays an important role in the pathogenesis of obesity. Leptin, which control energy metabolism, was derived from an adipocyte and may be associated with cardiovascular disease [11].

However, some reports have reported that there is an inverse relationship between obesity and clinical outcomes in patients with cardiovascular disease (Fig. 27.1). This paradoxical phenomenon, referred to as "obesity paradox," supports that overweight or obese patients with hypertension, heart failure (HF), and coronary heart disease tend to have more favorable outcomes. Furthermore, this finding has been identified in chronic disease such as chronic obstructive pulmonary disease, peripheral arterial disease, diabetes, chronic kidney disease, and malignancy as well as cardiovascular disease. One of the first studies to evaluate the obesity paradox was in the field of HF. Horwich et al. demonstrated that the best prognosis

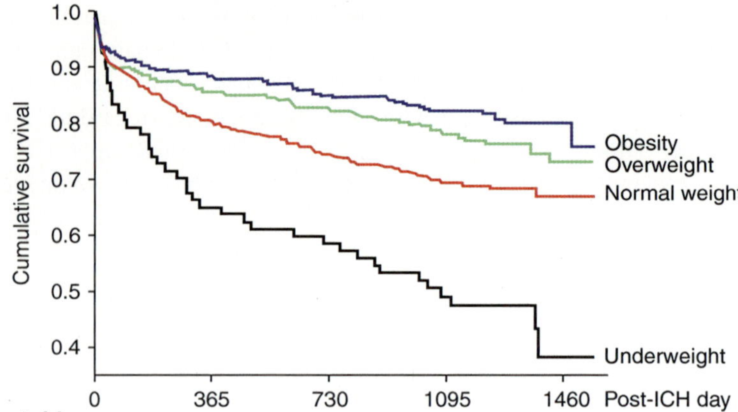

Patients at rirk:

	0	365	730	1095	1460
Obesity	345	305	293	224	22
Overweight	325	278	268	189	35
Normal weight	528	424	393	290	34
Underweight	77	50	45	31	5

Fig. 27.1 Survival rate after intracerebral hemorrhage. Kaplan-Meier curves showing mortality over 4 years of follow-up. Reproduced by permission of Neurology [14]

occurred in overweight group, followed by obese group, and the worst prognosis occurred in underweight HF patients by using body mass index (BMI) [12]. This paradoxical phenomenon was demonstrated in both IS and hemorrhagic stroke, as well. A nationwide, multicenter, prospective registry study in Korea analyzed 34,132 patients with acute IS and showed that stroke survivors whose BMI values were lower than the chosen reference level of 20–23 had 1.36-fold of increased risks of long-term mortality, whereas obese stroke patients had 0.83-fold of decreased risks of mortality [13]. In addition, another study in Korea, which analyzed 1356 patients with intracerebral hemorrhage, indicated that BMI was independently associated with a lower risk of long-term mortality (hazard ratio, 0.91 per 1-kg/m^2 increase; 95% confidence interval, 0.87–0.95) [14]. Previous study expanded on this observation by evaluating that the association between obesity and better outcome was also present by measuring percent body fat or waist circumference. The exact mechanisms were not elucidated yet. However, authors who support the obesity paradox suggested some potential reasons for proving this result. First, various cytokines of obese patients may be protective. Adipose tissue is known to make soluble tumor necrosis factor-alpha receptors, which neutralize the adverse effects of tissue necrosis factor-α (TNF-α). Second, obesity might be a great metabolic reservoir in some catastrophic events or chronic illness. Obese patients can endure more than underweighted individual who may exhaust energy more quickly. Third, a response of the rennin-angiotensin-aldosterone system was attenuated in obese patients. Fourth, there was some evidence that overweight or obese patients had lower levels of atrial natriuretic peptides and increased muscle mass compared with underweight or normal patients (Table 27.1) [12]. However, there are some critical issues in this theory. First, most data on obesity paradox came from observational studies and do not demonstrate a direct causal relationship between body composition and outcome. Second, diagnosis based on clinical criteria might be applied differently. For example, many of the studies used clinical criteria in addition to objective indicators to establish the diagnosis of HF. Furthermore, since the definition of obesity was not constant and fully reliable, multiple confounders such as age, sex, and race should be considered. Third, obese patients may more often use preventive drugs and be under control because of their cerebrovascular risk factors. Finally, underweight might be interpretated as nonpurposeful weight loss or cachexia. It was notable that in most studies, a U- or inverted J-shaped survival curve appears to have emerged. The negative impact of cachexia appeared to be the main reason for the inverse relation of obesity and outcome rather than the positive impact of obesity. Marked obesity does not show a clear protective effect [15]. Recent study suggested that obesity paradox might be an epiphenomenon in patients with IS (Fig. 27.2). Obese patients were more likely to have conventional vascular risk factors and to have mild stroke initially. Although patients with higher BMI had better short-term outcome after stroke, after adjusting for initial neurological severity, this association disappeared [16]. Long-term results from the Whitehall study support that "healthy obesity" is a transient phase moving toward glucometabolic abnormalities rather than a good state [17].

Table 27.1 Potential reasons for the obesity-stroke paradox

A. Protective cytokines
B. Greater metabolic reservoirs
C. Increased muscle mass
D. Nonpurposeful weight loss meaning cachexia
E. Attenuated response to renin-angiotensin-aldosterone system
F. Earlier symptom detection due to better medical consciousness
G. Inadequate measure of body composition

Reproduced by permission of JACC: Heart Failure [12]

Conclusion

In conclusion, although researches exploring this interesting paradox have been emerged in multiple disease categories, the exact pathomechanisms were not still identified yet. While the "paradox in stroke" seems to be a fascinating hypothesis, it might be a mere epiphenomenon or a transitional process toward disastrous clinical outcomes. Therefore, in considering unconfirmed limitations, physicians should carefully apply this hypothesis until more research is accumulated.

Suggestions from Current Clinical Practice Guidelines It is strongly recommended that active or passive smoking should be avoided in stroke patients. Regarding alcohol drinking, drinking greater than two drinks per day should be avoided. In terms of obesity, beneficial impact of weight reduction in obese stroke patients has not been explored, but weight reduction is still being recommended in body mass index ≥ 25 mg/m^2.

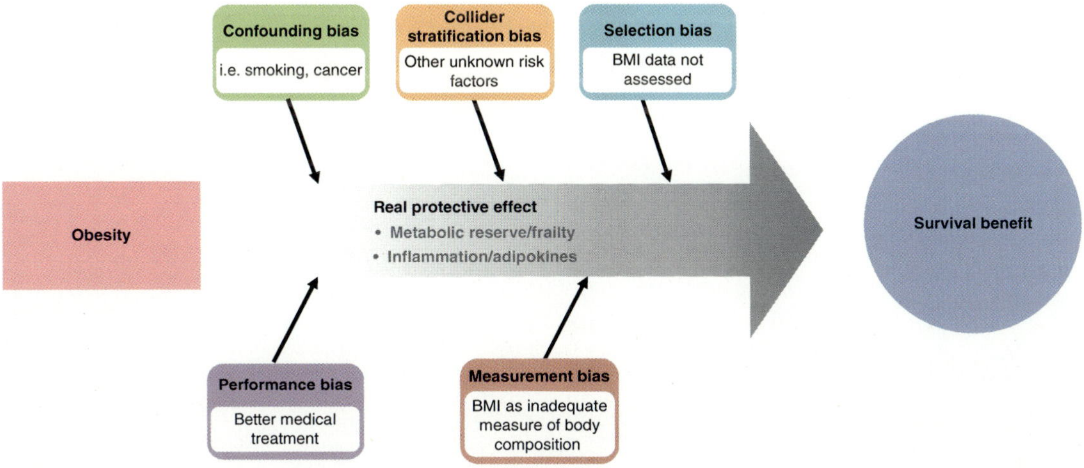

Fig. 27.2 Multiple biases in obesity-stroke paradox

References

1. Grines CL, Topol EJ, O'Neill WW, et al. Effect of cigarette smoking on outcome after thrombolytic therapy for myocardial infarction. Circulation. 1995;91:298–303.
2. Kirtane AJ, Martinezclark P, Rahman AM, et al. Association of smoking with improved myocardial perfusion and the angiographic characterization of myocardial tissue perfusion after fibrinolytic therapy for ST-segment elevation myocardial infarction. J Am Coll Cardiol. 2005;45:321–3.
3. Kufner A, Nolte CH, Galinovic I, et al. Smoking-thrombolysis paradox: recanalization and reperfusion rates after intravenous tissue plasminogen activator in smokers with ischemic stroke. Stroke. 2013;44:407–13.
4. Ovbiagele B, Saver JL. The smoking-thrombolysis paradox and acute ischemic stroke. Neurology. 2005; 65:293–5.
5. Zhang YJ, Iqbal J, van Klaveren D, et al. Smoking is associated with adverse clinical outcomes in patients undergoing revascularization with PCI or CABG: the SYNTAX trial at 5-year follow-up. J Am Coll Cardiol. 2015;65:1107–15.
6. Organization WH. Global status report on alcohol and health. Geneva: World Health Organization; 2014.
7. Gorelick PB. Alcohol and stroke. Stroke. 1987;18:268–71.
8. Hvidtfeldt UA, Frederiksen ME, Thygesen LC, et al. Incidence of cardiovascular and cerebrovascular disease in Danish men and women with a prolonged heavy alcohol intake. Alcohol Clin Exp Res. 2008;32:1920–4.
9. Lee SJ, Cho YJ, Kim JG, et al. Moderate alcohol intake reduces risk of ischemic stroke in Korea. Neurology. 2015;85:1950–6.
10. Thun MJ, Peto R, Lopez AD, et al. Alcohol consumption and mortality among middle-aged and elderly U.S. adults. N Engl J Med. 1997;337:1705–14.
11. Lavie CJ, Milani RV, Ventura HO. Obesity and cardiovascular disease: risk factor, paradox, and impact of weight loss. J Am Coll Cardiol. 2009;53:1925–32.
12. Lavie CJ, Alpert MA, Arena R, et al. Impact of obesity and the obesity paradox on prevalence and prognosis in heart failure. JACC Heart Fail. 2013;1:93–102.
13. Kim BJ, Lee SH, Jung KH, et al. Dynamics of obesity paradox after stroke, related to time from onset, age, and causes of death. Neurology. 2012;79:856–63.
14. Kim BJ, Lee SH, Ryu WS, et al. Paradoxical longevity in obese patients with intracerebral hemorrhage. Neurology. 2011;76:567–73.
15. Habbu A, Lakkis NM, Dokainish H. The obesity paradox: fact or fiction? Am J Cardiol. 2006;98:944–8.
16. Kim Y, Kim CK, Jung S, et al. Obesity-stroke paradox and initial neurological severity. J Neurol Neurosurg Psychiatry. 2015;86:743–7.
17. Bell JA, Hamer M, Sabia S, et al. The natural course of healthy obesity over 20 years. J Am Coll Cardiol. 2015;65:101–2.

Antithrombotics: Antiplatelet Drugs

28

Meng Lee and Bruce Ovbiagele

Abstract

Antiplatelet agents have been widely used in the treatment for noncardioembolic stroke or transient ischemic attack both in acute treatment and secondary prevention of stroke. Aspirin monotherapy is associated with reduction in the recurrence of ischemic stroke during acute stage and chronic stage. Other antiplatelet agents such as clopidogrel, cilostazol, and aspirin plus dipyridamole showed benefit for secondary prevention of stroke. Dual antiplatelet agents should be used with consideration of several clinical conditions for secondary prevention of stroke, because early, short-term, dual antiplatelet therapy (e.g., aspirin and clopidogrel) may have beneficial effect duration after minor ischemic stroke or transient ischemic attack. In addition, we could consider alternative antiplatelet agents for preventing recurrent stroke in the aspirin treatment failure.

Antiplatelet agents are a cornerstone of treatment for noncardioembolic stroke or transient ischemic attack (TIA) both in acute stage and secondary stroke prevention. Four antiplatelet drugs have been approved by the Food and Drug Administration (FDA) in the United States for the prevention of vascular events among patients with a stroke or TIA (i.e., aspirin, combination aspirin/dipyridamole, clopidogrel, and ticlopidine). While a fifth antiplatelet, cilostazol, has not been approved by the FDA for such indication, it has been approved by regulatory agencies in several Asian countries (e.g., Japan, Korea, and Taiwan) for secondary stroke prevention. Mechanisms of antiplatelet drugs are illustrated in Fig. 28.1.

M. Lee, M.D. (✉)
Department of Neurology, Chang Gung Memorial Hospital, Chang Gung University College of Medicine, Chiayi, Taiwan
e-mail: menglee5126@gmail.com

B. Ovbiagele, M.D., F.R.C.P.
Department of Neurology, Medical University of South Carolina, Charleston, SC, USA

S.-H. Lee (ed.), *Stroke Revisited: Diagnosis and Treatment of Ischemic Stroke*, Stroke Revisited, DOI 10.1007/978-981-10-1424-6_28

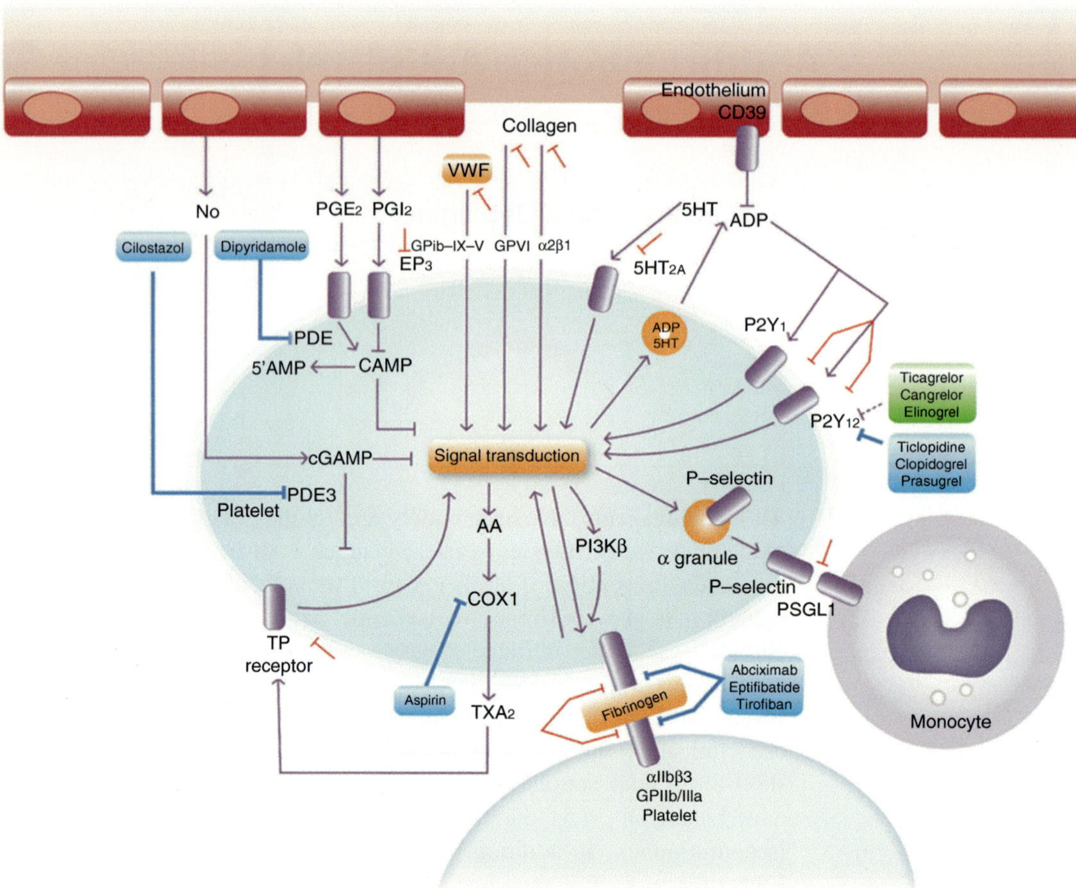

Fig. 28.1 Mechanisms of antiplatelet drugs

28.1 Antiplatelet Therapy of Acute Ischemic Stroke and TIA

28.1.1 Aspirin vs. Placebo

In the International Stroke Trial (IST), patients received aspirin 300 mg within 48 h of ischemic stroke, which was associated with significant reductions in the 2-week recurrence of ischemic stroke and combined outcome of nonfatal stroke or death [1]. In the Chinese Acute Stroke Trial (CAST), patients who received aspirin 160 mg daily, as compared to placebo, within 48 h of ischemic stroke had a 14% reduction in mortality at 4 weeks [2].

28.1.2 Ticagrelor vs. Aspirin

The ticagrelor was not superior to aspirin in reducing stroke, myocardial infarction, and death at 90 days in the SOCRATES trial enrolling ischemic stroke or TIA patients within 24 h of onset [3].

28.1.3 Combination Antiplatelet Therapy vs. Aspirin

The CHANCE trial randomly assigned Chinese patients within 24 h of onset of minor ischemic stroke or high-risk TIA to dual antiplatelet therapy with clopidogrel plus aspirin vs. aspirin [4].

There was a reduction in the risk of any stroke for the clopidogrel plus aspirin, as compared to aspirin. The rate of hemorrhagic stroke was not different between the two groups at 90 days. A meta-analysis of early dual antiplatelet therapy vs. monotherapy for noncardioembolic ischemic stroke or TIA patients showed significant reduction of recurrent stroke [5]. Ongoing trials, such as POINT [6] and TARDIS [7], are likely to provide more insights into the role and type of early antiplatelet treatment for acute ischemic stroke and TIA.

28.1.4 Prior Use of Antiplatelet Agent in Stroke Patients Receiving Intravenous tPA

Among ischemic stroke patients with prior use of antiplatelet agent, low-dose intravenous tPA (0.6 mg/kg), as compared to standard-dose intravenous tPA (0.9 mg/kg), showed a trend toward lower rates of death or disability [8].

28.2 Antiplatelet Therapy for Secondary Stroke Prevention

28.2.1 Aspirin vs. Placebo

Aspirin, the most commonly used antiplatelet agent, prevents recurrent stroke in patients with a history of recent stroke or TIA [9, 10]. A meta-analysis of 16 secondary prevention trials suggested that aspirin reduced the risk of recurrent ischemic stroke by 22% and any vascular event by 19% [11]. Several studies reported that Aspirin showed the strongest benefit effect for secondary stroke prevention in the early weeks after ischemic stroke or TIA patients [12]. Aspirin reduced the relative risk of recurrent ischemic stroke within the first 6 weeks by 58% [12]. The aspirin treatment benefit for secondary prevention was similar regardless of doses range (from 30 to 1300 mg) [9, 10], although the data for doses <75 mg were limited.

The gastrointestinal bleeding is a major complication of aspirin, and especially higher doses of aspirin are associated with greater risk [9, 10]. For patients who use lower doses of aspirin (≤325 mg), the annual risk of serious gastrointestinal bleeding is about 0.4%, which can lead to 2.5-fold increase in the risk compared with non-users [9, 10, 13]. Aspirin doses ≤200 mg daily were associated with a lower rate of major bleeding events compared with higher doses in a pooled analysis of 31 randomized controlled trials [14]. Despite aspirin therapy which is related to an increased risk of hemorrhagic stroke, the overall benefit of aspirin use on myocardial infarction and ischemic stroke may outweigh its adverse effects on the risk of hemorrhagic stroke in patients with vascular risks.

28.2.2 Clopidogrel vs. Aspirin

The CAPRIE trial randomly assigned patients with recent stroke, myocardial infarction, or peripheral artery disease to treatment with clopidogrel (75 mg/day) and aspirin (325 mg/day) [13]. The ischemic stroke, myocardial infarction, or vascular death occurred 5.3% patients per year in the clopidogrel group and 5.8% patients per year in the aspirin group (relative risk reduction 8.7%; 95% CI, 0.3% to 16.5%). Most of the benefit was observed in patients with peripheral artery disease, and the composite outcome was not different in patients with recent stroke. However, CAPRIE was not specifically designed to determine whether clopidogrel was superior to aspirin among stroke patients.

28.2.3 Aspirin Plus Dipyridamole vs. Aspirin

Two RCTs have investigated the effect of dipyridamole combined with aspirin vs. aspirin in patients with history of TIA or stroke [15, 16]. In ESPS-2 trial, combination therapy (aspirin 25 mg twice daily and dipyridamole 200 mg twice daily), as compared with aspirin alone (aspirin 25 mg twice daily), reduced the risk of stroke by 23% (P = 0.006). There was no significant bleeding event in the combination therapy group, but headache and gastrointestinal symptoms were more frequent in the combination group [16]. However, there are some concerns when interpreting the study results because the quality of reported data and a relatively low-dose (50 mg daily) aspirin treatment. The ESPRIT trial was a prospective, randomized, open-label, blinded auditing of outcome events; this was designed to compare aspirin (30–325 mg daily) plus dipyridamole (200 mg twice daily) with aspirin alone (30–325 mg daily) for the prevention of stroke, myocardial infarction, vascular death, or major bleeding among patients with a TIA or ischemic stroke within 6 months [16]. In the combination therapy groups, 83% of patients took the extended-release dipyridamole, and 17% of patients took the immediate-release dipyridamole. The primary outcome events were occurred in 13% of the combination therapy patients, and in 16% of the aspirin therapy patients for 3.5 years (HR, 0.80; 95% CI, 0.66–0.98). However, a limitation of this study was that the investigators did not report post-randomization risk factor management.

28.2.4 Aspirin Plus Extended-Release Dipyridamole vs. Clopidogrel

Among >20,000 patients with noncardioembolic ischemic stroke, stroke recurrence was 9.0% in the aspirin/dipyridamole group and 8.8% in the clopidogrel group over 2.5 years (HR, 1.01; 95% CI, 0.92–1.11) [17]. There were more major hemorrhagic events among aspirin plus extended-release dipyridamole recipients than among clopidogrel recipients (HR, 1.15; 95% CI, 1.00 to 1.32), including intracranial hemorrhage (HR, 1.42; 95% CI, 1.11 to 1.83) [17].

28.2.5 Aspirin Plus Clopidogrel vs. Aspirin

In the substudy of the CHARISMA trial, there was no significant benefit for cardiovascular events; however, the bleeding risk was higher in the combination therapy group compared with aspirin-alone group after a stroke or TIA event [18]. In the SPS3 trial, patients with lacunar stroke within 180 days were randomized to clopidogrel 75 mg combined with aspirin 325 mg daily versus aspirin 325 mg daily [19]. The recurrent ischemic stroke and intracranial hemorrhage rate were not significantly different between dual antiplatelet and aspirin monotherapy. The risk of major hemorrhage, primarily driven by an increased risk for gastrointestinal hemorrhage, and all-cause mortality were significantly higher in the combination therapy group [19].

28.2.6 Aspirin Plus Clopidogrel vs. Clopidogrel

The MATCH trial analyzed the effectiveness of the combination therapy of clopidogrel with aspirin compared with clopidogrel monotherapy for the prevention of vascular events among patients with a recent ischemic stroke or TIA [20]. During the 3.5-year follow-up period, there was no significant benefit of combination therapy for preventing cardiovascular events or death, readmission, and peripheral ischemic event compared to clopidogrel monotherapy. Life-threatening bleedings were higher in the group receiving aspirin and clopidogrel versus clopidogrel monotherapy [20].

A meta-analysis of completed clinical trials indicates that dual antiplatelet therapy, as compared to aspirin monotherapy, had a neutral effect on the prevention of recurrent stroke and intracranial hemorrhagic events [21]. Long-term dual antiplatelet therapy vs. clopidogrel monotherapy appeared to raise the risk of intracranial hemorrhage in people with a prior ischemic stroke or TIA and did not prevent recurrent ischemic events [21].

28.2.7 Cilostazol vs. Aspirin

The effectiveness of cilostazol compared with aspirin for secondary stroke prevention was examined by two major randomized controlled trials conducted in East Asia [22, 23]. One trial showed that cilostazol was associated with a nonsignificant reduction in any recurrent stroke during 12–18-month follow-up (HR, 0.62; 95% CI, 0.30–1.26) [22]. In a cilostazol for prevention of secondary stroke (CSPS 2), non-inferiority trial, the prevalence of recurrent ischemic stroke or hemorrhagic stroke was 2.76% in the cilostazol group and 3.71% in the aspirin group (HR, 0.74; 95% CI, 0.64–0.98) at 29-month follow-up [23]. Ischemic stroke was not reduced significantly by cilostazol compared to aspirin (2.43% per year versus 2.75% per year; HR, 0.89; 95% CI, 0.65–1.20). However, the cilostazol group was related to fewer intracranial and systemic hemorrhage compared with the aspirin group (0.77% versus 1.78% per year; HR, 0.46; 95% CI, 0.30–0.71). The cilostazol clinical studies were conducted in Asia, so it is uncertain whether this effect is applicable to other races. An ongoing trial, CSPS.com, is investigating the safety and efficacy of dual antiplatelet treatment involving cilostazol for secondary ischemic stroke prevention, in comparison with that of antiplatelet monotherapy.

28.2.8 Ticlopidine vs. Aspirin

Ticlopidine was superior to aspirin in one trial [24] and showed no benefit compared with aspirin in another trial [25]. Due to side effects, such neutropenia, as well as the availability of newer and relatively safer agents, ticlopidine is rarely used in current clinical practice.

28.3 Aspirin Treatment Failure

Patients with a history of ischemic stroke or TIA while taking aspirin monotherapy are frequently encountered in routine clinical practice. Although a modification of the antiplatelet regimen in such patients could be considered, the evidence of optimal antiplatelet therapy following an ischemic stroke or TIA while taking aspirin is still inconclusive. Several cohort studies or analyses of clinical trial subgroups have explored the best way to manage this situation.

In a nationwide cohort from Taiwan, switching to clopidogrel showed fewer recurrent vascular events than maintaining aspirin among patients with ischemic stroke while taking aspirin [26]. Moreover, prospective study using multicenter stroke registry database from Korea reported switching or adding alternative antiplatelet agents may have beneficial effect on preventing recurrent vascular events compared with maintaining aspirin in patients with history of an ischemic stroke while taking aspirin [27]. However, a substudy of SPS3 trial suggested that the addition of clopidogrel did not decrease the risk of vascular events compared with continuing aspirin monotherapy in patients with a lacunar stroke while taking aspirin [28]. Among patients on aspirin at the time of their index stroke or TIA in SOCRATES trial, those who were assigned to ticagrelor, as compared to aspirin, had a lower rate of major adverse cardiovascular events [3].

Conclusions

Antiplatelet therapy is essential in the management of noncardioembolic ischemic stroke and TIA. Aspirin monotherapy remains a valid treatment option for most patients with an initial noncardioembolic ischemic stroke or TIA. Early, short-term, dual antiplatelet therapy (e.g., aspirin plus clopidogrel) may be beneficial in patients with a minor ischemic stroke or TIA.

Suggestions from Current Clinical Practice Guidelines To prevent recurrence of vascular events in noncardioembolic stroke or transient ischemic attack (TIA), antiplatelet drugs are strongly recommended such as aspirin, clopidogrel, cilostazol, triflusal, and combination drugs of aspirin plus dipyridamole. Dual antiplatelet therapy of aspirin plus clopidogrel is recommended in two conditions as follows: (1) in a minor ischemic stroke or TIA for 21 days after stroke and (2) in recent stroke or TIA attributable to severe stenosis (≥70%) of a major intracranial artery for 90 days.

References

1. International stroke trial collaborative group. The international stroke trial (IST): a randomised trial of aspirin, subcutaneous heparin, both, or neither among 19435 patients with acute ischaemic stroke. Lancet. 1997;349:1569–81.

2. CAST (Chinese Acute Stroke Trial) collaborative group. CAST: randomised placebo-controlled trial of early aspirin use in 20,000 patients with acute ischaemic stroke. Lancet. 1997;349:1641–9.
3. Johnston SC, Amarenco P, Albers GW, et al. Ticagrelor versus aspirin in acute stroke or transient ischemic attack. N Engl J Med. 2016;375:35–43.
4. Wang Y, Wang Y, Zhao X, et al. Clopidogrel with aspirin in acute minor stroke or transient ischemic attack. N Engl J Med. 2013;369:11–9.
5. Wong KS, Wang Y, Leng X, et al. Early dual versus mono antiplatelet therapy for acute non-cardioembolic ischemic stroke or transient ischemic attack: an updated systematic review and meta-analysis. Circulation. 2013;128:1656–66.
6. Johnston SC, Easton JD, Farrant M, et al. Platelet-oriented inhibition in new tia and minor ischemic stroke (POINT) trial: rationale and design. Int J Stroke. 2013;8:479–83.
7. Bath PM, Robson K, Woodhouse LJ, et al. Statistical analysis plan for the 'triple antiplatelets for reducing dependency after ischaemic stroke (TARDIS) trial. Int J Stroke. 2015;10:449–51.
8. Anderson CS, Robinson T, Lindley RI, et al. Low-dose versus standard-dose intravenous alteplase in acute ischemic stroke. N Engl J Med. 2016;374:2313–23.
9. Farrell B, Godwin J, Richards S, et al. The United Kingdom transient ischaemic attack (UK-TIA) aspirin trial: final results. J Neurol Neurosurg Psychiatry. 1991;54:1044–54.
10. The Dutch TIA trial study group. A comparison of two doses of aspirin (30 mg vs. 283 mg a day) in patients after a transient ischemic attack or minor ischemic stroke. N Engl J Med. 1991;325:1261–6.
11. Antithrombotic Trialists' (ATT) Collaboration, Baigent C, Blackwell L, et al. Aspirin in the primary and secondary prevention of vascular disease: collaborative meta-analysis of individual participant data from randomised trials. Lancet. 2009;373:1849–60.
12. Rothwell PM, Algra A, Chen Z, et al. Effects of aspirin on risk and severity of early recurrent stroke after transient ischaemic attack and ischaemic stroke: time-course analysis of randomised trials. Lancet. 2016;388:365–75.
13. CAPRIE steering committee. A randomised, blinded, trial of clopidogrel versus aspirin in patients at risk of ischaemic events (CAPRIE). Lancet. 1996;348:1329–39.
14. Serebruany VL, Steinhubl SR, Berger PB, et al. Analysis of risk of bleeding complications after different doses of aspirin in 192,036 patients enrolled in 31 randomized controlled trials. Am J Cardiol. 2005;95:1218–22.
15. Diener HC, Cunha L, Forbes C, et al. European stroke prevention study. 2. Dipyridamole and acetylsalicylic acid in the secondary prevention of stroke. J Neurol Sci. 1996;143:1–13.
16. Group ES, Halkes PH, van Gijn J, et al. Aspirin plus dipyridamole versus aspirin alone after cerebral ischaemia of arterial origin (ESPRIT): randomised controlled trial. Lancet. 2006;367:1665–73.
17. Sacco RL, Diener HC, Yusuf S, et al. Aspirin and extended-release dipyridamole versus clopidogrel for recurrent stroke. N Engl J Med. 2008;359:1238–51.
18. Hankey GJ, Johnston SC, Easton JD, et al. Effect of clopidogrel plus asa vs. asa early after TIA and ischaemic stroke: a substudy of the CHARISMA trial. Int J Stroke. 2011;6:3–9.
19. Investigators SPS, Benavente OR, Hart RG, et al. Effects of clopidogrel added to aspirin in patients with recent lacunar stroke. N Engl J Med. 2012;367:817–25.
20. Diener HC, Bogousslavsky J, Brass LM, et al. Aspirin and clopidogrel compared with clopidogrel alone after recent ischaemic stroke or transient ischaemic attack in high-risk patients (MATCH): randomised, double-blind, placebo-controlled trial. Lancet. 2004;364:331–7.
21. Lee M, Saver JL, Hong KS, et al. Risk-benefit profile of long-term dual- versus single-antiplatelet therapy among patients with ischemic stroke: a systematic review and meta-analysis. Ann Intern Med. 2013;159:463–70.
22. Huang Y, Cheng Y, Wu J, et al. Cilostazol as an alternative to aspirin after ischaemic stroke: a randomised, double-blind, pilot study. Lancet Neurol. 2008;7:494–9.
23. Shinohara Y, Katayama Y, Uchiyama S, et al. Cilostazol for prevention of secondary stroke (CSPS 2): an aspirin-controlled, double-blind, randomised non-inferiority trial. Lancet Neurol. 2010;9:959–68.
24. Hass WK, Easton JD, Adams HP Jr, et al. A randomized trial comparing ticlopidine hydrochloride with aspirin for the prevention of stroke in high-risk patients. Ticlopidine aspirin stroke study group. N Engl J Med. 1989;321:501–7.
25. Gorelick PB, Richardson D, Kelly M, et al. Aspirin and ticlopidine for prevention of recurrent stroke in black patients: a randomized trial. JAMA. 2003;289:2947–57.
26. Lee M, Wu YL, Saver JL, et al. Is clopidogrel better than aspirin following breakthrough strokes while on aspirin? A retrospective cohort study. BMJ Open. 2014;4:e006672.
27. Kim JT, Park MS, Choi KH, et al. Different antiplatelet strategies in patients with new ischemic stroke while taking aspirin. Stroke. 2016;47:128–34.
28. Cote R, Zhang Y, Hart RG, et al. ASA failure: does the combination ASA/clopidogrel confer better long-term vascular protection? Neurology. 2014;82:382–9.

Antithrombotics: Anticoagulants Including NOACs

29

Jinkwon Kim

Abstract

Anticoagulants are a class of drugs that inhibit coagulation cascade and blood clotting. For many years, anticoagulants were widely used for the prevention of ischemic stroke and systemic thromboembolic events. Warfarin is the most commonly used anticoagulant inhibiting the synthesis of vitamin K-dependent clotting factors. Recently, a number of new oral anticoagulant were developed to overcome limitations of the conventional vitamin K antagonist. With increase of the aged population, the proportion of cardioembolic stroke consistently increased. Atrial fibrillation is a common cardiac arrhythmia and the most important cause of cardioembolic stroke. Proper anticoagulation dramatically reduces the thromboembolic events in patients at high risk for cardioembolic stroke. However, anticoagulation also increases the risk for bleeding complications compared to placebo or antiplatelet. Clinicians should consider both the benefits and risks from anticoagulation therapy. Therefore, anticoagulation is only recommended for patients with expected net clinical benefit, absolute reduction of thromboembolic risk, and low bleeding risk from anticoagulation. CHA_2DS_2-VASc and HAS-BLED scores are widely used risk stratification tool for thromboembolism and bleeding complication on oral anticoagulation, respectively. Here, we will discuss on commonly used anticoagulants, their antidote, indications which need anticoagulation, and specific clinical issues with anticoagulation.

Anticoagulants are class of drugs which inhibit coagulation pathway and formation of blood clot (Fig. 29.1). This class of drugs can be used for various interventional procedure with thrombotic risk, and long-term prevention of thromboembolism including ischemic stroke. Cardioembolic stroke is the major subtype of ischemic stroke,

J. Kim, M.D.
Department of Neurology, CHA Bundang Medical Center, CHA University, 59 Yatap-ro, Bundang-gu, Seongnam-si 13496, South Korea
e-mail: antithrombus@gmail.com; kimjinkwon@cha.ac.kr

S.-H. Lee (ed.), *Stroke Revisited: Diagnosis and Treatment of Ischemic Stroke*, Stroke Revisited, DOI 10.1007/978-981-10-1424-6_29

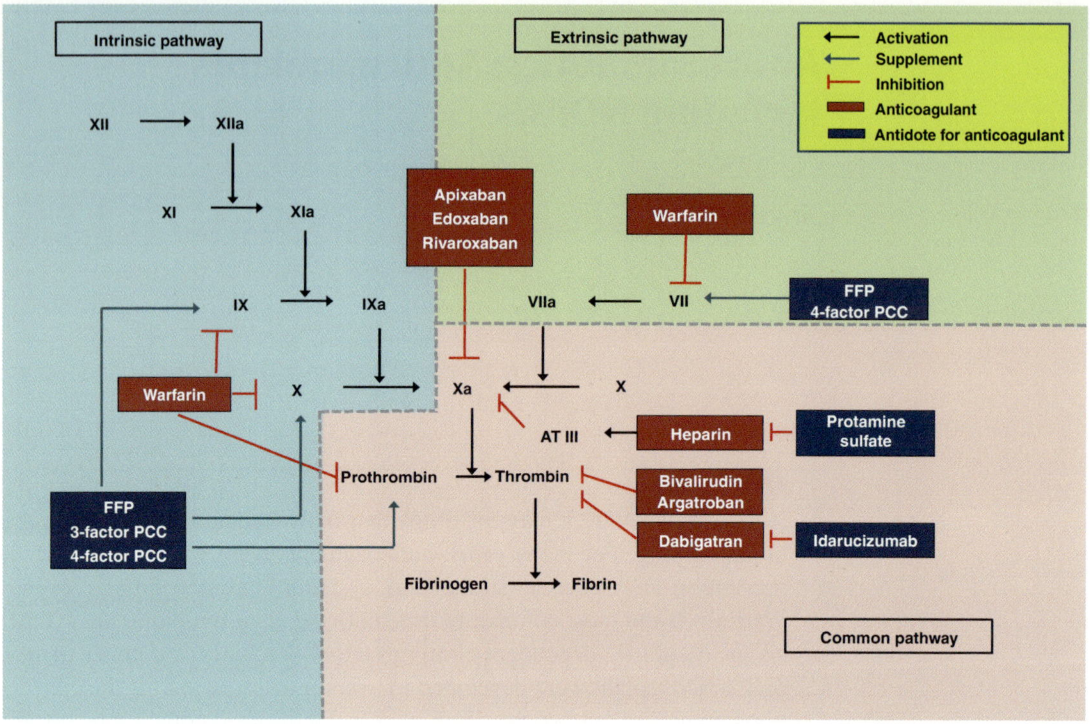

Fig. 29.1 Coagulation cascade with commonly used anticoagulants and their antidotes. *FFP* fresh frozen plasma, *PCC* prothrombin complex concentrates

and the incidence consistently increases with the growing proportion of elderly individuals. Of the patients with ischemic stroke who underwent cardiac evaluation, potential source of cardioembolism is identified in about 30%. Compared to other subtypes, cardioembolic stroke presents with more severe neurologic symptom and is associated with poor long-term functional outcome and high mortality. Because abnormal thrombus formation in the heart is the underlying mechanism of cardioembolic stroke, anticoagulants are widely used for the prevention and treatment of cardioembolic stroke. Proper use of oral anticoagulant leads to about 60% reduction of stroke risk in patients with non-valvular AF (AF) which is the most common cause of cardioembolic stroke. However, the risk for stroke is diverse with the potential source of cardioembolism and coexisting cardiovascular risk factors. In patients with congestive heart failure or patent foramen ovale, which are considered as potential source of cardioembolism, anticoagulation does not demonstrate clinical net benefit compared to antiplatelets [1]. Furthermore, many clinical trials have established that use of anticoagulation is significantly associated with increase of bleeding complication, even in recently developed new oral anticoagulants (NOAC). Therefore, not all patients with potential source of cardioembolism can get clinical benefits on anticoagulation. Some portion of patients with AF who do not have coexisting risk factor (lone AF) are considered as truly low-risk group for ischemic stroke and not recommended for long-term anticoagulation. In clinical practice, underuse of anticoagulation is also common due to the concern of bleeding and poor anticoagulation control. Anticoagulation for the prevention of stroke should be based on the underlying thromboembolic risk and bleeding tendency of the individuals. We should also know the characteristics of commonly used anticoagulants and clinical indications of them.

29.1 Anticoagulant Agents

29.1.1 Warfarin

Warfarin, also known as Coumadin, is a vitamin K antagonist inhibiting the synthesis of clotting factor II, VII, IX, and X. Vitamin K is an essential component for hepatic synthesis of clotting factor II, VII, IX, and X. Therefore, use of warfarin leads to deficiency of the vitamin K-dependent clotting factors and anticoagulation effect. The effective half-life of warfarin ranges from 20 to 60 h, and the anticoagulation effect lasts for two to 5 days. For decades, warfarin has been the most commonly used anticoagulants in the world. However, proper use of warfarin is frequently restricted by the narrow therapeutic range and need for permanent monitoring of anticoagulant activity by international normalized ratio (INR). Even in patients with well-controlled INR (2–3) on warfarin, INR should be monitored at least every 12 weeks, and out of therapeutic range is common. Warfarin also has multiple interactions with drugs and foods which interrupt maintenance within the narrow therapeutic range. The safety and effectiveness of warfarin are closely associated with the quality of anticoagulation. Low INR is ineffective for ischemic stroke, and bleeding risk significantly increases proportionally with international normalized ratio. In patients with AF taking warfarin, time in therapeutic range of INR (TTR) is commonly suboptimal and varied from 30 to 80% [2]. Both a highly variable INR and low TTR of INR are independent predictors of bleeding and thromboembolic complications. Mean TTR below 60% indicates that warfarin is inefficient, and consideration for a switch to one of the NOACs might be reasonable. Although warfarin has many clinical limitations, adjusted-dose warfarin significantly and efficiently reduces risk of ischemic stroke and systemic embolism in patients with atrial fibrillation (AF) (about 50–60% risk reduction compared to placebo). Compared to antiplatelet, warfarin reduces risk of ischemic stroke and systemic embolism to about one third. In clinical trials with warfarin and NOAC in non-valvular AF, subgroup patients with well-controlled warfarin therapy (TTR > 66%) were not significantly inferior for the prevention of thromboembolism to NOACs [3]. To improve INR control and therapeutic potential of warfarin treatment, validated decision support tools (paper nomogram or computerized dosing program) and patient self-test of INR using point-of-care system might be effective. One of the common misconceptions is that persons on warfarin should avoid taking foods containing vitamin K. However, warfarin therapy needs stable therapeutic level of INR derived by maintaining consistent dietary habit for vitamin K-containing foods which is balanced with dosage of warfarin intake. Avoidance of whole food containing vitamin K is impossible and not necessary.

29.1.2 New Oral Anticoagulant (NOAC)

To overcome the clinical limitations of vitamin K antagonist, a number of NOAC were developed. Currently four NOACs (dabigatran, rivaroxaban, apixaban, and edoxaban) got an approval from the European Medicines Agency (EMA) and US Food and Drug Administration (FDA) after clinical trials for the prevention of thromboembolism in patients with non-valvular AF. These NOACs have no interaction with food and have stable therapeutic effect with fixed dosage, and there is no need for routine monitoring of coagulation assay. Dabigatran is a selective inhibitor of factor IIa, and rivaroxaban, apixaban, and edoxaban are selective inhibitors of factor Xa. Because the underlying characteristics of study participants varied on each clinical trials with NOACs, direct compartment among the NOACs is impossible. Generally, NOACs for non-valvular AF have comparable preventive effect for ischemic stroke or systemic thromboembolism compared to conventional warfarin treatment and have relatively low bleeding complications especially in hemorrhagic stroke (Table 29.1). On review of the individual trials, apixaban and dabigatran 150 mg are superior to warfarin for the prevention of stroke or systemic thromboembolism. Dabigatran 150 mg bid is

Table 29.1 Characteristics and efficacy of new oral anticoagulant

Trials with new oral anticoagulants	Relative risk (95% confidence interval) compared with conventional warfarin treatment: Stroke or systemic embolic events	Ischemic stroke	Major bleeding[a]	All-cause death	Mean $CHADS_2$ score	TTR in warfarin treatment group
RE-LY: dabigatran 150 mg bid	RR 0.66 (0.53–0.82)	RR 0.76 (0.60–0.98)	RR 0.93 (0.81–1.07)	RR 0.88 (0.77–1.00)	2.1	64%
RE-LY: dabigatran 110 mg bid	RR 0.91 (0.74–1.11)	RR 1.11 (0.89–1.40)	RR 0.80 (0.69–0.93)	RR 0.91 (0.80–1.03)		
ROCKET AF: rivaroxaban 20 mg or 15 mg qd	HR 0.88 (0.74–1.03)	HR 0.94 (0.75–1.17)	HR 1.04 (0.90–1.20)	HR 0.85 (0.70–1.02)	3.5	55%
ARISTOLE: apixaban 5 mg or 2.5 mg bid	HR 0.79 (0.66–0.98)	HR 0.92 (0.74–1.13)	HR 0.69 (0.60–0.80)	HR 0.89 (0.80–0.99)	2.1	62%
ENGAGE AF: edoxaban 60 mg or 30 mg qd	HR 0.87 (0.73–1.04)	HR 1.00 (0.83–1.19)	HR 0.80 (0.71–0.91)	HR 0.92 (0.83–1.01)	2.8	68%
ENGAGE AF: edoxaban 30 mg or 15 mg qd	HR 1.13 (0.96–1.34)	HR 1.41 (1.19–1.67)	HR 0.47 (0.41–0.55)	HR 0.87 (0.79–0.96)		

RR risk ratio, *HR* hazard ratio, *TTR* time in therapeutic range of international normalized ratio
[a]The definition for major bleeding varied in each trial

the only NOAC which showed a significant reduction of risk of ischemic stroke compared to warfarin (RR 0.76, 95% CI 0.60–0.98). All-cause mortality is significantly reduced with apixaban (HR 0.89, 95% CI 0.80–0.99) and a low dose of edoxaban (HR 0.87, 95% CI 0.79–0.96). However, a low dose of edoxaban is inferior to warfarin therapy in preventing ischemic stroke. Major bleeding risk with NOACs is significantly low or comparable to the risk with warfarin, but there is concern for increase of GI bleeding with a high dose of edoxaban, dabigatran 150 mg, and rivaroxaban compared to warfarin. Because kidney function can influence drug metabolism and excretion of NOACs, kidney function should be considered before prescription of NOACs. Currently, all NOACs are contraindicated for patients with end-stage renal disease. For patients with reduced kidney function, dose adjustment is needed. Table 29.2 summarizes the recommended regimen of NOACs according to renal function. In subgroup analysis from the ENGAGE AF trial, the risk of ischemic stroke is higher than in warfarin in patients with creatinine clearance >95 mL/min; therefore, the FDA does not recommend edoxaban for patients with higher creatinine clearance.

29.1.3 Unfractionated Heparin and Low-Molecular-Weight Heparin

Unfractionated heparin has a binding capacity to antithrombin III (ATIII) and induces conformational change of ATIII. The heparin-enhanced ATIII leads to inactivation of thrombin and factor Xa, which induces anticoagulative effect. Unfractionated heparin also has some anticoagulation effect through inhibition of factor IXa, XIa, and XIIa. Unfractionated heparin has a half-life of 1–2 h and can reach therapeutic range immediately upon intravenous administration. Although unfractionated heparin is the most commonly used parenteral anticoagulant, it has a number of major limitations including a narrow therapeutic window and highly variable dose-response relation that requires laboratory monitoring of activated partial thromboplastin time and dose adjustment. Low-molecular-weight heparins

Table 29.2 Approved dosing of NOACs for patients with non-valvular atrial fibrillation according to renal function

Drug and indication	Normal CrCl ≥ 90 ml/min	Mild CrCl 60–89 ml/min	Moderate CrCl 30–59 ml/min	Severe CrCl 15–29 ml/min	End-stage renal disease CrCl < 15 ml/min
Dabigatran	150 mg bid	150 mg bid	EMA: 110 mg bid FDA: 150 mg bid	EMA: Contraindicated FDA: 75 mg bid	Contraindicated
Rivaroxaban	20 mg qd	20 mg qd	15 mg qd[a]	15 mg qd	Contraindicated
Apixaban	5 mg bid	5 mg bid	5 mg bid	2.5 mg bid[b]	Contraindicated
Edoxaban	60 mg qd[c]	60 mg qd	30 mg qd[d]	30 mg qd	Contraindicated

Reproduced by permission of Therapeutic Advances in Drug Safety [25]

FDA US Food and Drug Administration, *EMA* European Medicines Agency, *CrCl* creatinine clearance

[a]15 mg qd when CrCl 15–49 ml/min

[b]2.5 mg bid when patients had more than two factor in serum creatinine ≥1.5 mg/dl, age ≥ 80 years, or weight ≤ 60 kg

[c]FDA makes warning that do not use edoxaban in patients with CrCL > 95 mL/min

[d]30 mg qd when CrCl 15–50 ml/min

(LMWH) also bind to ATIII, but have more selective inhibitory effect on factor Xa than on IIa. With subcutaneous administration of LMWH, the peak level is reached at 2–4 h and the half-life is 3–4 h. LMWH has many merits compared to UFH including consistent dose-related anticoagulant response which leads to low bleeding complication and usage at fixed dose based on body weight; therefore, dose adjustment or monitoring of LMWH is not necessary except in patients with renal insufficiency. For many years, parenteral anticoagulation using heparin or low-molecular-weight heparin is commonly administrated for acute ischemic stroke patients for the prevention of secondary ischemic events. However, there is lacking evidence supporting the early use of parenteral anticoagulation even in patients with cardioembolic source. Some clinical data suggest parenteral anticoagulation may reduce early recurrent ischemic stroke, but there was significantly increased risk for symptomatic hemorrhage resulting in no net benefit [4]. Therefore, guidelines by the American Heart Association (AHA) and European Stroke Organization do not recommend the use of early parenteral anticoagulation for the treatment of patients with acute ischemic stroke. Even it is not for the prevention of stroke, LMWH can be recommended for prophylaxis of deep vein thrombosis to the immobilized patients with acute stroke.

29.1.4 Bivalirudin

Bivalirudin (commercial name: Angiomax) is a highly specific direct thrombin inhibitor which binds to both free and clot-bound thrombin resulting in inhibition of thrombin-mediated fibrin formation and thrombin-mediated platelet activation. Bivalirudin is primarily indicated for anticoagulants during percutaneous coronary intervention in place of heparin. By intravenous administration, bivalirudin has immediate anticoagulation effect with predictable dose response and short half-life time (about 30 min in normal renal function) without binding to plasma proteins. Therefore, bivalirudin has more predictable anticoagulative effect than unfractionated heparin and has low rate of bleeding complication in trials with percutaneous coronary intervention. Bivalirudin can be used for patients who were contraindicated with heparin due to heparin-induced thrombocytopenia or heparin-induced thrombosis–thrombocytopenia syndrome. Considering the more frequent intracranial hemorrhage during neuroendovascular procedure than percutaneous coronary intervention, bivalirudin might be an ideal alternative anticoagulant to heparin. However, there is insufficient data for the efficacy and safety of bivalirudin during the neuroendovascular procedures.

29.2 Common Indications Which Need Anticoagulation for Prevention of Ischemic Stroke

29.2.1 AF

AF is the most common cause of cardioembolic stroke and well-established indications which need long-term anticoagulation. In the USA, approximately 2% of people under the age of sixty-five have AF, and 9% of people over or equal to the age of sixty-five have AF [5]. As the prevalence of AF dramatically increases with age, the burden of AF and the AF-related stroke consistently increases. Without proper anticoagulation, AF increases the risk of stroke to about four to five times. If mitral valve stenosis is coexistent with AF, the risk increases up to 15-fold. AF is subdivided into paroxysmal or persistent by the duration of AF, but the stroke risk is considered similar between them. In the prior randomized trials, long-term oral anticoagulation with warfarin has been established as the effective management for the prevention of ischemic stroke rather than placebo (OR 0.34) or antiplatelet (OR 0.53) [6]. However, use of warfarin significantly increases systemic bleeding complication even in well-controlled therapeutic range. In AF patients, the absolute risk reduction with anticoagulation is dependent on the underlying thromboembolic risk; those with large risk have more absolute risk reduction with anticoagulation. For patients with low thromboembolic risk, routine use of anticoagulation is not recommended due to the low absolute risk reduction and expected bleeding complication. Therefore, risk stratification is essential for identification of candidates who get preventive benefit with long-term anticoagulation. $CHADS_2$ score is an established prediction tool for risk stratification in patients with non-valvular AF. The $CHADS_2$ scheme has a 0 to 6 score (each 1 point for congestive heart failure, hypertension, age ≥ 75 years, and diabetes mellitus and 2 points for prior stroke or transient ischemic attack), and there was approximately 2.0% increase of stroke rate for each 1 point increment of $CHADS_2$ score (Table 29.3) [5]. Based on the prior studies, non-valvular AF patients with

Table 29.3 $CHADS_2$ score and $CHADVAS_2$ score in patients with non-valvular atrial fibrillation

Definition and scores for $CHADS_2$ and CHA_2DS_2-VASc		Stroke risk stratification with the $CHADS_2$ and CHA_2DS_2-VASc	
$CHADS_2$ acronym	Score	Total score	Adjusted stroke rate (% per year)
Congestive HF	1	0	1.9
Hypertension	1	1	2.8
Age ≥ 75 years	1	2	4.0
Diabetes mellitus	1	3	5.9
Stroke/TIA/TE	2	4	8.5
Maximum score	6	5	12.5
		6	18.2
CHA_2DS_2-VASc acronym	Score		
Congestive HF	1	0	0
Hypertension	1	1	1.3
Age ≥ 75 years	2	2	2.2
Diabetes mellitus	1	3	3.2
Stroke/TIA/TE	2	4	4.0
Vascular disease (prior MI, PAD, or aortic plaque)	1	5	6.7
Age 65 to 74 years	1	6	9.8
Sex category (female)	1	7	9.6
Maximum score	9	8	6.7
		9	15.20

Reproduced by permission of Journal of the American College of Cardiology [5]

AF atrial fibrillation, *HF* heart failure, *LV* left ventricular, *MI* myocardial infarction, *PAD* peripheral artery disease, *TE* thromboembolic, *TIA* transient ischemic attack

$CHADS_2$ score ≥ 2 is indicated for long-term oral anticoagulation with the significant net benefit with prevention of stroke. All AF patients with history of ischemic stroke or transient ischemic attack ($CHADS_2$ score ≥ 2) should get long-term anticoagulation in the absence of major contraindication such as bleeding complication. $CHADS_2$ score is validated and a widely used risk assessment tool for the need of anticoagulation in non-valvular AF. However, $CHADS_2$ score has some limitations. Substantial portion of patients were classified as moderate risk ($CHADS_2$ score of 1) and it is uncertain whether anticoagulation or antiplatelet is better for them. $CHADS_2$ score has wide confidence intervals for each score and inadequate discrimination ability identifying truly low-risk patients who do not need neither anticoagulation nor antiplatelet. CHA_2DS_2-VASc score is a modified scoring system based on $CHADS_2$ score incorporating other common risk factors which provide better discrimination of truly low-risk and high-risk patients who need anticoagulation. The 2016 European Society of Cardiology (ESC) and 2014 American College of Cardiology (ACC)/AHA guidelines recommended the use of CHA_2DS_2-VASc score as the risk assessment tool in non-valvular AF [5, 7]. With non-valvular AF with CHA_2DS_2-VASc score ≥ 2, oral anticoagulation is recommended in the absence of major contraindications. If patients with AF and CHA_2DS_2-VASc score ≥ 2 are not suitable for anticoagulation, dual antiplatelet (aspirin plus clopidogrel) is recommended for the prevention of stroke. For non-valvular AF patients with CHA_2DS_2-VASc score of 1, optimal antithrombotic strategy is controversial, and recommendations varied between several guidelines for non-valvular AF (Table 29.4). The 2016 ESC guideline for AF management recommended oral anticoagulation for the patients with CHA_2DS_2-VASc score of 1. On the other hand, 2014 AHA/ACC guidelines for AF stated that no antithrombotic therapy or treatment with oral anticoagulation or aspirin may be considered for those with CHA_2DS_2-VASc score of 1 [5]. For the truly low-risk group with CHA_2DS_2-VASc score of 0, no antithrombotic therapy is more reasonable than the use of antiplatelet. The 2016 ESC guideline considered females with CHA_2DS_2-VASc score of 1 (no risk factor except female) as low-risk group which do not need antithrombotic therapy [7].

29.2.2 Sick Sinus Syndrome

Sick sinus syndrome (SSS) is a cardiac arrhythmia caused by a malfunction of the sinus node. Cardiac pacemaker implantation is recommended for the patients with SSS and to document symptoms concurrent with the dysrhythmia. Routine anticoagulation is generally not recommended for patients with SSS in normal sinus rhythm, but AF is the common tachydysrhythmia in the patients with SSS who are at increased risk for thromboembolism, which is most likely related to the associated AF. Although the risk and benefit of anticoagulation is not well established for the patient group, oral anticoagulation is recommended due to the high embolic risk in those with SSS and AF. Because atrial pacing does not prevent the occurrence of AF and asymptomatic AF is common, there is need for close monitoring for the development of AF which requires anticoagulation.

29.2.3 Mechanical Heart Valves or Valvular Heart Disease

All mechanical heart valves require lifelong anticoagulation [8, 9]. Currently warfarin is the only approved oral anticoagulant agents for valvular heart diseases and NOAC is not approved. The recommended target INR is 3.0 (2.5–3.5) for patients with mechanical mitral valve or patients with mechanical aortic value and risk factor (AF, prior thromboembolism, left ventricular dysfunction, or hypercoagulable state). For patients with mechanical mitral or aortic valves and low bleeding risk, additional use of low-dose aspirin is also recommended [9, 10]. Anticoagulation is also indicated in patients with (1) mitral valve stenosis and a prior embolic event or (2) mitral valve stenosis and a left atrial thrombus [9–11]. Currently, there is no conclusive data for the preventive benefit of long-term anticoagulation in the patients with nonrheumatic

Table 29.4 Summary of recommendations proposed by several guidelines for non-valvular atrial fibrillation

	High	Middle	Low	
Guidelines	$CHAD_2DS_2$-VASc ≥ 2	$CHAD_2DS_2$-VASc $= 1$	$CHAD_2DS_2$-VASc $= 0$	
ESC 2016	NOAC	NOAC	No Tx	
	Warfarin (alternative)			
APHRS 2013	OAC (D/R/A/W)	NOAC (D/A) W/R (alternative)	No Tx	
AHA/ACC/HRS 2014	OAC (D/R/A/W) (class I)	OAC (D/R/A/W) or no Tx or aspirin (can be considered) (class IIb)	No Tx	
NICE 2014	OAC (D/R/A/W)	Women: no Tx	No Tx	
		Men: OAC (D/R/A/W) (can be considered)		
	$CHADS_2 \geq 2$	$CHADS_2 = 1$	$CHADS_2 = 0$	
CCS 2012			• Age 65–74 • Female and vascular disease[a]	No risk factor
	OAC[b]	OAC[b] Aspirin (can be considered)	OAC[b]	No Tx
JCS 2014			Other risk factors[c]	No risk factor
	D/R/A/E/W[d]	D/A/R/E/W[d] (can be considered)	D/R/A/E/W[d] (can be considered)	No Tx

Reproduced by permission of Seminars in Thrombosis and Hemostasis [26]

Abbreviations: *A* apixaban, *AHA/ACC/HRS* American Heart Association/American College of Cardiology/Heart Rhythm Society, *APHRS* Asia Pacific Heart Rhythm Society, *CCS* Canadian Cardiovascular Society, *CHA_2DS_2-VASc score* congestive heart failure, hypertension, age ≥ 75 years (double), diabetes mellitus, previous thromboembolism (double), vascular disease, age 65–74 years, and female gender, *$CHADS_2$ score* congestive heart failure, hypertension, age ≥ 75 years, diabetes mellitus, and previous stroke/transient ischemic attack (double), *D* dabigatran, *E* edoxaban, *ESC* European Society of Cardiology, *JCS* Japanese Circulation Society, *NICE* National Institute for Health and Care Excellence, *NOAC* non-VKA oral anticoagulants, *OAC* oral anticoagulation, *R* rivaroxaban, *W* warfarin

[a]Either female **or** vascular disease is recommended with aspirin

[b]NOACs (D, R, A) > warfarin

[c]Cardiomyopathy, 65–74 years of age, or vascular disease

[d]Age < 70 INR 2.0–3.0, age ≥ 70 INR 1.6–2.6

mitral valve regurgitation, mitral valve prolapse, or aortic stenosis without AF. For patients with bioprosthetic value, antiplatelet is recommended in the absence of other indication for anticoagulation [9]. However, for patients with bioprosthetic value who have TIA, stroke, or thromboembolism despite of proper antiplatelet therapy, anticoagulation might be considered as preventive management [11].

29.2.4 Acute Myocardial Infarction

Acute myocardial infarction is a significant risk factor for ischemic stroke. A meta-analysis for population-based studies found that 11.1 ischemic strokes occurred per 1000 MI hospitalization [10, 12]. In another meta-analysis with acute myocardial infarction, oral anticoagulation reduced the risk of stroke (OR 0.75, 95% CI 0.63–0.89), but increased major bleeding (OR 2.03, 95% CI 1.56–2.64) [13]. Treatments with warfarin significantly reduced the risk of left ventricular thrombus which is a strong predictor for thromboembolism. Therefore, for patients with ST-elevated myocardial infarction accompanied by left ventricular mural thrombi or anterior apical wall motion abnormalities (akinesis/dyskinesis), anticoagulation might be reasonable [10]. Although the optimal duration of anticoagulation for LV thrombus is not well established, the 2014 AHA/American Stroke Association (ASA) guideline for the secondary prevention of stroke recommended for 3 months of VKA for patients with ischemic stroke or TIA in the setting of acute MI complicated by LV thrombus [11]. Currently, there is insufficient data for the preventive efficacy of new oral anticoagulant in patients with acute myocardial infarction. Therefore, vitamin K antagonist remains the standard anticoagulation therapy for them.

29.2.5 PFO with Deep Vein Thrombosis

Patent foramen ovale (PFO) is a structural defect in the interatrial septum resulted from incomplete closure of atrial tissue. Many observational data suggested that PFO is associated with increased risk of ischemic stroke. However, there is controversy over whether PFO is a real risk factor for ischemic stroke and closure of PFO can reduce the risk of ischemic stroke. Current AHA/ASA guidelines for stroke prevention do not prefer anticoagulation over than antiplatelet for PFO [10, 11]. However, in the patients with venous embolic source such as deep vein thrombosis, PFO can be the conduit for an embolism. Therefore, for patients with ischemic stroke or TIA who have both PFO and venous embolic source, anticoagulation is recommended for the secondary prevention [11].

29.2.6 Cerebral Venous Thrombosis

Cerebral venous thrombosis (CVT) is an uncommon form of stroke derived by thrombosis of the dural sinus of cerebral veins. Underlying thrombophilic condition or medical history is commonly present in patients with cerebral venous thrombosis (provoked CVT). As an initial treatment and long-term prevention of CVT, anticoagulation is the principal therapy. As initial treatment, adjusted-dose UFH or weight-based LMWH is reasonable, and substantial change to warfarin is recommended for long-term prevention. The optimal duration of anticoagulation is unknown. The AHA guidelines for CVT recommended warfarin use for 3 to 6 months to provoked CVT and 6 to 12 months to unprovoked CVT [14].

29.2.7 Stroke with Hypercoagulable State

When ischemic stroke patients had established coagulopathy or inherited thrombophilias (protein C deficiency, protein S deficiency, antithrombin III deficiency, factor V Leiden mutation, etc.), anticoagulation might be reasonable for further prevention of thromboembolism. Antiphospholipid syndrome is an autoimmune disorder that is characterized by excessive clotting of blood by the presence of antiphospholipid antibody. Young patients with ischemic stroke and antiphospholipid syndrome are at high risk of recurrence, and anticoagulation with warfarin may be beneficial. However, there is little evidence for clinical benefits of long-term anticoagulation for these indications.

29.2.8 Conditions of Uncertain Beneficial Effect with Anticoagulation

Dissection of cerebral artery is an important cause of ischemic stroke and embolism. Currently, there is lack of data for the optimal antithrombotic strategy to prevent stroke in patients with arterial dissection [11]. There are many clinical conditions associated with increased risk of ischemic stroke including heart failure, intracranial atherosclerosis, aortic atheroma, and so on, but the therapeutic efficacy of anticoagulation in these cases are not established compared to placebo or antiplatelet which has lower risk of bleeding. Therefore, routine use of anticoagulation is not recommended for the conditions. Cardiac tumor (myxoma and papillary fibroelastomas) is rare but highly thrombogenic and could become an embolic source. Anticoagulation might be helpful as the preventive management for patients, but anticoagulation for cardiac tumor is not established, and surgical resection should be the treatment of choice.

Stroke is a frequent complication of infectious endocarditis, but use of anticoagulation is not recommended for patients with infectious endocarditis due to high risk of intracranial bleeding.

29.3 Management of Bleeding Complication on Anticoagulant

Bleeding complication is the most serious and frequent complication with anticoagulation even in patients maintaining proper therapeutic ranges. The risk of major bleeding on oral anticoagulation ranged from 2 to 13% during a mean duration of follow-up of 6 to 30 months [15]. The HAS-BLED score is a risk prediction tool developed for estimating the 1-year risk for major bleeding in patients on anticoagulation with AF (Table 29.5) [16]. The management strategy for bleeding is dependent on the severity and origin of bleeding and underlying medical conditions of the patients. For patients with minor bleeding or only abnormal coagulopathy profile without bleeding, conservative management including cessation of antithrombotics, simple compression of bleeding site, and close monitoring might be enough. However, for major bleeding patients, antidote for anticoagulant, if available, should be immediately administrated (Table 29.6).

29.3.1 Warfarin

In the major bleeding with prolonged INR on warfarin, vitamin K should be administrated immediately (5–10 mg, intravenous infusion). Anaphylactic reactions with vitamin K are possible and slow dilute infusion is recommended. Because producing clotting factor from vitamin K takes time, the effect of vitamin K is not apparent for several hours. Therefore, administration of plasma derivatives containing clotting factor (fresh frozen plasma or prothrombin complex concentrates) should be indicated simultaneously. Conventional dose for reversal of warfarin-induced anticoagulation is 15 mL/kg for fresh frozen plasma (FFP, 1 unit = 250 mL) and 25–50 units/kg for prothrombin complex concentrates (PCC), but the dosage depends on the prolonged INR level. In the absence of active bleeding, administration of plasma derivatives is not recommended. For major bleeding with severely prolonged INR, large volume of FFP is

Table 29.5 Clinical characteristics comprising the HAS-BLED bleeding risk score

Letter	Clinical characteristic	Points	HAS-BLED score (Total points)	Bleeds per 100 patient-years
H	Hypertension	1	0	1.13
A	Abnormal renal and liver function (1 point each)	1 or 2	1	1.02
S	Stroke	1	2	1.88
B	Bleeding tendency or predisposition	1	3	3.74
L	Labile INRs	1	4	8.70
E	Elderly (age > 65 years)	1	5 to 9	Insufficient data
D	Drugs (concomitant use of antiplatelet agents or NSAIDs) or alcohol abuse (1 point each)	1 or 2		

"Hypertension" is defined as systolic blood pressure >160 mm Hg. "Abnormal kidney function" is defined as the presence of chronic dialysis or renal transplantation or serum creatinine ≥200 μmol/L. "Abnormal liver function is defined as chronic hepatic disease (e.g., cirrhosis) or biochemical evidence of significant hepatic derangement (e.g., bilirubin >2× upper limit of normal, in association with aspartate transaminase/alanine transaminase/alkaline phosphatase >3× upper limit normal). "Bleeding" refers to previous bleeding history or predisposition to bleeding (e.g., bleeding diathesis, anemia). "Labile INRs" refer to unstable/high international normalized ratios or poor time in therapeutic range (e.g., <60%). Drugs/alcohol use refers to concomitant use of drugs, such as antiplatelet agents and nonsteroidal anti-inflammatory drugs

Reproduced by permission of American Journal of Medicine [16]

Table 29.6 Antidotes and their usage for reversal of anticoagulants

Anticoagulant	Half-life	Antidote	Comment
Warfarin	20 to 60 h	Vitamin K (5–10 mg IV) plus [PCC (25–50 units/kg) or FFP (15 ml/kg or 4 unit)]	PCC is preferred over FFP
Unfractionated heparin	1–2 h	1 mg protamine sulfate per 80–100 units of UFH administered in the 2 h prior to reversal	Protamine sulfate should be given slower than 5 mg/min Maximum dose of protamine sulfate is 50 mg
Low-molecular-weight heparin	Enoxaparin: 4.5 h Dalteparin: 2 h Tinzaparin: 4 h	1 mg protamine per (1 mg of enoxaparin, 100 units of dalteparin, 100 units of tinzaparin) administered 8 h prior to reversal	Protamine cannot reverse whole efficacy of LMWH Protamine should be given slower than 5 mg/min
Bivalirudin	25 min	No available antidote	
Dabigatran	12–17 h	Idarucizumab (5 g, IV)	Indicated for (1) emergency surgery/urgent procedures and (2) life-threatening or uncontrolled bleeding
Rivaroxaban	7–11 h	No antidote is approved	Two candidate agents are under development: andexanet alfa, ciraparantag
Apixaban	9–14 h		
Edoxaban	9–11 h		

FFP fresh frozen plasma, *PCC* prothrombin complex concentrate, *IV* intravenous, *LMWH* low-molecular-weight heparin

needed for INR correction, and the INR reversal is frequently incomplete. Therefore, many guidelines recommended PCC over FFP (10 mL of PCC is equivalent to 600 mL of FFP) [17, 18]. Before transfusion of FFP, ABO compatibility should be checked but Rh compatibility or cross-match is not necessary. There were two PCC products available for warfarin reversal, three-factor PCC and four-factor PCC. Both types of PCC contain coagulation factors II, IX, and X, but the three-factor PCC has minimal amounts of factor VII. There is insufficient comparative data on the efficacy of them for warfarin reversal, but there are more clinical evidences for the effectiveness of the four-factor PCC. Cryoprecipitate is a frozen blood product prepared from plasma containing factor VIII, vWF, fibrinogen, and factor XIII. Cryoprecipitate is a poor source of vitamin K-dependent factors; thus cryoprecipitate alone should not be used for reversal of warfarin-induced coagulopathy. Currently, therapeutic use of recombinant factor VIIa, another clotting factor derive, is not recommended for warfarin reversal due to lack of clinical evidence and concern for the increase in thromboembolic risk.

29.3.2 Unfractionated Heparin and Low-Molecular Weight Heparin

Unfractionated heparin can be rapidly reversed with protamine sulfate. The dosage of protamine sulfate is calculated from the administrated dose of heparin in the prior 2 h, and 1 mg of protamine sulfate neutralizes about 80–100 units of unfractionated heparin. Protamine sulfate also can cause allergic reaction; intravenous administration should be given slower than 5 mg/min. Protamine sulfate also can be used for reversal of LMWH, but the anti-factor Xa activity by LMWH is not completely neutralized with protamine (maximum about 60%).

29.3.3 New Oral Anticoagulants

Idarucizumab (Praxbind) is approved as specific treatment to reverse the anticoagulant effect of dabigatran by FAD and the European Commission. Dabigatran has relatively low plasma protein binding (35%); thus hemodialysis might be effective for reducing the plasma concentration of dabigatran in active bleeding. Currently, there is no approved agents for the reversal of factor Xa inhibitors. Andexanet alfa and ciraparantag are specific antidotes under development for reversing factor Xa inhibitors. Gastric lavage with activated charcoal can reduce gastrointestinal absorption of NOACs if the last dose was taken within 2–3 h. Although there is only limited data, use of four-factor PCC might be considerable for patients with NOAC-related major bleeding [7].

29.4 Specific Practical Issues with Clinical Use of Anticoagulation for Stroke Prevention

29.4.1 Optimal timing for the initiation of anticoagulation in acute ischemic stroke

If a patient with acute ischemic stroke is candidate for long-term anticoagulation, there is no conclusive data on proper timing for the initiation of anticoagulation. There is need of consideration for severity of ischemic insult, risk for hemorrhagic transformation, and recurrent stroke. The AHA/ASA guidelines for secondary prevention recommended initiation of oral anticoagulation within 14 days after stroke onset [11]. Some advocate the consensus opinion of "1–3–6–12-day rule"; anticoagulation is initiated on patients with transient ischemic attack after 1 day, with small, non-disabling infarct after 3 days, with a moderate stroke after 6 days, while large infarcts will be treated not before 2 (or even 3) weeks [7, 19]. Before reaching the therapeutic range on oral anticoagulant, bridging therapy with heparin or LMWH is usually not required.

29.4.2 Change from Warfarin to a New Oral Anticoagulant

When change from warfarin with NOAC is needed, NOAC can be initiated if INR < 2.0. If the INR is 2.0–2.5, initiation of NOAC at the next day might be reasonable. In case of INR > 3.0, rechecking of INR is reasonable.

29.4.3 New Oral Anticoagulants for Tube Feeding

Dabigatran is capsuled, which is required for adequate absorption; thus dabigatran capsules should not be altered or administrated by feeding tube. Rivaroxaban and apixaban can be crushed for oral administration via enteral feeding tube. The label of edoxaban acknowledged that no data are available regarding the bioavailability upon crushing and mixing of edoxaban tablets into food and liquids or administration through feeding tubes.

29.4.4 Combined Anticoagulation and Antiplatelet Therapy

Some proportions of patients who need long-term anticoagulation have coexisting indications for antiplatelet therapy. However, prior clinical studies have demonstrated that long-term combined use of anticoagulation and antiplatelet is not superior in the prevention of ischemic event than anticoagulation only. Furthermore, concurrent use of anticoagulant and antiplatelet is strongly associated with increased risk for fatal and nonfatal bleeding complication regardless of controlled therapeutic range of anticoagulation. Therefore, combined anticoagulation and antiplatelet therapy should be avoided in clinical practice [20]. As an exception, patients with mechanical prosthetic value may have beneficial effect with warfarin plus aspirin [9]. Another indication for antiplatelet and antiplatelet is AF patients with acute coronary syndrome or undergoing coronary stent who have a need for maintaining dual antiplatelet to prevent thrombotic complication including stent thrombosis. The antithrombotic regimen and duration of combined therapy should be selected based on the stability of coronary artery disease, stent type (bare metal vs drug eluting), thrombotic risk, and bleeding tendency of individuals [7, 21]. After the minimal maintaining period (3–12 months) with combined therapy for the patients with acute coronary syndrome or stent implantation, anticoagulation monotherapy is usually enough as long-term management. These recommendations for combined therapy are mainly based on prior studies with warfarin and antiplatelet. NOACs have relatively low bleeding risk than warfarin; therefore, the benefit and risk of combined therapy with NOACs and antiplatelet should be further evaluated.

29.4.5 Perioperative Management on Anticoagulation

When patients on anticoagulation undergo surgery or an invasive procedure, there is need for interrupting anticoagulation to prevent bleeding complication. The interruption of anticoagulation can increase the risk of thromboembolism; on the other hand, continuing anticoagulation increases the risk of bleeding during the invasive procedures. Therefore, the management of anticoagulation is challenging to prevent both bleeding and thromboembolic complications. Principally, the decision for anticoagulation depends on the individual patient's risk for thromboembolism, bleeding tendency, and invasiveness of the procedure. If the procedure has minimal risk for serious bleeding, oral anticoagulation can be continued during the procedure such as cataract extract and minimal dental procedure (Table 29.7) [22]. During the implantation of a cardiac electronic device or catheter ablation, continuation of oral anticoagulant (warfarin or NOAC) is recommended. For patients at low thromboembolic risk who need interventions with high bleeding risk,

Table 29.7 Classification of elective surgical interventions according to bleeding risk

Interventions not necessarily requiring discontinuation of anticoagulation
Dental interventions
Extraction of 1–3 teeth
Periodontal surgery
Incision of abscess
Implant positioning
Ophthalmology
Cataract or glaucoma intervention
Endoscopy without surgery
Superficial surgery (e.g., abscess incision, small dermatologic excisions, etc.)
Interventions with low bleeding risk
Endoscopy with biopsy
Prostate or bladder biopsy
Electrophysiological study or radio-frequency catheter ablation for supraventricular tachycardia (including left-sided ablation via single transseptal puncture)
Angiography
Pacemaker or implantable cardioverter defibrillator implantation (unless complex anatomical setting, e.g., congenital heart disease)
Interventions with high bleeding risk
Complex left-sided ablation (pulmonary vein isolation; VT ablation)
Spinal or epidural anesthesia; lumbar diagnostic puncture
Thoracic surgery
Abdominal surgery
Major orthopedic surgery
Liver biopsy
Transurethral prostate resection
Kidney biopsy

Reproduced by permission of Europace [19]

Table 29.8 Last intake of new oral anticoagulant before elective surgical intervention

	Dabigatran		Apixaban		Edoxaban		Rivaroxaban	
	No important bleeding risk and/or adequate local hemostasis possible: perform at trough level (i.e., ≥12 h or 24 h after last intake)							
Bleeding risk with surgery	Low risk	High risk	Low risk	High risk	Low risk	High risk	Low risk	High risk
CrCl ≥ 80 ml/min	≥24 h	≥48 h	≥24 h	≥48 h	No data	No data	≥24 h	≥48 h
CrCl 50–80 ml/min	≥36 h	≥72 h	≥24 h	≥48 h	No data	No data	≥24 h	≥48 h
CrCl 30–50 ml/min b	≥48 h	≥96 h	≥24 h	≥48 h	No data	No data	≥24 h	≥48 h
CrCl 15–30 ml/min b	Not indicated	Not indicated	≥36 h	≥48 h	No data	No data	≥36 h	≥48 h
CrCl < 15 ml/min	No official indication for use							

Reproduced by permission of Europace [19]
CrCl creatinine clearance

transient interruption of anticoagulation and no bridging therapy is recommended. For patients at high risk for thromboembolism, bridging anticoagulation with unfractionated heparin or LMWH might be helpful, but the benefit of bridging therapy is not established, and one recent randomized trial stated against the use of bridging therapy due to significant increase of bleeding and no reduction of thromboembolism [23]. If temporary discontinuation of anticoagulation is needed for intervention with high bleeding risk, warfarin is stopped approximately 5 days before intervention. For patients taking NOAC, the time for discontinuation of NOAC should be individualized according to the kidney function of the patient (Table 29.8). If there is adequate hemostasis after procedures, resuming of warfarin after 12–24 h is reasonable. After invasive procedure with high bleeding risk, the optimal time of restarting of NOAC is not well established.

29.4.6 Thrombolysis for Patients on Anticoagulation

For intravenous thrombolysis, patients who satisfied other indications and with INR < 1.7 is considered acceptable, but those with INR > 1.7 is not recommended. If patients who received unfractionated heparin within 48 h resulting in abnormally elevated aPTT or LMWH within the previous 24 h, intravenous alteplase is not recommended [24]. As the plasma half-life of NOACs range between 8 and 17 h, intravenous alteplase is not recommended within 48 h after the last administration of NOAC [19, 24]. Endovascular mechanical thrombectomy might be considerable for the patients who are contraindicated for intravenous thrombolysis with the use of anticoagulants, although the safety and clinical efficacy of endovascular mechanical thrombectomy is unknown for the patients.

Suggestions from Current Clinical Practice Guidelines Vitamin K antagonist such as warfarin is strongly recommended in all types of cardioembolic stroke or transient ischemic attack (TIA) to prevent further cardioembolic events. However, both vitamin K antagonist and new oral anticoagulants (NOAC) are equally recommended in non-valvular atrial fibrillation, because NOAC use is supported by several randomized controlled trials on non-valvular atrial fibrillation. Usefulness of NOAC in other causes of cardioembolic stroke such as valvular atrial fibrillation or heart failure is being tested in large trials for now.

References

1. Homma S, Thompson JLP, Pullicino PM, et al. Warfarin and aspirin in patients with heart failure and sinus rhythm. N Engl J Med. 2012;366:1859–69.
2. Wan Y, Heneghan C, Perera R, et al. Anticoagulation control and prediction of adverse events in patients

with atrial fibrillation: a systematic review. Circ Cardiovasc Qual Outcomes. 2008;1:84–91.
3. Ruff CT, Giugliano RP, Braunwald E, et al. Comparison of the efficacy and safety of new oral anticoagulants with warfarin in patients with atrial fibrillation: a meta-analysis of randomised trials. Lancet. 2014;383:955–62.
4. Sandercock PAG, Counsell C, Kane EJ. Anticoagulants for acute ischaemic stroke. Cochrane Database Syst Rev. 2015:CD000024.
5. January CT, Wann LS, Alpert JS, et al. 2014 AHA/ACC/HRS guideline for the management of patients with atrial fibrillation a report of the American College of Cardiology/American heart association task force on practice guidelines and the heart rhythm society. J Am Coll Cardiol. 2014;64:e1–e76.
6. Aguilar MI, Hart R. Oral anticoagulants for preventing stroke in patients with non-valvular atrial fibrillation and no previous history of stroke or transient ischemic attacks. Cochrane Database Syst Rev. 2005:CD001927.
7. Kirchhof P, Benussi S, Kotecha D, et al. 2016 ESC guidelines for the management of atrial fibrillation developed in collaboration with EACTS. Eur Heart J. 2016:ehw210.
8. Authors/Task Force Members, Vahanian A, Alfieri O, et al. Guidelines on the management of valvular heart disease (version 2012): the joint task force on the Management of Valvular Heart Disease of the European Society of Cardiology (ESC) and the European Association for Cardio-Thoracic Surgery (EACTS). Eur Heart J. 2012;33:2451–96.
9. Nishimura RA, Otto CM, Bonow RO, et al. 2014 AHA/ACC guideline for the management of patients with valvular heart disease: a report of the American College of Cardiology/American heart association task force on practice guidelines. J Am Coll Cardiol. 2014;63:e57–185.
10. Meschia JF, Bushnell C, Boden-Albala B, et al. Guidelines for the primary prevention of stroke a statement for healthcare professionals from the American Heart Association/American stroke association. Stroke. 2014;45:3754–832.
11. Kernan WN, Ovbiagele B, Black HR, et al. Guidelines for the prevention of stroke in patients with stroke and transient ischemic attack a guideline for healthcare professionals from the American Heart Association/American stroke association. Stroke. 2014;45:2160–236.
12. Witt BJ, Ballman KV, Brown RD, et al. The incidence of stroke after myocardial infarction: a meta-analysis. Am J Med. 2006;119:354.e1–9.
13. Haq SA, Heitner JF, Sacchi TJ, et al. Long-term effect of chronic oral anticoagulation with warfarin after acute myocardial infarction. Am J Med. 2010;123:250–8.
14. Saposnik G, Barinagarrementeria F, Brown RD, et al. Diagnosis and management of cerebral venous thrombosis a statement for healthcare professionals from the American Heart Association/American stroke association. Stroke. 2011;42:1158–92.
15. Crowther MA, Warkentin TE. Bleeding risk and the management of bleeding complications in patients undergoing anticoagulant therapy: focus on new anticoagulant agents. Blood. 2008;111:4871–9.
16. Lip GY. Implications of the CHA2DS2-VASc and HAS-BLED scores for thromboprophylaxis in atrial fibrillation. Am J Med. 2011;124:111–4.
17. Makris M, Van Veen JJ, Tait CR, et al. Guideline on the management of bleeding in patients on antithrombotic agents. Br J Haematol. 2013;160:35–46.
18. Hemphill JC, Greenberg SM, Anderson CS, et al. Guidelines for the management of spontaneous intracerebral hemorrhage a guideline for healthcare professionals from the American Heart Association/American stroke association. Stroke. 2015;46:2032–60.
19. Heidbuchel H, Verhamme P, Alings M, et al. European heart rhythm association practical guide on the use of new oral anticoagulants in patients with non-valvular atrial fibrillation. Europace. 2013;15:625–51.
20. Jauch EC, Saver JL, Adams HP, et al. Guidelines for the early management of patients with acute ischemic stroke a guideline for healthcare professionals from the American Heart Association/American stroke association. Stroke. 2013;44:870–947.
21. Lip GYH, Windecker S, Huber K, et al. Management of antithrombotic therapy in atrial fibrillation patients presenting with acute coronary syndrome and/or undergoing percutaneous coronary or valve interventions: a joint consensus document of the European Society of Cardiology Working Group on thrombosis, European heart rhythm association (EHRA), European Association of Percutaneous Cardiovascular Interventions (EAPCI) and European Association of Acute Cardiac Care (ACCA) endorsed by the Heart Rhythm Society (HRS) and Asia-Pacific Heart Rhythm Society (APHRS). Eur Heart J. 2014;35:3155–79.
22. Douketis JD, Spyropoulos AC, Spencer FA, et al. Perioperative management of antithrombotic therapy: antithrombotic therapy and prevention of thrombosis, 9th ed: American college of chest physicians evidence-based clinical practice guidelines. Chest. 2012;141:e326S–50S.
23. Douketis JD, Spyropoulos AC, Kaatz S, et al. Perioperative bridging anticoagulation in patients with atrial fibrillation. N Engl J Med. 2015;373:823–33.
24. Demaerschalk BM, Kleindorfer DO, Adeoye OM, et al. Scientific rationale for the inclusion and exclusion criteria for intravenous alteplase in acute ischemic stroke a statement for healthcare professionals from the American Heart Association/American stroke association. Stroke. 2016;47:581–641.
25. Vílchez JA, Gallego P, Lip GY. Safety of new oral anticoagulant drugs: a perspective. Ther Adv Drug Saf. 2013; doi:10.1177/2042098613507945.
26. Senoo K, Lip GYH. Comparative efficacy and safety of the non-vitamin K antagonist oral anticoagulants for patients with nonvalvular atrial fibrillation. Semin Thromb Hemost. 2015;41:146–53.

Carotid Endarterectomy Versus Carotid Angioplasty and Stenting for Stroke Prevention

30

Tae Jung Kim and Seung-Hoon Lee

Abstract

In the current clinical situation, no surgery or procedure has been authorized for the treatment for intracranial artery stenosis, and hence, the importance of treatment methods for extracranial carotid atherosclerosis cannot be overstated. Moreover, as two methods—carotid endarterectomy (CEA) and carotid angioplasty and stenting (CAS)—have been concurrently developing, confusion often arises as to the selection of appropriate approach to be used in each case. In this chapter, we analyze the results of clinical trials on CEA and CAS used to treat carotid stenosis and present information essential to the understanding of the current state of research in this field, in conjunction with experience-based treatment suggestions.

Carotid artery stenosis is a major cause of ischemic stroke or transient ischemic attack, comprising 15–20% of all cases. Annually, ischemic stroke recurs in 10% of patients with symptomatic carotid stenosis and 2–4% of those with asymptomatic carotid stenosis [1, 2]. Carotid artery stenosis is a disease caused by atherosclerosis of the artery walls. Atherosclerotic plaques of the carotid arteries mainly occur where the common carotid artery bifurcates into the internal and external carotid arteries, as atheroma frequently occurs in this area due to disruptions in laminar flow and conditions of low shear stress. If the size of the atheromatous plaque increases, the artery lumen narrows, decreasing blood flow in the carotid artery, which can result in hemodynamic infarction due to hypoperfusion. Additionally, ischemic stroke may be caused by sudden thrombosis following platelet activation due to plaque rupture, surface erosion, calcification of nodules, etc. [2]. Therefore, in order to prevent carotid artery stenosis, it is essential to prevent and manage risk factors such as hyperlipidemia, diabetes mellitus, obesity, hypertension, and smoking, among others. If carotid stenosis has already occurred, carotid revascularization is highly recommended [2–4].

T.J. Kim • S.-H. Lee, M.D. Ph.D., F.A.H.A. (✉)
Department of Neurology, Seoul National University Hospital, 101 Daehak-ro, Jongno-gu, Seoul 03080, South Korea
e-mail: sb0516@snu.ac.kr

S.-H. Lee (ed.), *Stroke Revisited: Diagnosis and Treatment of Ischemic Stroke*, Stroke Revisited, DOI 10.1007/978-981-10-1424-6_30

30.1 Evaluation of Carotid Artery Stenosis

30.1.1 Diagnosis of Carotid Artery Stenosis

In cases of carotid artery stenosis, it is important to assess the degree and location of the stenosis as well as the nature of plaques in developing a plan for future treatment. Major noninvasive modalities used to evaluate extracranial large artery stenosis include carotid duplex ultrasound (CDU), computed tomography angiography (CTA), and magnetic resonance angiography (MRA). If such noninvasive modalities are insufficient for evaluating the degree of stenosis, or if carotid artery revascularization is indicated due to the severity of carotid artery stenosis, conventional angiography may also be performed [2, 3]. CDU is widely utilized because it is safe and can be used at bedside for preliminary evaluation of flow velocity, plaque nature, etc. However, CDU is limited in that the results can vary depending on the skill level of the testing clinician. Furthermore, it is difficult to develop a treatment plan based on CDU results alone, and the method is thus regarded as a simple screening test (Fig. 30.1a). Although CTA is an excellent modality for the evaluation of carotid stenosis, the accuracy of this method is slightly lower in

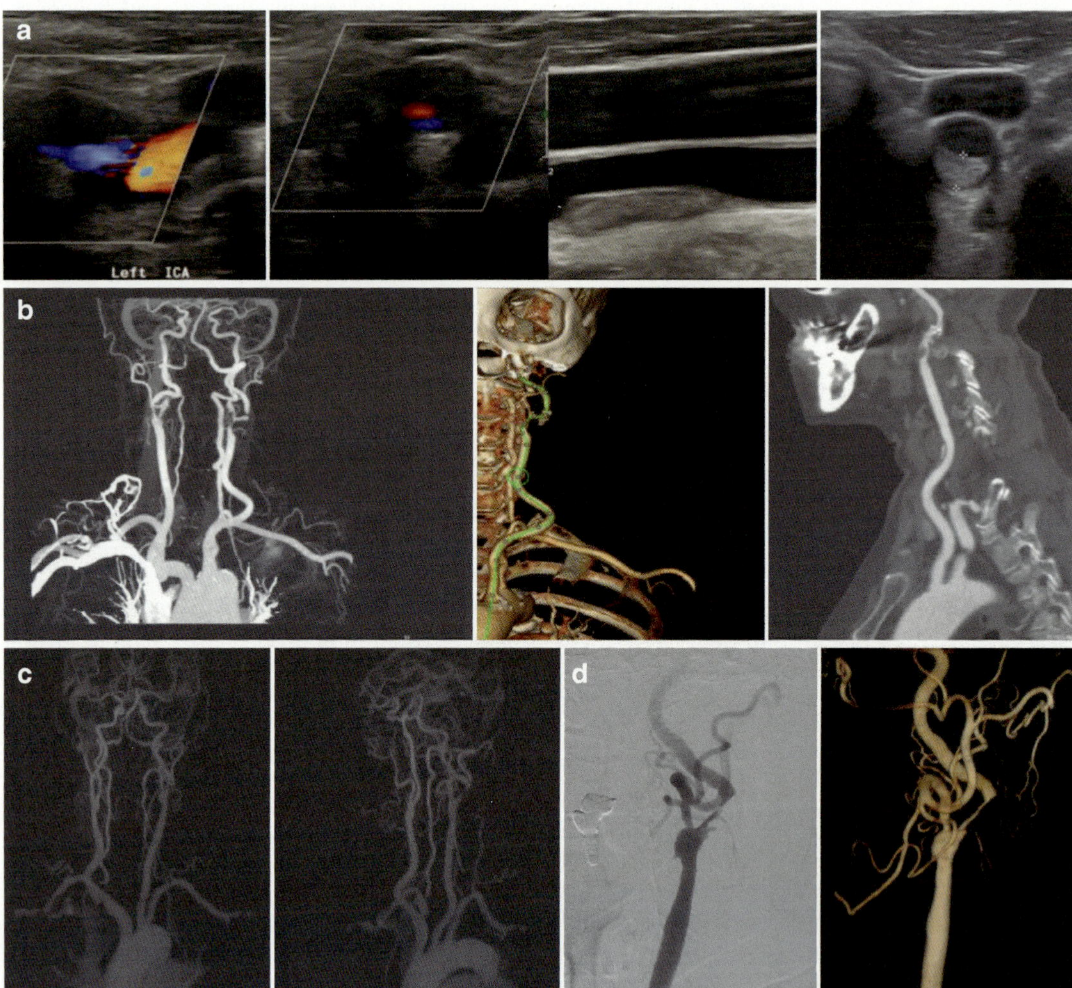

Fig. 30.1 Diagnosis modalities of carotid artery stenosis: (**a**) carotid Doppler ultrasound, (**b**) computed tomography angiography, (**c**) magnetic resonance angiography, (**d**) conventional angiography

cases of severe stenosis, and there are risks of nephropathy and radiation exposure due to the contrast agent used in the test (Fig. 30.1b). MRA is relatively accurate in the evaluation of the degree of carotid artery stenosis, and there is no risk of radiation exposure because no contrast agent is required. However, care should be taken when interpreting MRA results, as artifacts may arise in the presence of metallic foreign bodies and because this method is contraindicated in patients with a pacemaker (Fig. 30.1c) [2, 3]. Accordingly, a preliminary test method should be selected by considering each patient's individual medical history. Conventional angiography is performed when noninvasive evaluations yield inconclusive results or when carotid revascularization is indicated. While conventional angiography can accurately assess stenosis in patients with carotid disease, the procedure is expensive and invasive, and there is risk of radiation exposure and risk due to the use of a contrast agent (Fig. 30.1d) [2]. Therefore, patients should first undergo evaluation with noninvasive modalities, followed by conventional angiography, in order to develop the most appropriate treatment plan for each patient.

30.1.2 Evaluating the Degree of Stenosis

It is essential to accurately assess the degree of carotid artery stenosis in deciding whether to perform revascularization. Although there has been much confusion because two clinical trials—i.e., NASCET (North American Symptomatic Carotid Endarterectomy Trial) [5] and ECST (European Carotid Surgery Trial) [6]—have been conducted to evaluate carotid endarterectomy (CEA) using different methods to assess the degree of stenosis, the NASCET method is currently the most widely utilized (Fig. 30.2a, b). The NASCET method more accurately reflects hemodynamic features, whereas the ECST method more accurately reflects plaque burden around the stenosis. However, the accuracy of the ECST method is lower because measurements are obtained by drawing an imaginary line over the carotid bulb, and thus it is highly likely for different testers to

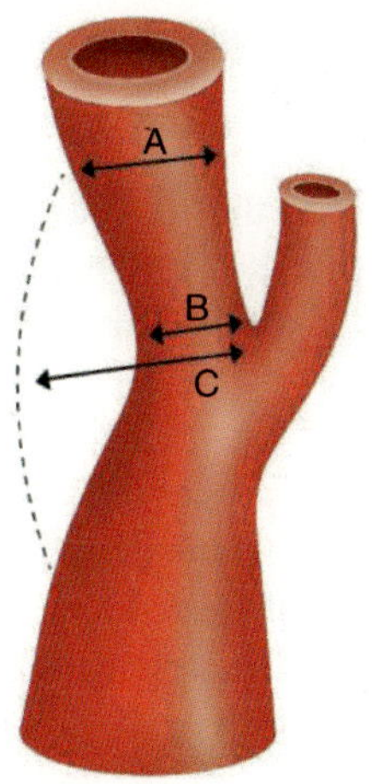

$$\text{a NASCET} \quad \frac{A-B}{A} \qquad \text{b ECST} \quad \frac{C-B}{C}$$

Fig. 30.2 Evaluating the degree of carotid artery stenosis

obtain different measurement results. For this reason, the ECST method may produce exaggerated assessment results with regard to stenosis when compared with the NASCET method [7, 8]. Based on the NASCET measurement method, carotid artery stenosis can largely be classified into no stenosis, mild stenosis (<50% stenosis), moderate stenosis (50–69% stenosis), severe stenosis (>70% stenosis), and occlusion, and the treatment approach can be determined according to the degree of stenosis [7, 8].

30.2 Treatment of Carotid Artery Stenosis

In patients who have experienced an ischemic stroke due to significant carotid artery stenosis, CEA or carotid artery stenting (CAS) should be considered. Because there are two methods that can be used in such patients, the physician should select the most optimal method for each patient by analyzing previous clinical trial results objectively and in detail and by applying the results appropriately to the treatment center where the physician is working. Below, we analyze and summarize important clinical trial findings regarding CEA and CAS and make recommendations for treatment based upon these findings.

30.2.1 CEA in Symptomatic Carotid Stenosis

In the NASCET, the first large-scale study that compared methods of treatment in patients with symptomatic carotid artery stenosis, CEA reduced 2-year stroke recurrence by 17.0% in patients with stenosis of 70% or more and reduced 5-year stroke recurrence by 6.5% in patients with moderate stenosis (50–69%), compared to medical management [5, 7, 9]. The ECST study conducted in the EU reported a very similar finding: three-year stroke recurrence was reduced by 12.9% in patients with stenosis of 70% or more. The findings of these clinical trials suggest that CEA rather than medical management should be considered in patients with symptomatic carotid stenosis of 50% or more [6, 7, 9].

30.2.2 Timing of CEA in Symptomatic Carotid Stenosis

No independent clinical trial has been conducted to investigate when CEA should be performed after ischemic stroke due to symptomatic carotid stenosis. A secondary analysis of previous studies (including the NASCET, ECST, etc.) revealed that the risk of stroke and death for 5 years was decreased by 30% if CEA was performed in patients with symptomatic carotid artery stenosis within 2 weeks after an ischemic event versus later (2–4 weeks: 18%, 4–12 weeks: 11%, and 12 weeks or more: 9%) [10]. Subsequently, many guidelines have recommended that CEA be performed within 2 weeks after the occurrence of an ischemic stroke [4], although clear evidence for the safety and efficacy of such treatment remains lacking, as no large-scale studies have been conducted to examine the effect of surgery timing. Accordingly, the appropriate timing of surgery should be determined based upon the individual characteristics of each treatment center and patient.

30.2.3 Asymptomatic Carotid Stenosis: CEA

Large-scale studies have been conducted to investigate the treatment effect of CEA not only in patients with symptomatic carotid stenosis but also in those with asymptomatic carotid stenosis. In the ACAS (Asymptomatic Carotid Atherosclerosis Study) [11] and ACST (Asymptomatic Carotid Surgery Trial) [12], CEA decreased 5-year stroke recurrence by approximately 6% in patients with significant asymptomatic carotid stenosis of 60% or more, and thus it is recommended that CEA should be considered as the primary treatment for patients with significant asymptomatic carotid artery stenosis as well (Table 30.1) [9]. However, criterion

Table 30.1 Randomized clinical trial for ipsilateral stroke prevention in patients with carotid artery stenosis of carotid endarterectomy and medical treatment

Study	Degree of stenosis (%)	Medical treatment	Stroke in CEA	Stroke in medical treatment	ARR (%)	Follow-up
Symptomatic population						
NASCET	70–99	Aspirin 1300 mg daily	9.0	24.5	15.5	2-year
NASCET	50–69	Aspirin 1300 mg daily	15.7	22.2	6.5	5-year
ECST	70–99	Not specified	7.0	19.9	12.9	3-year
Asymptomatic population						
ACAS	60–99	Aspirin325 mg daily	5.1	11.0	5.9	5-year
ACST	60–99	Antiplatelet drugs	6.4	11.8	5.4	5-year

Reproduced by permission of European Heart Journal [9]

NASCET North American Symptomatic Carotid Endarterectomy Trial, *ECST* European Carotid Symptomatic Trial, *ACAS* Asymptomatic Carotid Atherosclerosis Study, *ACST* Asymptomatic Carotid Surgery Trial, *CEA* carotid endarterectomy of CEA recommendation for asymptomatic carotid stenosis is 60%, which is higher than the criterion for symptomatic stenosis (50%) [4, 9, 13].

30.2.4 CEA Versus CAS: Symptomatic Stenosis

To date, most studies that have compared the treatment effects of CEA and CAS were designed and conducted for the purpose of demonstrating the non-inferiority of CAS versus CEA in patients with symptomatic carotid artery stenosis. The results are summarized below (Table 30.2):

1. CAVATAS (Carotid and Vertebral Artery Transluminal Angioplasty Study): The study was conducted with 504 patients with carotid stenosis, revealing that CAS treatment had similar major risks and effectiveness in preventing stroke for 3 years compared with CEA [14].
2. SPACE (Stent-Protected Percutaneous Angioplasty of the Carotid Artery vs. Endarterectomy): The study compared the effects of CAS and CEA on stroke recurrence and periprocedural complication rates up to 30 days following the procedure in 1183 patients with symptomatic carotid stenosis. However, it failed to indicate the non-inferiority of CAS compared with CEA with regard to the periprocedural complication rate [15].
3. EVA-3S (Endarterectomy vs. Angioplasty in Patients with Symptomatic Severe Carotid Stenosis) [16] and ICSS (International Carotid Stenting Study) [17]: These studies compared the effects of CEA and CAS on stroke recurrence and complication rates during pre- and post-procedure in patients with symptomatic carotid stenosis. In both studies, the effect of CEA was superior: short-term (within 30 days) stroke recurrence or death and long-term stroke rate were all higher in CAS groups than in CEA groups. Particularly in the ICSS, the MRI sub-analysis revealed that patients in the CAS group were three times more likely to develop a new ischemic lesion than those in the CEA group (50% in CAS vs. 17% in CEA) [18].

30.2.5 CEA Versus CAS: Symptomatic Plus Asymptomatic Stenosis

Large-scale studies involving patients with both asymptomatic and symptomatic carotid artery stenosis have been conducted to investigate the effects of CEA and CAS treatment. In both SAPPHIRE and CREST studies, the use of

Table 30.2 Randomized clinical trial for any stroke prevention in patients with carotid artery stenosis of carotid endarterectomy and carotid artery stenting

Study	Study population (CEA/CAS)	EPDs (%)	30-days any stroke (%)	Long-term any stroke (%)	Benefit of CEA vs. CAS in long-term effect	Follow-up
SPACE	595/605	27	6.2/7.5	10.1/10.9	CEA≒CAS	2-year
CAVATAS	253/251	0	6.0/6.0[a]	14.2/14.3[a]	CEA≒CAS	3-year
ICSS	858/855	72	3.3/7.0	9.4/15.2	CEA ≥ CAS	5-year
EVA-3S	262/265	91.9	3.5/9.2	3.4/9.1	CEA ≥ CAS	4-year
SAPPHIRE	167/167	100	3.1/3.6	9.0/9.0	CEA≒CAS	3-year
CREST	1240/1262	96.1	2.3/4.1	7.9/10.2	CEA ≥ CAS	4-year
CREST-S	653/668	96.1	3.2/5.5	6.4/7.6[b]	CEA≒CAS	4-year

CEA carotid endarterectomy, *CAS* carotid artery stenting, *SPACE* Stent-Protected Percutaneous Angioplasty of the Carotid Artery vs. Endarterectomy, *CAVATAS* Carotid and Vertebral Artery Transluminal Angioplasty Study, *EVA-3S* Endarterectomy vs. Angioplasty in Patients with Symptomatic Severe Carotid Stenosis, *SAPPHIRE* Stenting and Angioplasty with Protection in Patients at High Risk for Endarterectomy, *ICSS* International Carotid Stenting Study, *CREST* Carotid Revascularization Endarterectomy vs. Stenting Trial, *CREST-S* Carotid Revascularization Endarterectomy vs. Stenting Trial, symptomatic group

[a]Death or disabling stroke

[b]All periprocedural strokes or postprocedural ipsilateral stroke

embolic protection devices (EPD) was mandatory for the CAS procedure. The CREST study ensured that the surgeon performing CAS had undergone sufficient training and was highly experienced. Nonetheless, the study failed to show the non-inferiority of CAS compared to CEA in stroke recurrence (Table 30.2).

1. The SAPPHIRE (Stenting and Angioplasty with Protection in Patients at High Risk for Endarterectomy) study examined the treatment effect of CEA and CAS in a high-risk CEA patient group among symptomatic (>50% stenosis) or asymptomatic patients (>80% stenosis). Significantly better results were obtained for the CAS group with regard to rates of 1-year death, stroke, and myocardial infarction (12.2% in the CAS group and 20.1% in the CEA group). However, no significant difference was observed between the groups when only rates of stroke occurrence were compared. Furthermore, an analysis of only patients with symptomatic carotid stenosis revealed that the recurrence rate of long-term stroke was 6.6% in the CAS group and 5.4% in the CES group, resulting in no between-group differences [19].
2. The CREST (Carotid Revascularization Endarterectomy vs. Stenting Trial) also compared the treatment effect of CEA and CAS in symptomatic (>50%) or asymptomatic patients (>60% stenosis). The overall occurrence rate of long-term death, stroke, myocardial infarction, and any ipsilateral stroke was similar between the two groups, although the occurrence rate of long-term stroke was lower in the CEA group. Additionally, during pre- and post-procedure, myocardial infarction occurred more frequently in the CEA group (2.3% vs. 1.1%), whereas stroke occurred more frequently in the CAS group (4.1% vs. 2.3%) [20].

30.2.6 CAS Is Never Superior to CEA: No Use of EPD?

Care should be taken when interpreting and applying the findings of individual clinical trials to clinical practice, and it is difficult to consider CAS as a treatment that can sufficiently replace CEA. Most studies argue that CAS did not show non-inferiority compared to CEA because the use of EPD was not mandatory when CAS was performed. However, when the rate of EPD was considered in each of the studies (Table 30.2), there was no clear trend in treatment effect between studies with lower EPD use and those with higher EPD use [1, 9]. Thus, the impact of EPD on the findings of large-scale studies remains controversial, and evidence is lacking because a large-scale study has not yet been conducted to investigate the effect of EPD.

Both SPACE and CAVATAS studies found no difference in the treatment effects of CEA and CAS, while the EVA-3S and ICSS reported that CEA was associated with significantly greater reduction in the rate of stroke recurrence when compared to CAS. While all four of these studies were conducted in Europe, the SAPPHIRE and CREST studies were mainly conducted in the USA [14–17, 19, 20]. The SPACE, CAVATAS, EVA-3S, and ICSS studies did not require the use of EPD during CAS procedures and were conducted in a general clinical practice environment without specifying the qualifications of the CAS operator; these procedural aspects are likely to have contributed to the null finding that CAS was not as effective as CEA in stroke recurrence. In contrast, SAPPHIRE and CREST mandated the use of EPD, and the CREST was conducted with the specification that experienced operators should perform CAS. Probably due to this effort, CAS was associated with better outcomes for vascular events in the SAPPHIRE study, although no difference in stroke was noted [19, 20]. Despite such efforts, however, the CREST study—the largest of the clinical trials—did not reveal the superiority of CAS [20].

30.2.7 CEA Versus CAS: Suggestion

In summary, the results of the aforementioned clinical trials indicate that CEA, rather than CAS, should generally be considered the gold standard treatment for the prevention of ischemic stroke. However, we may be neglecting an important aspect. Until now, we have focused on CEA and CAS as mainly competing rather than as complementary treatment methods. CEA is a procedure in which the lining of the carotid artery is completely removed and is thus beneficial in treating a lesion with many vulnerable plaques, for which a high embolic risk exists. In such case, the vulnerability of atheromatous plaque is a more important than the degree of stenosis itself. In contrast, CAS does not eliminate an atheromatous plaque but pushes it out in the direction of the arterial wall using the force of a balloon and stent. Because the procedure purposefully induces plaque rupture, it is highly likely for plaque debris to embolize to the brain if EPD is not used. Accordingly, CAS is likely to be appropriate in patients with a high risk of hemodynamic stroke due to hypoperfusion associated with a high degree of stenosis than in those with a high risk of embolic stroke. However, previous clinical trials have not considered the benefits and characteristics of each treatment in application [1, 9]. Moreover, it is impossible to reexamine the characteristics of patients included in these trials, even via a secondary analysis. Therefore, selection of either CEA or CAS should be based upon a consideration of the comparative risk of each patient for embolic stroke and hemodynamic stroke, even in cases in which the degree of stenosis seems similar.

Presently, the guidelines recommend that CEA should primarily be considered for patients with significant symptomatic carotid artery stenosis (>50%) whose risk of complications (stroke, mortality) due to surgery is under 6%, in order to prevent the recurrence of ischemic stroke. CAS is recommended as a second treatment method for patients in whom CEA may be too risky [4]. In addition, prophylactic CEA or CAS can be recommended for patients with asymptomatic carotid artery stenosis (>60% in conventional angiography or 70% in CDU) whose risk of complication (stroke, mortality) due to surgery or procedure is under 3%, though CEA is often recommended as the primary treatment in such cases [13].

30.3 Patient Selection for CEA or CAS

As previously described, CEA should be utilized prior to CAS. Furthermore, when the mechanism of stroke is taken into account, CEA is more appropriate for the treatment of large, vulnerable plaques with a high embolic risk, while CAS is more appropriate for large, stable plaques with a high risk of hemodynamic stroke. However, other factors may be relevant when considering either CEA or CAS.

When classifying patients with high CEA risk, the medical and anatomical conditions of each patient should largely be considered. It is first necessary to determine whether the location is accessible using each surgical procedure. CAS should be considered if the location of carotid artery stenosis is difficult to access surgically (above C2 level, above mandible level, or below clavicle level). CAS can also be considered for patients for whom general anesthesia is considered risky owing to heart failure, coronary artery disease, chronic pulmonary disease, etc., as the procedure can be performed on patients under light sedation or during the awake state. Additionally, CEA may be difficult to perform in patients with a history of radiation therapy, restenosis following CEA, a history of neck surgery, or contralateral carotid occlusion [9, 19, 21].

CAS is advantageous compared to CEA in that it is a less invasive procedure and can be used in patients with comorbidities for which general anesthesia is contraindicated, as it is performed with local anesthesia. However, performing CAS can be difficult in patients whose lesions are difficult to access during the procedure or in those with anatomical factors that render stenting difficult. For example, CAS is difficult to perform in patients with a steep aortic arch or severe tortuosity in the common carotid artery, as it is difficult to access the lesion area of the carotid artery with a guidewire or a stent [9]. This point was also reflected in the previous findings of the CREST, SPACE, and ICSS studies: CAS was associated with a lower rate of stroke occurrence relative to CEA in patients under age 70, whereas CAS was associated with higher stroke occurrence than

CEA in patients over 70. These results may be reflective of the observation that older adults are more likely to have carotid artery tortuosity and calcification. Accordingly, these clinical trials present evidence for the priority of CEA over CAS in a selection between the two procedures for older patients (>70 years) [3, 21, 22].

30.4 Techniques of CEA and CAS and Periprocedural Monitoring

30.4.1 CEA Technique and Monitoring

CEA can be performed in a relatively short time and is associated with a relatively short recovery period following the procedure. During surgery, however, care should be taken to remove the plaque without injuring the surrounding structures and to minimize the risk of events such as embolic stroke. Patients who undergo CEA are treated with aspirin 100–325 mg/day prior to surgery and typically receive general anesthesia rather than local anesthesia [4, 9, 23]. Presenting the surgical techniques in detail is not appropriate here, and we hope that Fig. 30.3A can aid the reader in developing a general understanding of these methods. During carotid artery cross-clamping, optimal cerebral blood flow should be maintained using electrocardiography, pulse oximetry, and intra-arterial arterial pressure monitoring in order to prevent cerebral ischemia and reduce cardiac stress [23]. In addition, changes in wave amplitude should be monitored via electroencephalography (EEG) or somatosensory-evoked potentials (SSEP), while the total cerebral clamp time should also be monitored. Currently, 16-channel EEG is more frequently used than SSEP, although both methods are reported to have an accuracy level over 95% in monitoring cortical cerebral perfusion. Inadequate cerebral perfusion should be suspected if high-frequency

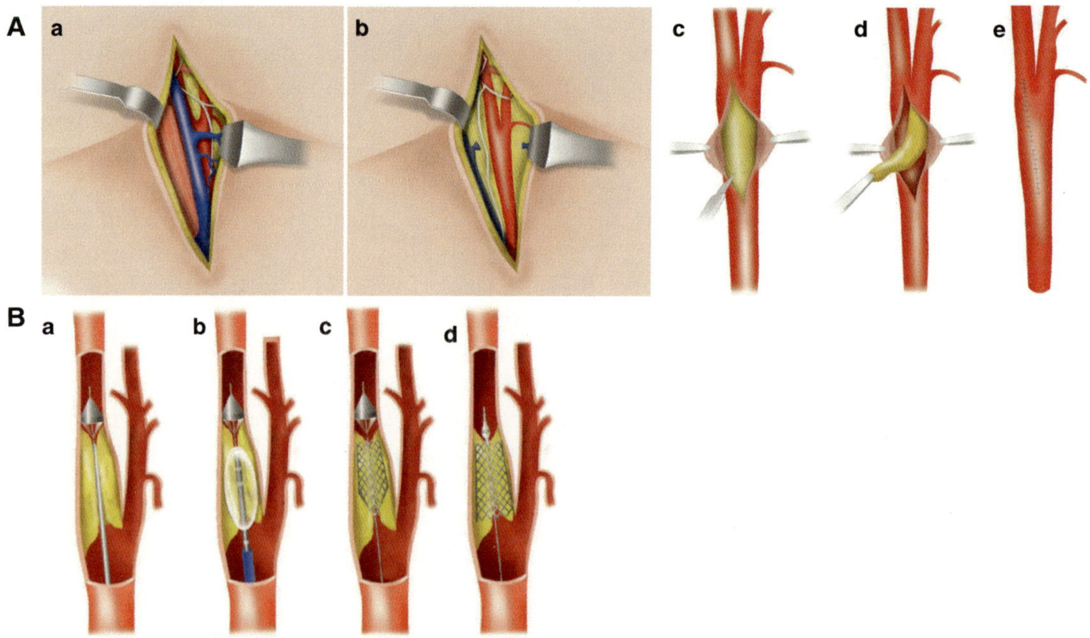

Fig. 30.3 Techniques of carotid endarterectomy and carotid artery stenting. (**A**) Carotid endarterectomy: a. incision down anterior border of sternocleidomastoid muscle; b. exposure of the carotid artery; c. clamping common carotid artery, internal carotid artery, and external carotid artery; d. removal of plaque in carotid artery; e. repair. (**B**) Carotid artery stenting: a. deploying filter in the internal carotid artery, b. inflation of balloon for angioplasty, c. deploying stent, d. removal of filter

amplitude or low-frequency activity is present ipsilaterally or bilaterally in EEG during carotid clamping or if there is a reduction over 50% in P25 amplitude (N20/P25 complex) of the cortex in SSEP [23].

30.4.2 Carotid Artery Stenting Technique and Monitoring

By convention, dual antiplatelet therapy with aspirin and clopidogrel is often administered to patients who undergo CAS. We suggest the readers review the techniques of the CAS procedure presented in Fig. 30.3B. CAS is typically performed while the patient is under light sedation or awake, and thus, intensive monitoring is not necessarily required. However, it is necessary to continually monitor the neurological status of the patient, as embolic events may still occur. Electrocardiography, pulse oximetry, and blood pressure monitoring should also be performed, as bradycardia or hypotension can occur during stenting due to baroreceptor stimulation in the carotid bulb [9, 23].

30.5 Complications of CEA and CAS

A major intraoperative complication of CEA is ischemic stroke, which occurs in approximately 2.1–5.5% of patients. Cardiovascular complications such as acute coronary syndrome, which occurs in 0.5–2.3% of patients and is mainly caused by hemodynamic disturbances due to CEA in patients with existing coronary artery disease, may also develop. Accordingly, an abrupt change in blood pressure, coughing, etc. should be avoided in patients with the relevant risk factors. Direct injury to the cranial nerves (most frequently the hypoglossal nerve) during CEA procedures is reported to occur in approximately 5.1% of patients during retraction or vascular resection. In addition, neck hematoma is reported to occur approximately in 1.7–1.9% of patients following surgery [3, 4, 23].

In contrast, CAS is associated with complications such as embolic stroke, which occurs in 5.5–9.2% of patients, as well as bradycardia and hypotension, which occur in 20–30% of patients during the stenting procedure. Although rare, hematoma, infection, puncture site complications, contrast-related complications, etc. have also been reported as complications of CAS [3, 24].

Hyperperfusion syndrome is a complication that may occur during CEA and CAS. It is reported to occur in 0.2–19% of patients following CEA and in 0.4–11.7% following CAS. Typically, ipsilateral cerebral blood flow increases by 20–40% from the baseline either post CEA or post CAS, although hyperperfusion syndrome can occur if it increases by 100% or more. Hyperperfusion syndrome can induce ipsilateral headache, seizure, focal neurological deficits, hemorrhage, etc. and has been reported to typically occur between 3–4 and 7 days after the procedure, although symptoms can occur as late as 4 weeks after the procedure. The main mechanism underlying hyperperfusion syndrome is the reduction in cerebrovascular reactivity due to an impairment in the cerebral autoregulatory mechanism associated with increased cerebral blood flow. Major risk factors of hyperperfusion syndrome include high-grade carotid artery stenosis, old age, poor collateral flow, contralateral carotid occlusion, increased intraoperative cerebral blood flow, post CEA/CAS systemic hypertension, etc. Therefore, such patients should be managed with special caution against postoperative hypertension [23, 25].

30.6 Follow-Up After CEA or CAS

30.6.1 Post-Revascularization Medical Treatment

Antiplatelet agents such as aspirin should be administered after CEA. Aside from aspirin, clopidogrel and low-dose aspirin plus extended-release dipyridamole can be administered. It is necessary to maintain dual antiplatelet therapy (aspirin plus clopidogrel) in patients who undergo CAS for at least 1 month before and after the procedure [3, 4].

30.6.2 Follow-Up After Revascularization

Following carotid revascularization treatment, restenosis can occur in 6–10.7% of patients treated with CAS and in 5–7% treated with CEA [1, 4]. In principle, a Doppler ultrasound is used for follow-up evaluation of restenosis. MR angiography imaging is ineffective due to the influence of stent artifacts. CT angiography can identify restenosis relatively accurately, though this method requires unnecessary exposure to radiation hazards and contrast agents. Therefore, follow-up monitoring is conducted using Doppler ultrasound for several years at an interval of 6 months to a year [1, 4].

Conclusion

Many articles and textbooks have discussed the superiority of either CEA or CAS, resulting in much confusion for readers. As illustrated in Fig. 30.4, important points to understand, however, can be summarized as follows: (1) the NASCET method is mainly used to examine the degree of carotid stenosis; (2) revascularization is considered if symptomatic carotid stenosis is over 50% or asymptomatic stenosis is over 60%; (3) in general, CEA is superior to CAS, though this may differ depending on the characteristics of the treatment center, the mechanism of stroke for each patient, etc.; (4) CEA may be more appropriate in the treatment of embolic stroke, while CAS may be more appropriate for hemodynamic stroke; (5) hyperperfusion syndrome should be carefully monitored following revascularization; (6) Doppler ultrasound should be performed at each follow-up.

Suggestions from Current Clinical Guidelines Carotid endarterectomy (CEA) is recommended in patients with recent symptomatic stroke or transient ischemic attack (within 6 months) and ipsilateral carotid stenosis more than 50%. Perioperative morbidity and mortality should be estimated to be less than 6%. Carotid angioplasty and stenting (CAS) is just an alternative method to CEA. In asymptomatic stenosis more than 70%, CEA is also reasonable if the perioperative morbidity and mortality is less than 3%.

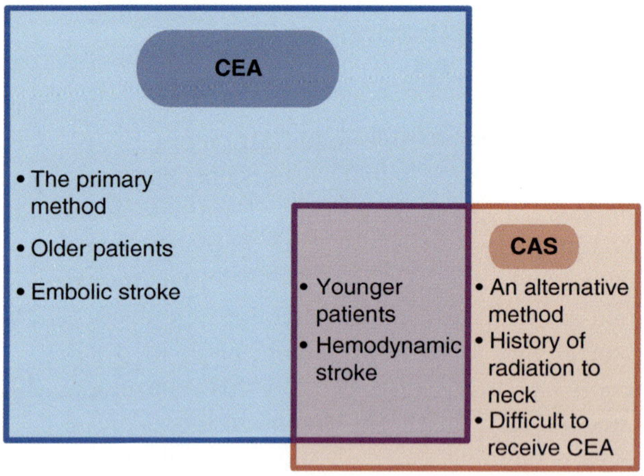

Fig. 30.4 A schematic diagram showing application of CEA or CAS

References

1. Gahremanpour A, Perin EC, Silva G. Carotid artery stenting versus endarterectomy: a systematic review. Tex Heart Inst J. 2012;39:474–87.
2. Hall HA, Bassiouny HS. Pathophysiology of carotid atherosclerosis. In: Nicolaides A, et al., editors. Ultrasound and carotid bifurcation atherosclerosis. Heidelberg: Springer; 2011. p. 27–39.
3. Brott TG, Halperin JL, Abbara S, et al. 2011 ASA/ACCF/AHA/AANN/AANS/ACR/ASNR/CNS/SAIP/SCAI/SIR/SNIS/SVM/SVS guideline on the management of patients with extracranial carotid and vertebral artery disease: executive summary. A report of the American College of Cardiology Foundation/American Heart Association task force on practice guidelines, and the American Stroke Association, American Association of Neuroscience Nurses, American Association of Neurological Surgeons, American College of Radiology, American Society of Neuroradiology, Congress of Neurological Surgeons, Society of Atherosclerosis Imaging and Prevention, Society for Cardiovascular Angiography and Interventions, Society of Interventional Radiology, society of NeuroInterventional surgery, Society for Vascular Medicine, and Society for Vascular Surgery. Circulation. 2011;124:489–532.
4. Kernan WN, Ovbiagele B, Black HR, et al. Guidelines for the prevention of stroke in patients with stroke and transient ischemic attack: a guideline for healthcare professionals from the American Heart Association/American Stroke Association. Stroke. 2014;45:2160–236.
5. Collaborators NASCET. Beneficial effect of carotid endarterectomy in symptomatic patients with high-grade carotid stenosis. N Engl J Med. 1991;325:445–53.
6. European Carotid Surgery Trialists' Collaborative Group. MRC European carotid surgery trial: interim results for symptomatic patients with severe (70–99%) or with mild (0–29%) carotid stenosis. Lancet. 1991;337:1235–43.
7. Rothwell P, Eliasziw M, Gutnikov S, et al. Analysis of pooled data from the randomised controlled trials of endarterectomy for symptomatic carotid stenosis. Lancet. 2003;361:107–16.
8. Oates C, Naylor A, Hartshorne T, et al. Joint recommendations for reporting carotid ultrasound investigations in the United Kingdom. Eur J Vasc Endovasc Surg. 2009;37:251–61.
9. Roffi M, Mukherjee D, Clair DG. Carotid artery stenting vs. endarterectomy. Eur Heart J. 2009;30:2693–704.
10. Rothwell P, Eliasziw M, Gutnikov S, et al. Endarterectomy for symptomatic carotid stenosis in relation to clinical subgroups and timing of surgery. Lancet. 2004;363:915–24.
11. Walker MD, Marler JR, Goldstein M, et al. Endarterectomy for asymptomatic carotid artery stenosis. JAMA. 1995;273:1421–8.
12. Group MACSTC. Prevention of disabling and fatal strokes by successful carotid endarterectomy in patients without recent neurological symptoms: randomised controlled trial. Lancet. 2004;363:1491–502.
13. Meschia JF, Bushnell C, Boden-Albala B, et al. Guidelines for the primary prevention of stroke: a statement for healthcare professionals from the American Heart Association/American Stroke Association. Stroke. 2014;45:3754–832.
14. Brown M, Rogers J, Bland J. Endovascular versus surgical treatment in patients with carotid stenosis in the carotid and vertebral artery Transluminal angioplasty study (CAVATAS): a randomised trial. Lancet. 2001;357:1729–37.
15. Eckstein H-H, Ringleb P, Allenberg J-R, et al. Results of the stent-protected angioplasty versus carotid endarterectomy (SPACE) study to treat symptomatic stenoses at 2 years: a multinational, prospective, randomised trial. Lancet Neurol. 2008;7:893–902.
16. Mas J-L, Chatellier G, Beyssen B, et al. Endarterectomy versus stenting in patients with symptomatic severe carotid stenosis. N Engl J Med. 2006;355:1660–71.
17. Investigators ICSS. Carotid artery stenting compared with endarterectomy in patients with symptomatic carotid stenosis (international carotid stenting study): an interim analysis of a randomised controlled trial. Lancet. 2010;375:985–97.
18. Bonati LH, Jongen LM, Haller S, et al. New ischaemic brain lesions on MRI after stenting or endarterectomy for symptomatic carotid stenosis: a substudy of the international carotid stenting study (ICSS). Lancet Neurol. 2010;9:353–62.
19. Yadav JS, Wholey MH, Kuntz RE, et al. Protected carotid-artery stenting versus endarterectomy in high-risk patients. N Engl J Med. 2004;351:1493–501.
20. Brott TG, Hobson RW, Howard G, et al. Stenting versus endarterectomy for treatment of carotid-artery stenosis. N Engl J Med. 2010;363:11–23.
21. Economopoulos KP, Sergentanis TN, Tsivgoulis G, et al. Carotid artery stenting versus carotid endarterectomy: a comprehensive meta-analysis of short-term and long-term outcomes. Stroke. 2011;42:687–92.
22. Collaboration CST. Short-term outcome after stenting versus endarterectomy for symptomatic carotid stenosis: a preplanned meta-analysis of individual patient data. Lancet. 2010;376:1062–73.
23. Erickson K, Cole D. Carotid artery disease: stenting vs endarterectomy. Br J Anaesth. 2010;105(suppl 1):i34–49.
24. Nicosia A, Nikas D, Castriota F, et al. Classification for carotid artery stenting complications: manifestation, management, and prevention. J Endovasc Ther. 2010;17:275–94.
25. van Mook WN, Rennenberg RJ, Schurink GW, et al. Cerebral hyperperfusion syndrome. Lancet Neurol. 2005;4:877–88.

Post-Stroke Management: Emotional Disturbances and Pain

31

Jong S. Kim

Abstract

Patients with stroke often have sequelae such as motor dysfunction, ataxia, visual field defect, etc. However, there still are disturbances that are not apparent and frequently unnoticed by physicians. They include cognitive dysfunction, mood and emotional disturbances, and pain or paresthesia. In this chapter, post-stroke emotional disturbances and pain are described. Post-stroke mood and emotional disturbances are frequent and diverse in their manifestations and can be categorized as post-stroke depression, post-stroke emotional incontinence, post-stroke anger proneness, and post-stroke fatigue. These symptoms are distressing for both the patients and their caregivers and negatively influence the patient's quality of life. Post-stroke pain includes nociceptive pain, central pain, and headache and is equally distressing for patients. Fortunately, these mood/emotional disturbances and pain syndromes can be treated or prevented by various methods, including pharmacological therapy. To administer the appropriate therapy, we have to understand the phenomenology and the similarities and differences in the pathophysiological mechanisms associated with these phenomena.

31.1 Post-Stroke Mood and Emotional Disturbances

Mood and emotional disturbances are frequent symptoms in stroke survivors and include post-stroke depression (PSD), post-stroke anxiety, post-stroke emotional incontinence (PSEI), post-stroke anger proneness (PSAP), and post-stroke fatigue (PSF). Underlying factors and pathophysiologic mechanisms of these emotional disturbances partially overlap, but are still different [1].

J.S. Kim, M.D., Ph.D.
Stroke Center and Department of Neurology, University of Ulsan College of Medicine, Asan Medical Center, Songpa-gu, Seoul 138-736, South Korea
e-mail: jongskim@amc.seoul.kr

S.-H. Lee (ed.), *Stroke Revisited: Diagnosis and Treatment of Ischemic Stroke*, Stroke Revisited, DOI 10.1007/978-981-10-1424-6_31

These emotional disturbances have negative impacts on patients' clinical outcomes. PSD, for example, negatively influences later functional outcomes after stroke, decreases quality of life, leads to less efficient use of rehabilitation services, and increases mortality. Patients with PSF are more often unemployed and fail to return to previous jobs than those without PSF. Although the overall negative impacts of PSEI and PSAP are less marked than those of PSD, they still lead to distress and embarrassment and impair patients' quality of life. These post-stroke mood and emotional disturbances can be treated by various methods, including pharmacological therapy.

31.1.1 Depression and Depressive Mood

The symptoms of post-stroke depression or depressive symptoms include depressed mood, anhedonia, loss of energy, decreased concentration, and psychic retardation. Although somatic symptoms, such as decreased appetite and insomnia are common, they may in part be attributed to the stroke itself or comorbid diseases. Guilty feelings and suicidal ideations are less common than in primary depression.

The fifth US Diagnostic and Statistical Manual of Mental Disorders has been used for the diagnosis of PSD. It defines depressed mood or anhedonia (loss of interest or pleasure) for 2 weeks or longer, in addition to the presence of at least four of the following symptoms: substantial weight loss or gain, insomnia or hypersomnia, psychomotor agitation or retardation, fatigue or loss of energy, worthlessness or inappropriate guilt, diminished concentration, and indecisiveness. However, it remains controversial whether this tool can be used in stroke patients, especially in the acute setting. Thus, other depression screening instruments are also used that include the nine-item Patient Health Questionnaire, the Center of Epidemiological Studies-Depression Scale, the Hospital Anxiety and Depression Scale, the Hamilton Depression Rating Scale, the Beck Depression Inventory, and the Montgomery-Asberg Depression Scale [1].

The prevalence of PSD varies widely (5–67%) due to different study settings, time since stroke, and the different criteria/methods used to diagnose PSD [2]. Generally, the prevalence of depression decreases over time along with the improvement of neurological deficits. Demographic characteristics (age and sex), the side of the lesion, and pathological subtype are not consistently associated with PSD. A history of depression before stroke and cognitive impairment appears to be associated with PSD.

The most consistent factors associated with PSD are severe stroke and early or late physical disability. It seems that patients' acute depressive symptoms are related to physical dysfunction, while PSD at the chronic stage has an additional psychosocial component [3]. Although Robinson emphasized the role of left frontal lesions in producing PSD [4], others have shown heterogeneous results. One study found that the association between left anterior cortical stroke and PSD was apparent at the acute stage, but not the subacute or chronic stages. Higher lesion volumes, cerebral atrophy, silent infarcts, and white matter lesions may also be associated with a higher risk of PSD.

The close relationship between PSD and neurological deficits suggests that PSD may be a psychological, reactive depressive symptom associated with sudden functional deficits. The chronic PSD may be related with persistent functional deficits, patients' personality traits, and environmental factors, such as social support, economic matters, job stability, etc. In addition, alterations in neurotransmitter systems, such as serotonergic, adrenergic, and dopaminergic systems, may play a role.

The Cochrane review of treatment trials involving 1655 subjects showed that drugs such as selective serotonin reuptake inhibitors (SSRI) or tricyclic antidepressant drugs improve depressive symptoms, but they may be associated with gastrointestinal and central nervous system side effects [5]. For old stroke patients, SSRI is a more appropriate drug for initial use because its side effect is less serious than that of tricyclic antidepressants. There was no evidence for effectiveness of psychological therapies alone for the treatment of PSD. It remains unclear whether administration of antidepressants prevents development of depression or depressive symptoms. European and American guidelines recommend pharmaceutical treatment for patients with PSD, along with monitoring for effectiveness and side effects. It is recommended that treatment be continued for at least 6 months after initial recovery.

31.1.2 Emotional Incontinence

In 1924, Wilson described patients with uncontrollable outbursts of involuntary laughing or crying and called this phenomenon as "pathologic laughing and crying." Afterwards, similar emotional displays have been described variably: pseudobulbar affect, emotionalism, emotional lability, emotional incontinence, and involuntary emotional expression disorder [6].

Typically, patients show sudden, uncontrollable, excessive, or inappropriate crying or laughing without apparent motivating stimuli or in response to stimuli that would not normally evoke such responses. In clinical practice, milder symptoms that are triggered by appropriate and congruent stimuli are actually more common. Thus, a broad term "PSEI" will be used in this chapter. Depending upon the characteristics of patients and diagnostic criteria, PSEI prevalence has been reported to vary from 6 to 34%. One report indicates that the prevalence of PSEI is 15% one month post-stroke, 21% at 6 months, and 11% at 12 months post-stroke.

Severe motor/neurologic dysfunction and the presence of depression are reported to be related to PSEI [7]. The anterior cortex-internal capsule/basal ganglia-ventral brainstem circuitry is closely related to PSEI. Patients with lesions in the thalamus or cerebellum also occasionally exhibited PSEI [7]. It seems that a complex cortico-limbic subcortical-thalamic-ponto-cerebellar system contributes to the expression of emotions, and any deficit in this system may lead to PSEI [6].

Studies have shown the important role of serotonergic fibers in producing these symptoms that ascends from the brainstem raphe nuclei to limbic forebrain structures and then projects through the basal ganglia to the frontal cortex [7]. Other neurotransmitters that may also be involved include dopamine and glutamine, which may have roles in regulating the influence of the motor cortex on the brainstem laughing/crying centers [6].

SSRIs are generally quite effective in reducing the frequency and severity of PSEI. Although less well studied, tricyclic antidepressants also seem to be effective. SSRIs are a better option for PSEI treatment, because they are better tolerated in stroke patients and more rapidly alleviate PSEI symptoms than tricyclic antidepressants. Dextromethorphan/quinidine (Nuedexta®, Avanir) is another potentially useful drug for the treatment of PSEI. Dextromethorphan, a sigma-1 receptor agonist, may modulate the serotonergic system as activation of sigma-1 receptor agonists increases the serotonergic function of the dorsal raphe nucleus.

31.1.3 Post-Stroke Aggression and Anger Proneness

Stroke patients may show aggressive behaviors including hitting or hurting others, kicking, biting, throwing objects, cursing, and screaming. This overt aggression is usually observed during the acute stage of stroke. However, if carefully examined, simple anger proneness or inability to control anger and aggression is a much more common than overt aggression. After stroke, patients become more irritable, impulsive, hostile, and less tolerable and generous; they easily express anger at their spouses and children regarding trivial matters [8]. Therefore, these symptoms may collectively be described as post-stroke anger proneness (PSAP).

The PSAP has been studied using various tools, such as the Spielberger Trait Anger Scale, Present State Examination, NEO Personality Inventory Revised, and the Emotional Behavior Index. PSAP is found to be present in 15–35% of patients during the acute or subacute stage depending on the definition of PSAP and characteristics of patients.

Neurologic dysfunction, motor dysfunction, dysarthria, previous stroke, premorbid neuroticism personality trait, depression, and low monoamine oxidase A activity have been reported to be associated with PSAP [8, 9]. It seems that the lesion location responsible for PSAP is fronto-lenticulocapsular-brainstem pontine base area [8]. Similar to PSEI, serotonergic dysfunction seems to play a role in the development of PSAP. At least some of the PSAP is a manifestation of depression or frustration. Thus, PSAP may be a multifactorial phenomenon related to reactive behavioral changes associated with functional deficits and repeated strokes, serotonergic dysfunction due to brain damage, and genetic trait [9].

For treatment, SSRIs such as fluoxetine and escitalopram are of benefit in the treatment of aggressive behavior or anger proneness in patients with personality disorder, dementia, and stroke [10]. Beta adrenergic antagonists and lithium may reduce aggressiveness in patients with brain injury, but have not been studied in stroke patients.

31.1.4 Post-Stroke Fatigue

Stroke patients often develop fatigue. The PSF can be further distinguished by its onset as "fatigue during the acute stage vs. chronic, persistent fatigue," and by its different constructs: exertion vs. mental fatigue. Although there is no fatigue scale that fully considers the complex nature of PSF, previous studies have used: the Fatigue Assessment Scale, the Fatigue Impact Scale, the Checklist of Individual Strength, the visual analogue scale, the Chalder fatigue scale, the Multidimensional Fatigue Symptom Inventory, and the Fatigue Severity Scale. Depending on the definition of PSF, the time elapsed since stroke, and the characteristics of patients, the prevalence of PSF varies widely, from 23 to 75%. The frequency of PSF tends to decrease with time after stroke [1].

Neurologic deficit is one of the most important factors related to PSF. However, the association may at least in part be attributed to associated depression. Studies have shown that the significant association between disability and PSF in the subacute state is lost after controlling for the effects of depression during the chronic stage. Medical comorbidities such as hypertension, medications, eating problems (dysphagia, decreased appetite, etc.), and sleep disturbances may result in PSF. In addition, post-stroke pain and pre-stroke fatigue have been reported to be associated with PSF [11].

Although PSF is closely associated with depression, many PSF patients do not have depression. Unlike depressive patients, PSF patients rarely express worthlessness and hopelessness. The impact of depression on PSF may differ according to the stage of stroke. While neurologic disability leads to exertional fatigue during the early stage of stroke, depression seems to play a more important role in chronic and mental fatigue. Impairments in some domains of cognition, such as attention deficits, slow mental processing, and memory dysfunction, seem to be associated with mental fatigue [11]. Studies have shown that PSF is related to damage to the medial prefrontal cortex, basal ganglia, and the brainstem/thalamic reticular formation, suggesting that alterations in neurotransmitters such as dopamine or adrenaline may lead to PSF. However, more recent MRI-based studies have found no association between PSF and lesion location. Chronic inflammation, altered immune responses after stroke, and genetic trait (i.e, MAO-A) may also be involved in the pathogenesis of PSF. Given the diverse causes of PSF, physicians should identify potentially treatable medical causes of PSF, such as anemia, hypotension, drug overdose, eating disturbances, depression, etc. Generally, SSRIs are not effective for improving PSF. A recent clinical trial using modafinil, a drug originally used for patients with hypersomnia or narcolepsy, showed equivocal result.

31.1.5 Summary of Post-Stroke Mood and Emotional Syndromes

Post-stroke mood and emotional disturbances manifest in diverse manners. The phenomenology, predicting factors, pathophysiology, and response to pharmacological treatments are different, although there also are overlapping factors. PSD is associated with complex pathophysiological mechanisms involving both psychological/psychiatric problems associated with patients' functional deficits as well as neurochemical changes secondary to brain damage. Therefore, although antidepressants, especially SSRIs, are considered to be the treatment of choice, their benefits are not robust. PSEI is more closely associated with lesion location and consequent alterations in neurotransmitters, notably serotonin. Thus, PSEI tends to respond more to SSRIs compared to PSD. Although PSAP is also a complex phenomenon, it seems to have better responsiveness to SSRIs than PSD. Although PSF is closely associated with PSD, it is also causally related to multiple factors. Thus, the benefits of pharmacological therapy are unproven, and treatments have to be individualized according to the causative factors present in each patient. The different aspects of post-stroke emotional syndrome are shown in Fig. 31.1. Undoubtedly, more researches are needed to improve the management of post-stroke mood and emotional disturbances.

31.2 Post-Stroke Pain

One of the most troublesome sequelae of stroke is pain, which occurs in 19–74% of patients. The wide variation of pain incidence is due to differences in the characteristics of subjects, the time of assessment, and the definition of "pain" [12]. According to a study investigating stroke patients using the visual analogue scale (VAS), moderate to severe pain (defined by VAS 40–100) was reported in 32% after 4 months post-stroke (median VAS = 60) and 21% at 16 months. The factors related to pain included younger age, female sex, higher NIHSS score, and elevated

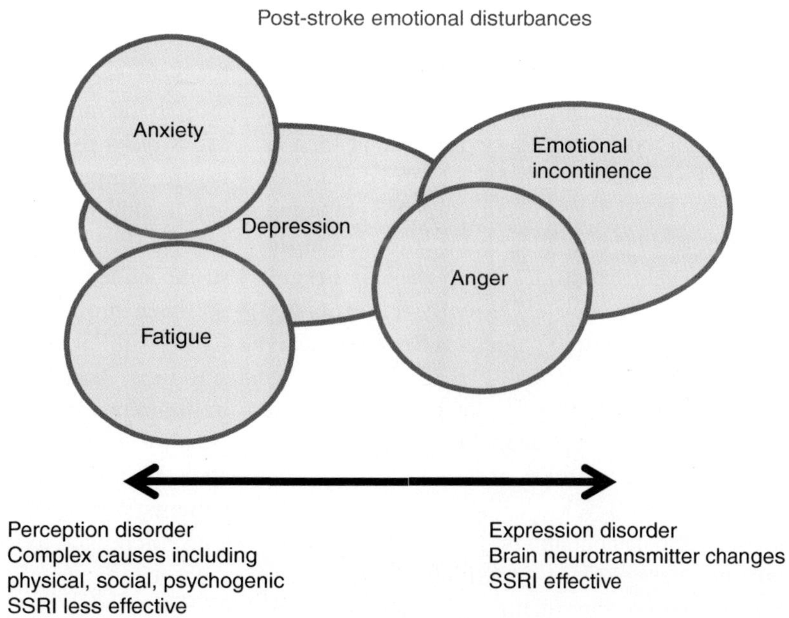

Fig. 31.1 Diagram explaining the different manifestations of post-stroke mood and emotional disturbances

HbA1c at stroke onset. Pain disturbed sleep in 58%, and 40% required rest for relief of pain. However, another controlled, population-based study assessing stroke patients with 2 years of follow-up, development of chronic pain after stroke was only slightly more common than that of sex- and age-matched control group: 39.0 versus 28.9%. In this study, novel headache, shoulder pain, and pain from increased muscle stiffness were more common in stroke patients, whereas joint pain was equally common in the two groups.

The most common location of post-stroke pain is the shoulder, which has a prevalence ranging from 11 to 40%. The shoulder pain is usually due to immobilization and contraction of the shoulder muscles in patients with severe upper arm paresis. In addition, spasticity, bed sores, arthropathy associated with chronic abnormal weight bearing, diabetic neuropathy, depression, and anxiety are causally associated with post-stroke pain. Aside from the pain due to peripheral problems, another important cause of pain in stroke patients is that due to the brain lesion itself. Although this phenomenon was initially described as "thalamic syndrome" or "thalamic pain," it is now widely recognized that strokes occurring anywhere in the sensory tract can produce central pain. Therefore, the term central post-stroke pain (CPSP) is now generally used, although many patients describe the symptoms as "burning," "cold," or "squeezing" rather than as pain. CPSP occurs in 1–8% of stroke patients. However, the delayed occurrence of symptoms, the lack of objective diagnostic criteria, and the fluctuations in symptom severity make it difficult to assess the prevalence. Currently, it is estimated that more than 30,000 patients suffer from CPSP in the USA.

CPSP may start at stroke onset, but more often its onset is delayed, usually within 6 months after stroke onset. The symptoms almost always develop within the area of initial sensory impairment and may be restricted to distal or, less often, proximal body parts. Spinothalamic abnormalities, particularly temperature-sensory ones, are frequently associated with CPSP. Dysesthesia and allodynia are frequent. CPSP is frequently aggravated by a cold environment, psychological stress, heat, fatigue, or body movement. The pathogenesis of CPSP remains unknown, but suggested mechanisms include hyperexcitation in the damaged sensory pathways, damage to the central inhibitory pathways, or a combination of the two. It is highly likely that various neurotransmitters, i.e., adrenergic, serotonin, and glutaminergic, are involved in this process.

Management of post-stroke pain is challenging. The type of pain should be carefully investigated, and treatment should be individualized according to the nature and severity of pain. Because muscle stiffness and spasticity are associated with pain, physical therapy, occupational therapy, aquatics, and splints are often applied. Application of analgesics, topical cream, injection, and repetitive transcranial magnetic stimulation (rTMS) may be of help. Drugs such as diazepam, dantrolence, baclofen, clonidine, and gabapentin are used to relieve spasticity. Botulinum toxin injection works in some patients.

For CPSP, many drugs capable of modulating the CNS neurochemicals have been developed. Amitriptyline was the first drug that was found to improve CPSP in a double-blind, placebo-controlled, crossover study [13]. Amitriptyline is cheap and has been considered the first-line drug in the management of CPSP. However, it is often only partially effective in patients with severe symptoms, and the side effects, such as dry mouth, urinary retention, somnolence, and confusion, are frequently intolerable in aged stroke patients. Although their efficacies have not been properly investigated in patients with CPSP, similar antidepressants with adrenergic activities, such as nortriptyline, desipramine, imipramine, doxepin, and venlafaxine, are occasionally used when amitriptyline is not tolerated. Various antiepileptics have been tried in patients with CPSP under the assumption that CPSP is related to neuronal hyperexcitability in the sensory system. Although the efficacy of carbamazepine and phenytoin on CPSP was not proven, lamotrigine, a novel antiepileptic drug that presynaptically inhibits sodium channels and suppresses glutamate release, was reported to be moderately effective for CPSP in a double-blind, placebo-controlled study.

Recently, gabapentin, a structural analogue of GABA, has received special attention because it acts on presynaptic voltage-sensitive calcium channels, which modulate the release of multiple neurochemicals. Gabapentin was found to be effective in relieving neuropathic pain due to peripheral nerve disease and central pain caused by spinal cord lesions. Unfortunately, there has been no clinical trial that examined the efficacy of gabapentin in patients with CPSP. A closely related drug, pregabalin, was also found to be effective in the treatment of various neuropathic pains, including central pain due to spinal cord lesion. Recently, a 13-week, randomized, double-blind, placebo-controlled study using pregabalin was conducted in patients with CPSP [14]. The benefit of pregabalin on the primary outcome, the mean pain score on the Daily Pain Rating Scale over the last 7 days, was not proven. However, the conclusion should be cautiously interpreted because pregabalin produced significantly greater pain relief up to 8 weeks versus placebo, and no loss of pain reduction was seen thereafter. Moreover, pregabalin resulted in significant improvements in the secondary endpoints that included sleep disturbances, anxiety, and the clinician global impression of change. There are no universally accepted treatment guidelines for CPSP. Figure 31.2 describes one of the typical approaches used to treat CPSP patients [15].

Non-pharmacological treatment such as deep brain stimulation (DBS), electrical motor cortex stimulation (MCS), and high-frequency repetitive transcranial magnetic stimulation (rTMS) of the motor cortical area are occasionally used in some parts of the world. There is a need for larger and rigorously designed studies that examine the efficacy of these methods. Until more data are obtained, non-pharmacological therapies should be reserved only for medically intractable cases and be performed in centers with sufficient experience [15].

Suggestions from Current Clinical Practice Guidelines
There are no recommended guidelines on these issues.

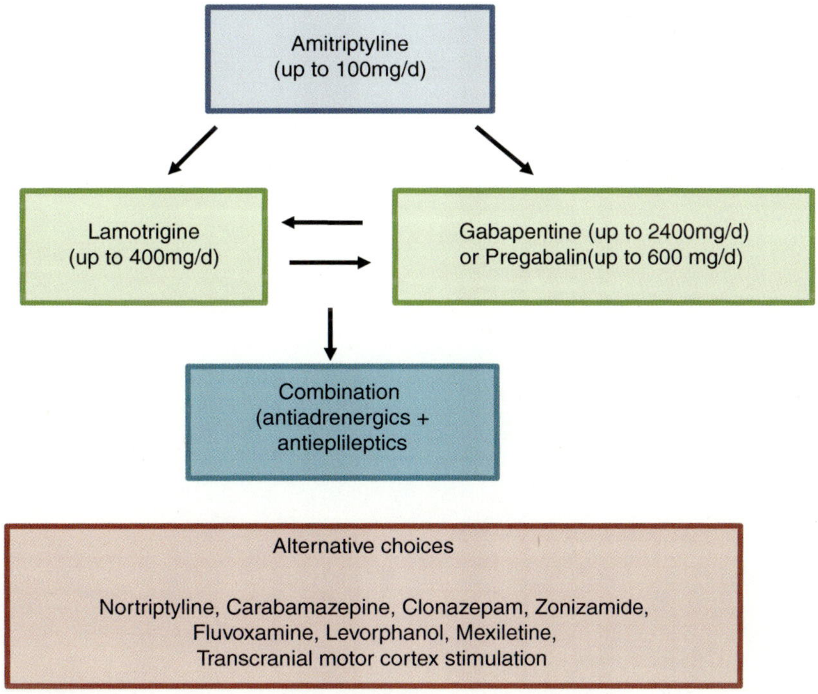

Fig. 31.2 Current approach of medical treatment for central post-stroke pain

References

1. Hackett ML, Kohler S, O'Brien JT, et al. Neuropsychiatric outcomes of stroke. Lancet Neurol. 2014;13:525–34.
2. Ferro JM, Caeiro L, Santos C. Poststroke emotional and behavior impairment: a narrative review. Cerebrovasc Dis. 2009;27(Suppl 1):197–203.
3. Gainotti G, Marra C. Determinants and consequences of post-stroke depression. Curr Opin Neurol. 2002;15:85–9.
4. Robinson RG, Jorge RE. Post-stroke depression: a review. Am J Psychiatry. 2016;173:221–31.
5. Hackett ML, Anderson CS, House A, et al. Interventions for treating depression after stroke. Cochrane Database Syst Rev. 2008;4:CD003437.
6. Kim JS, Choi-Kwon S. Disturbances in the voluntary control of emotional expression after stroke. In: Ferro JM, editor. Neuropsychiatric symptoms of cerebrovascular diseases. Heidelberg: Springer; 2013. p. 131–60.
7. Kim JS, Choi-Kwon S. Poststroke depression and emotional incontinence: correlation with lesion location. Neurology. 2000;54:1805–10.
8. Kim JS, Choi S, Kwon SU, et al. Inability to control anger or aggression after stroke. Neurology. 2002;58:1106–8.
9. Choi-Kwon S, Han K, Cho KH, et al. Factors associated with post-stroke anger proneness in ischaemic stroke patients. Eur J Neurol. 2013;20:1305–10.
10. Choi-Kwon S, Han SW, Kwon SU, et al. Fluoxetine treatment in poststroke depression, emotional incontinence, and anger proneness: a double-blind, placebo-controlled study. Stroke. 2006;37:156–61.
11. Choi-Kwon S, Kim JS. Poststroke fatigue: an emerging, critical issue in stroke medicine. Int J Stroke. 2011;6:328–36.
12. Klit H, Finnerup NB, Jensen TS. Central post-stroke pain: clinical characteristics, pathophysiology, and management. Lancet Neurol. 2009;8:857–68.
13. Leijon G, Boivie J. Central post-stroke pain—a controlled trial of amitriptyline and carbamazepine. Pain. 1989;36:27–36.
14. Kim JS, Bashford G, Murphy TK, et al. Safety and efficacy of pregabalin in patients with central post-stroke pain. Pain. 2011;152:1018–23.
15. Kim JS. Pharmacological management of central post-stroke pain: a practical guide. CNS Drugs. 2014;28:787–97.

Identification of Vascular Cognitive Impairment

32

Jae-Sung Lim

Abstract

Vascular cognitive impairment (VCI) is the second most common neurocognitive disorder followed after Alzheimer's dementia (AD). Recently, the vascular contribution to AD pathogenesis has garnered attention, of which might shed light on the implications for the treatment. Moreover, recent advances in neuroimaging techniques deepened understanding of pathogenesis of VCI; thus, this progress might be a basis for future therapeutic trials. Recently, there were continuing effort and collaborations to standardize neuropsychological evaluation protocol and diagnostic criteria in patients with VCI. In this paper, we will overview clinical characteristics, diagnostic criteria, neuropsychological evaluations, and neuroimaging biomarkers along with pathophysiological perspectives in VCI.

Vascular cognitive impairment (VCI) is the second most common neurocognitive disorder followed after Alzheimer's dementia (AD). Post-stroke dementia (PSD), which is one of distinctive clinical syndrome in VCI, is known to be accompanied in about 10% first-ever stroke and 30% in recurrent stroke [1]. In patients with intracerebral hemorrhage, the incidence of new-onset dementia was observed in 14.2% in 1 year, 28.3% at 4 years after hemorrhage [2]. However, the prevalence and incidence might vary according to time intervals between index-stroke and cognitive evaluations and research setting such as community- or hospital-based study [1]. Another major cause of VCI is subcortical VCI, which might be represented by diffuse and confluent small vessel disease (SVD) in neuroimaging. It was suggested that the attributable risks at death of cerebrovascular diseases in patients with dementia are 12% by SVD, 9% by multiple vascular pathology, and 7% by cerebral amyloid angiopathy [3]. These findings shed light on the therapeutic potentials in dementia field not only VCI but also neurodegenerative dementia [2]. Risk factors for PSD are

J.-S. Lim, M.D.
Department of Neurology, Hallym University Sacred Heart Hospital, Anyang, South Korea
e-mail: jaesunglim@hallym.ac.kr

S.-H. Lee (ed.), *Stroke Revisited: Diagnosis and Treatment of Ischemic Stroke*, Stroke Revisited, DOI 10.1007/978-981-10-1424-6_32

mostly non-modifiable factors: age, education, lesion extent, lesion location, index-stroke severity, and amyloid imaging positivity. Modifiable risk factors during both acute stroke and chronic stage still remained to be investigated.

32.1 Definition and Diagnostic Criteria of VCI

Cognitive impairment is an inclusive concept of both dementia and mild cognitive impairment. VCI refers to cognitive impairment caused by vascular lesions such as cerebral infarction, intracerebral hemorrhage, subcortical diffuse ischemic changes, amyloid angiopathy, etc. Mild cognitive impairment denotes that one can show objective cognitive impairment in neuropsychological tests but preserve activities of daily living.

There were various proposals for definition, classification, and diagnostic criteria for VCI. Until now, the National Institute of Neurological Disorders and Stroke and Association Internationale pour la Recherche et l'Enseignement en Neurosciences (NINDS-AIREN) criteria have been the most commonly used criteria in practice and researches [4]. According to the criteria, impairment of memory and of two or more cognitive domains is required for the diagnosis of vascular dementia. Cerebrovascular disease should be accompanied, which is defined by the presence of focal signs on neurologic examination consistent with stroke, and evidence of relevant cerebrovascular disease by brain imaging (CT or MRI) including multiple large vessel infarcts or a single strategically placed infarct as well as multiple basal ganglia and white matter lacunes or extensive periventricular white matter lesions, or combinations thereof. In addition, a relationship between the above two disorders should be manifested or inferred by the presence of one or more of the following: (1) onset of dementia within 3 months following a recognized stroke; (2) abrupt deterioration in cognitive functions; or (3) fluctuating, stepwise progression of cognitive deficits. Like this criteria, classical diagnostic criteria should be accompanied by memory deficit. Due to accumulating evidences about clinical characteristics of VCI, the preferential decline in attention/frontal executive function was emphasized in early diagnosis of VCI. These findings incorporated in the recently proposed diagnostic criteria such as American Heart Association-American Stroke Association statement, VasCog statement, and Diagnostic and Statistical Manual of Mental Disorders, Fifth Edition (DSM-5) criteria [5]. According to AHA-ASA criteria, vascular dementia is defined as cognitive impairment of at least two cognitive domains regardless of memory deficit along with imaging evidence of cerebrovascular disease and a clear temporal relationship between a vascular event and onset of cognitive deficit or clear relationship in the severity and pattern of cognitive impairment and the presence of diffuse, subcortical cerebrovascular disease pathology [5]. Cognitive tests should include a minimum of four cognitive domains: executive/attention, memory, language, and visuospatial functions.

In addition to AHA-ASA criteria, the recently proposed DSM-5 also removed the prerequisites of memory impairment for diagnosis of VCI in contrast with former DSM-IV criteria. Looking further ahead, VasCog statement extended the concept of vascular dementia defining it as cognitive deficits in only one cognitive domain if activities of daily living are impaired [6]. Besides that, VasCog statement further specified the criteria for cognitive impairment as below −2 standard deviation from age-, education-adjusted norm. Until now, other diagnostic criteria did not specify the threshold of cognitive impairment; thus, several criteria of −1.5 SD, −2 SD, and −10 percentile have been used by clinicians and researchers.

32.2 Clinical Characteristics and Classifications of VCI

Vascular dementia might be classified as two distinctive clinical syndromes, PSD and subcortical vascular dementia (sVaD). PSD is further classified as multi-infarct dementia and strategic infarct dementia [7]. PSD could develop early (3 months) or delayed (several years) after index stroke. Their pathophysiology is known to be different according to temporal profile; early PSD was associated with index-stroke-related factors, and delayed PSD was with superimposed amyloid pathology (Fig. 32.1) [8]. Stroke survivors with positive amyloid imaging showed poor cognitive trajectories compared to those without amyloid positivity. These interactions shed light on the pathophysiology of delayed cognitive decline after index stroke. These findings might give perspective to future therapeutic trials, and new classification systems might incorporate these interactions between vascular insult and amyloid process within the scheme. However, it was not thoroughly investigated yet that stroke might accelerate neurodegenerative process.

Multi-infarct dementia is dementia syndrome caused by recurrent and multiple infarctions, and stroke lesion extent and severity determined the neuropsychological construct. In contrast, strategic infarct dementia is caused by relatively small lesion, which is strategically located in functionally important location such as the anterior limb or genu of internal capsule, caudate nucleus, thalamus, medial frontal lobe, inferomedial temporal lobe, and angular gyrus.

These syndromes are caused by clinically evident stroke, and patients with PSD had suffered from relatively abrupt cognitive decline after stroke, and location and extent of stroke lesions might affect to the development of cognitive impairment.

In contrast, subcortical vascular dementia (sVaD) is difficult to be distinguished from other neurodegenerative dementia syndromes. It showed more gradual decline in cognition compared to other vascular dementia syndromes. It accompanied diffuse subcortical ischemic lesions without clinically evident stroke. It was known to account for major proportion of VCI in epidemiological studies [9]. Slowly progressive memory deficit as well as impairment of processing speed and frontal executive function is a characteristic feature of sVaD. It is difficult to be differentiated with AD; detailed neuroimaging studies might help differentiate these syndromes. Subcortical VaD could be further classified according to the presence of underlying positivity of amyloid imaging. Pure sVaD denotes patients who had confluent white matter hyperintensities without amyloid positivity and consisted of about 68.9% of sVaD patients

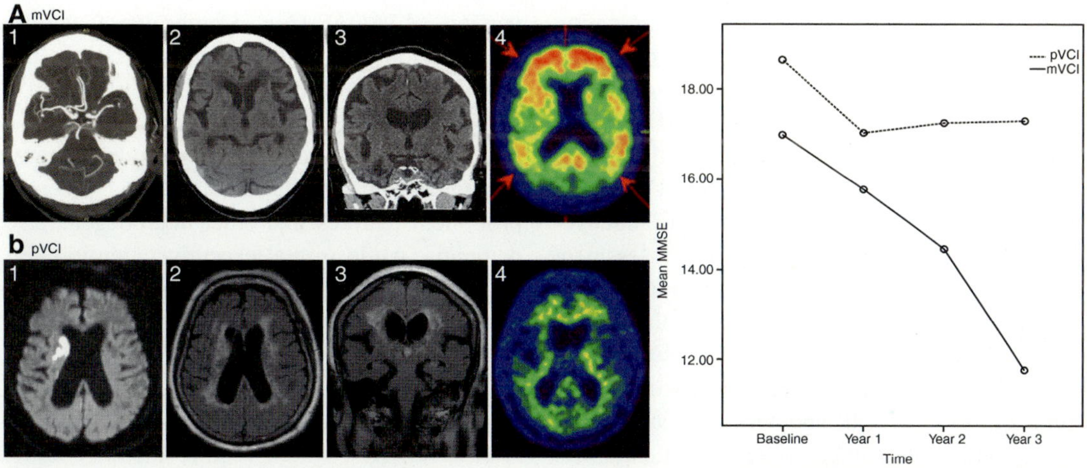

Fig. 32.1 Contribution of amyloid PET positivity to longitudinal cognitive trajectory after stroke [8]. Mixed VCI (mVCI) is characterized by positivity amyloid PET finding (A-4) and delayed decline in MMSE scores during 4-year follow-up. In contrast, patients with pure VCI (pVCI) showed negative amyloid PET imaging, and his MMSE score remained stable. Reproduced by permission of Stroke [8]

who aged around 70s [10]. They showed better performances in the delayed recall of both the verbal and visual memory test compared to those with mixed subcortical VCI [10].

32.3 Clinical Evaluation in Patients with VCI

For proper evaluations of VCI, somewhat different approach is needed compared to those in patients with AD. Most stroke survivors have stroke sequelae such as hemiparesis and dysarthria; these neurologic deficits might affect the proper neuropsychological evaluations. For the diagnosis of dementia, determination of activities of daily living impairment is important. However, due to abovementioned stroke sequelae, impairment of activities of daily living should be based on solely cognitive deficit, not based on physical barriers. Furthermore, most diagnostic criteria did not give any specific cutoff values for "cognitive impairment"; thus, various cutoffs, such as below −1.5 SD or 10 percentile from age-, education-adjusted mean, have been adopted in previous studies. Recently, VasCog statement and DSM-5 have suggested below −2 SD as proper criteria for "cognitive impairment."

There are various tools to briefly evaluate cognitive function. Firstly, the most representative screening tool is Mini-Mental State Examination (MMSE). It can be conducted within 5 or 10 min and has many supporting evidences of which have used it as cognitive screening tool. However, it has shortcomings that frontal function could not be assessed properly, because MMSE has focused on orientation, memory, and language-related functions. Montreal Cognitive Assessment (MoCA) is another brief screening tool, and it could be conducted in around 15 min. It had alternating trail making, cube, and clock tasks, which improve sensitivity to detect frontal dysfunction. Both MMSE and MoCA require intact motor and visual function. Thus, patients with hemiparesis or visual field defect could not complete the test properly. Several tests, which are 5-min National Institute of Neurological Disorders and Stroke-Canadian Stroke Network protocol and Six-Item Screener, are consisted of only verbally conducted tasks and are capable to be conducted in those with dominant hand weakness and visual field defect.

In cases of below age-, educated-adjusted norm in brief screening test, detailed neuropsychological tests are required to identify domain-specific cognitive impairment and magnitude of deficits. For those with VCI, National Institute of Neurological Disorders and Stroke-Canadian Stroke Network has proposed the Vascular Cognitive Impairment Harmonization Standards—Neuropsychological Protocol (VCIHS-NP) as standard tests to evaluate cognitive function [11]. It is consisted of 5-, 30-, and 60-min protocol, and 5-min protocol is a constellation of subtests of MoCA. Detailed test of each protocol is listed in Table 32.1.

VCIHS-NP was proposed as a reliable evaluation tool for multinational, multicenter trials and was consisted of sensitive and proper tests for patients with VCI, and many countries have published local norm and validation data. In addition, Alzheimer's Disease Assessment Scale-Cognitive (ADAS-Cog) and Consortium to Establish A Registry for Alzheimer's Disease (CERAD) which are usually used in patients in degenerative dementia have been used for cognitive evaluation for VCI. VDAS-Cog, a modified version of ADAS-Cog, Cambridge Cognition Examination (CAMCOG), and several computerized cognitive evaluation tools are also used.

Neuropsychological construct of VCI is different from that of other neurodegenerative dementia. Memory decline is one of the most prominent features like other neurodegenerative dementia, while frontal executive/attention deficit, decline of processing speed, is also the earliest feature in patients with VCI. Recent diagnostic criteria, AHA-ASA, VasCog statement, and DSM-5 criteria, have adopted those characteristic features in the criteria compared to NINDS-AIREN criteria, which require memory deficit for the diagnosis. Furthermore, patients with VCI might accompany behavioral and emotional problems in early phase of diseases.

Table. 32.1 Vascular cognitive impairment harmonization standards—Neuropsychological protocol [11]

5-Minute Protocol
MoCA subtests
5-Word Memory Task (registration, recall, recognition)
6-Item Orientation
1-Letter Phonemic Fluency
30-Minute Test Protocol
Semantic Fluency (Animal Naming)
Phonemic Fluency (Controlled Oral Word Association Test)
Digit Symbol-Coding from the Wechsler Adult Intelligence Scale, Third Edition
Hopkins Verbal Learning Test
Center for Epidemiologic Studies Depression Scale
Neuropsychiatric Inventory, Questionnaire Version (NPI-Q)
Supplemental: MMSE, Trail Making Test
60-Minute Test Protocol
Executive/Activation
Animal Naming (Semantic Fluency)
Controlled Oral Word Association Test
WAIS-III Digit Symbol-Coding
Trail Making Test
List Learning Test Strategies
Future Use: Simple and Choice Reaction Time
Language/Lexical Retrieval
Boston Naming Test, Second Edition, Short Form
Visuospatial
Rey-Osterrieth Complex Figure Copy
Supplemental: Complex Figure Memory
Memory
Hopkins Verbal Learning Test-Revised
Alternate: California Verbal Learning Test–2
Supplemental: Boston Naming Test Recognition
Supplemental: Digit Symbol-Coding Incidental Learning
Neuropsychiatric/Depressive Symptoms
Neuropsychiatric Inventory, Questionnaire Version
Center for Epidemiological Studies Depression Scale
Others
Informant Questionnaire on Cognitive Decline in the Elderly, Short Form
MMSE

32.4 Prognosis and Natural Course

Longitudinal studies showed various trajectories in VCI. One study showed that 78% patients were stable, 14% were aggravated, and 8% were improved [12]. However, another study showed longitudinal trajectories were different according to cognitive domains: aggravation mainly in memory and executive function and relatively preservation in visuospatial function and language [13]. Likewise, prognosis of VCI might show various characteristics according to evaluation time and tools.

Effect of stroke occurrence for longitudinal cognitive trajectories was identified in recent research published in JAMA in 2016. It has followed up 23,572 subjects who were aged over 45 years during 6.1 years [14]. In this study, stroke has caused abrupt decline in global cognition, new learning, and verbal memory at stroke onset, and cognitive decline has been accelerated in global cognition and frontal executive function compared with pre-stroke slopes.

Based on current evidences of longitudinal researches, stroke might cause abrupt decline of cognitive function and thereafter showed relatively stable course. However, there are some patients who showed continuous cognitive decline after stroke, and it might be caused by superimposed amyloid pathology or other premorbid neurodegenerative process. Recent study showed that age, diabetes mellitus, and severity of white matter hyperintensities and medial temporal lobe atrophy are associated with delayed cognitive decline after stroke during 4-year follow-up [15].

32.5 Neuroimaging Biomarkers and Pathophysiological Perspectives

Recent advances in neuroimaging technique shed light on the pathophysiology of VCI. In addition to traditional neuroimaging biomarkers such as medial temporal lobe atrophy and small vessel diseases, the multimodal imaging including diffusion tensor imaging and resting-state functional MRI gave an insightful data. Dysfunctions in neurovascular unit dysfunction and blood-brain barriers, cortical microinfarction, and cerebral amyloid angiopathy are also intriguing topics in recent neuroimaging research fields.

Acute stroke in specific region might cause system-wide consequences. In previous study using resting-state functional MRI, the resting activity of default mode network was altered in patients with acute stroke compared to control group, and this alteration was correlated with cognitive test score and line cancellation test score [16]. Lesion-mapping study also showed that strategically located lesions located at the major hubs of default mode network might increase the risk of PSD [17]. These studies suggest the importance of large-scale functional neural network for the pathophysiology and as a biomarker of PSD.

Small vessel disease is also thoroughly investigated for its pathophysiological role for VCI. In previous studies, the extent of white matter hyperintensities, the presence and number of lacunar infarction, and cerebral microbleeds were associated with cognitive function including processing speed and memory. Recently, intriguing studies of SVD broaden our understanding of complex interactions among chronic ischemic pathology, neurodegenerative process, and human cognitive function. Quantification of cholinergic pathway disruption by strategically located white matter hyperintensities was proposed by Bocti et al. [18]. In another study, subcortical cholinergic pathway disruption was associated with the development of post-stroke dementia and impairs the frontal cognitive function [17, 18].

Furthermore, several studies investigating the multimodal imaging in patients with cerebral autosomal dominant arteriopathy with subcortical infarcts and leukoencephalopathy (CADASIL), one could get an insight for the longitudinal associations between white matter hyperintensities and lacunar infarction. Circulatory insufficiency in the periphery of deep medullary artery in brain parenchyma may aggravate the white matter hyperintensities, and newly developed lacunar infarctions were frequently observed in the distal part of these arteries [19]. In addition, lacunar infarction located in the anterior thalamic radiation and forceps minor caused the regional atrophy of corresponding cortical regions and finally frontal executive dysfunction (Fig. 32.2) [20]. These sequential processes might give us a glimpse of how subcortical vascular dementia and

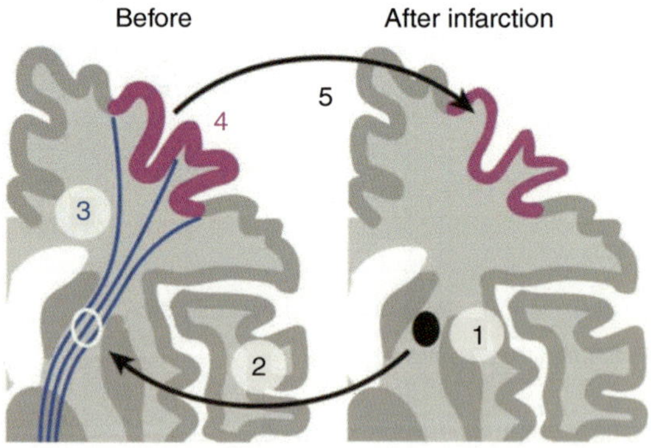

Fig. 32.2 Pathophysiological perspective of strategic infarct dementia and subcortical vascular dementia [20]. Stroke lesion located at the anterior limb of internal capsule (1) might disrupt (2) the ipsilateral thalamocortical fibers (3) and eventually lead to the cortical atrophy of the corresponding regions. (4, 5) Reproduced by permission of Neurology [20]

strategic infarct dementia could be developed by incident ischemic lesions.

Superimposed amyloid pathology also showed complex interactions with vascular lesions. Patients with mixed VCI, who had positive amyloid imaging by amyloid PET at index stroke, had followed up for 3 years after stroke. They showed poor cognitive outcome assess by MMSE or MoCA compared to patients with pure VCI who did not have amyloid pathology by imaging [8].

Conclusion

For understanding of VCI, its pathophysiological process was illustrated in Fig. 32.3. Identification of cognitive impairment in stroke survivors requires a thorough knowledge about clinical characteristics as well as risk factors of VCI. Recently revised diagnostic criteria, standardized neuropsychological evaluation tools should be kept in mind to evaluated patients properly. Advanced multimodal imaging studies might shed light on the pathophysiology of VCI. Modifiable risk factors should be investigated to halter this devastating cognitive sequela of vascular insults.

Clinical Practice Guideline There are no recommended guidelines on these issues.

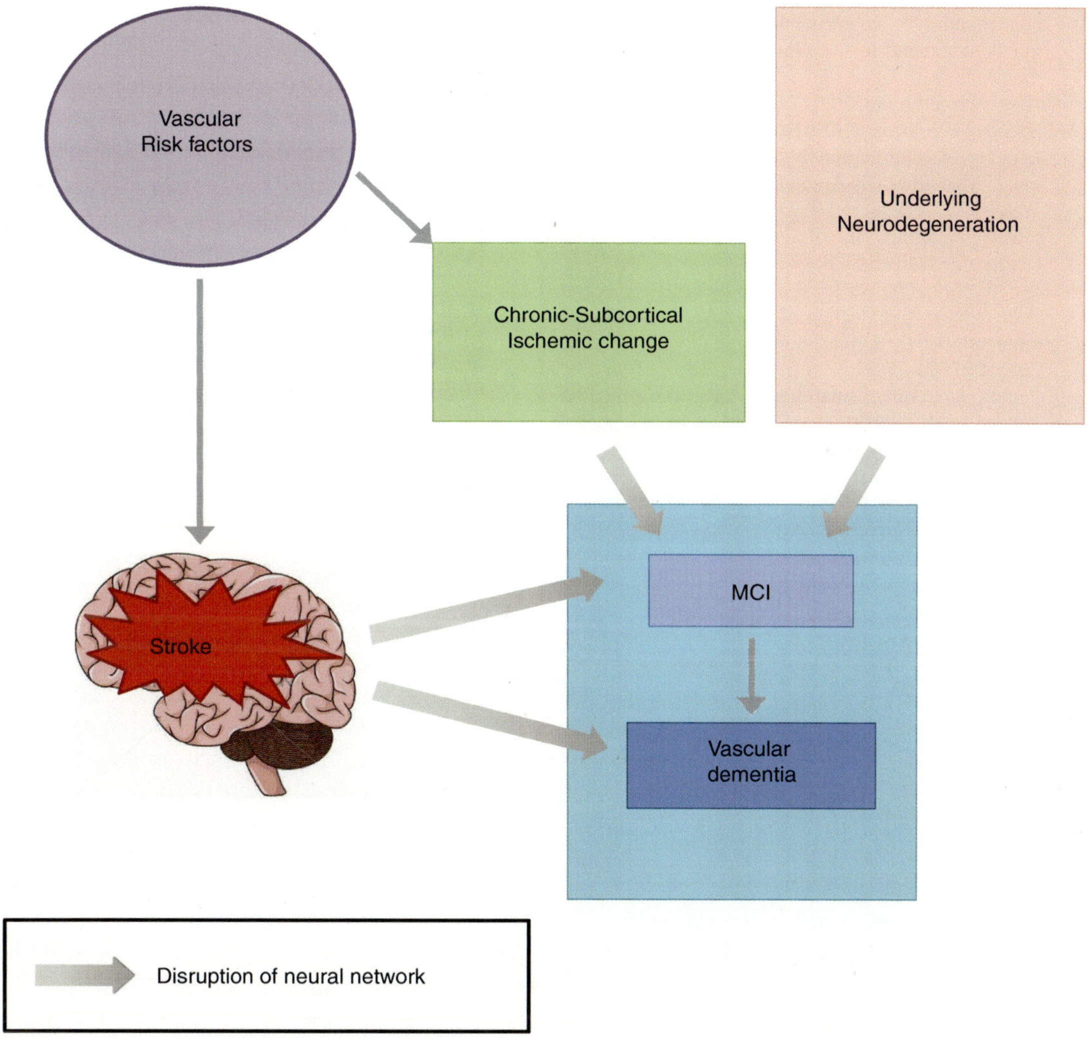

Fig. 32.3 A schematic illustration of VCI pathophysiology

References

1. Pendlebury ST, Rothwell PM. Prevalence, incidence, and factors associated with pre-stroke and post-stroke dementia: a systematic review and meta-analysis. Lancet Neurol. 2009;8:1006–18.
2. Moulin S, Labreuche J, Bombois S, et al. Dementia risk after spontaneous intracerebral haemorrhage: a prospective cohort study. Lancet Neurol. 2016;15: 820–9.
3. Matthews FE, Brayne C, Lowe J, et al. Epidemiological pathology of dementia: attributable-risks at death in the Medical Research Council cognitive function and ageing study. PLoS Med. 2009;6:e1000180.
4. Roman GC, Tatemichi TK, Erkinjuntti T, et al. Vascular dementia: diagnostic criteria for research studies. Report of the NINDS-AIREN international workshop. Neurology. 1993;43:250–60.
5. Gorelick PB, Scuteri A, Black SE, et al. Vascular contributions to cognitive impairment and dementia: a statement for healthcare professionals from the American Heart Association/American Stroke Association. Stroke. 2011;42:2672–713.
6. Sachdev P, Kalaria R, O'Brien J, et al. Diagnostic criteria for vascular cognitive disorders: a Vascog statement. Alzheimer Dis Assoc Disord. 2014;28:206–18.
7. Wahlund L, Erkinjuntti T, Gauthier S. Vascular cognitive impairment in clinical practice. New York: Cambridge University Press; 2009.
8. Liu W, Wong A, Au L, et al. Influence of amyloid-beta on cognitive decline after stroke/transient ischemic attack: three-year longitudinal study. Stroke. 2015;46:3074–80.
9. Pantoni L. Cerebral small vessel disease: from pathogenesis and clinical characteristics to therapeutic challenges. Lancet Neurol. 2010;9:689–701.
10. Lee JH, Kim SH, Kim GH, et al. Identification of pure subcortical vascular dementia using 11c-Pittsburgh compound B. Neurology. 2011;77:18–25.
11. Hachinski V, Iadecola C, Petersen RC, et al. National institute of neurological disorders and stroke-Canadian stroke network vascular cognitive impairment harmonization standards. Stroke. 2006;37:2220–41. doi:10.1161/01.STR.0000237236.88823.47
12. del Ser T, Barba R, Morin MM, et al. Evolution of cognitive impairment after stroke and risk factors for delayed progression. Stroke. 2005;36:2670–5.
13. Ballard C, Rowan E, Stephens S, et al. Prospective follow-up study between 3 and 15 months after stroke: improvements and decline in cognitive function among dementia-free stroke survivors >75 years of age. Stroke. 2003;34:2440–4.
14. Da L, Galecki AT, Langa KM, et al. Trajectory of cognitive decline after incident stroke. JAMA. 2015;314:41–51.
15. Yang J, Wong A, Wang Z, et al. Risk factors for incident dementia after stroke and transient ischemic attack. Alzheimers Dement. 2015;11:16–23.
16. Dacosta-Aguayo R, Grana M, Iturria-Medina Y, et al. Impairment of functional integration of the default mode network correlates with cognitive outcome at three months after stroke. Hum Brain Mapp. 2015;36:577–90.
17. Lim JS, Kim N, Jang MU, et al. Cortical hubs and subcortical cholinergic pathways as neural substrates of poststroke dementia. Stroke. 2014;45:1069–76.
18. Bocti C, Swartz RH, Gao FQ, et al. A new visual rating scale to assess strategic white matter hyperintensities within cholinergic pathways in dementia. Stroke. 2005;36:2126–31.
19. Duering M, Csanadi E, Gesierich B, et al. Incident lacunes preferentially localize to the edge of white matter hyperintensities: insights into the pathophysiology of cerebral small vessel disease. Brain. 2013;136:2717–26.
20. Duering M, Righart R, Csanadi E, et al. Incident subcortical infarcts induce focal thinning in connected cortical regions. Neurology. 2012;79:2025–8.

33 Rehabilitation in Subacute and Chronic Stage After Stroke

Han-Young Jung

Abstract

Despite advancing rehabilitation programs, stroke is the most prevalent disease to cause disablement. With the increase of the elderly population, the number of stroke patients increases as well. Although stroke patients at an early stage depend on a stroke unit in the acute hospital, their functional recovery and long-term health status are more affected by subacute rehabilitation hospital. Moreover, a stroke patient's initial evaluation is crucial for prognosis and establishment of rehabilitation training strategies. The earlier stroke patients start their rehabilitation treatment, the better results they can attain; the recovery from stroke occurs within 3 months after the onset of stroke. Similarly, while neurological and functional recovery occurs in the acute and subacute stages, sometimes, it occurs 6 months after the onset of stroke or in the chronic stage. There are two main mechanisms of neurological recovery. The first is activity-dependent neuroplasticity in the injured cortical representation area, and second is vicariation, which is an operating mechanism as a substitute for the injured brain function in the remnant cortical area, outside of the damaged brain area. This stroke recovery is affected by many factors that influence reorganization of the damaged brain and early rehabilitation; furthermore, intensive rehabilitation and organized enriched environments also significantly affect recovery. In addition, there are substantial researches about new rehabilitation treatment, likely rTMS, tDCT, robotic therapies, mirror therapy, virtual reality, and drug augmentation; therefore, the results of these studies are expected to highlight promising rehabilitation treatments for stroke in the future.

Despite advancing rehabilitation programs, stroke is the most prevalent disease to cause disablement. With the increase of the elderly population, the number of stroke patients increases as well. While from 50 to 70% of stroke patients to

H.-Y. Jung
Department of Rehabilitation Medicine, Inha University Medical School, Incheon, South Korea
e-mail: rmjung@inha.ac.kr

S.-H. Lee (ed.), *Stroke Revisited: Diagnosis and Treatment of Ischemic Stroke*, Stroke Revisited, DOI 10.1007/978-981-10-1424-6_33

be independent, 15–30% chronic disability and, especially, 10–20% of stroke patients live in institutional facilities supported by other persons. Although stroke patients at an early stage depend on the specialized stroke unit in the acute hospital, their functional recovery and long-term health status are more affected by subacute rehabilitation hospital and caregivers. Therefore, rehabilitation is one of the most important aspects in the stroke patient care. Scientific evidence is available that rehabilitation treatment of subacute stroke in well-organized comprehensive stroke rehabilitation units both decreases disability, increases cost-effective benefits, and leads to shortening of the length of hospital stay. Moreover, a stroke patient's initial evaluation is crucial for prognosis and establishment of rehabilitation training strategies. Depending on the evaluation results, patients can be discharged early, get medical treatment with rehabilitation treatment, or be transferred to a rehabilitation ward or other medical facilities. The earlier stroke patients start their rehabilitation treatment, the better results they can attain; the recovery from stroke occurs within 3 months after the onset of stroke. Similarly, while neurological and functional recovery occurs in the acute and subacute stages, sometimes, it occurs 6 months after the onset of stroke or in the chronic stage (Fig. 33.1) [1].

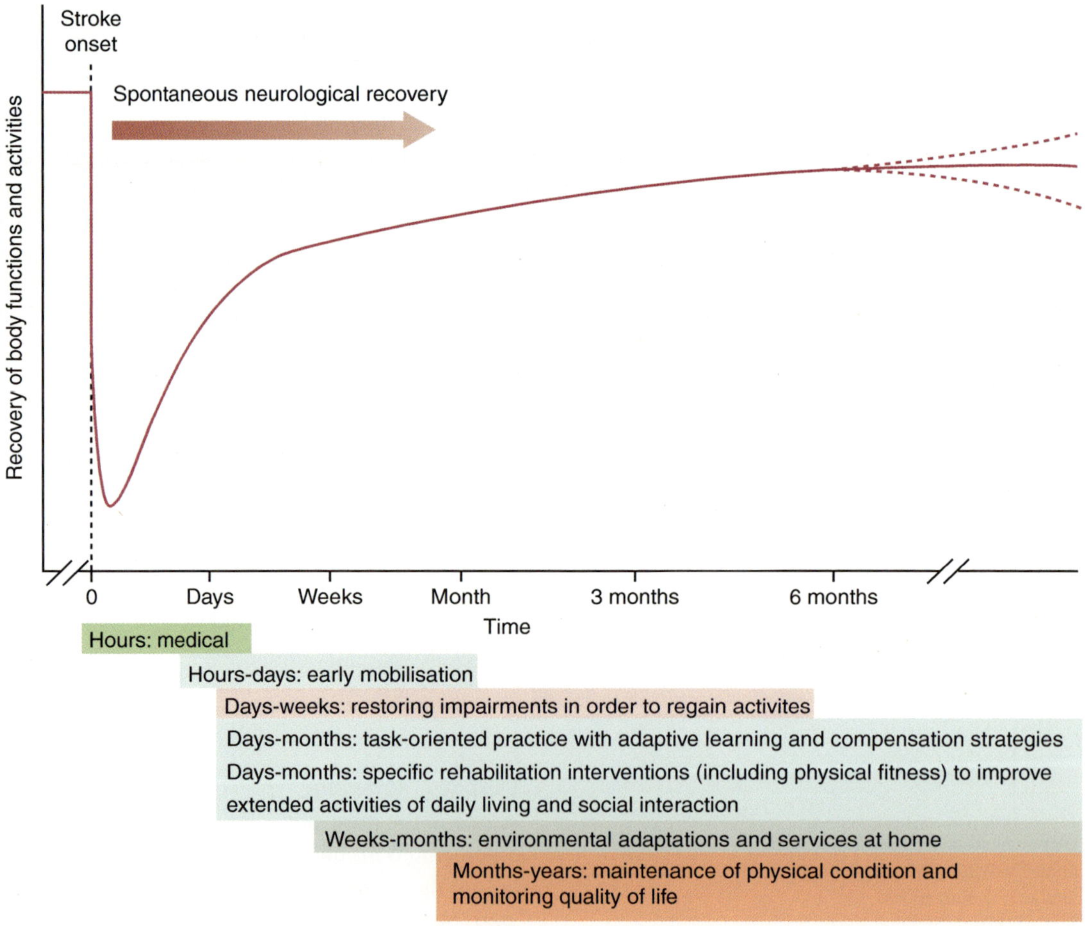

Fig. 33.1 Hypothetical pattern of recovery after stroke with timing of intervention strategies. Reproduced by permission of Lancet [1]

There are two main mechanisms of neurological recovery. The first is activity-dependent neuroplasticity in the injured cortical representation area, which is the underlying mechanism of task-oriented repetitive training, like the constraint-induced movement therapy, and robotic-assisted gait or arm training. Second is vicariation, which is an operating mechanism as a substitute for the injured brain function in the remnant cortical area, outside of the damaged brain area. This appears in the early stage of stroke or in the severe cerebral infarction stage. This stroke recovery is affected by many factors that influence reorganization of the damaged brain-nervous system and early rehabilitation; furthermore, intensive rehabilitation and organized enriched environments also significantly affect recovery. In addition, there is a substantial body research about new rehabilitation treatment, including repetitive transcranial magnetic stimulation (rTMS), transcranial direct current therapy (tDCT), robotic therapies, mirror therapy, virtual reality training, and drug augmentation.

33.1 Evolutional Time Course for Stroke Rehabilitation: From the Acute, Subacute Stages to the Chronic Stage

After the onset of stroke, treatment should be different at each stage [2]. The acute phase is the time when disease treatment should be focused on according to the critical path specific to the pathophysiology of acute stroke. In the subacute or convalescent phase, rehabilitation programs should be the focus in order to treat several impairments, including hemiplegia, aphasia, neglect, and shoulder subluxation, as well as to manage activity limitations, such as walking, feeding, transferring, etc. In the chronic phase, compensatory rehabilitation programs, such as house reconstruction, transfer system, caregiver education with the view of quality life, and control of environmental factors, should be prioritized. Likewise, depending on the time of the onset, several experts or care facilities are involved in damage from disease, shift from disease to impairment, and, furthermore, quality of life. To make these things systematic, the stroke liaison critical path for stoke is needed [2].

Peak neurologic recovery of stroke occurs within 1–3 months after the onset of stroke. From this time to 6 months, recovery slows down and 5% of the patients, especially those who show severe functional damage at the early stage, continuously recover up to 1 year after the onset. Also, functional recovery mostly occurs 3 months after the onset, suggesting that functional recovery is strongly related to neurologic severity. According to the Copenhagen Stroke Study, the patients with a mild case recover within 8.5 weeks after the onset, while the patients with a severity case recover within 13 weeks and the patients with an advanced case get better within 17–20 weeks [3]. However, functional recovery or communication skills could continuously progress and reduce activity limitations, even in cases when neurological impairment would not recover anymore. This means that the correlation between impairments and activity limitations is not linear, which was obtained by the use of technical aid for the affected limb and/or compensatory use of the unaffected limb. It can be helpful for the patients who cannot recover from neurological impairment anymore in order to reduce activity limitations and participation restriction using some compensatory strategies. Therefore, these comprehensive multidisciplinary rehabilitation programs are considered to be major stroke management strategies.

33.2 Assessment of Stroke Patients for Rehabilitation

33.2.1 Meaning and Time Schedules of Stroke Assessment

There are four stages in rehabilitation for stroke patients. The first is an assessment of the patient's functional status and his/her requirement of rehabilitation. The second is setting a realizable, optimizing rehabilitation goal. The third is a rehabilitation program to achieve the goal. The last is a reassessment of the rehabilitation process and goal achievement.

Patient assessment is categorized into global assessment and specific assessment. With the acute phase, radiologic imaging study and assessment of global neurological impairment, consciousness, muscle power, and pain are performed to figure out the neurological status within 24–48 h after hospitalization. Based on these parameters, the necessity of early rehabilitation or intensive rehabilitation is determined. With the subacute phase, an assessment of the global activity limitation, balance, hand function, and swallowing function is performed to establish the patient's functional status. In order to perform these various assessments, multidisciplinary comprehensive approaches with a rehabilitation specialist, physical therapist, occupational therapist, speech therapist, clinical psychologist, social worker, and caregiver are needed. That is why a comprehensive rehabilitation stroke unit is required. With the chronic phase, an assessment is performed from the point of view related to the stroke patient's quality of life at home or in an institution and maintenance of ADL. In addition, all assessment tools should be standard tools with reliability and validity and should be performed by experts. To hospitalize in a stroke rehabilitation unit, a patient should be in medically stable and have some functional impairment. Also, the patient should have a cognitive ability to communicate to some degree and be able to maintain in the sitting position on a wheelchair to actively participate in one session of the rehabilitation training for about 20–30 min.

33.2.2 Goal Setting and ICF-Based Stroke Assessment

In order to explain chronic disease that constantly affects humans, the World Health Organization International Classification of Functioning, Disability and Health (WHO ICF 2001) introduced new concepts of human functioning. There are three parts of functioning, namely, body structure and function, activity, and participation. Both individual and environmental factors interact with functioning here. WHO wanted to make a kind of a frame to collect the data commonly available in the world [4]. However, what constitutes ICF was so large-scale that WHO made several comprehensive core sets and brief core sets; clinically brief core sets are more likely to be used [5]. A brief core set for stroke consists of 18 components: six related to body functions, two to body structures, seven to activities and participation, and three to environmental factors. With an objective and scientific assessment of a stroke patient using the ICF stroke core set, his/her functioning or disabilities make it possible to recognize neurological impairment, individual activity limitation, interpersonal and social participation restriction, and the information about nearby medical facilities, family members, and house structure. The global neurological impairment assessments include National Institutes of Health Stroke Scale (NIHSS), Mini-Mental State Examination (MMSE), and Glasgow Coma Scale (GCS), among others. The global assessments for activity limitations are Modified Barthel Index (MBI), Functional Independence Measure (FIM), and modified Rankin Scale (mRS); also for participation restriction, there are Europal-5D, SF-18, etc. (Table 33.1).

33.2.3 Comprehensive Stroke Rehabilitation Units

Comprehensive stroke rehabilitation units should consist of well-organized team members who work in different professional fields and have sufficient experience on rehabilitation. They should manage stroke patients' complications and/or comorbidities with evidence-based practice. Furthermore, each stroke patient should be provided with individualized, different rehabilitation programs depending on the severity of stroke through a multidisciplinary systematic evaluation [6]. Stroke patients with more moderate severity have an opportunity to be admitted into comprehensive stroke rehabilitation units. Once a week, every member should attend a conference for patients and pay attention to family, caregivers, and sociopsychological factors. In report on the systematically randomized comparative trials for the patients hospitalized in comprehensive stroke

Table 33.1 ICF stroke core set-based functional evaluation for stroke patients

( ): Negativity		ICF: Functioning or disability		
ICF domains	Disease (Pathology)	Body function and structure (Impairment)	Activity (Limitation)	Participation (Restriction)
Modification of ICF stroke core set	Cerebral infarct ICH SAH Others	Conscious functions Orientation functions Muscle power Mental functions of language Attention functions Memory functions Structure of brain Structure of upper and lower extremity	Walking Speaking Toileting Eating Washing Dressing Communication	Driving Return to work, gainful employment
Evaluation tools	Brain CT or MRI SPECT, PET Doppler TMS SEP	NIHSS or GCS FMA MMSE MAS WAB	MBI FIM mRS BBS	Euroqol-5D SF-18 SIP

Abbreviations: *ICF* International Classification of Functioning, *ICH* intracranial hemorrhage, *SAH* subarachnoid hemorrhage, *SPECT* single-photon emission computed tomography, *PET* positron emission tomography, *TMS* transcranial magnetic stimulation, *SEP* somatosensory evoked potential, *NIHSS* National Institutes of Health Stroke Scale, *FMA* Fugl-Meyer Assessment, *GCS* Glasgow Coma Scale, *MMSE* Mini-Metal State Examination, *MAS* modified Aschowers scale, *WAB* Western Aphasia Battery, *MBI* Modified Barthel Index, *FIM* Functional Independence Measure, *mRS* modified Rankin scale, *BBS* Berg Balance Scale, *SF-18* Short-Form Health Survey, *SIP* Stroke Impact Profile

rehabilitation units or in a general ward, Stroke Unit Trialists' Collaboration reported that the patients who were hospitalized in comprehensive stroke rehabilitation units had a more functional recovery, lower death rate, shorter length of hospital stay, and severe stroke patients' lower rate of admission in a long-term care institution [2].

33.3 Stroke Recovery Mechanism

33.3.1 General Principles of Functional Stroke Recovery

Functional impairment after stroke onset is due to neural loss of the injured area as well as to the decrement of the neural function of another area connected to the injured area. The degree of diaschisis, which is a malfunction in the opposite area connected to the damaged brain tissue, represents the degree of brain nerves' damage, and reversal of diaschisis is an indicator of functional recovery. The mechanism of recovery after a stroke is not exactly known; however, the mechanism of early functional recovery is mainly known as (1) reversal of diaschisis, (2) hyperactivity of the existing neuronal pathway, and (3) neuroplasticity developed by the relearning process. Let us examine neuroplasticity, which is the main mechanism of functional recovery by rehabilitation.

33.3.2 Neurological Recovery

Brain plasticity is a broad term connected to adapting characteristics of the human brain after environment, experience, and brain injury. The adaptability in a changing environment is the basic attribution and basic element of learning. This occurs in several levels, from molecules to cortical reorganization in brain cells [7].

Neurological reorganization is a major mechanism of functional restoration after stroke, and this is more important, because neurological reorganization is affected by rehabilitation training. The stroke patient's neurological reorganization occurs in the damaged brain tissue, as well as in the surrounding intact cortical tissue; further, it occurs in the remote area structurally connected to the damaged area [7]. In an animal experiment, Nudo reported that synaptogenesis or increased long-term potentiation in synaptic strength during motor learning is similar to the phenomenon of recovery from stroke [8]. Through this phenomenon, neuroplasticity is considered a major underlying mechanism to explain neurological recovery after stroke rehabilitation. This neuroplasticity, or neurological reorganization, can be assessed through various types of advanced medical equipment, such as transcranial magnetic stimulation (TMS), functional magnetic resonance imaging (fMRI), and diffusion tensor imaging (DTI).

33.3.3 Functional Recovery

Functional recovery can be understood as a recovery of activity of daily living (ADL), such as hand grasping or ambulation, which is closely related to the improvement of neurological impairment. Final functional recovery occurs with the improvement of neurological impairment, as well as with a combination of the body parts which have no neurological impairment. Therefore, functional recovery is affected by rehabilitation training using the holistic use of all body parts. Motor impairment after stroke is one of the important elements in stroke recovery, especially in gait disturbance; however, this does not completely determine functional recovery. Functional recovery for ADL is affected by the coordinated movement of hands, apraxia, sensory deficit, limitation of range of motion, communication problems, cognition impairment, as well as by other factors including the unaffected body parts.

In older adults, premorbid general weakness deteriorates as lengthening of duration of bed rest after stroke onset. Mixed muscle training, including aerobic exercise and strengthening exercise, helps recovery of muscle strength of disuse weakness and balance, hemiplegic weakness, as well as promotes the improvement of cardiovascular function, control of body weight, and diabetes. Recently, it has been reported that moderate intensity of aerobic exercise stimulates secretion of neurotrophic factors, such as BDNF in the brain, accelerating neuroplasticity, neurogenesis, and enhancing cognitive function as well. It also stimulates secretion of neurotransmitter of dopamine and serotonin, helping control of cognition, depression, and anxiety [9].

33.3.4 Compensatory Recovery

Compensatory recovery is possible without neurological or functional recovery, which can be another key factor of rehabilitation training. Appropriate prescription and education of supportive devices or changes of external environment improve a patient's ADL. Wearing ankle-foot orthosis (AFO) on the hemiplegic ankle can improve the ambulatory function preventing foot drop and assisting knee extensor power, while the application of a shoulder sling on the hemiplegic shoulder can partly prevent progression of subluxation of the shoulder [10]. In addition, wearing a footplate and a functional electrical stimulator (FES) on the peroneal nerve under the knee joint of the hemiplegic leg can improve ambulatory function [11], while making a chair higher can help the function of the extensor muscle in the paralyzed knee when standing from the chair sitting. Likewise, a stroke patient's quality of life (QOL) can be improved through appropriate use of supportive devices or a change of the surrounding environment.

33.4 Time Course of Stroke Rehabilitation

33.4.1 Rehabilitation in the Acute Stage of Stroke

It is medically valuable to treat an acute phase stroke patient in a stroke unit, which is the most suitable for management of stroke. The attention to a very early rehabilitation in a stroke unit is nowadays increasing. The reason is that bed rest has a negative effect on the musculoskeletal, cardiovascular, respiratory, emotional condition and immobilization and related complications often occur, which might delay recovery in the acute stage of stroke. Recently, A Very Early Rehabilitation Trial (AVERT) study has been conducted several times. According to the latest study, depending on the patient's status within 24 h after stroke onset, if a stroke patient performs the set amount of ADL and task-oriented exercises within a certain period, the study group recovers more than the control group in terms of functional improvements 3 months after the onset [12]. After the onset of stroke, in the case of medically stable condition, the early intensive rehabilitation can make the best functional recovery in the long term. Although there is no consensus about the critical period for stroke rehabilitation treatment, according to animal experiments, a promising period can be within 3 weeks after the onset of stroke [13].

33.4.2 Rehabilitation in the Subacute Stage of Stroke

In order to manage functional impairment from stroke, subacute stroke rehabilitation is crucial. Since this is the time when neurological and functional recovery is very active, task-oriented, intensive, and repetitive training is needed. For that purpose, it is recommended that stroke patient should be transferred or admitted to a comprehensive stroke rehabilitation unit where a multidisciplinary approach is available [14]. Overall, task-oriented repetitive intensive training and conventional rehabilitation programs, including physical and occupational therapy, endurance and strengthening exercises, and flexibility, balance, and coordination training, are performed in the subacute stage of stroke. Furthermore, speech/language therapy for aphasia and dysarthria and occupational therapy for dysphagia are added depending on the patient's need. In addition, multimodal sensory stimulation and noninvasive transcortical stimulation are added depending on expert opinion. First, treadmill training with or without body weight support, robotic therapy for arm/hand and gait training, and constraint-induced movement therapy are used for a task-oriented intensive rehabilitation treatment. This intensive training selectively affects the cortical representation area specific to the training arm or leg. Second, a multimodal sensory stimulation approved through animal experiments in an enriched environment is introduced as mirror therapy, action observation, motor imagery, and virtual reality training. Third, noninvasive cortex stimulation methods have recently started to be introduced, and these include repetitive transcranial magnetic stimulation (rTMS) [15] and transcranial direct current stimulation (tDCT) [16]. In expert opinion, these are one of the relevant treatment options for motor impairment, cognitive impairment, language problems, pain, and depression.

33.4.3 Rehabilitation for the Chronic Stage of Stroke

Stroke patients in the acute or subacute phase are mainly managed in hospitals; however, a patient's quality of health and life in the chronic phase can be an important concern in the family or community for a longer time. From 6 months to 1 year after the onset of stroke, it reaches the chronic phase in the event of no more functional recovery. Three years after that time, the patient maintains average functions or his/her ability to adapt in everyday life gets better [17]. However, 4–5 years after the onset of stroke, as physical condition deteriorates, more caregiver's support may be needed and more patients could go into nursing facilities or a long-term institution. Furthermore, the patient's socialization, or leisure activity, reduces, while his/her emotional instability or depression increases. Therefore, family or community members should pay more attention to the patient to maintain his/her quality of life.

After a discharge from the hospital, every chronic stroke patient with a functional impairment needs to be trained in a community-based rehabilitation center or by visiting therapists depending on the functional status of the patient. Mostly, there are several basic trainings such as endurance training that reduces general fatigue, balance training to prevent failing accident, and stretching to prevent contracture of both joint and muscle. At the same time, one-to-one individualized training programs require 2–3 days a week. In addition, remodeling the house or the surrounding environment, such as stairs or a wrong load, depending on the patient's functional severity is necessary [1].

33.5 Several Promising Techniques for Stroke Rehabilitation

33.5.1 Neuromodulation

In numerous recent studies, a noninvasive method to stimulate the brain, likely repetitive transcranial magnetic stimulation (rTMS) and transcranial direct current stimulation (tDCS), has been introduced; these can do neuromodulation, such as strengthening plasticity of brain neurons during a stroke rehabilitation treatment, especially in motor and cognitive rehabilitation fields [18]. rTMS can affect excitation or inhibition at certain specific areas of the cerebral cortex depending on stimulation frequency, duration of stimulation, strength of magnetic field, and shape of coil. tDCT is known to induce change in the neuronal cell membrane by transferring the activated current to the cerebral cortex. The change in the cerebral cortical excitability lasts for a considerable period of time and can induce brain plasticity. By using these latest treatments to the part of the ipsilesional brain or the contralesional brain after stroke, getting physical therapy or occupational therapy at the same time, a patient's recovery get better in motor and cognitive function (Fig. 33.2) [16]. However, even though more studies are needed because there are ambiguous opinions, such as the absence of control group,

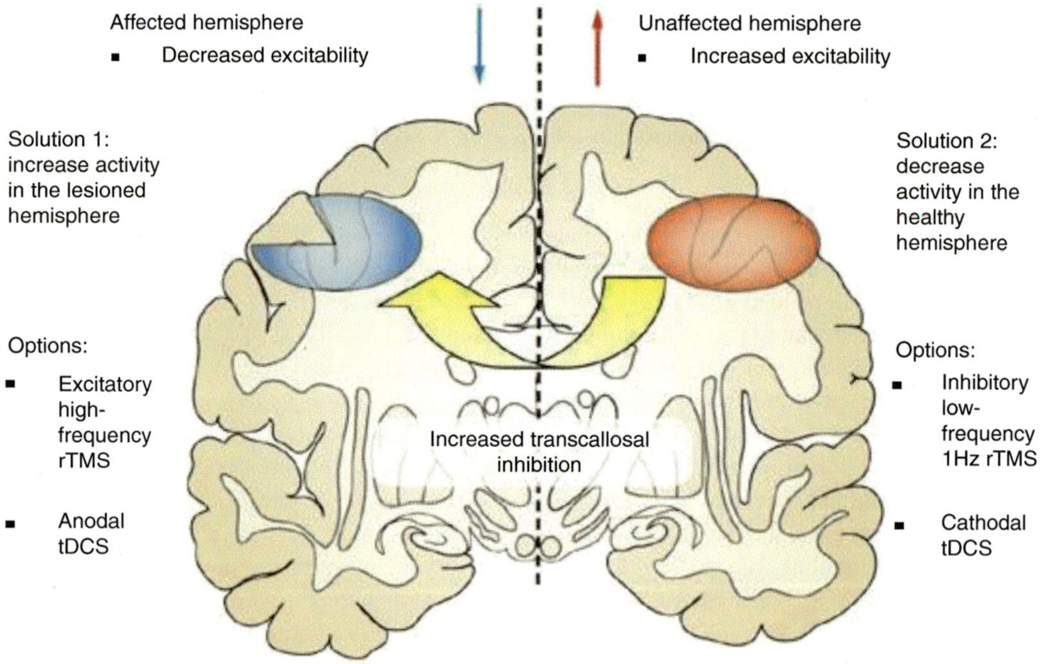

Fig. 33.2 Noninvasive brain stimulation in stroke. After a stroke, there is increased activity in the unaffected hemisphere (*red area*) and decreased activity in the affected hemisphere (*blue area*) as a result of increased transcallosal inhibition (*yellow arrow*) from the unaffected to the affected hemisphere. In this type of case, enhancing the excitability of the affected hemisphere (with high-frequency rTMS or anodal tDCS) or suppressing the unaffected hemisphere (with low-frequency rTMS or cathodal tDCS) can promote recovery of motor function. Note, however, that specific brain regions might need to be targeted and that the effects of stimulation might differ between patients and brain areas depending on the nature and site of the initial insult. *Abbreviations*: *rTMS* repetitive transcranial magnetic stimulation, *tDCS* transcranial direct current stimulation. Reproduced by permission of Nature Clinical Practice Neurology [16]

non-consensus of the initiation time, treatment duration, and specific treatment mode, these are expected to be promising new advanced techniques in the future.

33.5.2 Multimodal Sensory Stimulation

In many animal experiments, it has been reported that, as compared to the animals trained in the normal environment, stroke animals have a much better neuroplasticity in an enriched environment where animals can simultaneously get cognition, sensation, and movement. These environments in animal experiments are similar to the concepts like multimodal sensory stimulation in the human case. There are some new rehabilitation strategies based on these theoretical backgrounds, which are mirror therapy, action observation, motor imagery, and virtual reality training. Mirror therapy seeks to create an illusion that makes a paralyzed hand move well, putting a paralyzed hand behind the mirror, and looking at a healthy hand movement in front of the mirror. This therapy is reported to be very effective with stroke patients in the subacute phase [19]. Virtual reality training offers a considerably higher level of sensory stimulus close to the patient's real situation by offering a multimodal, interactive, and/or realistic virtual environment [20]. Recent times, a simple level of virtual reality training has been applied to stroke patients, and it is believed to be a promising new technique in the future.

33.5.3 Pharmacological Intervention for Brain Plasticity in Stroke

Changes in synaptic interaction or cortical excitability are affected by the CNS neurotransmitter. Therefore, numerous studies have focused on strengthening brain plasticity using this neurotransmitter such as glutamate, acetylcholine, noradrenaline, dopamine, etc. Amphetamine and fluoxetine showed an improvement of the motor function of stroke patients, while memantine improved spontaneous speech production in aphasia [21, 22]. There have been studies on levodopa, D-amphetamine, methylphenidate, donepezil, and several antidepressants. Besides, central depressant agents making some decrement of a patient's arousal state such as benzodiazepine, haloperidol, and clonidine have negative effects on rehabilitation treatment due to lowering the excitability of cerebral cortex. Therefore, these agents should be carefully used.

33.6 Prognostic Factors for Stroke Functional Recovery

Functional recovery and prognosis after stroke onset are determined by the lesion site and size of stroke as well as by the presence of appropriate rehabilitation treatment. The difference in the recovery mechanism by the lesion size of stroke depends on the change in the remaining remnant intact cortex surrounding the lesion area in the case of a small size of stroke; however, in other cortical regions, such as contralesional cerebral cortex in the case of a large size of stroke, the phenomenon is partially affected by rehabilitation treatment.

There are external environmental factors to affect the stroke outcome during rehabilitation treatment, namely, (1) early rehabilitation, (2) optimal goal setting by a well-organized rehabilitation team, (3) learning-dependent process, (4) task-oriented intensive rehabilitation, (5) good motivation, and (6) family or caregiver support [14]. In the case of a stroke patient's individual factors, the patient with BDNF val66met polymorphism in the BDNF genotype has less effect on motor learning and brain plasticity than the patient without it. This can negatively affect stroke recovery. Likewise, the recovery mechanism of stroke is not simple; it is affected by heterogeneous factors.

Suggestions from Current Clinical Practice Guidelines
To improve functional outcome in stroke patients, it is generally recommended that early rehabilitation after stroke be provided by multidisciplinary stroke care team. However, the timing of initiation of rehabilitation is yet to be clarified.

References

1. Langhorne P, Bernhardt J, Kwakkel G. Stroke rehabilitation. Lancet. 2011;377:1693–702.
2. Tsuji T. Considerations for establishing community liaison for stroke: from a rehabilitation perspective. JMAJ. 2010;53:311–8.
3. Jørgensen HS, Nakayama H, Raaschou HO, et al. Outcome and time course of recovery in stroke. Part II: time course of recovery. The Copenhagen stroke study. Arch Phys Med Rehabil. 1995;76:406–12.
4. Jette AM. Toward a common language for function, disability, and health. Phys Ther. 2006;86:726–34.
5. Geyh S, Cieza A, Schouten J, et al. ICF core sets for stroke. J Rehabil Med. 2004;44(Suppl):135–41.
6. Chan DK, Cordato D, O'Rourke F, et al. Comprehensive stroke units: a review of comparative evidence and experience. Int J Stroke. 2013;8:260–4.
7. Wieloch T, Nikolich K. Mechanisms of neural plasticity following brain injury. Curr Opin Neurobiol. 2006;16:258–64.
8. Nudo RJ. Adaptive plasticity in motor cortex: implications for rehabilitation after brain injury. J Rehabil Med. 2003;41(Suppl):7–10.
9. Cotman CW, Berchtold NC. Exercise: a behavioral intervention to enhance brain health and plasticity. Trends Neurosci. 2002;25:295–301.
10. Tyson SF, Sadeghi-Demneh E, Nester CJ. A systematic review and meta-analysis of the effect of an ankle-foot orthosis on gait biomechanics after stroke. Clin Rehabil. 2013;27:879–91.
11. Knutson JS, Fu MJ, Sheffler LR, et al. Neuromuscular electrical stimulation for motor restoration in hemiplegia. Phys Med Rehabil Clin N Am. 2015;26:729–45.
12. AVERT Trial Collaboration group, Bernhardt J, Langhorne P, et al. Efficacy and safety of very early mobilisation within 24 h of stroke onset (AVERT): a randomised controlled trial. Lancet. 2015;386:46–55.
13. Biernaskie J, Chernenko G, Corbett D. Efficacy of rehabilitative experience declines with time after focal ischemic brain injury. J Neurosci 2004;24:1245–54.
14. Lindsay P, Bayley M, Hellings C, et al. Canadian best practice recommendations for stroke care (updated 2008). CMAJ. 2008;179:S1.
15. Kang N, Summers JJ, Cauraugh JH. Transcranial direct current stimulation facilitates motor learning post-stroke: a systematic review and meta-analysis. J Neurol Neurosurg Psychiatry. 2016;87:345–55.
16. Fregni F, Pascual-Leone A. Technology insight: noninvasive brain stimulation in neurology-perspectives on the therapeutic potential of rTMS and tDCS. Nat Clin Pract Neurol. 2007;3:383–93.
17. Kwon SY, Hong SE, Kim EJ, et al. Monitoring of functioning status in subjects with chronic stroke in south Korea using WHODAS II. Ann Rehabil Med. 2016;40:111–9.
18. Hummel FC, Cohen LG. Non-invasive brain stimulation: a new strategy to improve neurorehabilitation after stroke? Lancet Neurol. 2006;5:708–12.
19. Yavuzer G, Selles R, Sezer N, et al. Mirror therapy improves hand function in subacute stroke: a randomized controlled trial. Arch Phys Med Rehabil. 2008;89:393–8.
20. Fu MJ, Knutson JS, Chae J. Stroke rehabilitation using virtual environments. Phys Med Rehabil Clin N Am. 2015;26:747–57.
21. Berthier ML, Green C, Lara JP, et al. Memantine and constraint-induced aphasia therapy in chronic post stroke aphasia. Ann Neurol. 2009;65:577–85.
22. Chollet F, Tardy J, Albucher JF, et al. Fluoxetine for motor recovery after acute ischemic stroke (FLAME): a randomized placebo-controlled trial. Lancet Neurol. 2011;10:123–30.

Part V

Clinical Practice Guidelines

History, Purpose, and Use of Clinical Practice Guidelines for Stroke

34

Jeong-Min Kim

Abstract

The major objectives of medical guidelines are typically intended for clinicians to help them take better care of patients. However, there are many other guideline users in the healthcare system. Although clinical practice guidelines are suggestions rather than rules, insurance company or administrators often use guidelines to set standards on quality assessment and payment for care. There is a widespread effort to deal with rising costs and the need for the quality improvement by implementing guidelines. Lawyers may use well-accepted guidelines in the litigation of medical practice. In this chapter brief history of modern clinical practice guideline and requirement of trustworthy guideline will be illustrated, which would be useful for clinicians to understand the merits and limitations of clinical practice guideline.

In modern healthcare systems, doctors are frequently faced with clinical practice guidelines in performing medical procedures. So far, as of 2016, there are more than 6000 guidelines registered in the Guideline International Network, which is a global network founded in 2002 to support evidence-based healthcare and to reduce inappropriate variations in medical practice. There even exist guidelines for the production of guidelines, as well as several standardized protocols for grading guidelines according to their quality. The Institute of Medicine from the National Academies of Science/Engineering/Medicine in the United States, now known as the Health and Medicine Division, defined clinical practice guidelines as "statements that include recommendations intended to optimize patient care that are informed by a systematic review of evidence and an assessment of the benefits and harms of alternative care options" (2011) [1].

The current spread of clinical guidelines might be explained by two aspects. First, guidelines have been imposed on physicians by politicians and administrators to deal with increasing healthcare spending. This effort may not always be successful, because a growing body of evidence

J.-M. Kim
Department of Neurology, Chung-Ang University Hospital, Seoul, South Korea
e-mail: bellokim1@gmail.com

S.-H. Lee (ed.), *Stroke Revisited: Diagnosis and Treatment of Ischemic Stroke*, Stroke Revisited, DOI 10.1007/978-981-10-1424-6_34

suggests that guidelines actually increase the use of medications and healthcare expenditure. Another way of explanation is that physicians themselves have prepared most of the guidelines to preserve their professional autonomy in the face of administrative pressures or as a way for groups to compete in the marketplace. However, it is more reasonable to conclude that the proliferation of guidelines is the product of multiple groups of actors in the medical system rather than a simple dichotomy between the needs of physicians and administrators [2].

The guidelines in general have two parts: the foundational part is a systematic review of the current research evidence bearing on a clinical question, focused on the strength of evidence, and second part a set of recommendations, harboring both the evidence and value judgment regarding benefits and harms of alternative care options, addressing how patients with that condition should be managed, considering everything else being equal [1]. "Good" practice guidelines should be based on a systematic evidence review, developed by a panel of multidisciplinary experts, provide a clear explanation of the logical relationships between alternative care options and health outcomes, and provide ratings of both the quality of evidence and the strength of the recommendations. In this chapter we will cover the history and purpose of clinical practice guidelines and how to use them appropriately.

34.1 History of Clinical Practice Guideline

Before the 1970s, medical actions were at most regulated by the training and credentials guaranteed by organized profession, which might have started from medieval times. Individual physicians were assumed to be competent enough to determine the appropriate medical procedures once they completed their education and acquired a medical qualification. Beginning in the 1970s, the pressure on the standardization of medical procedures had increased due to several reasons [2]. First, public health standards evolved as preventive medicine which effectively repressed epidemic diseases such as sexually transmitted disease, cholera, tuberculosis, as well as established control programs against cancer and cardiovascular disease [2]. To deal with these medical issues, organized or standardized medical procedures should have been established before implementing to general population. Hospitals also generated demands for standardized organizational structures, practices, and data collection due to its increasing size and complexity. Second, the results of medical research greatly advanced and complicated medical practice [2]. Effort to determine the efficacy of new diagnostic and therapeutic procedures warranted the standardize classification of disease categories, instruments, measurement procedures and units, and also research protocols. Advanced medical research especially after both world wars produced many new and sophisticated procedures that cannot be performed effectively and safely without standardized protocol (think about intravenous thrombolysis protocol or endovascular thrombectomy procedure for acute ischemic stroke treatment). Third, bureaucratic control, rationality, and knowledge on medical procedures have been increased more than ever [2]. After World War II, the government's influence on the medical system has been grown extensively both as a provider and a purchaser, which means that private medical practice enters the public domain. Complex mechanisms to monitor, evaluate, and improve healthcare system demanded elaborate guideline which convince both consumers and producers of medical service. In this circumstance, practice variation can easily be regarded as lack-of-scientific evidence [2].

The first effort toward the standardization of medical service stems from the standardization of terminology rather than standardization of the procedures themselves [2]. It is conceivable that the production of practice guideline might not be possible without sufficiently developed terminological and outcome standards. During the 1850s a series of conferences produced an international nomenclature system of causes of death, which is essential for creating accurate and comparable mortality statistics. The first international classification of disease, called the International List of Causes of Death, was adopted by the International Statistical Institute in 1893 [2]. This nomenclature system is now followed by World Health Organization as International Classification of Disease, and the 11th revised version will be available by 2018. This international effort has maintained by the early twentieth century, and several standardized systems of cancer classification and nomenclature were published. In the United Kingdom, the administrative influence was greater in developing and implementing standardized protocol than in the United States [2]. The British government controlled the distribution of radium to the hospitals which adopted proposed standards of diagnostic process and therapeutic practice of cancer by establishing the Radium Trust and the Radium Commission in 1929 [2]. Standardization efforts of the American College of Surgeons produced the guidelines for organizing cancer services in hospital and manual of fracture care in 1931 [2]. The first standard blood pressure measurement protocol was produced in 1941 by the collaboration of private American and British organization [2].

Such efforts are an essential part for the development of clinical practice guidelines, although there are obstacles to overcome. Attempts to reach collective conclusions that would direct medical practice often provoked hostile mood among medical professionals because they challenge individual medical autonomy [2]. Individualizing therapy for each patient case had been traditionally regarded as the art of medicine, and medical procedure should not be directed by so called "cookbook medicine" (it would be even worse if there would not be enough recipes in such a book). Another obstacle is a lack of high-quality evidence sufficient enough to persuade majority of medical society. In this circumstance the consensus derived from a small professional group can be easily ignored by another opinion leader or by a group of stakeholders from a different community of specialists [2].

The history of randomized controlled trials in medicine started in the 1940s when a British epidemiologist-statistician named Austin Bradford Hill devised a clinical trial with a complete random allocation scheme [3]. In 1948 the first randomized clinical trial was performed by the British Medical Research Council which studied streptomycin for the treatment of tuberculosis [3]. This new study design was an urgently needed tool for investigating the effectiveness of new medical procedures, which gained great popularity in research community [3]. When the Congress in the United States passed Kefauver-Harris Amendments to the Food, Drug, and Cosmetic Act in 1962, the randomized clinical trial became a mandatory methodology by which the Food and Drug Administration could require pharmaceutical manufacturers to demonstrate therapeutic safety and efficacy before granting drug approval [3]. Nowadays, the randomized controlled clinical trial has been regarded as a gold standard for evaluating new therapies, and medical practices different from results validated from RCT are not a correct one [4].

The evidence-based approach is often impossible in the areas of greatest uncertainty due to lack of evidence. To provide recommendations in such circumstances, an explicit methodology is needed to ensure that a credible process is undertaken and that rigorous, reliable advice is provided [5]. The Delphi method is a structured communication technique or method originally developed as a systematic interactive forecasting method which relies on a panel of experts, which was developed in 1959 by Olaf Helmer to forecast the technology development of military weaponry [6]. The Delphi method or modified Delphi method can provide a structured transparent process to obtain anonymous feedback from multiple experts, but lacking a face-to-face engagement of participants, which might be useful in resolving disagreements [5].

From the 1980s, guidelines were produced in many different countries. Each nation's guidelines remain the product of complex relationships among multiple stakeholders. European countries have succeeded in placing guideline production authorities under the influential power of national agencies and in bringing together professional and administrative actors as well as experts in various disciplines [2]. These organizations include the National Institute for Clinical

Excellence (NICE) in the United Kingdom, the Scottish Intercollegiate Guidelines Network (SIGN) in Scotland, the Arztliches Zentrum fur Qualitat in der Medizin (AZQ) in Germany, the Dutch College of General Practitioners in the Netherlands, and the Haute Autorite de sante in France [2]. In the United States the government power was not as strong as in Europe and rather fragmented, which delayed to develop centralized institutions facilitating widespread implementation of clinical practice guideline [2]. The National Guidelines Clearinghouse created in 1990 by the Agency for Healthcare Research and Quality (AHRQ) of the US Department of Health and Human Services serves limited role as a clearinghouse of guideline. This phenomenon might be associated with duplicated guidelines from several specialty groups and rapidly escalating medical costs due to inappropriate or unnecessary medical procedures. Military medicine, especially healthcare division for veterans, was a sector in which bureaucratic power made the progression of early guidelines regarding tuberculosis and cancer treatment [2]. This standardization effort was followed by the "evidence-based medicine" beginning in the 1990, which aims to facilitate the conscientious and judicious use of current best evidence from clinical care research in the management of individual patients [2].

34.2 What Are the Requirements of Trustworthy Clinical Practice Guideline?

The Grading of Recommendations, Assessment, Development, and Evaluation (GRADE) system is a scoring system of guidelines by two components: the strength of the recommendation and the level of evidence. A high-quality level of evidence is derived from well-conducted randomized controlled trials, whereas low-quality evidence typically comes from nonsystematic observations or expert opinion (Fig. 34.1). A strong recommendation is dictated when the benefits clearly outweigh the risks for nearly all patients. A weak recommendation is made when the difference between the risks and benefits is uncertain. Not all guidelines are on the same quality. Several basic elements for the development of high-quality guidelines are illustrated in Table 34.1.

First of all, credible guidelines should be evidence based, which is derived from a systematic review of identified published researches by scientific strength and level of evidence [1]. However, high-quality evidence is often not possible, and a considerable area in medical care is left with scientific uncertainty. For example, previous analysis showed that nearly half of the recommendations of the American/Heart Association/American College of Cardiology guidelines were based on the lowest level of evidence [1]. The situation might be more serious in developing countries, where high-quality scientific evidence focusing on domestic medical issues may be scarce. In that case, most part of the guidelines would be derived from adaptation and translation of clinical practice guidelines from developed countries (mostly from the United States or European countries) or from expert consensus.

A multidisciplinary approach is essential in developing practice guideline because a collaboration of experts representing the full range of expertise regarding the clinical question is more likely to avoid the blind spots of members from a single specialty [1]. These panels could include primary and subspecialty physicians, representatives from allied health sciences, public health specialists, economists, consumers, and ethicists. This process requires a considerable time. The evidence-based guidelines developed by the National Clinical Clearing Center for implementation in the National Health Service are processed for 2.5 years from inception to release. The clinical practice guidelines produced by single-specialty group are frequently involved with a narrower spectrum of interest which may be limited to members in the relevant society.

The guidelines, once produced, should be renovated and revised regularly; otherwise it may be out of date [1]. A study of 100 quantitative systematic reviews found that new findings with impact on the reviews found that the median time for the survival of an analysis was 5.5 years,

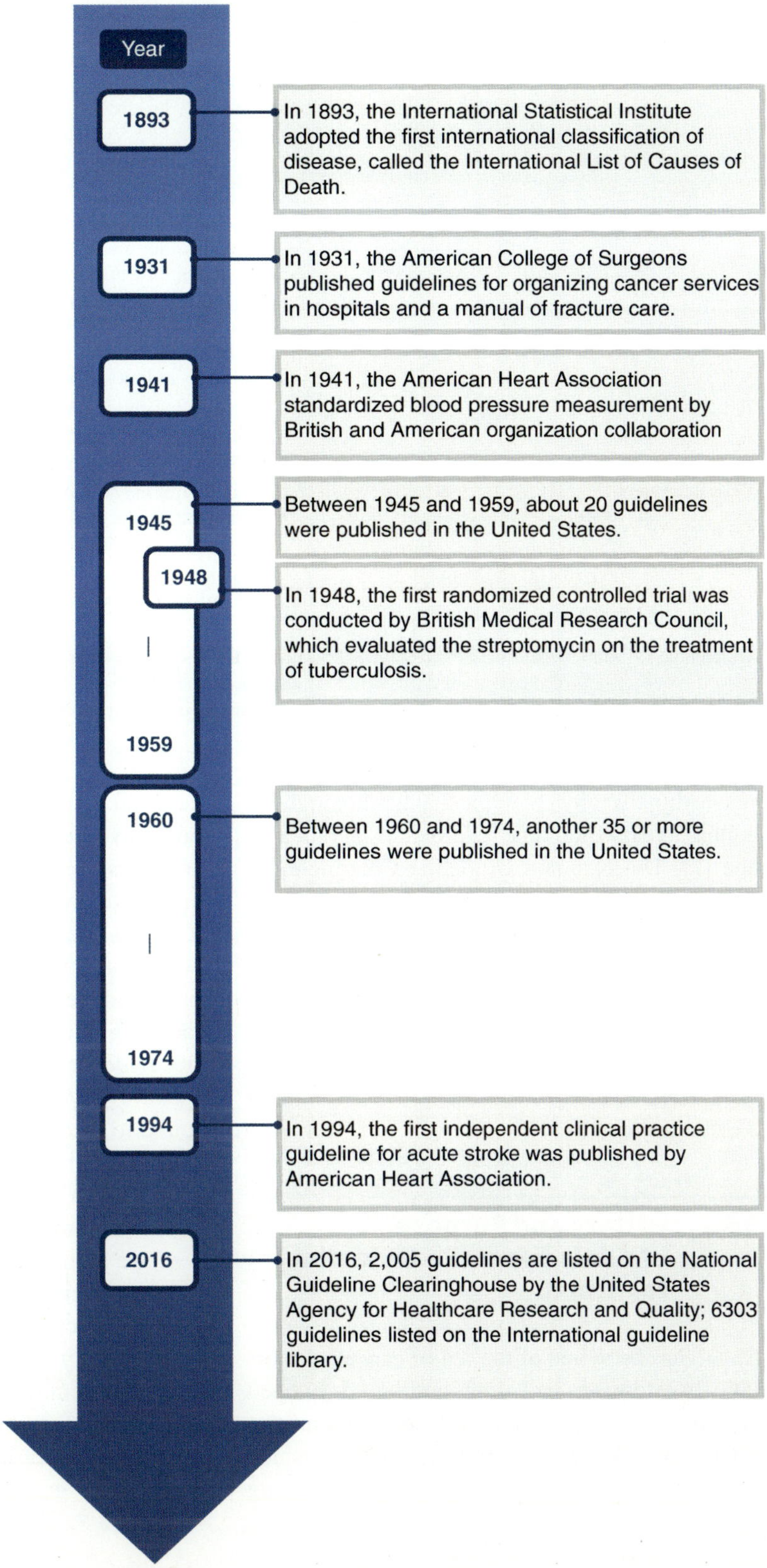

Fig. 34.1 The hierarchy of research design according to the level of scientific evidence. The scientific evidence increased according to the ability to control for bias and to demonstrate cause and effect in human, although the greater relevance, the fewer available literature

Table 34.1 The requirements for the trustworthy guidelines

Participation of multidisciplinary specialists	The guideline editing team should be multidisciplinary and balanced, including a patient or consumer, of populations expected to be affected by the guideline
Review of past literature	The guideline should be based on systematic reviews of the literature and consider quality, quantity, and consistency of the available evidence
Strength of evidence	The guideline should summarize evidence about potential benefits and harms. Each recommendation should be accompanied by discussion of the scientific rationale, the evidence and its quality, the contribution of values and experience, ratings of the level of confidence in the evidence and the strength of the recommendation, and the differences of opinion regarding recommendations
Recommendation	The guideline should precisely state the recommended actions, when they should be performed, and how they could be measured for evaluation of compliance
Outside review	The guidelines should be reviewed by the full spectrum of relevant stakeholders. The general public should have an opportunity to review the guidelines before they are final
Escape from bias, benefit, and conflict	The guidelines should include an explicit description of process and funding to minimize bias, distortion, and conflict of interests
Immediate revision	Guidelines should state their date of publication and the date of the evidence reviewed. Guideline should be updated when new, clinically important evidence is available

suggesting that any guideline that has not updated within 5 years should be regarded as an outdated one [7]. The National Guideline Clearinghouse requires evidence that a guideline has been developed, reviewed, or revised within 5 years for inclusion of the guideline in their listing. Lastly, each member of the panel involved in the guideline production should report conflicts of interest, and no one with a relevant conflict of interest should decide the overall direction or strength of a recommendation [1].

34.3 History and Purpose of Clinical Practice Guideline for Stroke

Stroke has been one of the major causes of mortality worldwide, including both in developed and in developing countries. Stroke victims are often confronted with neurological deficits which limit everyday quality of life while increasing healthcare expenditure as well as the emotional burden to be carried by their family members or caregivers. Many nations have been trying to derive effective treatment guideline to suppress the rising incidence of cerebrovascular disease and to distribute medical resource for valid diagnostic and treatment modalities. Stroke clinical practice guideline is intended to provide scientific evidence and effective treatment strategy based on a systematic review of scientific background to medical doctors who are dealing with stroke patient care [8, 9]. Developed countries such as the United States, Japan, Canada, and European countries as well as developing countries have established and implemented their own clinical practice guidelines. It is important to develop clinical practice guideline of their own because every country would have a distinct medical system, available resources, and urgent issues in stroke management.

In the United States, the first independent management guidelines for acute stroke were published by the American Heart Association in 1994 [10]. These guidelines provided information about the management strategy for acute stroke especially within 24 h; and they emphasized the evidence-based medicine [10]. At that time there had been no breakthrough treatment for stroke such as thrombolysis, but the societal burden of stroke was already considerable [11]. Several guidelines from Western countries have been published thereafter and early 2000s by the European Stroke Society or Canadian Stroke Consortium. The most recent early stroke management guideline from the American Heart Association and American Stroke Association was published in 2013. These emphasize the relentless effort to reduce the stroke incidence worldwide by integrated approach and are based on a rather optimistic view due to the recent decline of stroke mortality from the 3rd to the 4th in the United States [10]. Regarding the early management of stroke patients, an update of endovascular thrombectomy and scientific rationale for the inclusion and exclusion criteria for intravenous thrombolysis were additionally published thereafter [12].

Conclusion

As with other clinical practice guidelines, the evidence-based, carefully developed guidelines for stroke provide synthesis of the literature by the experts in various fields including neurologists, neurosurgeon, neuro-interventionist, rehabilitation specialist, and so on, clear recommendations for translating the scientific evidence into clinical application to promote the best practice, and opportunities to evaluate the outcomes of implementation in the real-world setting [9]. However several potential limitations exist in clinical practice guideline such as the potential for inappropriate use of guidelines as tools for restrictive administrative or legal purposes, the potential for conflict of interests, applying guidelines developed to address specific condition to a patient with multiple comorbidities, and difficult accessibility at the point of care [13]. The doctors must know the potentials and caveats of clinical practice guideline to wisely use it in the best possible way.

References

1. Shekelle P. Overview of clinical practice guidelines. In: Uptodate. 2016. https://www.uptodate.com/contents/overview-of-clinical-practice-guidelines. Accessed 21 Aug 2016.
2. Weisz G, Cambrosio A, Keating P, et al. The emergence of clinical practice guidelines. Milbank Q. 2007;85:691–727.
3. Bothwell LE, Greene JA, Podolsky SH, et al. Assessing the gold standard – lessons from the history of RCTs. N Engl J Med. 2016;374:2175–81.
4. Bothwell LE, Podolsky SH. The emergence of the randomized, controlled trial. N Engl J Med. 2016;375:501–4.
5. Loblaw DA, Prestrud AA, Somerfield MR, et al. American society of clinical oncology clinical practice guidelines: formal systematic review-based consensus methodology. J Clin Oncol. 2012;30:3136–40.
6. RAND corporation. Delphi method. 2016. http://www.rand.org/topics/delphi-method.html. Accessed 21 Aug 2016.
7. Shojania KG, Sampson M, Ansari MT, et al. How quickly do systematic reviews go out of date? A survival analysis. Ann Intern Med. 2007;147:224–33.
8. European Stroke Organisation (ES) Executive Committee. Guidelines for management of ischaemic stroke and transient ischaemic attack 2008. Cerebrovasc Dis. 2008;25:457–507.
9. Jauch EC, Saver JL, Adams HP Jr, et al. Guidelines for the early management of patients with acute ischemic stroke: a guideline for healthcare professionals from the American Heart Association/American Stroke Association. Stroke. 2013;44:870–947.
10. Adams HP Jr, Brott TG, Crowell RM, et al. Guidelines for the management of patients with acute ischemic stroke. A statement for healthcare professionals from a special writing group of the stroke council, American Heart Association. Circulation. 1994;90:1588–601.
11. Biller J, Love BB. Nihilism and stroke therapy. Stroke. 1991;22:1105–7.
12. Powers WJ, Derdeyn CP, Biller J, et al. 2015 American Heart Association/American Stroke Association focused update of the 2013 guidelines for the early management of patients with acute ischemic stroke regarding endovascular treatment: a guideline for healthcare professionals from the American Heart Association/American Stroke Association. Stroke. 2015;46:3020–35.
13. Pronovost PJ. Enhancing physicians' use of clinical guidelines. JAMA. 2013;310:2501–2.

Discrepancy and Pitfalls of Clinical Practice Guideline

35

Seung-Hoon Lee and Han-Gil Jeong

Abstract

The popularization of clinical practice guideline (CPG) provided an opportunity for the active sharing of medical information and the improvement of the medical standard. Unlike the initial phase, however, the problems due to the overcredulity on CPG have currently become a major issue. Most of the problems resulted from either the overcredulity on the results of the randomized clinical trials (RCT) or the overambitious intention of making the recommendations despite the lack of RCT evidence. Efforts to bring out the best in CPG and compensate for its weakness via real-world evidence are deemed necessary. Furthermore, the authors of CPG and other clinicians in various fields need to know the strength and weakness of CPG and make an effort to improve it.

The previous and current roles of clinical practice guideline (CPG) are described in detail in Chap. 6.1. To put it simply, CPG is not designed to introduce the most recent innovative treatment, but to provide resources that can be used by almost all of the centers worldwide. In other words, CPG is based on a systematic review of clinical evidence by various scholars to offer recommendations about the medical procedures that are needed to be performed at the centers in deprived areas with questionable medical quality than that of the centers with the best equipment and medical team. In this regard, the primary purpose of CPG is to raise the quality of primary and secondary care to above average. For example, every clinician knows that magnetic resonance imaging (MRI) is better than computed tomography (CT) for the diagnosis of stroke. However, most of the CPGs recommended to use brain imaging (e.g., CT or MRI), which reflects the primary purpose of CPG. High-level CPG takes one step further and eliminates the unnecessary questions on the diagnosis and treatment process, simplifies the decision-making process,

S.-H. Lee, M.D., Ph.D., F.A.H.A. (✉)
Clinical Division, Department of Neurology, Seoul National University Hospital, 101 Daehak-ro, Jongno-gu, Seoul 03080, South Korea
e-mail: sb0516@snu.ac.kr

H.-G. Jeong, M.D., M.Sc.
Public Health Doctor, Ministry of Health and Welfare, Seoul, South Korea

S.-H. Lee (ed.), *Stroke Revisited: Diagnosis and Treatment of Ischemic Stroke*, Stroke Revisited, DOI 10.1007/978-981-10-1424-6_35

and helps in selecting the right procedure within a very short timeframe. Many CPGs actually improved the overall quality of care in various countries and helped many doctors to make evidence-based decisions in practice. Recently, however, CPG often causes unnecessary conflicts over treatment in some situations. In this case, CPG occasionally becomes the source of legal or insurance dispute over proper treatment beyond the individual patient level. However, CPG is by no means a one-size-fits-all guideline similar to a panacea. The overcredulity on CPG might cause huge problems to the doctors, patients, and insurance companies. In some cases, CPG does not describe at all or describe overcautiously about the entirely predictable conflict between the doctor and the patient. In other words, with some exaggeration, CPG infringes upon minor issues, but manages to evade important legal issues. We need to fully understand the "yin and yang" of CPG. We would like to identify several problems regarding the CPG description and recommendations and discuss how to improve CPG in the future.

35.1 Problems of CPG Writing Process

35.1.1 On What Issues Are Randomized Clinical Trials (RCTs) Conducted?

Are the results of the RCT significantly effective on CPG writing? Yes. Then is it right? We need to think about it. The cost of a properly conducted RCT is immense. Investigators can design study subjects and methods as many as the investigators want, according to their clinical needs. However, it is realistically impossible to conduct the RCT by the investigators only due to the costs. Therefore, the RCT often moves toward the desired direction of funders. Multinational pharmaceutical companies have the most influence as funders of RCT, and it is inevitable that there will be more RCTs to evaluate their new drugs. Although this is not always a wrong direction, RCT on new drugs or secondary analyses on RCT are conducted much more than clinical needs, which may overestimate the effect of the new drugs.

Example 1 The use of statin to lower cholesterol in order to prevent atherothrombotic stroke has become common knowledge. However, there were only 8 sponsor-initiated trials (SITs) of lovastatin and 23 SITs of pravastatin, as compared to 166 SITs of atorvastatin, 88 SITs of rosuvastatin, and 122 SITs of simvastatin (data were analyzed from the web site: clinicaltrials.gov).

35.1.2 Was Most Appropriate Drug Selected for RCT?

It is natural that when pharmaceutical companies have the initiative, they prioritize their new patented drugs for RCT. Therefore, there is very little chance that pharmaceutical companies would like to perform RCT on off-patent drugs or popular drugs that have been used for a long time, even if another excellent efficacy has been recently verified because they discovered that off-patent drugs lacked marketability. It is very common in a capitalistic society, so these researches need to be done by the government or an organization that manages the public fund. The problem is that the standpoint on pharmaceutical industries by the government officials is usually more focused on industrial and economic revival than welfare. As a result, the investment on drugs without marketability or exclusivity might be difficult. However, there are some differences of varying degrees among the countries.

Example 2 AstraZeneca developed an antioxidant agent called NXY-059 as a neuroprotectant in the early stage of acute ischemic stroke. The manufacturer sponsored the Phase 3 clinical trials (SAINT I and II trials) twice worldwide [1, 2]. Although the result of the SAINT I trial showed a marginally significant neuroprotective effect [1], the SAINT II trial failed to reproduce the same result [2]. Therefore, this agent could not make it to the market and disappeared in the mists of history. Then, there was a very famous drug named minocycline, which was a neuroprotective agent in the basic stroke research field. This drug was developed 30 years ago, and there were more than 100 statistically significant reports of its effectiveness in animal models of stroke. However, this drug has never been tested via clinical trials. Why was NXY-059 able to undergo Phase 3 clinical trials twice with an astronomical amount of money spent on them, despite the fact that minocycline has much more evidence and superior reliability on drug efficacy? This is due to the multinational pharmaceuticals, patent, and marketability.

35.1.3 Absolute Acceptance of Past RCTs Conducted Via Inadequate Methods

The overcredulity on RCT often leads to a blind faith with regard to the results of the previous RCTs that were conducted prior to an evolved methodology. In particular, the results of RCTs on off-patent drugs or drugs unrelated to patency were conducted inconsiderately in the past, and they were easily accepted. There must be some way to verify with similar methods or discover the positive aspects of drugs with other methods.

Example 3 The use of steroid to reduce vasogenic edema in order to improve the prognosis of patients with intracerebral hemorrhage (ICH) is theoretically a reasonable and logical strategy that had been popular in the past. However, there was only one clinical trial that was properly conducted, although it was published in 1987 [3]. This study was conducted in order to compare the study group (steroid use) and the control group in supratentorial ICH patients, but it was discontinued due to the adverse effects when only 93 participants were enrolled. There were 13 patients who had infection in a study group of 46 patients, and there were 6 patients who had infection in a control group of 47 patients. However, there were no differences in mortality rates between the groups. Do you think this result is acceptable at the present time? Even though it is an RCT, there were only 93 participants, and those patients were only observed during the early phase. Moreover, the study might not have the excellent supportive medical care that we have nowadays. Would this result be the same if we selected a sufficient number of participants with present knowledge, dosage control, and steroid use duration? Nonetheless, this study has not yet been verified, and the use of steroid in any type of ICH is never currently recommended.

35.1.4 Acceptance of RCT Results Conducted Under Impossible Circumstances

Even with the recently presented RCTs, there are some studies presenting the results collected up to the point when the study was discontinued. The design of the RCT was impossible to conduct from the very beginning, so they have given up before making any progress. This is the case when a study could not proceed properly due to various situations of the investigators, problems with patient enrollment, or flaws with the design. They discontinued the study and presented the early terminated results. However, such studies are occasionally published on highly respected journals because of their RCT format and some authority of authors. In this case, the authors of CPG are not likely to disregard these issues, so they are included in the recommendations after selecting them even as high-level evidence. Reevaluation is practically impossible because the clinical trials for the verification are not conducted for the same reason as that of the discontinued studies.

Example 4 The GIST-UK study is the only clinical trial conducted on the effects of hypoglycemia correction in patients with acute stroke [4]. This study started in 1998 with funds from the Stroke Association and NHS executives in the UK. However, during the course of the study, they realized that the target recruitment could not be achieved within the existing routine of the NHS clinical practice, existing financial resources, or proper period of time. In 2005, this study was discontinued, and the result prior to the time of discontinuation was presented to the Lancet Neurology. The result of the discontinued study showed that it was difficult to verify the greater effect of hyperglycemia correction in patients with stroke, and this study has remained the only study on hyperglycemia correction for stroke patients. This study is contrary to the study result of correcting hyperglycemia with insulin in critically ill patients, who are admitted in the intensive care unit. However, reverification is still not possible. At present, there is no firm recommendation on hyperglycemia control in stroke patients, only a vague statement.

Example 5 The FASTER study is conducted in order to prevent the relapse of stroke with the administration of clopidogrel or simvastatin within 24 hours of stroke onset (a two-by-two study design in the baseline treatment of aspirin) [5]. The results were highly anticipated at that time, but the trial was discontinued early due to the failure to recruit patients at the prespecified minimum enrollment rate as a result of the increased use of statins. It was presented as inconclusive, because all of the results were not statistically significant. The early effect of clopidogrel addition to aspirin was examined in the following CHANCE trial later [6]. However, the early effect of statin has not yet been tested.

Example 6 The COSS study is a clinical trial that is conducted in order to examine the effectiveness of the extracranial-intracranial (EC-IC) bypass surgery in patients with internal carotid artery (ICA) occlusion [7]. It was designed to perform positron emission tomography (PET) in order to select proper patients. However, PET is too expensive equipment to be installed in every center. Accordingly, there was a significant problem on patient enrollment because of issues with regard to PET facility location for a real study even if there were suitable patients. Although this study started in 2002, the researchers enrolled only 49 patients in 18 centers until 2010, and it was discontinued due to ineffectiveness. Even with critical problems in patient enrollment, this study published the results in JAMA, thereby stating that the EC-IC bypass was ineffective. What would CPG recommend while considering that there were almost no clinical studies and one failed study even utilizing PET? It is, of course, "the EC-IC bypass should not be used." Is the EC-IC bypass not beneficial to the patients at all? The EC-IC bypass is not allowed to be conducted on any patient under this circumstance. If we see a 50-year-old patient with hemodynamic infarction due to ICA occlusion presenting with a significantly decreased perfusion on imaging tests, is the antiplatelet therapy sufficient? Do we have to give up the effectiveness of this surgical procedure because of the only clinical trial conducted on 49 patients over the span of 9 years?

35.1.5 Excluded from the Recommendations Due to the Reason of Not Having RCT on Logically Reasonable Therapy

Are clinical trials required to examine whether the soldiers on high-altitude jump training from an airplane need parachutes or not? Since CPG is the final product of an evidence-based medicine, it is often quite conservative even to the obvious therapies that do not require RCT.

Example 7 The STICH trial showed that there were no significant differences between the medical treatment group and the surgical treatment group in the ICH [8]. Based on this study result, it was confirmed that not every ICH patient needs an emergency surgery. In this study, however, patients who needed surgery from the start were excluded from the analysis, while the patients in the medical treatment group, who underwent surgery while admitted to the hospital in accordance with the doctor's decision, remained in the medical treatment group. Therefore, this study result must not be overinterpreted as medical treatment is better for all the ICH patients. Can we put off surgery if we suspect an impending herniation or brainstem compression? Can we hold the surgery even if we knew that the situation would be worsened, such as a suspected ongoing bleeding due to a WFR-induced bleeding in the case of a large-sized lobar hemorrhage or relatively larger edema around the hemorrhage? CPG needs to strongly emphasize the importance of surgery when it is required. However, there are very limited information or recommendation on cases that require surgery because most of the researchers involved in CPG are neurological physicians.

Example 8 Do we want to know whether the decompression surgery is needed in patients with malignant middle cerebral artery (MCA) infarction or not? Even clinicians with little experience know that the patients in this case might die without a surgery. Is an RCT required to find out the effect of surgery? Then, RCTs were indeed performed at three different places [9]. The result was obvious, in that surgery improved the survival rate and the rate of disability. Currently, CPG strongly recommends surgery on patients diagnosed with malignant MCA infarction. Were RCTs really needed to prove this hypothesis?

35.1.6 Overgeneralization or Wrong Conclusion from Other Evidence

Although this is not a common mistake in CPG, it is something that happens and cannot be easily corrected. Because it is not possible to know the background information and history only through reading the CPG, these mistakes are often found by clinicians with many years of clinical experience. The problem is that the mistakes regarding these drugs have been already generalized as established medical knowledge, and it is too late to verify or change it. Examples are shown below.

Example 9 Heparin is a broad-spectrum anticoagulant that effectively inhibits the activation of clotting factor in a fast and powerful manner. Unfractionated heparin (UFH) has been used for a very long time. Administration via intravenous (IV) route is a very cheap and prompt way of urgent anticoagulation. Therefore, it has been commonly used in various urgent situations of systemic thromboembolism and stroke. However, as fast as its effectiveness, the drug concentration changes rapidly. It also changes in activated partial thromboplastin time (aPTT), which reflects the anticoagulation status. As a result, it is recommended to regularly measure the aPTT throughout the day. In fact, there are no clinical trials on UFH in stroke, even though it has been used effectively for a very long time. Only clinical trials on new low-molecular-weight heparin (LMWH) drugs have been conducted, even though they might have been expected to less effective than UFH. It was because of the financial power of the pharmaceutical companies manufacturing the new drugs. Nevertheless, most of the LMWH studies unpredictably failed to prove the effectiveness on the prevention of relapse in stroke patients. However, CPG strictly recommended all types of heparin to be contraindicated, just after combining the LMWH study results. UFH did not undergo any clinical trial for acute stroke, and the UFH with an IV-adjusted dose showed an instant and strong effectiveness, as compared to the LMWH. Would the prohibition of UFH, based on the LMWH study failure, be appropriate without the clinical trials of UFH?

Example 10 It is well understood that the CAPRIE trial results were erroneous [10]. This study very unusually enrolled participants—stroke, myocardial infarction (MI), and peripheral artery disease (PAD) patients—all together from the beginning stage and defined the endpoint event if any of these three recurred. This study was conducted as SIT, and it is more appropriate to consider its goal of pharmaceutical company as to receive indications for all three diseases from one study was strongly reflected, rather than a certain academic purpose. This study showed that clopidogrel is slightly superior than aspirin in the prevention of the composite events of these three diseases after randomly administering aspirin or clopidogrel to these patients. Then, clopidogrel was indicated to patients with each stroke, MI, and PAD based on this result. Upon closer inspection of the study result, the superior efficacy of clopidogrel was not significant in patients with MI or stroke. The superior efficacy of clopidogrel in all PAD patients was extremely strong. After combining all data on three events, the superior efficacy of clopidogrel in all patients was yielded. Is clopidogrel indeed superior to aspirin in stroke patients? It is not easy to conduct RCTs on this issue again, and the superiority of clopidogrel is not established in stroke. Fortunately, clopidogrel was produced at the right time.

35.1.7 Evidence Extraction with Intended Manner

In some cases, CPG tends to lean toward national benefit or benefit of the industry in the country because it does not have a verification process by another country or organization.

Example 11 There are some drugs (e.g., ozagrel and edaravone) recommended in Japan that are not mentioned in other countries. While RCTs on these drugs have not been conducted in other countries, there are many basic studies and several clinical studies conducted in Japan. However, it is difficult to generalize the results because all the results only came from Japan with relatively small numbers of participants. Furthermore, these drugs were manufactured in Japan. Likewise, CPG in Korea recommends triflusal and cilostazol for stroke prevention. Triflusal is a Spanish drug and cilostazol is a Japanese drug. Why was this recommendation included, even though there had been no multinational RCTs? These drugs have something in common, in which they have been actively marketed by the Korean pharmaceutical companies. These characteristics of CPG by country may show a kind of support to benefit of the industries in their countries. Certainly, there were some RCT evidences on these drugs, but the quality of RCTs needs to be discussed with caution.

35.1.8 Passive Attitude Toward Legally Sensitive Matters

CPG needs to be more actively engaged on legally sensitive matters because it can prevent the formation of future legal issues by explaining the previous evidence in detail on a questionable medical situation. CPGs with detailed description on such matters might reduce unnecessary conflicts between the patients and the medical team and even protect both parties. However, these sensitive issues are not likely to be mentioned. The CPG authors do not want to be involved in unnecessary lawsuits, but neglecting the legal positions that are required of doctors and researchers might be cowardly.

Example 12 It is very common for patients with stroke or its high risks to undergo surgery due to other problems or cardiovascular problems. Lawsuits because of developed stroke or deterioration of cognitive functions after surgery are numerous in any country. However, there is no CPG stating the types of diagnostic tests, which are required in advance, risks involved, process of prescribing medications, and process of preparing preoperative and postoperative procedures in these patients. Even the title of this issue is rarely mentioned. Although there are some manuals or protocols from some hospitals, they are limited for use as legal basis. Although the level of evidence may not be regarded as high, why are the CPGs not interested in these issues at all? It is obvious. They do not want to face individual lawsuits. Then, why does the CPG recommend treatment methods for individual patients? Why, especially, are the recommendations on new drugs of pharmaceutical companies promptly addressed?

35.2 Problems with the Application Process of CPG

35.2.1 Misconception Due to Lack of Understanding of Stroke Subtype

The importance of a stroke subtype is already described in detail in Chap. 2.8. In an ischemic stroke, it is safe to say that the large artery atherosclerosis, small vessel occlusion, and cardioembolism are totally different diseases due to their completely different pathophysiology.

Nowadays, therefore, many clinical trials tend to be conducted on targeted subtypes. CPGs use the expression of "recommend to certain subtype only" from these study results, and general readers are not easy to fully understand these recommendations. In particular, treatments with recommendations tend to be applied excessively. We need to properly understand the CPG's recommendation.

Example 13 Atorvastatin is verified as an effective treatment on the secondary prevention of stroke and cardiovascular diseases via the SPARCL trial [11]. However, other results, hemorrhagic stroke with 66% of hazard ratio increase by atorvastatin, were also identified. Further, numerous cohort studies previously suggested the high association between low serum cholesterol and hemorrhagic stroke, and there is no reason why statin should be actively used in hemorrhagic stroke patients or SVO patients. In addition, the main mechanism of statin is to prevent the progression or aggravation of atherosclerosis by lowering the cholesterol level. Then, statin use needs to be focused on LAA. The CPG of AHA/ASA recommends statin to be used in "atherothrombotic TIA or stroke." There is a question as to whether any physicians can easily recognize the term "atherothrombotic" or not. Without mentioning the phrase, "do not use in SVO or hemorrhagic stroke," this "atherothrombotic" terminology does not stand out. It could be due to the vague expression of CPG that many physicians use statin regardless of stroke subtype.

35.2.2 Uniformity of Treatment Due to CPG

Every clinical manifestation and pathophysiology of patients visiting the hospital is almost different from one another, but the CPGs for each condition are made by categorized patients according to mechanism or conditions to help communications between the medical teams, education, and convenience of treatment. Nonetheless, using the CPG like a cookbook in order to easily categorize the characteristics of the patients is one of the most unwanted consequences due to CPG. Let us see the problems related to uniformity in treatment if the CPGs are applied as such.

First, consistent practice pattern and reduced variation can cause a decrease in the tailored treatment of patients who required a special approach. There are real clinical situations that are much more various and complex to cover with only CPG, and stroke, in particular, often shows a variety of subtypes and progress. CPGs do not reflect the clinical situations of individual patients with flexibility without thoughtful consideration on various characteristics of each individual and the consequential heterogeneity. In a difficult clinical situation, experienced specialists can make a series of tailored decision-making after putting together the individual situation of the patient, as well as the past history of the patient and previous evidence. However, a treatment strategy from a clinician's own experience might be misunderstood as inappropriate because of attitude of simple use of CPGs.

Second, the specialty of the medical team might be disregarded by the CPG. Auditors or hospital administrators may interpret the quality of care arbitrarily after simply acquiring the contents of the CPGs. This means that the quality of care of the center would be assessed not by evaluating the care on an individual patient's situation, but by simply calculated measures, such as the application rate of a certain treatment. Furthermore, if the CPG is cited unreasonably in lawsuits on individual malpractice or regulatory methods of medical expenses, the quality of care of every clinician might eventually be standardized downward to become more passive and safer.

Third, there are some possibilities that many promising tries might be regulated inappropriately because of CPG recommendations. This will not be good to future medical research and scientific progress. The funding bodies might not support tries considering different aspects of the treatments that the CPGs concluded evidence of benefit is lacking.

35.3 How Do We Solve the Problems of CPG?

35.3.1 Overcredulity on CPGs Should Be Avoided

There is little chance of improving these situations, despite the appeals for better CPGs. CPGs by individual academic society is often made in context with the characteristics of the academic society and situation, and many complex invisible profits are involved. How do we properly handle these problems on CPG?

The most sensible and definite way is to ovoid overcredulity on CPG. In the medical field, the most ideal way of practice is for the experienced clinicians and specialists to completely learn about CPG and its background and then provide optimal treatment to each patient separately. However, in a real clinical world, not all clinicians treat CPGs with wisdom. The quality of care assessors simply evaluate the quality of treatment by the CPG. If the members of society related to medicine fully understand the pros and cons of CPGs, communicate well, and try to use it properly in their own society, the present shortcomings of CPGs may be resolved considerably.

35.3.2 Support of CPG in Other Way: Real-World Evidence (RWE)

The primary purpose of CPG is to effectively educate the local centers with insufficient medical quality. However, CPG became a dinosaur with the overwhelming influence on every medical society, including the specialist medical team. If going back to the primary purpose is not realistic, we need to make an effort to improve as much as possible. The core problems of CPGs stated above are (1) to make recommendations even with little or no evidence and (2) to make recommendations with the wrong information, even though it is almost impossible to gather evidence. Less than 30% of clinically conducted treatments have evidences from RCTs. CPGs unreasonably became a judgment tool on all cases in these circumstances. CPGs need to accept cases without sufficient evidences "with open-minded attitude." Where do we get new evidence? Wouldn't it incur a new cost because it will require a new study methodology for research?

The most appropriate direction for CPG improvement is to accept data from real-world practice as evidence and modify the recommendations. The root of all problems was the gap between CPG and real-world practice. Therefore, its solution also may be found in real-world practice. Currently, this data from real-world practice is called real-world data (RWD), and the evidence from RWD is called RWE. RWD includes all data from almost all real-world practices. RWE is the data gathered from various and inhomogeneous patients with insurance claims data and electronic health record. What are the roles of the RWE? (1) RWE enables the testing of RCT data on safety and efficacy of new drugs or medical devices in real-world practice. (2) RWE also enables the identification of already-authorized drugs regarding its value to the patients or clinicians in the real world. For example, RWE enables the precise decision on safety issues in a post-marketing situation. In addition, it allows the verification of a heterogeneous response, which is difficult to see in the RCTs, and this enables the identification of the subgroups with more benefit, effectiveness on patients with various complex comorbidities, and equivalent effectiveness in various clinical practice situations. (3) It enables a longer term of longitudinal study. The RWE collects data from patient visits or insurance claim submissions. Therefore, identifying a long-term study of patient outcomes and healthcare utilization is less expensive. (4) Hypothesis generation, wherein the analysis of the RWD may contribute largely toward making research hypothesis and questions on medications or treatment in randomized trials in the future. (5) Patient recruitment, wherein the RWD sources can be utilized to expedite the identification and recruitment of patients for clinical research.

RWE is not merely a big data, but rather, it is an integration of multiple sources of data (e.g., clinical data, genomic data, and socioeconomic data). This will better represent the individual characteristics of the patients and enable tailored treatment. However, RWD does not always mean data included in a big data research. RWD may include

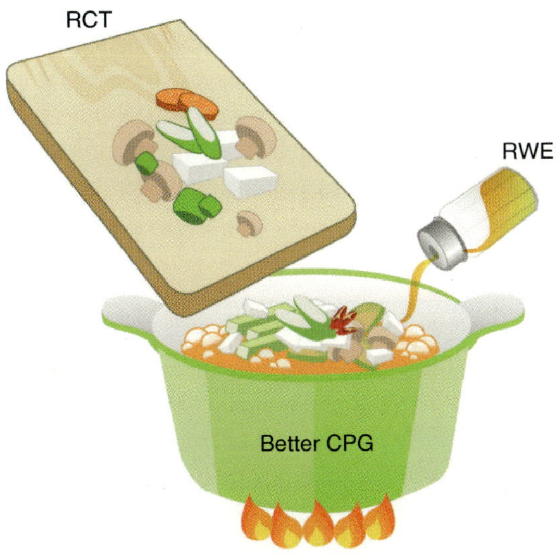

Fig. 35.1 A backup strategy of real-world evidences to make a better clinical practice guidelines by resolving current problems of randomized controlled trials. *RCT* randomized controlled trial, *CPG* clinical practice guideline, *RWE* real-world evidence

even case series or a single center-based hospital study. If the realm of evidence of CPG is expanded in this manner, collect evidence of issues that are not solved in the previous RCTs, and modify the recommendations logically; the previously stated problems of CPG will be resolved considerably. If the stroke field makes full use of RWD to get more evidence, there will be more rooms that the CPG answers logically (Fig. 35.1).

Conclusion

CPG has a lot of advantages, but it clearly has disadvantages as well. CPGs that were made by the government or payer to control the cost might be effective as a public policy, but it might seriously infringe on autonomy of clinicians and patients. CPGs that were made by specialist organizations might have a self-serving bias and might not be helpful to clinicians on general practice. CPGs that were made with firm rules without flexibility might transform a very sophisticated and inhomogeneous medicine to cookbook medicine. A critical understanding of the advantages and limitations of CPG will prevent poor decisions to cause harm on the patients, clinicians, and healthcare system. The most important thing would be to gather more high-quality evidence from the RWE or to enhance RCT with RWD. It is necessary to develop a support system for decision making after considering all conditions at an individual level rather than a population level. Medical practice in real world needs to become science and art based on CPGs and RWE.

Suggestions from Current Clinical Practice Guidelines
Not applicable to this chapter.

References

1. Lees KR, Zivin JA, Ashwood T, et al. NXY-059 for acute ischemic stroke. N Engl J Med. 2006;354:588–600.
2. Shuaib A, Lees KR, Lyden P, et al. NXY-059 for the treatment of acute ischemic stroke. N Engl J Med. 2007;357:562–71.
3. Poungvarin N, Bhoopat W, Viriyavejakul A, et al. Effects of dexamethasone in primary supratentorial intracerebral hemorrhage. N Engl J Med. 1987;316:1229–33.
4. Gray CS, Hildreth AJ, Sandercock PA, et al. Glucose-potassium-insulin infusions in the management of post-stroke hyperglycaemia: the UK Glucose Insulin in Stroke Trial (GIST-UK). Lancet Neurol. 2007;6:397–406.
5. Kennedy J, Hill MD, Ryckborst KJ, et al. Fast assessment of stroke and transient ischaemic attack to prevent early recurrence (FASTER): a randomised controlled pilot trial. Lancet Neurol. 2007;6:961–9.
6. Wang Y, Wang Y, Zhao X, et al. Clopidogrel with aspirin in acute minor stroke or transient ischemic attack. N Engl J Med. 2013;369:11–9.
7. Powers WJ, Clarke WR, Grubb RL Jr, et al. Extracranial-intracranial bypass surgery for stroke prevention in hemodynamic cerebral ischemia: the carotid occlusion surgery study randomized trial. JAMA. 2011;306:1983–92.
8. Mendelow AD, Gregson BA, Fernandes HM, et al. Early surgery versus initial conservative treatment in patients with spontaneous supratentorial intracerebral haematomas in the International Surgical Trial in Intracerebral Haemorrhage (STICH): a randomised trial. Lancet. 2005;365:387–97.
9. Vahedi K, Hofmeijer J, Juettler E, et al. Early decompressive surgery in malignant infarction of the middle cerebral artery: a pooled analysis of three randomised controlled trials. Lancet Neurol. 2007;6:215–22.
10. Steering Committee CAPRIE. A randomised, blinded, trial of clopidogrel versus aspirin in patients at risk of ischaemic events (CAPRIE). Lancet. 1996;348:1329–39.
11. Amarenco P, Bogousslavsky J, Callahan A 3rd, et al. High-dose atorvastatin after stroke or transient ischemic attack. N Engl J Med. 2006;355:549–59.

Printed by Printforce, the Netherlands